Congenital Cardiac Anesthesia

Congenital Cardiac Anesthesia

A Case-Based Approach

Edited by

Laura K. Berenstain
Professor of Clinical Anesthesiology, Cincinnati Children's Hospital Medical Center

James P. Spaeth
Professor of Clinical Anesthesiology, Cincinnati Children's Hospital Medical Center

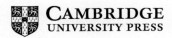

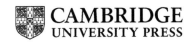

Shaftesbury Road, Cambridge CB2 8EA, United Kingdom

One Liberty Plaza, 20th Floor, New York, NY 10006, USA

477 Williamstown Road, Port Melbourne, VIC 3207, Australia

314–321, 3rd Floor, Plot 3, Splendor Forum, Jasola District Centre,
New Delhi – 110025, India

103 Penang Road, #05–06/07, Visioncrest Commercial, Singapore 238467

Cambridge University Press is part of Cambridge University Press & Assessment,
a department of the University of Cambridge.

We share the University's mission to contribute to society through the pursuit of
education, learning and research at the highest international levels of excellence.

www.cambridge.org
Information on this title: www.cambridge.org/9781108494168
DOI: 10.1017/9781108657341

Original drawings (Figures 2.1 to 2.4, 4.1, 5.1, 5.2, 6.1, 7.1, 9.1, 14.1, 19.2, 20.2, 21.1,
23.1, 25.1, 26.1 to 26.3, and 27.1) for this text were provided by Ryan A. Moore, MD,
MSc and Matt Nelson, BFA. Dr. Moore and Mr. Nelson are part of Cincinnati
Children's Media Lab, a digital arts and medical animation studio within Cincinnati
Children's Hospital, directed by Ken Tegtmeyer, MD and lead animator Jeff
Cimprich, BFA. Illustrations created for this textbook were inspired by the 3D heart
models the team has created for the Heartpedia app, Surgical Animate pp, and
accompanying animations.

© Cambridge University Press & Assessment 2021

First published 2021 (version 2, September 2023)

Printed in Great Britain by CPI Group (UK) Ltd, Croydon CR0 4YY, September 2023

A catalogue record for this publication is available from the British Library

ISBN 978-1-108-49416-8 Hardback

Cambridge University Press & Assessment has no responsibility for the persistence
or accuracy of URLs for external or third-party internet websites referred to in this
publication and does not guarantee that any content on such websites is, or will
remain, accurate or appropriate.

Every effort has been made in preparing this book to provide accurate and up-to-date
information that is in accord with accepted standards and practice at the time of
publication. Although case histories are drawn from actual cases, every effort has been
made to disguise the identities of the individuals involved. Nevertheless, the authors,
editors, and publishers can make no warranties that the information contained herein
is totally free from error, not least because clinical standards are constantly changing
through research and regulation. The authors, editors, and publishers therefore
disclaim all liability for direct or consequential damages resulting from the use of
material contained in this book. Readers are strongly advised to pay careful attention
to information provided by the manufacturer of any drugs or equipment that they
plan to use.

To Michael, whose belief in me makes everything possible, and to Katharine, Cecile, and Emily – you are my world. My sincere thanks to all who have contributed so generously to this project.

L. K. B.

To Christine, for your unwavering patience and support, without which an endeavor such as this would not be possible. My sincere gratitude to mentors and colleagues alike who instilled in me and continue to drive my passion for congenital cardiac care.

J. P. S.

Contents

Contents

Contributors

Adam C. Adler, MD, MS, FAAP, FASE
Department of Anesthesiology, Perioperative and Pain Medicine, Baylor College of Medicine, Texas Children's Hospital, Houston, TX

M. Iqbal Ahmed, MBBS, FRCA
Professor, Department of Anesthesiology and Pain Management, University of Texas Southwestern Medical Center, and Children's Health, Dallas, TX

Stephen Alcos, DO
Pediatric Cardiac Anesthesiologist, Valley Anesthesiology Consultants, Phoenix Children's Hospital, Phoenix, AZ

Lori A. Aronson, MD
Professor of Clinical Anesthesiology and Pediatrics, University of Cincinnati College of Medicine, Department of Pediatric Anesthesiology, Cincinnati Children's Hospital Medical Center, Cincinnati, OH

Wenyu Bai, MD
Clinical Assistant Professor, Department of Anesthesiology, University of Michigan Medical School, Section of Pediatric Anesthesiology, Ann Arbor, MI

Rahul G. Baijal, MD
Associate Professor of Anesthesiology and Pediatrics, Departments of Anesthesiology, Perioperative and Pain Medicine and Pediatrics, Baylor College of Medicine, and Arthur S. Keats Division of Pediatric Cardiovascular Anesthesiology, Texas Children's Hospital, Houston, TX

Laura K. Berenstain, MD, FASA
Professor of Clinical Anesthesiology, University of Cincinnati College of Medicine, Division of Pediatric Cardiac Anesthesia, Cincinnati Children's Hospital Medical Center, Cincinnati, OH

Jaime Bozentka, MD
Assistant Professor of Anesthesiology, Northwestern Feinberg School of Medicine, Division of Pediatric Cardiac Anesthesia, Ann & Robert H. Lurie Children's Hospital, Chicago, IL

Matthew Careskey, MD
Assistant Professor of Clinical Anesthesiology, University of Cincinnati College of Medicine, Department of Pediatric Anesthesiology, Cincinnati Children's Hospital Medical Center, Cincinnati, OH

Destiny F. Chau, MD, FAAP
Professor of Anesthesiology, University of Arkansas for Medical Sciences, Arkansas Children's Hospital, Little Rock, AR

Kelly Chilson, MD
Associate Professor, Department of Anesthesiology, Washington University School of Medicine, and Director, Pediatric Cardiac Anesthesiology, St. Louis Children's Hospital, St. Louis, MO

Vannessa Chin, MBBS, DM
Assistant Professor, Department of Anesthesiology and Pain Medicine, University of Toronto, and Pediatric Cardiac Anesthesiologist, The Hospital for Sick Children, University of Toronto, Toronto, Ontario, Canada

Arpa Chutipongtanate, MD
Ramathibodi Hospital, Mahidol University, Bangkok, Thailand, and Cincinnati Children's Hospital Medical Center, Cincinnati, OH

Erin Conner, MD
Assistant Professor of Anesthesiology and Pediatrics, Oregon Health and Science University, Portland, OR

Nina Deutsch, MD
Associate Professor of Anesthesiology and Pediatrics, George Washington University School of Medicine and Health Sciences; Vice Chief of Academic Affairs; Director, Cardiac Anesthesiology, Division of Anesthesiology, Sedation and Perioperative Medicine, the Children's National Hospital, Washington, DC

Nicole Dobija, DDS, MD
Clinical Assistant Professor, Department of Anesthesiology, University of Michigan Medical School, Section of Pediatric Anesthesiology, Ann Arbor, MI

Michael J. Eisses, MD
Associate Professor, Department of Anesthesiology and
Pain Medicine, University of Washington School of
Medicine, and Seattle Children's Hospital, Seattle, WA

Ana Maria Manrique Espinel, MD
Assistant Professor of Anesthesiology and Critical Care
Medicine, Perelman School of Medicine at the University
of Pennsylvania, Division of Cardiac Anesthesiology, The
Children's Hospital of Philadelphia, Philadelphia, PA

Kelly Everhart, MD, MS
Fellow in Pediatric Anesthesiology, Seattle Children's
Hospital, University of Washington School of Medicine,
Seattle, WA

David Faraoni, MD, PhD
Department of Anesthesiology, Perioperative and Pain
Medicine, Baylor College of Medicine, and Arthur S. Keats
Division of Pediatric Cardiovascular Anesthesiology,
Texas Children's Hospital, Houston, TX

James Fehr, MD
Anesthesiologist-in-Chief, Lucile Packard Children's
Hospital, Stanford University School of Medicine,
Stanford, CA

Neil M. Goldenberg, MD, PhD, FRCPC
Department of Anesthesiology and Pain Medicine, The
Hospital for Sick Children, University of Toronto,
Toronto, Ontario, Canada

Mikel Gorbea, MD
Assistant Instructor, Department of Anesthesiology and
Pain Management, University of Texas Southwestern
Medical Center, Dallas, TX

Stephanie N. Grant, MD
Assistant Professor, Departments of Anesthesiology and
Pediatrics, Emory University School of Medicine, and
Division of Pediatric Cardiovascular Anesthesiology,
Children's Healthcare of Atlanta, Atlanta, GA

Kelly L. Grogan, MD
Assistant Professor of Anesthesiology and Critical Care
Medicine, Perelman School of Medicine at the University
of Pennsylvania, Division of Cardiac Anesthesiology, The
Children's Hospital of Philadelphia, Philadelphia, PA

Bishr Haydar, MD
Clinical Associate Professor, Department of
Anesthesiology, University of Michigan Medical School,
Section of Pediatric Anesthesiology, Ann Arbor, MI

Anna E. Jankowska, MD, FASA
Assistant Professor, Department of Anesthesiology,
Perioperative Care and Pain Medicine, NYU Langone
Health, NYU Robert I. Grossman School of Medicine, New
York, NY

Denise C. Joffe, MD
Professor, Department of Anesthesiology and Pain
Medicine, University of Washington School of Medicine,
University of Washington Medical Center and Seattle
Children's Hospital, Seattle, WA

Anna Kaiser, MD
Assistant Professor, Departments of Anesthesiology and
Pediatrics, Emory University School of Medicine, and
Division of Pediatric Cardiovascular Anesthesiology,
Children's Healthcare of Atlanta, Atlanta, GA

Amanpreet S. Kalsi, MBBS, FRCA, BSc
Clinical Assistant Professor, Department of
Anesthesiology, University of Michigan Medical School,
Section of Pediatric Anesthesiology, Ann Arbor, MI

Nicholette Kasman, MD
Associate Professor of Clinical Anesthesiology, University
of Cincinnati College of Medicine, Division of Pediatric
Cardiac Anesthesia, Cincinnati Children's Hospital
Medical Center, Cincinnati, OH

Zachary Kleiman, MD
Clinical Assistant Professor of Anesthesiology, Stanford
University School of Medicine, Palo Alto, CA

Ramesh Kodavatiganti, MD
Assistant Professor of Anesthesiology and Critical Care
Medicine, Perelman School of Medicine at the University
of Pennsylvania, Division of Cardiac Anesthesiology, The
Children's Hospital of Philadelphia, Philadelphia, PA

Kirk Lalwani, MD, FRCA, MCR
Professor of Anesthesiology and Pediatrics, Oregon Health
and Science University, Portland, OR

Jennifer E. Lam, DO
Associate Professor of Clinical Anesthesiology and
Pediatrics, University of Cincinnati College of Medicine,
Division of Pediatric Cardiac Anesthesia, Cincinnati
Children's Hospital Medical Center, Cincinnati, OH

Andrés Bacigalupo Landa, MD
Fellow in Pediatric Cardiovascular Anesthesiology, Baylor
College of Medicine, Texas Children's Hospital,
Houston, TX

Leah Landsem, MD
Fellow in Pediatric Cardiac Anesthesiology, Department of Anesthesiology and Pain Medicine, University of Washington School of Medicine, and Seattle Children's Hospital, Seattle, WA

Gregory J. Latham, MD
Professor, Department of Anesthesiology and Pain Medicine, University of Washington School of Medicine; and Director, Pediatric Cardiac Anesthesiology, Seattle Children's Hospital, Seattle, WA

Erica P. Lin, MD
Associate Professor of Clinical Anesthesiology, University of Cincinnati College of Medicine, Division of Pediatric Cardiac Anesthesia, Cincinnati Children's Hospital Medical Center, Cincinnati, OH

Andreas W. Loepke, MD, PhD, FAAP
Professor of Anesthesiology and Critical Care Medicine and Professor of Pediatrics, Perelman School of Medicine at the University of Pennsylvania; Chief, Division of Cardiac Anesthesiology, The Children's Hospital of Philadelphia, Philadelphia, PA

Joseph McSoley, MD
Assistant Professor of Clinical Anesthesiology, University of Cincinnati College of Medicine, Department of Pediatric Anesthesiology, Cincinnati Children's Hospital Medical Center, Cincinnati, OH

Bruce E. Miller, MD
Associate Professor, Departments of Anesthesiology and Pediatrics, Emory University School of Medicine, Children's Healthcare of Atlanta, Atlanta, GA

Wanda C. Miller-Hance, MD
Professor of Anesthesiology and Pediatrics, Departments of Anesthesiology, Perioperative and Pain Medicine and Pediatrics, Baylor College of Medicine, and Arthur S. Keats Division of Pediatric Cardiovascular Anesthesiology, Texas Children's Hospital, Houston, TX

Matthew P. Monteleone, MD
Associate Professor of Clinical Anesthesiology, University of Cincinnati College of Medicine, Division of Pediatric Cardiac Anesthesia, Cincinnati Children's Hospital Medical Center, Cincinnati, OH

Viviane G. Nasr, MD
Associate Professor of Anaesthesia, Harvard Medical School, and Department of Anesthesiology, Critical Care and Pain Medicine, Boston Children's Hospital, Boston, MA

Jennie Ngai, MD
Associate Professor, Department of Anesthesiology, Perioperative Care and Pain Medicine; and Associate Director, Division of Cardiothoracic Anesthesiology, NYU Langone Health, NYU Robert I. Grossman School of Medicine, New York, NY

Susan C. Nicolson, MD
Professor of Anesthesiology and Critical Care Medicine, Perelman School of Medicine at the University of Pennsylvania, and Division of Cardiac Anesthesiology, The Children's Hospital of Philadelphia, Philadelphia, PA

Joanna Rosing Paquin, MD
Associate Professor of Clinical Anesthesiology, University of Cincinnati College of Medicine, Division of Pediatric Cardiac Anesthesia, Cincinnati Children's Hospital Medical Center, Cincinnati, OH

Bridget Pearce, MD
Clinical Assistant Professor, Department of Anesthesiology, University of Michigan Medical School, Section of Pediatric Anesthesiology, Ann Arbor, MI

J. Nick Pratap, MA, MBBCh, MRCPCH, FRCA
Associate Professor of Clinical Anesthesiology, University of Cincinnati College of Medicine, Division of Pediatric Cardiac Anesthesia, Cincinnati Children's Hospital Medical Center, Cincinnati, OH

Joseph P. Previte, MD, FAAP
Professor of Anesthesiology, University of Cincinnati College of Medicine, Department of Pediatric Anesthesiology, Cincinnati Children's Hospital Medical Center, Cincinnati, OH

Sheila M. Rajashekara, MD
Clinical Assistant Professor, Department of Anesthesiology, Division of Pediatric Anesthesia, Stanford University School of Medicine, Stanford, CA

Chandra Ramamoorthy, MD
Professor, Department of Anesthesiology, Division of Pediatric Anesthesia, Stanford University School of Medicine, Stanford, CA

Lori Q. Riegger, MD
Clinical Associate Professor, Department of Anesthesiology, University of Michigan Medical School, Section of Pediatric Anesthesiology; and Director, Congenital Cardiac Anesthesiology, Ann Arbor, MI

Katie J. Roddy, MD
Assistant Professor, Departments of Anesthesiology and Pediatrics, Emory University School of Medicine, Division of Pediatric Cardiovascular Anesthesiology, Children's Healthcare of Atlanta, Atlanta, GA

Maricarmen Roche Rodriguez, MD
Instructor of Anaesthesia, Harvard Medical School, Department of Anesthesiology, Critical Care and Pain Medicine, Boston Children's Hospital, Boston, MA

Deborah A. Romeo, MD
Assistant Professor, Department of Anesthesia and Perioperative Medicine, Division of Pediatric Anesthesia, Medical University of South Carolina, Charleston, SC

Faith J. Ross, MD, MS
Assistant Professor, Department of Anesthesiology and Pain Medicine, University of Washington School of Medicine, and Seattle Children's Hospital, Seattle, WA

Rita Saynhalath, MD
Assistant Professor, Department of Anesthesiology and Pain Management, University of Texas Southwestern Medical Center, and Children's Health, Dallas, TX

Annette Y. Schure, MD, DEAA, FAAP
Assistant Professor of Anaesthesia, Harvard Medical School, and Senior Associate in Cardiac Anesthesia, Department of Anesthesiology, Critical Care and Pain Medicine, Boston Children's Hospital, Boston, MA

Jamie McElrath Schwartz, MD
Assistant Professor of Anesthesia and Critical Care Medicine, The Johns Hopkins University School of Medicine; Division Chief, Pediatric Critical Care Medicine, and Co-Director, Blalock-Taussig-Thomas Pediatric and Congenital Heart Center, Johns Hopkins Children's Center, Baltimore, MD

James P. Spaeth, MD
Professor of Clinical Anesthesiology and Pediatrics, University of Cincinnati College of Medicine; and Director, Division of Pediatric Cardiac Anesthesia, Cincinnati Children's Hospital Medical Center, Cincinnati, OH

Timothy D. Switzer, MBBCh, FCAI
The Hospital for Sick Children, Toronto, Ontario, Canada

Maxwell Teets, MD
Clinical Assistant Professor, Department of Anesthesiology, Perioperative Care and Pain Medicine, NYU Langone Health, NYU Robert I. Grossman School of Medicine, New York, NY

Premal M. Trivedi, MD
Assistant Professor of Anesthesiology, Baylor College of Medicine, and Arthur S. Keats Division of Pediatric Cardiovascular Anesthesiology, Texas Children's Hospital, Houston, TX

Sana Ullah, MBChB, FRCA
Associate Professor, Department of Anesthesiology and Pain Management, University of Texas Southwestern Medical Center, and Children's Medical Center, Dallas, TX

Chinwe Unegbu, MD
Assistant Professor of Anesthesiology and Pediatrics, George Washington University School of Medicine and Health Sciences, Division of Anesthesiology, Sedation and Perioperative Medicine, the Children's National Hospital, Washington, DC

Elizabeth R. Vogel, MD, PhD
Department of Anesthesiology, Critical Care and Pain Medicine, Division of Cardiac Anesthesia, Boston Children's Hospital, Boston, MA

Andrew T. Waberski, MD
Assistant Professor of Anesthesiology and Pediatrics, George Washington University School of Medicine and Health Sciences, Division of Cardiac Anesthesiology, the Children's National Hospital, Washington, DC

Rajeev Wadia, MD
Assistant Professor of Anesthesia and Critical Care Medicine, The Johns Hopkins University School of Medicine, Division of Pediatric Anesthesia and Critical Care Medicine, Johns Hopkins Children's Center, Baltimore, MD

Lisa Wise-Faberowski, MD, MS, FAAP
Associate Professor, Med Center Line, Department of Anesthesiology, Perioperative and Pain Medicine, Stanford University Medical Center, Stanford University, Stanford, CA

Luis M. Zabala, MD
Professor, Department of Anesthesiology and Pain Management; and Medical Director of Pediatric Cardiac Anesthesia, University of Texas Southwestern Medical Center and Children's Health, Dallas, TX

Katherine L. Zaleski, MD
Assistant Professor of Anaesthesia, Harvard Medical School, and Department of Anesthesiology, Critical Care and Pain Medicine, Boston Children's Hospital, Boston, MA

Introduction

Congenital heart disease (CHD) is unfortunately quite common, occurring in just under 1% of live births. With the continuing evolution of treatment modalities for patients with CHD, both in the cardiac operating rooms and cardiac catheterization suites, the survival of these patients has significantly improved, albeit with varying degrees of physiologic impairment and/or sequelae. In fact, the population of adults with CHD is growing at a rate of approximately 5% per year. Multiple studies have illustrated that children with CHD are at higher risk for perioperative cardiac arrest compared to the general population during anesthesia and surgery. Additionally, children with CHD also experience increased morbidity, mortality, and increased length of hospital stay.

The ever-growing population of patients with CHD means that these patients are presenting with increasing frequency for a wide variety of non-cardiac-related surgeries and imaging studies. It is not uncommon for pediatric anesthesia practitioners, often without specific cardiac training, to be asked to care for patients ranging from neonates to adults with unrepaired, repaired, and palliated CHD in a variety of venues, including diagnostic imaging, the general operating rooms, and interventional radiology. Indeed, as this patient population continues to grow, it will become the "new normal" for many patients with some form of CHD to receive care from non-cardiac-trained anesthesia care providers. We hope to address this growing need with this book, by offering both an organized approach to analyzing and understanding CHD as well as strategies for assessing and caring for these patients. Our aim is to provide a useful educational resource for anesthesia residents, fellows, nurse anesthetists, nurse anesthesia students, and anesthesiologists who do not routinely care for patients with CHD.

We have chosen to use a case-based approach for a number of reasons. Case presentations emphasize the practical aspects of perioperative care and allow the reader to be actively involved in analyzing information and formulating an appropriate care plan. Cases of varying complexity are offered to facilitate an understanding of the diverse nature of CHD and provide learning for readers with varying levels of experience. Visual aids are used to assist in understanding the anatomy and physiology of the different congenital lesions. An understanding of the underlying physiologic abnormalities allows the practitioner to develop an appropriate anesthetic plan for each patient.

Each chapter contains **Key Objectives**, **Questions and Answers**, **Clinical Pearls**, and **Suggested Readings**. Chapters are further divided into two sections: "**Pathophysiology**" wherein the cardiac lesion is defined and analyzed, and "**Anesthetic Implications**," which then discusses the specific concerns related to the particular cardiac lesion which will affect formation of the perioperative plan. Chapters vary greatly in complexity. In part, this is to allow the reader to appreciate the diversity that exists even within a given anomaly, meaning that the anesthetic plan might vary considerably depending on the child's individual pathology. Second, this is to accommodate those readers with a particular interest and knowledge of CHD and to allow them to continue to enrich their knowledge base. It is our hope that the more complicated scenarios will prove useful for those training to provide care for this patient population. We have also included multiple scenarios in the cardiac catheterization laboratory, in recognition of the fact that anesthesia staffing in this particular location varies from institution to institution.

Our hope is that this case-based book will allow readers to better understand the vast array of congenital heart defects and assist them in understanding the key principles which guide safe perioperative management. There is rarely a single "right way" to provide an anesthetic for a patient with CHD; instead, the key is to understand the hemodynamic goals that should guide decision making during the perioperative course. We hope that this book will be a practical guide for anesthesia care providers in all regions of the world and will in some small way have a positive impact on the anesthetic care of patients with congenital heart disease.

A Congenital Heart Disease Primer

Laura K. Berenstain and James P. Spaeth

The ability to interpret cardiac data to determine an individual patient's cardiac anatomy and physiology is paramount in developing a safe plan for anesthesia or sedation. Although cardiac lesions can be placed into broad diagnostic categories, within each category and for each lesion significant variation can exist. For example, infants with tetralogy of Fallot (TOF) may have obstruction to pulmonary blood flow ranging from minimal to severe; if obstruction is minimal, they may exhibit signs and symptoms of pulmonary overcirculation or if severe, they may be overtly cyanotic. Patients who have been described as "pink tets" at home may, during the stress imposed by anesthesia and surgical manipulation, exhibit significant tet spells. Wide pathophysiologic variability exists even within a given lesion and each patient must be considered on an individual basis, rather than being defined by his or her diagnosis. Patients who have undergone corrective surgeries, although "repaired," often have important residua or sequelae that must be noted. It should also be emphasized that the effects of the patient's underlying cardiac disease on other organ systems must be taken into account as well.

The anesthesia practitioner must be able to efficiently assimilate data including the patient's current history, physical examination, pertinent imaging studies, and cardiac catheterization data in order to develop an accurate assessment of the individual patient's pathophysiology prior to surgery. Are there intracardiac shunts, elevated pressures in specific cardiac chambers and/or volume overload, or reduced ventricular function? Are there rhythm abnormalities that might lead to a reduction in cardiac output? These factors may all impact the perioperative and anesthetic plan. This chapter is dedicated to outlining major principles useful in guiding preoperative analysis of the patient with congenital heart disease (CHD).

Basic Concepts

When referring to cardiac chambers, the terms "right" and "left" refer to morphologic characteristics and the terms "right-sided," "left-sided," "anterior," and "posterior" give a spatial frame of reference. When referencing structures other than cardiac chambers, such as the vena cavae, the terms "right" and "left" refer to spatial positioning in the thorax.

- The **segmental approach** to analysis of congenital cardiac lesions offers a framework for assessment and analysis of the path of blood flow through the heart. The three major segments or building blocks considered are the **atria,** the **ventricles**, and the **great arterial trunks**, along with the connections between each of them. The segmental approach begins by determining the position of the heart in the thorax, the direction of the cardiac apex, and the situs of the thoracic and abdominal organs. Visceral situs, or sidedness, may be *solitus* (normal arrangement), *inversus* (liver on the left, stomach on the right), or *ambiguous* (indeterminate). Abnormal arrangements of the viscera, heart, and lungs are seen in heterotaxy syndromes and are associated with a high likelihood of CHD.
- The **physiologic approach** considers classification of lesions according to the presence of **shunts, obstruction**, or **combinations** of the two.

Shunting may be described as anatomic or physiologic. *Physiologic* shunting is defined as venous return from one circulatory system recirculating through the arterial outflow of the same circulatory system. *Anatomic* shunts are communications between two circulations, either at the atrial, ventricular, or great arterial level. Physiologic shunts are often the result of anatomic shunts, but they can also occur in the absence of an anatomic shunt. An example of physiologic shunting without anatomic shunting may be seen in transposition of the great arteries, where systemic venous return travels to the right atrium, the right ventricle, to the aorta, and then again returns to the right atrium.

Effective blood flow is defined as the quantity of venous blood from one circulation that reaches the arterial system of the other circulation. Therefore, effective pulmonary blood flow is the quantity of systemic venous return that reaches the pulmonary arterial system. Effective pulmonary blood flow and effective systemic blood flow are *always equal*. Effective blood flow is the flow necessary to maintain life.

Total blood flow is the sum of both effective blood flow to a circulation and recirculated blood flow. Total systemic blood flow and total pulmonary blood flow are *not equal* even in normal patients, as a small amount of physiologic shunting always exists. Recirculated or physiologic shunt flow can be thought of as the extra noneffective blood flow added to effective blood flow, together yielding total blood flow to a circulation.

Anatomic shunts may additionally be characterized as simple or complex. In **simple shunts** the degree of shunting is determined by the size of the orifice. With a small orifice, the size of the opening determines the amount of shunting. For large or nonrestrictive orifices (**dependent shunt**), the quantity and direction of shunting is determined by the outflow resistances, or the ratio between the pulmonary vascular resistance (PVR) and systemic vascular resistance (SVR). This ratio is known as the Q_p:Q_s. As the direction and magnitude of shunting are determined by the relationship between PVR and SVR, the effects of hemodynamic and ventilatory manipulations on these resistances during an anesthetic assume great importance.

Obstruction(s) may exist to either systemic or pulmonary blood flow at one or multiple levels. Infants with critical obstruction to either circulatory system frequently require prostaglandin E_1 infusions to maintain ductal patency and flow to the obstructed circulation until a surgical or catheter-based therapeutic intervention can take place. **Complex shunts** occur when obstruction exists along with a shunt. The degree of shunting in a complex shunt is determined by the degree of obstruction along with the PVR or SVR; the more significant the obstruction, the less the PVR and/or SVR will impact shunting. Obstructions may be either *fixed* or *dynamic* in nature. In a lesion such as tetralogy of Fallot it is common for elements of both fixed and dynamic obstruction to be present and to impact the direction and magnitude of shunting through the ventricular septal defect. For example, a child with TOF has a large ventricular septal defect (VSD) frequently accompanied by significant fixed and/or dynamic subvalvular right ventricular outflow tract (RVOT) obstruction as well. For this child, the degree and direction of shunting at the level of the VSD is determined primarily by the degree of RVOT obstruction; therefore left-to-right shunting decreases as RVOT obstruction increases with a tet spell, resulting in a decrease in shunting or even reversal of shunting. Although increases in PVR will contribute to the total right ventricular outflow resistance for the patient with TOF, the role of PVR is not as significant in this scenario compared to a child who has an isolated large or nonrestrictive VSD and no RVOT obstruction.

> **Clinical Pearl**
>
> *Shunting occurs when venous blood from one circulatory system (either pulmonary or systemic) returns or recirculates through the arterial outflow of the same circulatory system, completely bypassing the other circulation. In a nonrestrictive or dependent shunt, as shunting is determined by the relationship between pulmonary and systemic vascular resistances, the effects of hemodynamic and ventilatory manipulations during an anesthetic assume great importance.*

Another important concept in understanding complex CHD involves the concept of **series** versus **parallel circulations**. In general, the normal systemic and pulmonary circulations are in series, with blood traveling through each circulation once, without mixing of deoxygenated and oxygenated blood (excepting the bronchial veins). An example of parallel circulations is unrepaired dextro (d)-transposition of the great arteries, where blood travels only to the pulmonary or systemic circulation. Mixing at the atrial, ventricular, or great arterial level (patent ductus arteriosus) is essential to allow mixing of oxygenated and deoxygenated blood and maintain life. (See Figure 1.1.) Another example of a parallel circulation is the child with single ventricle physiology, with both pulmonary and systemic circulations dependent on the same pump. Manipulations affecting resistance or flow in either circulation will therefore affect the performance of the other circuit. This is often referred to as "balancing" circulations and will be discussed in several chapters.

Imaging

Cardiac Catheterization

Cardiac catheterization in patients with CHD may be performed for diagnostic or therapeutic/interventional indications. Echocardiography has become the gold standard for initial diagnosis and ongoing assessment, particularly because in most patients it avoids the need for sedation or general anesthesia and for invasive vascular access. Fewer cardiac catheterizations are now performed solely for diagnostic indications. Conversely, interventional applications for cardiac catheterization have continued to grow in importance and include percutaneous implantation of valves and hybrid procedures utilizing both surgical and catheterization techniques. Most children require general anesthesia for cardiac catheterization, particularly when interventional procedures are anticipated. Unless extenuating circumstances exist, all efforts are made to utilize an FiO_2 of 0.21 and to maintain

Table 1.1 Calculations and Normal Values

	Calculation	Normal Value
Ejection fraction (EF) (%)	(SV/EDV) × 100	54%–75%
Shortening fraction (SF) (%)	(EDD − ESD)/EDD × 100	30%–40%
Cardiac output (CO)	SV × HR	0.8–1.3 L/m (neonate/infant) 1.3–3.0 L/m (child) 4–8 L/m (adolescent/adult)
Cardiac index (CI)	CO/BSA	4.0–5.0 L/m/m^2 (neonate/infant) 3.0–4.5 L/m/m^2 (child) 2.5–4.0 L/m/m^2 (adolescent/adult)
Oxygen content	(O$_2$ sat × 1.36 × 10 × hemoglobin concentration)	
Pulmonary blood flow (Q_p)	VO$_2$ (mL/min)/PV O$_2$ conc − PA O$_2$ conc	
Systemic blood flow (Q_s)	VO$_2$ (mL/min)/ SA O$_2$ conc − MV O$_2$ conc	
Q_p:Q_s (simplified)	SA sat − MV sat/PV sat − PA sat	
SVR	(MAP − CVP) × 80/CO	10–15 iWu (infants) 15–20 iWu (1–2 years) 15–30 iWu (child)
PVR	(mPAP − mLAP) × 80/CO	8–10 iWu (<8 weeks) 1–3 iWu (>8 weeks)
TPG	mPAP − LAP	

BSA, body surface area; CVP, central venous pressure; EDD, end-diastolic diameter; EDV, end-diastolic volume; ESD, end-systolic diameter; HR, heart rate; iWu, indexed Wood units; MAP, mean arterial pressure; mLAP, mean left atrial pressure; mPAP, mean pulmonary artery pressure; MV, mixed venous; MV sat, mixed venous saturation; PA sat, pulmonary artery saturation; PV sat, pulmonary venous saturation; PVR, pulmonary vascular resistance; Q_p:Q_s, ratio of total pulmonary blood flow to total systemic blood flow; SA, systemic artery; SA sat, systemic arterial saturation; SV, stroke volume; SVR, systemic vascular resistance; TPG, transpulmonary gradient; VO$_2$, oxygen consumption.

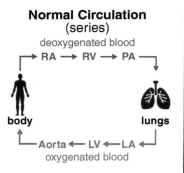

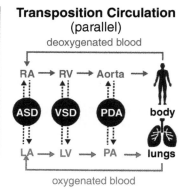

Figure 1.1 Comparison of the normal circulation, which is in series, with that in transposition of the great arteries (TGA), which is in parallel. In the normal circulation (left), deoxygenated blood from the body enters the right-sided circulation, then is oxygenated by the lungs and then distributed to the body via the left side of the heart. In the transposition circulation (right), the potential sites of mixing are shown: atrial septal defect (ASD), ventricular septal defect (VSD), and patent ductus arteriosus (PDA). The circulation is in parallel, so deoxygenated blood from the body enters the right side of the heart, but because of the anomalous connection, it is recirculated to the body via the aorta. Similarly, the oxygenated blood from the lungs enters the left heart but is recirculated to the lungs via the PA (pulmonary artery). RA, right atrium; RV, right ventricle. From McEwan A. and Manolis M. *Anesthesia for Transposition of the Great Arteries.* In Andropoulos D. B., Stayer S., Mossad E. B., et al. eds. *Anesthesia for Congenital Heart Surgery,* 3rd ed. John Wiley & Sons; 2015: 542–66. With permission.

ventilatory and hemodynamic parameters that parallel awake conditions, at least while initial hemodynamic parameters are measured. Any changes should be discussed with the cardiologist, as these changes will impact both the measured values that are obtained as well as calculated values.

The following data may be appreciated from a catheterization report. (See Table 1.1.)

- **Anatomic diagnosis:** The child's anatomy, including the effect of any interventions, is documented and assessed.
- **Saturation data:** Saturation data can be used to calculate Q_p:Q_s ratios and to document shunts via "step-ups" or "step-downs" in saturation between vessels and chambers. They may also help differentiate intracardiac shunting from ventilation/perfusion mismatch or intrapulmonary shunting.

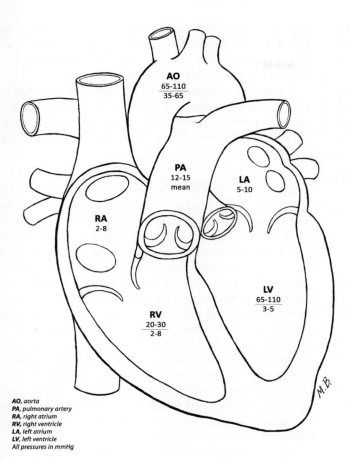

Figure 1.2 Normal cardiac pressures.

AO
65-110
35-65

PA
12-15
mean

LA
5-10

RA
2-8

LV
65-110
3-5

RV
20-30
2-8

M.B.

AO, aorta
PA, pulmonary artery
RA, right atrium
RV, right ventricle
LA, left atrium
LV, left ventricle
All pressures in mmHg

- **Angiography**: Cineangiography may be used to demonstrate blood flow patterns and ventricular function.
- **Pressures**: Right and left intracardiac pressures as well as vascular pressures are measured, along with pressure gradients. (See Figure 1.2.) Pressure gradients may be reported as either peak or mean gradients. Gradients may vary according to cardiac output: the higher the output, the higher the gradient. Thus a gradient can appear decreased with decreased cardiac output.
- **Shunts**: The direction and magnitude of shunts are recorded. The ratio of pulmonary to systemic blood flow is calculated and is an important piece of information to obtain prior to anesthetizing a child with CHD. (See Chapter 2, $Q_p:Q_s$.)
- **Resistances**: Resistance is measured as change in pressure divided by flow and is reported in Wood units (Wu). Systemic and pulmonary vascular resistances may be calculated and are most often normalized or indexed to body surface area. Notations for indexed pulmonary vascular resistance (PVR) can thus appear

as "PRVI," "PVRi," or "iWu." In children with pulmonary hypertension it is important to note not only the initial PVR but also the response after any vasoreactivity testing or initiation of drug therapies.
- **Cardiac output**: Cardiac output (CO) for children is often indexed to body surface area and reported as cardiac index (CI). In measuring CO, either thermodilution or the Fick determination can be used; when utilizing the Fick determination, estimates of oxygen consumption (VO_2) based on body surface area or heart rate and age may be referenced for children. Maintaining the patient's FiO_2 at room air during cardiac catheterization is important while gathering this information in order to allow the dissolved oxygen component of the equation to be ignored.

Echocardiography

Echocardiography is the gold standard of diagnosis and ongoing assessment for most patients with CHD. Whenever possible, echo reports should be compared to previous reports to assess the progression of pathophysiology, and it is also useful to note in the cardiology evaluation the frequency of echocardiographic assessment for a particular patient. In patients with complex CHD echocardiographic reports may list a multitude of findings, and echocardiographic findings often prove useful to roughly sketch the heart, beginning with systemic venous return to the heart and adding each diagnosis as listed in the report. This heightens appreciation of the sources of pulmonary and systemic blood flow, as well as the presence of any shunts or obstructions, and aids immeasurably in understanding the patient's physiology and developing an appropriate anesthetic plan.

The following important parameters may be appreciated from an echocardiographic report:

- **Ventricular function**: The **ejection fraction** (EF) is defined as the fraction of blood ejected by the ventricle relative to its end-diastolic volume. It is important to note that EF assesses systolic function of the ventricle, and that diastolic dysfunction may exist in the face of a normal EF. The **shortening fraction** is calculated utilizing the percentage of change in ventricular diameter during the cardiac cycle and is dependent on preload and afterload.
- **Gradients**: The degree of obstruction across semilunar valves and outflow tracts may be estimated using the peak and/or mean instantaneous gradients.
- **Regurgitant lesions**: These are generally classified as mild, moderate, or severe and can best be appreciated by evaluating trends in the reported data.
- **Pressure data**: Information regarding right ventricular systolic pressure can be estimated by utilizing peak velocity of a tricuspid regurgitant jet.
- **Measurement of chamber sizes**: The size and thickness of the interventricular septum, the chamber dimensions of the ventricles, and information regarding valve annular sizes are reported. The "**z-score**" reported along with the values establishes a reference representing standard deviations of the measured value from the mean in a comparative population.

Other Imaging Modalities

Cardiac magnetic resonance imaging (CMRI) is noninvasive and avoids the use of ionizing radiation. It can provide excellent assessment of ventricular volumes, intracardiac anatomy, valvular regurgitation, blood flow through the heart, and extracardiac vascular anatomy. It is frequently utilized for ongoing assessment of right ventricular volume, ejection fraction, and pulmonary regurgitant fraction in patients who have undergone repair of TOF, and for

serial assessment of coronary artery aneurysms in patients with Kawasaki disease. Use of CMRI often requires sedation or general anesthesia for pediatric populations, particularly for patients under the age of 8 years.

Computed tomography (CT), although it involves ionizing radiation exposure, is an important modality for assessment of CHD, particularly extracardiac vasculature, and is the gold standard for assessment of coronary artery disease.

High-Risk Patient Populations

Within the wide spectrum of patients with CHD who require noncardiac surgery, several groups have been specifically defined as having higher risk during the perioperative period. As studies have documented increased risk, they have also aided in delineating those patients and diagnostic categories at higher risk for adverse events, cardiac arrest, and/or mortality. Younger age, higher American Society of Anesthesiologists physical status, and need for emergent surgery have been shown to contribute to increased risk. Not surprisingly, analysis of outcome data for noncardiac surgeries in adult CHD patients also reveals increased mortality when compared with a cohort of patients without CHD. Significantly, Maxwell et al. identified that the number of procedures being performed in this patient population was increasing over time, and many were performed outside of teaching hospitals [1].

Specific categories or lesions have also been identified as follows:

- **Pulmonary hypertension**, particularly with systemic or suprasystemic right ventricular pressures
- **Single ventricle physiology**, particularly patients with shunt-dependent physiology, significant atrioventricular valve regurgitation, and the failing Fontan
- **Severe ventricular dysfunction**, including cardiomyopathies
- **Severe left-sided obstructive lesions** (aortic stenosis (gradient >60 mm Hg), subaortic stenosis, mitral stenosis)
- **Williams syndrome**

Mortality in children with and without heart disease has recently been evaluated using the American College of Surgeons National Surgical Quality Improvement Program database. Children with heart disease were assessed and divided into groups with minor, major, or severe residual lesion burden and functional status. Using this strategy, children with minor CHD were found to have no greater risk than the general population for overall mortality or adverse events, while children with major or severe CHD had a higher mortality [2]. Therefore, utilizing the expertise of colleagues with specific training in cardio-vascular anesthesia, as well as consultation with colleagues in pediatric cardiology, is always recommended when caring for patients who meet the above criteria or when other specific high-risk factors are identified.

References

1. Maxwell B. G., Wong J. K., Kin C., et al. Perioperative outcomes of major noncardiac surgery in adults with congenital heart disease. *Anesthesiology* 2013; **119**: 762–69.

2. Faraoni D., Zurakowski D., Vo D., et al. Post-operative outcomes in children with and without congenital heart disease undergoing noncardiac surgery. *J Am Coll Cardiol* 2016; **67**: 793–801.

Suggested Reading

Del Castillo-Beaupre S., Frazier, J. A., Nelson D. P., et al. *Edwards' Critical Care Education, Quick Guide to Pediatric Cardiopulmonary Care*. Irvine, CA: Edwards Lifesciences Corporation, 2015.

Ramamoorthy C., Haberkern C. M., Bhananker S. M., et al. Anesthesia-related cardiac arrest in children with heart disease: data from the pediatric perioperative cardiac arrest (POCA) registry. *Anesth Analg* 2010; **110**: 1376–82.

Taylor D. and Habre W. Risk associated with anesthesia for noncardiac surgery in children with congenital heart disease. *Pediatr Anesth* 2019; **29**: 426–34.

Tharakan J. A. Admixture lesions in congenital cyanotic heart disease. *Ann Pediatr Cardiol* 2011; **4**: 53–59.

Chapter

2

Ventricular Septal Defect

Maxwell Teets and Adam C. Adler

Case Scenario

A 6-month-old child weighing 3.7 kg presents from home for bilateral inguinal hernia repair and circumcision. He was recently seen in the emergency room for an incarcerated hernia that was manually reduced. He was born at 26 weeks estimated gestational age with a birth weight of 1100 grams. He was intubated for 3 weeks and weaned from high-flow nasal cannula to room air prior to discharge from the neonatal intensive care unit at 34 weeks postconceptional age. The parents say that in the neonatal unit the baby was diagnosed with a "hole in his heart" and that he takes medicine for it every day.

Current vital signs are heart rate 140 beats/minute, respiratory rate 45 breaths/minute, blood pressure 70/38 mm Hg and SpO_2 98% on room air.

The patient has been scheduled for same-day surgery and the parents are requesting a spinal anesthetic, as they are concerned about neonatal apnea with general anesthesia.

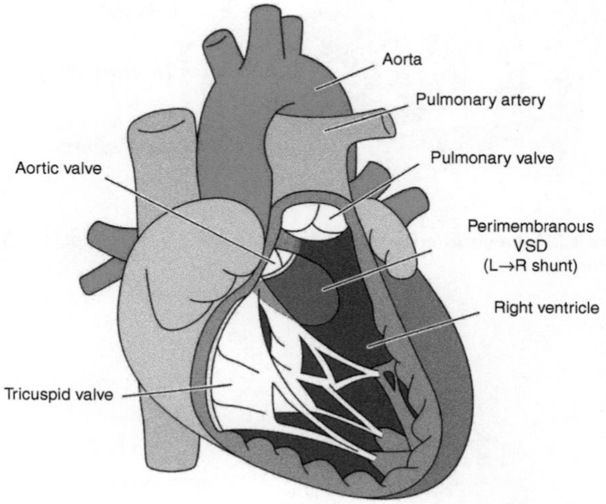

Figure 2.1 Perimembranous ventricular septal defect. Drawing by Ryan Moore, MD, and Matt Nelson.

Key Objectives

- Understand the physiology of a left-to-right shunt.
- Describe the preoperative workup and perioperative management of a premature infant with a ventricular septal defect.
- Identify an anesthetic plan in the context of balancing pulmonary vascular resistance and systemic vascular resistance.
- Outline postoperative management and appropriate discharge planning.

Pathophysiology

How are VSDs characterized?

Ventricular septal defects (VSDs) are the most common congenital heart defect, occurring in 50% of patients with congenital heart disease (CHD). It is estimated that 75%–80% of VSDs are *perimembranous* (see Figure 2.1), indicating the communication between ventricles occurs adjacent

to the very small membranous septum. *Inlet* VSDs, also known as canal type, are located posteriorly beneath the septal leaflet of the tricuspid valve. (See Figure 2.2.) *Muscular* VSDs may occur anywhere within the muscular wall of the interventricular septum and can also exist as part of other more complex cardiac defects. (See Figure 2.3.) *Subarterial* (also called subpulmonary, supracristal, conal, or infundibular) VSDs lie beneath the pulmonary valve within the outlet septum. (See Figure 2.4.) A VSD can also be present in many other forms of CHD as part of a constellation of defects.

What are the hemodynamic effects of a VSD?

An isolated VSD results in the ability to shunt blood between the left and right ventricles. The size of the defect and pulmonary vascular resistance (PVR) determine the blood flow across the VSD. Left-to-right (L-to-R) shunting generally occurs predominantly during systole and this shunting results in an increased volume load to both ventricles.

9

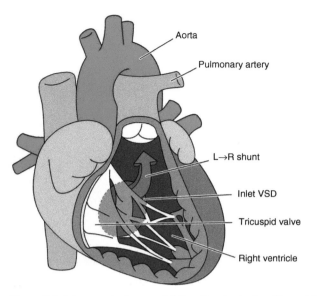

Figure 2.2 **Inlet ventricular septal defect.** Drawing by Ryan Moore, MD, and Matt Nelson.

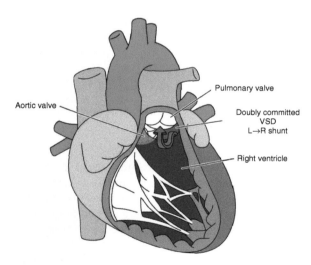

Figure 2.4 **Subarterial ventricular septal defect.** Drawing by Ryan Moore, MD, and Matt Nelson.

What is the difference between a restrictive and a nonrestrictive VSD?

The term "nonrestrictive" implies that the size of the VSD approximates the size of the aortic annulus, allowing equalization of pressures in the right and left ventricles. In reality, small pressure gradients may exist due to the relative resistances of the systemic and pulmonary vascular beds.

Infants with nonrestrictive VSDs often display signs and symptoms of congestive heart failure (CHF) as the

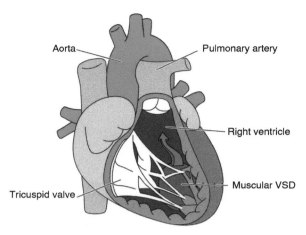

Figure 2.3 **Muscular ventricular septal defect.** Drawing by Ryan Moore, MD, and Matt Nelson.

PVR falls in the first postnatal months and the degree of L-to-R shunting increases. Nonrestrictive VSDs should be closed in the first 2 years of life to avoid the development of pulmonary vascular changes that can lead to the development of pulmonary vascular occlusive disease (PVOD) and Eisenmenger's syndrome. Given the history of prematurity this infant is at increased risk for early development of such changes. A patient's symptomatology depends on his age, the size of the VSD, the degree of L-to-R shunting, and other factors impacting PVR, such as a history of prematurity.

> **Clinical Pearl**
>
> *A patient's symptomatology depends on his age, the size of the VSD, the degree of L-to-R shunting, and other factors impacting PVR, such as a history of prematurity.*

What is the Q_p:Q_s ratio and what is its significance?

The Q_p:Q_s ratio is the ratio of the pulmonary blood flow (Q_p) to systemic blood flow (Q_s) and denotes the magnitude of a cardiovascular shunt. Normally this ratio equals 1, with the entire preload to the RV eventually becoming the preload to the LV. In cardiac lesions with a L-to-R shunt the Q_p:Q_s is >1, and in lesions with a resultant R-to-L shunt the Q_p:Q_s is <1.

In lesions with the capability for intracardiac shunting it is important to determine the percentage of recirculating blood. Often this ratio is calculated by comparing blood saturation levels obtained during cardiac catheterization.

The following formula may be utilized to calculate the ratio of pulmonary to systemic blood flow:

$$Q_p{:}Q_s = \text{Ao sat} - \text{MV sat}/\text{PV sat} - \text{PA sat},$$

where *Ao sat* is aortic oxygen saturation; *MV sat* is mixed venous oxygen saturation; *PV sat* is pulmonary venous saturation; and *PA sat* is pulmonary arterial saturation. Small VSDs will have a $Q_p{:}Q_s$ ratio of <1.5:1, medium VSDs a $Q_p{:}Q_s$ of 2–3:1, and large VSDs can have $Q_p{:}Q_s$ ratios exceeding 3:1.

Clinical Pearl

While it is not essential to know the $Q_p{:}Q_s$ ratio for an isolated VSD, the $Q_p{:}Q_s$, if available, can provide valuable information to assess the degree of shunting occurring with a VSD. A larger $Q_p{:}Q_s$ is indicative of greater pulmonary overcirculation.

What factors influence the $Q_p{:}Q_s$ ratio and the degree of shunting?

The $Q_p{:}Q_s$ ratio is affected by changes in pulmonary and systemic vascular resistance (PVR and SVR).

Acidemia, hypercarbia, hypoxemia, hypothermia, and pain are known to elevate PVR, thereby decreasing pulmonary blood flow (PBF). Additionally, significant atelectasis or high inspiratory pressures and/or tidal volumes can contribute to reductions in PBF.

Conversely, increased FiO_2, hyperventilation, alkalosis, and the use of inhaled nitric oxide (iNO) can reduce PVR and promote PBF. Nitric oxide should be available in the operating room for high-risk patients with evidence of pulmonary hypertension.

Is there a "typical" age for repair of an isolated VSD?

Timing for the surgical repair of a VSD varies based on patient age and symptomatology as well as the size and location of the lesion. Most nonrestrictive VSDs are closed within the first few years of life to avoid long-term pulmonary sequelae that can lead to eventual shunt reversal and cyanotic R-to-L shunting (Eisenmenger syndrome). If the patient is <6 months old and has failure to thrive and CHF refractory to medical management, then surgical repair of the VSD is generally considered. If medical management allows continued growth and appropriate milestone acquisition, surgery is often delayed until the child is older to avoid cardiopulmonary bypass during infancy.

Clinical Pearl

Poor weight gain and continued tachypnea and dyspnea, particularly with exertion or feeding, often signify pulmonary overcirculation.

Should the cardiac lesion be repaired prior to the hernia surgery?

Ventricular septal defects may decrease in size over the first year of life and may become relatively asymptomatic. Spontaneous closure of small perimembranous and muscular VSDs occurs in up to 50% of patients. With careful surveillance and medical management some patients may be able to avoid surgical intervention altogether. However, the incidence of inguinal hernias is much higher in low birthweight and premature infants compared to full term infants, affecting up to 30% of preterm infants. Overall, it is also thought that risk of incarceration is much higher in this population. As hernias can compromise intestinal blood supply, repair should be performed on a semielective basis to avoid the risk of emergency surgery should the hernia become incarcerated. In this case scenario, the patient has already experienced one episode of incarceration and should therefore undergo definitive hernia sac closure to prevent a potentially life-threatening recurrence.

Anesthetic Implications

What are the important preoperative considerations for this child?

History The focus of the preoperative evaluation should center on this patient's current medical status as related to his major concerns of prematurity and an unrepaired VSD. While failure to thrive may be noted in infants for a variety of reasons, the most likely etiology in this patient is the presence of the VSD, resulting in chronic pulmonary overcirculation. In addition to history from the parents, efforts should be made to review the most recent cardiology evaluation and echocardiogram, chest radiograph, and electrocardiogram.

Due to this patient's prolonged neonatal intubation it is important to identify airway concerns, including any known or suspected airway stenosis. The results of any prior evaluation of the airway by otolaryngology should be reviewed. Additionally, significant prematurity can also predispose patients to laryngotracheomalacia. The patient history should elucidate episodes of noisy breathing or stridor.

Physical Examination On physical examination the presence of increased work of breathing and/or significant chest retractions at baseline should be noted along with the rate and character of respirations. Recent symptoms of any recent respiratory infections should be elicited, as these would place the child at increased anesthetic risk due to potential increases in airway irritability and PVR. Preoperative baseline hemoglobin–oxygen saturation should be noted. Signs and symptoms of CHF may be present, including hepatomegaly and pulmonary congestion.

Laboratory A preoperative hemoglobin/hematocrit should be obtained as anemia may place this baby at increased risk for postoperative apneic events. If significant anemia is present, it may be prudent to obtain a type and screen. Since the infant is taking furosemide it may be appropriate to obtain an electrolyte panel as well.

Regarding this child's cardiac condition, what other information should be sought?

The current medication regimen, compliance with medications, and the response to therapy should be evaluated. The presence of tachypnea, especially with feeding and/or poor weight gain, can signify chronic pulmonary overcirculation and CHF. Additionally, severely preterm infants are at risk for bronchopulmonary dysplasia due to failure of arborization of distal alveoli and their vasculature. This is a common cause of elevated pulmonary vascular pressures in formerly preterm children and can lead to varying degrees of pulmonary hypertension. Generally, these patients are seen relatively frequently by the pediatrician and cardiologist to ensure adequacy of medical management. If a change in symptoms is noted during the preoperative evaluation, this should raise concerns that the patient's medical management is not currently optimized.

The most recent cardiology evaluation should be reviewed along with recent echocardiographic findings. Echocardiographic findings to review include

- Type, number, location, and size of VSDs
- Estimates of pulmonary artery pressure and signs of RV hypertension
- The presence of any valvular abnormalities/regurgitance
- Biventricular function
- Presence of other cardiac anomalies

What potential perioperative issues exist for a patient on diuretic therapy?

Diuretics are frequently used to medically manage symptoms associated with CHF. The goal of treatment is euvolemia achieved by fluid restriction and diuretic therapy. Diuretics such as furosemide may result in electrolyte disturbances and/or preoperative hypovolemia, particularly in a patient who has been nil per os (NPO) for an extended time period.

What are the effects of anesthesia on systemic and pulmonary vascular resistances?

An understanding of factors impacting PVR and SVR is vital to the anesthetic management of the patient with a large VSD. Most anesthetic agents will decrease SVR to a greater degree than PVR, especially during induction and prior to surgical stimulation. This imbalance may initially reduce L-to-R shunting through the VSD, particularly if pulmonary vascular pressure is elevated. With the initiation of surgery an increase in SVR may augment L-to-R shunting through the VSD.

The optimal anesthetic is one in which PVR and SVR are relatively balanced with respect to the patient's preoperative baseline. Both PVR and SVR are impacted by multiple factors including ventilation strategy, anesthetic agents used, and the depth of anesthesia. A ventilation strategy utilizing a low FiO_2, mild hypercarbia, and acidosis (pH 7.30) is the primary modality used to limit pulmonary overcirculation during anesthesia and surgery. It is important to remember common causes of hypotension and oxygen desaturation during anesthesia. In addition to issues with airway management, the differential diagnosis for hypoxemia in a patient with a large VSD should include increases in PVR and an awareness of the factors that can adversely impact PVR. It is important to recognize that the use of phenylephrine to treat hypotension may actually increase the degree of L-to-R shunting by increasing SVR, and although systemic blood pressure may increase, there may be a reduction in systemic cardiac output.

Clinical Pearl

The use of phenylephrine to treat hypotension may actually increase the degree of L-to-R shunting by increasing SVR, and although systemic blood pressure may increase, there may be a reduction in systemic cardiac output.

If the surgeon prefers a laparoscopic approach, what are the physiologic implications for this patient?

Laparoscopic abdominal insufflation increases intraabdominal pressure and may reduce preload. In turn, the pressures required to maintain adequate ventilation increase, as does the degree of atelectasis. Additionally, insufflation with carbon dioxide raises $PaCO_2$. When taken together, this cascade tends to reduce PBF and the degree of L-to-R shunting through the VSD which may be beneficial for this patient. Release of the pneumoperitoneum (i.e., insufflation) at the end of the laparoscopy can lead to a sudden increase in L-to-R shunting and should be monitored closely. Treatment may consist of elevating PVR by reducing minute ventilation or anesthetic depth. If at any point during the laparoscopic approach the hemodynamics become compromised, there should be a discussion with the surgeon regarding conversion to an open surgical approach.

What is an appropriate anesthetic plan for this patient?

In the absence of poor ventricular function, pulmonary hypertension, or other major comorbidities, most patients with isolated VSDs can safely undergo an inhalational induction if appropriately NPO and without risk factors necessitating a rapid sequence induction of anesthesia. However, as this patient has a history of prematurity, vascular access could prove challenging and this should be factored into decision-making regarding the appropriate method of anesthetic induction.

Assuming this patient does not currently have symptoms of heart failure or evidence of pulmonary hypertension, it would be appropriate to proceed with a laparoscopic approach. Although spinal anesthesia is successfully used in some centers, this technique is dependent on surgeon and institutional preference and the surgical approach chosen. A spinal block is not generally used for a laparoscopic approach given the impact of insufflation on the child's ventilatory status and a general anesthetic with endotracheal intubation is appropriate.

A caudal block is helpful to minimize both intraoperative anesthetic requirements and to promote postoperative pain control while minimizing the need for opioids. Young children undergoing regional or neuraxial anesthesia do not experience the sympathectomy seen in adults, and therefore concern for preload reduction is not warranted. While a penile block and/or bilateral ilioinguinal blocks would be reasonable, a caudal block will provide analgesia to all surgical sites. The patient's weight of 3.7 kg in this case precludes multiple blocks due to the limited maximum allowable local anesthetic dosage that can be used.

Fluid management is a final major anesthetic consideration. Intravenous fluids should be administered judiciously, as excessive volume loading may promote postoperative symptoms of CHF and pulmonary edema.

Clinical Pearl

Intravenous fluids should be administered judiciously as excessive volume loading may promote postoperative symptoms of CHF and pulmonary edema.

Can this patient be discharged following an uncomplicated repair?

This patient is at risk for apnea of prematurity which is known to occur more commonly in premature infants (<60 weeks postconceptional age [PCA]) and those with anemia (hemoglobin <10 g/dL). Apnea can be centrally or peripherally mediated, although most cases at this age are of mixed etiology. At-risk patients should be observed following surgery and have at least 12 apnea-free hours prior to discharge. Institutional guidelines may vary regarding the precise PCA required for discharge.

If a spinal anesthetic is performed, it does not obviate the need for postoperative monitoring for apnea. This patient's PCA is approximately 50 weeks, and he should be admitted postoperatively to a unit with the capability to continuously monitor heart rate and pulse oximetry.

Where should the patient be monitored postoperatively and for how long?

The patient may be monitored in the post-anesthesia care unit provided he has an uneventful operative course. Postoperative admission for observation due to the concern for apnea of prematurity is required and should, at minimum, include continuous heart rate and pulse oximetry monitoring. Home medications and diet should be resumed as soon as possible, and unnecessary administration of intravenous fluids should be avoided.

Suggested Reading

Abdulhai S. A., Glenn I. C., and Ponsky T. A. Incarcerated pediatric hernias. *Surg Clin North Am* 2017; **97**: 129–45.

Corno A. F. and Festa P. Ventricular septal defect. In *Congenital Heart Defects: Decision Making for Cardiac Surgery. Volume 3: CT Scan and MRI*. Heidelberg: Steinkopff, 2003; 49–55.

Latham G. J. and Yung D. Current understanding and perioperative management of pediatric pulmonary hypertension. *Pediatr Anesth* 2019; **29**: 441–56.

Minette M. S. and Sahn D. J. Ventricular septal defects. *Circulation* 2006; **114**: 2190–7.

Rosenthal D. N. and Hammer G. B. Cardiomyopathy and heart failure in children: anesthetic implications. *Pediatr Anesth* 2011; **21**: 577–84.

Taylor D. and Habre W. Risk associated with anesthesia for noncardiac surgery in children with congenital heart disease. *Pediatr Anesth* 2019; **29**: 426–34.

Chapter 3

Double-Outlet Right Ventricle

Ramesh Kodavatiganti

Case Scenario

A 2-year-old child weighing 12.3 kg with a history of double-outlet right ventricle, large ventricular septal defect, and pulmonary stenosis presents as an outpatient for elective surgical repair of bilateral strabismus. She was palliated with a right-sided modified Blalock–Taussig shunt shortly after birth. Her parents report that she is active but has been taking more "breathing breaks" lately. Her current medications include aspirin and multivitamins. She sees her cardiologist regularly and complete repair of her cardiac lesion is planned in the forthcoming year. Her parents would prefer to take her home after surgery and would like to know if that is safe.

Vital signs include blood pressure 86/39 mm Hg, respiratory rate 22 breaths/minute, heart rate 127 beats/minute, and SpO_2 86% on room air.

Recent echocardiography findings include:

- *Dynamic subpulmonary obstruction, peak gradient 65 mm Hg through the outflow tract and pulmonary valve*
- *No branch pulmonary artery stenosis*
- *Normal biventricular function*
- *Subaortic ventricular septal defect*

Key Objectives

- Identify anatomic subtypes of double-outlet right ventricle.
- Review the pathophysiology and clinical presentation of double-outlet right ventricle.
- Understand the physiology of a ventricular septal defect combined with severe pulmonary stenosis.
- Formulate a safe anesthetic plan for children with unrepaired double-outlet right ventricle.

Pathophysiology

What is double-outlet right ventricle?

Double-outlet right ventricle (DORV) includes a variety of anatomic arrangements wherein both great arteries, the aorta and pulmonary artery, associate primarily with the right ventricle (RV). Children with DORV nearly always have a ventricular septal defect (VSD). The incidence of DORV is estimated at 1 in 10,000 live births and comprises approximately 1.0% of congenital heart disease (CHD) defects.

Double-outlet right ventricle has many anatomic subtypes depending on the relationship of the VSD to the great arteries and the presence or absence of other coexisting cardiac anomalies. Morphologically DORV lies between VSD with overriding aorta and transposition of the great arteries (TGA). In most cases the great arteries are normally related to each other (aorta posterior and to the right of the pulmonary trunk), but they can be positioned in any configuration in relationship to one another. The VSD is usually unrestrictive and can be variably positioned beneath the great arteries or, less commonly, be remote from the great arteries. Understanding the child's specific cardiac anatomy aids in determining the physiologic implications and guides planning for either surgical palliation or correction.

Clinical Pearl

The clinical presentation of patients with DORV depends on the relationship of the VSD to the great arteries, the variable relationship of the great arteries to each other, and the presence or absence of other coexisting cardiac anomalies.

What additional cardiac defects can be associated with DORV?

The following cardiac defects may be seen in association with DORV:

- Multiple VSDs
- Atrioventricular canal defects
- Atrioventricular valve abnormalities, stenosis, or atresia
- Right ventricular outflow tract obstruction: infundibular, valvular, and/or hypoplasia of pulmonary arteries

- Subaortic stenosis, aortic arch anomalies, or coarctation of the aorta
- Ventricular hypoplasia
- Transposition of the great arteries
- Coronary artery anomalies

Double-outlet right ventricle can also be associated with trisomy 13, 18, and 21 as well as 22q11 deletion.

> **Clinical Pearl**
>
> *Patients with newly diagnosed DORV should undergo thorough evaluation for the existence of associated cardiac and noncardiac anomalies.*

What anatomic features determine the pathophysiology displayed by an individual patient?

The pathophysiology displayed in DORV is a result of the intracardiac shunting that occurs. This varies according to the following anatomic features:

- The size of the VSD and its relationship to the great arteries
- The relationship of the great arteries to one another
- The presence of outflow tract obstruction, either right or left
- The presence of other associated coexisting cardiac anomalies

How may the relationship of the VSD to the great arteries be described anatomically?

The anatomic relationship of the VSD to the great arteries provides the primary basis for the four different subtypes of DORV. Importantly, these descriptions do not imply that the VSD moves within the intraventricular septum, but rather they emphasize the highly variable relationship of the great arteries to each other. (See Figure 3.1.)

Ventricular septal defect–great artery relationships may be described as

- Subaortic VSD (most common)
- Subpulmonic VSD
- Noncommitted VSD: apical or muscular, remote from the great arteries
- Doubly committed VSD (least common)

Double-outlet right ventricle with subaortic VSD (with or without PS) accounts for approximately 50% of DORV presentations, while DORV with subpulmonic VSD accounts for 30%.

> **Clinical Pearl**
>
> *Descriptions of the VSD and its relationship to the great arteries do not imply that the VSD moves within the intraventricular septum, but rather the descriptions emphasize the highly variable relationship of the great arteries to each other.*

What are the physiologic subtypes of DORV?

Double-outlet right ventricle subtypes are a result of the variations that can exist in ventriculoarterial alignment, ranging from concordant or normally related great vessels to discordant relationships or transposition-type relationships. The "VSD-type" and "tetralogy of Fallot (TOF)-type" subtypes are seen with concordant great vessel relationships while the "Taussig–Bing" or "transposition of the great arteries" (TGA) subtype is seen with discordant great vessel relationships (aorta anterior and leftward of pulmonary artery).

Based on the physiologic subtypes of DORV, what clinical presentations are seen?

Double-outlet right ventricle physiology can result in clinical presentations ranging from pulmonary overcirculation and congestive heart failure to cyanosis and pulmonary hypoperfusion.

Double-outlet right ventricle with subaortic VSD: The great vessels are normally related. Two thirds of patients with DORV and a subaortic VSD also have PS in varying degrees. (See Figure 3.1a.)

- *Double-outlet right ventricle, subaortic VSD without PS presents with VSD-type physiology.* These patients will have excessive pulmonary blood flow (PBF) and signs of congestive heart failure as PVR falls after birth.
- *Double-outlet right ventricle, subaortic VSD with PS presents with TOF–type physiology,* with signs of diminished PBF due to the PS. The degree of PS determines the severity of clinical symptoms and signs. The infant will present with a systolic murmur and varying degrees of cyanosis depending on the degree of PS. If pulmonary stenosis is severe or near-critical, additional flow from a patent ductus arteriosus (PDA) may be necessary to ensure adequate PBF. Patients with severe PS may require urgent institution of a prostaglandin (PGE_1) infusion to maintain ductal patency. However, if PS is less severe, with adequate antegrade flow via the right ventricular outflow tract and a balanced systemic and pulmonary circulation, the child could present later in infancy or childhood.

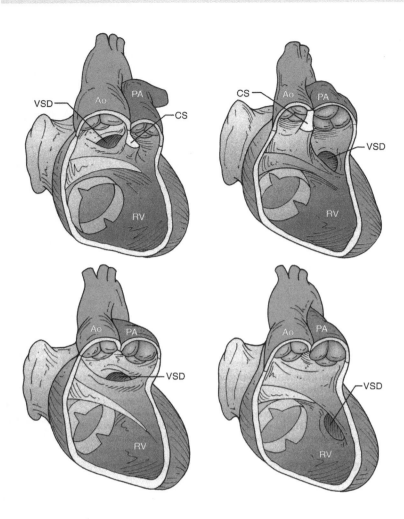

Figure 3.1 Double-outlet right ventricle subtypes according to ventricular septal defect location. Upper left, subaortic VSD. Upper right, subpulmonary VSD. Lower left, doubly committed VSD. Lower right, noncommitted VSD. From Bichell D. Double-outlet right ventricle. In Ungerleider R. M., Meliones J. N., McMillan K. N., et al., eds. *Critical Heart Disease in Infants and Children*, 3rd ed. Elsevier; 2019: 694–704. With permission.

Double-outlet right ventricle with subpulmonic VSD: Because the pulmonary artery (PA) is more closely associated with the LV in this variant, physiology more closely resembles transposition of the great arteries and is known as *TGA-type*. (See Figure 3.1b.) In the Taussig–Bing anomaly, the great arteries are levo-malposed with no PS, and coronary artery and aortic arch anomalies are common. A parallel circulation exists because the LV primarily ejects oxygenated blood through the VSD into the PA while RV-to-aorta flow streams deoxygenated blood into the aorta. Infants with this subtype of DORV present in the neonatal period with cyanosis due to inadequate mixing of oxygenated and deoxygenated blood and may require a balloon atrial septostomy to improve intracardiac mixing and inotropic support to augment cardiac output.

Double-outlet right ventricle with doubly committed VSD can present as *VSD-type* physiology *or TOF-type physiology* depending on the presence or absence of PS

or right ventricular outflow tract obstruction (RVOTO). A large component of the LV output is ejected through the VSD into the closely situated aortic valve. The amount of RV output (deoxygenated blood) directed to the aorta determines the oxygen saturation. Due to the high pulmonary vascular resistance (PVR) at birth these infants present with cyanosis of varying degrees. However, as PVR decreases pulmonary overcirculation may ensue. The infant then develops symptoms of congestive heart failure with tachypnea and failure to thrive. Medical management and optimizing caloric intake are mainstays of therapy until surgical intervention. (See Figure 3.1c.)

Double-outlet right ventricle with noncommitted VSD: Muscular or apical VSDs are more remote from the great arteries and therefore described as noncommitted. These patients have physiology that resembles a complete atrioventricular canal defect. (See Figure 3.1d.)

What are the cardiac surgical treatment options for patients with DORV?

The goal of surgical treatment for DORV is complete anatomic repair, with closure of the VSD and connection of the RV to the pulmonary artery and the LV to the aorta. Timing of surgical repair is dependent on the patient's symptomatology and associated cardiac anomalies.

- *VSD-type DORV*: An intraventricular baffle is placed to close the VSD and direct LV flow through the VSD into the aorta.
- *TOF-type DORV*: Pulmonary stenosis can range from relatively mild to severe and may be valvular, subvalvular, or supravalvular. If PS is severe, the child may be surgically palliated via placement of a modified Blalock–Taussig (mBT) shunt (right subclavian or innominate artery to pulmonary artery) to improve PBF and allow growth while awaiting definitive repair. Corrective surgery will utilize an intraventricular baffle to close the VSD and either a patch to enlarge the RVOT or a right ventricle-to-pulmonary artery (RV–PA) conduit.
- *TGA-type DORV*: An arterial switch procedure is performed along with a baffle closure of the VSD to the PA.

If patients have associated anomalies such as unbalanced ventricular size or straddling atrioventricular valve chordae that render the size of the ventricles or atrioventricular valves inadequate for a two-ventricle repair, they may need to undergo a staged single ventricle palliative approach.

Anesthetic Implications

What is expected clinically for this patient?

The clinical picture resembles that of TOF, with decreased PBF and resultant right-to-left (R-to-L) shunting due to PS. Even though this patient underwent an mBT shunt placement early in life, she may still be at risk for hypercyanotic spells. Most mBT shunts utilize a GOR-TEX® graft, which is not able to grow with the child, thus leading to progressively worsening cyanosis. At 2 years of age with an unrepaired DORV, this child is likely to have symptoms consistent with reduced PBF evidenced by her inability to keep up with her siblings, frequent stopping at play and squatting, and baseline oxygen saturation of 86% on room air. On physical examination central and peripheral cyanosis with clubbing of digits may be evident.

What information is relevant in the preoperative anesthesia assessment?

A detailed clinical history including previous anesthetic issues, current physical status, allergies, and current medications should be obtained. Her last report from her cardiologist should be reviewed as well, and he or she should be made aware of the impending surgery. The pediatric cardiology evaluation should outline the congenital cardiac anomaly, latest echocardiogram report and important current hemodynamic issues and management plans. It is important to understand the cardiac anatomy and pathophysiology by reviewing the echocardiogram and any other available imaging data. A review of the latest electrocardiogram to screen for arrhythmias is important. A discussion between cardiology and ophthalmology should occur regarding the patient's use of aspirin in the perioperative period.

What are some of the perioperative concerns and risks associated with anesthesia?

The perioperative anesthetic management of the patient with DORV, VSD, and PS is similar to that of patients with classic TOF. Physiologic goals include maintaining adequate PBF and baseline oxygen saturations. Increases in heart rate and contractility should be avoided if hyperdynamic components of RVOTO are present. Systemic hypotension should be avoided and systemic vascular resistance (SVR) maintained. Adequate preload should be assured by minimizing fasting time and judicious use of intravenous (IV) fluids. (See Chapters 7, 8, and 47.)

In view of the patient's cardiac physiology particular care should be taken to avoid additional risk factors that might require surgical postponement, such as recent upper or lower respiratory infections.

Is premedication appropriate for this patient?

Children with DORV, VSD, and PS are predisposed to cyanotic spells. Preoperative events such as prolonged fasting duration, acquisition of IV access, and agitation due to separation anxiety may affect the incidence of or provoke cyanotic spells. A preoperative premedication (either midazolam, or a combination of midazolam and ketamine) to decrease the patient's anxiety and enhance compliance with acquisition of IV access is generally beneficial. Alternatively, if the patient already has IV access, dexmedetomidine is an excellent choice as well.

Considering that this child has had an mBT shunt, what precautions should be observed?

In children with a palliative shunt, it is important to maintain adequate hydration, minimize fasting time, avoid stimuli that can provoke preoperative cyanotic spells, and reduce hypotension during all phases of anesthesia. Dehydration can reduce systemic blood pressure and blood flow through the shunt and increase viscosity, which may promote shunt thrombosis.

Most patients with an mBT shunt are maintained on oral anticoagulation or antiplatelet therapy to prevent shunt thrombosis. The pros and cons of withholding anticoagulants in these patients should be discussed with the surgeon and primary cardiology team. In all cases, a plan to restart or bridge anticoagulation for the perioperative period should be in place. The cardiology team should be consulted in cases where the patient is admitted postoperatively.

Clinical Pearl

In patients with mBT shunts, cessation of anticoagulation should be carefully considered and a plan for perioperative management discussed with the cardiologist and surgeon. If anticoagulation is stopped for a procedure, it should be stopped for a minimal amount of time and resumed as soon as possible.

What perioperative monitoring is appropriate for this patient?

Monitoring during strabismus surgery should follow the American Society of Anesthesiologists standard guidelines. Standard noninvasive monitoring is ideal for surgical procedures with minimal blood loss and minimal hemodynamic aberrations. The surgical procedure to be performed along with expected blood loss and fluid shifts often dictates the need for invasive access, particularly arterial blood pressure monitoring. In this case strabismus surgery is unlikely to result in dramatic hemodynamic changes and invasive monitoring is not warranted. Preoperative

baseline hemoglobin-oxygen saturations should be noted and maintained throughout surgery.

What anesthetic considerations are specific to this case?

The occurrence of significant bradycardia and even asystole may occur during ocular manipulation via the oculocardiac reflex. Although anticholinergic premedication (atropine or glycopyrrolate) will help delay and decrease the occurrence of bradycardia, it will not abolish the reflex bradycardia during ocular surgery. In addition, anticholinergic premedication may cause significant tachycardia, which can reduce PBF in the patient with TOF-type physiology. If bradycardia secondary to the oculocardiac reflex does occur, it is best to withhold further surgical stimulation until the heart rate recovers spontaneously. If significant bradycardia persists with the absence of surgical eye manipulation, then treatment with anticholinergics may be warranted.

For this procedure, a laryngeal mask airway may be appropriate, avoiding the depth of anesthesia required for endotracheal intubation. Additionally, analgesia, either topical or by formal ocular block, may be requested from the surgeon and can reduce hemodynamic changes associated with strabismus surgery. Topical medications instilled into the eyes should be discussed with the anesthesiologist and announced prior to administration as they often have systemic absorption.

Clinical Pearl

All ophthalmic medications should be discussed with the anesthesiologist as their systemic absorption can affect cardiac physiology.

What are important intraoperative considerations?

Intraoperative systemic hypotension should be avoided as it will exaggerate the amount of R-to-L shunting and thereby the degree of cyanosis. Patients with a palliative shunt are at risk of shunt occlusion during hypotensive episodes and prolonged fasting periods. A good clinical practice is to auscultate the chest for a shunt murmur over the right parasternal area, assessing mBT shunt flow. This should be done periodically intraoperatively and postoperatively.

The approach to avoiding intraoperative cyanotic spells includes avoiding dehydration, optimizing IV hydration once access is obtained, and optimizing analgesia during surgery. During anesthetic induction it is important to recognize that significant reductions in SVR will increase R-to-L shunting. Should significant cyanosis occur, treatment includes IV fluid boluses, administration of 100% oxygen, and prompt treatment with vasopressors such as phenylephrine.

> **Clinical Pearl**
>
> *Significant reductions in SVR should be avoided as they will increase R-to-L shunting and cyanosis.*

Should sudden changes in oxygenation and hemodynamics occur, what are most likely causes?

Changes in the quality of the shunt murmur along with abrupt changes in blood pressure, oxygen saturation and/ or end-tidal CO_2 should be immediately evaluated and aggressively treated to exclude shunt occlusion as an etiology for decreased PBF. Increasing blood pressure with a systemic vasoconstrictor such as phenylephrine should increase blood pressure and improve oxygen saturations. If the decrease in oxygen saturations persists despite the administration of fluids and phenylephrine, a high probability of shunt occlusion should be assumed and the patient should be given intravenous heparin as an anticoagulant to attempt to reestablish shunt flow and an echocardiogram should immediately be performed to assess the flow characteristics of the mBT shunt.

> **Clinical Pearl**
>
> *A sudden change in hemodynamics, with a decrease in oxygen saturation that is nonresponsive to fluid administration or phenylephrine, should prompt the anesthesia provider to consider the possibility of a shunt occlusion.*

How should extubation of this patient be managed?

Aside from the standard extubation criteria, avoidance of excessive coughing and bucking is crucial to avoid significant intrathoracic pressure elevation and cyanotic episodes. Titration of dexmedetomidine to achieve a smooth and stable emergence while preserving airway patency is often a useful approach.

What are some concerns for postoperative recovery in this patient?

This patient should be observed postoperatively in a monitored setting with providers able to recognize and treat cyanotic spells. The patient should be monitored for the maintenance of an appropriate heart rate and rhythm, blood pressure, and oxygen saturations. In the patient with a palliative mBT shunt it is important that the cardiology team see the child postoperatively and that anticoagulant therapies be resumed as soon as possible unless an alternate plan is already in place.

If the patient presented as an outpatient, what are the criteria for discharge home?

In many cardiac centers a patient with an mBT shunt is monitored in the hospital overnight even after an uneventful anesthetic and surgery. These patients are still at risk for postoperative pain and poor oral intake, which could increase the risk for shunt thrombosis or a hypercyanotic spell. In the patient with an mBT shunt it is important that anticoagulation medications are resumed prior to discharge home.

Suggested Reading

Aoki M., Forbess J. M., Jonas R. A., et al. Results of biventricular repair for double-outlet right ventricle. *J Thorac Cardiovasc Surg* 1994; **107**: 338–49.

Kotwani M., Rayaburg V., and Tendolkar B. A. Anaesthetic management in a patient of uncorrected double outlet right ventricle for emergency surgery. *Indian J Anaesth* 2017; **61**: 87–8.

Spaeth J. P. Perioperative management of DORV. *Semin Cardiothorac Vasc Anesth* 2014; **18**: 281–9.

Walters H. L., Mavroudis C., Tchervenkov C. I., et al. Congenital heart surgery nomenclature and database project: double outlet right ventricle. *Ann Thorac Surg* 2000; **69**: S249–63.

Transitional Atrioventricular Septal Defect

Ana Maria Manrique Espinel and Adam C. Adler

Case Scenario

A 4-year-old child weighing 14 kg arrives to the emergency department after being attacked by a dog. He ate lunch shortly before the incident occurred. The child presents with multiple facial lacerations resulting in significant loss of tissue around his nose and upper lip and is scheduled for urgent debridement, washout, and repair.

His family recently emigrated from Central America and he presented to the pediatrician several weeks ago with shortness of breath. Cardiology evaluation included a chest radiograph that was remarkable for cardiomegaly and increased pulmonary markings.

Transthoracic echocardiogram revealed the following:

- *Large ostium primum atrial septal defect with a left-to-right (L-to-R) shunt*
- *Moderate left-sided atrioventricular valve regurgitation*
- *Restrictive ventricular septal defect*
- *Dilated right atrium and ventricle with preserved function*

The child was diagnosed with a transitional atrioventricular septal defect and started on furosemide.

Examination reveals a mildly tachypneic child who is comfortable after receiving morphine. Auscultation reveals a splitting of the second heart sound along with a holosystolic murmur radiating from the apex to the base. Bibasilar rhonchi are present. Vital signs are respiratory rate 42 breaths/minute, blood pressure 80/39 mm Hg, and SpO$_2$ 100% on room air.

Key Objectives

- Identify the anatomic subtypes of atrioventricular septal defects.
- Review the pathophysiology and clinical presentation for atrioventricular septal defects.
- Formulate an anesthetic plan for children with atrioventricular septal defects.

Pathophysiology

What are the common anatomic characteristics of atrioventricular septal defects?

Atrioventricular septal defects (AVSDs) are common congenital heart defects affecting the interatrial and interventricular septa as well as the atrioventricular valves (AVV). There are three common "types" or descriptions for AVSD defects: partial, transitional, and complete. (See Figure 4.1.) An ostium primum type atrial septal defect (ASD) exists in all types of AVSD defects. (See Chapter 5.)

Atrioventricular septal defects occur due to the failure of endocardial cushions to properly develop and migrate to septate the heart during embryonic development; therefore they are also referred to as *endocardial cushion defects*. The atrial septum primum begins to develop at around day 28 of gestation, growing from the superior portion of the common atrium toward the central endocardial cushions. The septum secundum develops as an atrial infolding to the right of the septum primum. The inferior segment of the atrial septum is an upward extension of the endocardial cushions. It is this inferior segment that fails to extend, leading to the type of ASD found in patients with AVSD defects.

In addition, there is an abnormal, common level of insertion of the AVVs, as well as an elongation of the left ventricular outflow tract (LVOT) due to the anterior displacement of the aortic valve. The anatomic defects associated with the various subtypes of AVSDs are summarized and compared in Table 4.1.

What are the physiologic differences between partial, transitional, and complete AVSD defects?

The physiologic implications of a *partial AVSD* are dependent on the patient's age, the size of the atrial defect, and the presence and degree of other medical issues. Isolated partial AVSD defects will, over time, lead to right-sided overcirculation (L-to-R shunting) and pulmonary overload. In the

Table 4.1 Anatomic Defects Associated with Subtypes of Atrioventricular Septal Defects

Atrioventricular Septal Defect Type	Defect Location	Associated Issues
Partial AV septal defect	**Atrial:** Primum ASD **AVV:** Cleft anterior mitral valve leaflet Two distinct AVV orifices	Tricuspid valve often abnormal Mitral regurgitation due to cleft leaflet
Transitional AV septal defect	**Atrial:** Primum ASD **AVV:** Cleft anterior mitral valve leaflet AV valve anomaly *Ventricular:* VSD (restrictive)	Mitral regurgitation due to cleft leaflet
Complete AV septal defect	**Atrial:** Primum ASD **AVV:** Common AV Valve *Ventricular:* VSD (nonrestrictive)	Mitral regurgitation due to cleft leaflet Classified according to Rastelli types A, B, C

Adapted from Adler A. C., Chandrakantan A., and Litman R. S. (eds.), *Case Studies in Pediatric Anesthesia*, 1st ed. Cambridge University Press. With permission.

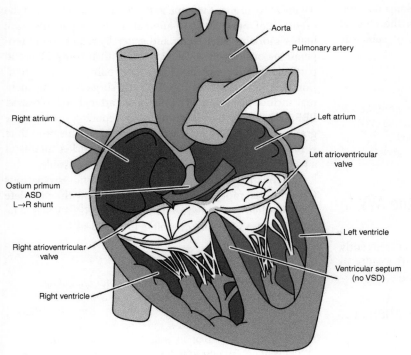

Aorta
Pulmonary artery
Right atrium
Left atrium
Left atrioventricular valve
Ostium primum ASD L→R shunt
Right atrioventricular valve
Left ventricle
Ventricular septum (no VSD)
Right ventricle

Figure 4.1 Partial atrioventricular septal defect.
Drawing by Ryan Moore, MD, and Matt Nelson.

presence of pulmonary hypertension or right ventricular outflow tract (RVOT) obstruction, the degree of L-to-R shunting may be reduced or eliminated. (See Figure 4.1.)

In addition to a partial AVSD defect, ***transitional AVSDs*** include a small and restrictive VSD that is occluded by chordal attachments. Generally, a transitional AVSD is not associated with physiologic implications of greater significance than those seen with a partial AVSD. The right

atrium and ventricle are typically enlarged and, with time, the increased pulmonary blood flow (PBF) may produce changes in the pulmonary vasculature. As a response to prolonged and excessive PBF, changes occur in the pulmonary vascular musculature that can result in pulmonary vascular occlusive disease (PVOD). If untreated, flow reversal ultimately occurs when right-sided pressures exceed left-sided pressures. This is known as Eisenmenger syndrome and patients become cyanotic due to the right-to-left (R-to-L) shunting.

In *complete AVSD* the VSD is large and unrestrictive, and therefore significant L-to-R shunting occurs at both the atrial and ventricular levels, with right ventricular and pulmonary artery pressures that are the same as systemic pressures. This produces symptoms earlier in the course of disease and hastens both diagnosis and need for treatment.

What cardiac anomalies of the AV valves and LVOT are associated with AVSD defects?

In patients with AVSDs the left and right AVV have the same level of insertion. This occurs due to a downward displacement of the left AV valve to the level of the septal leaflet of the right AV valve. Secondary to this, the distance between the cardiac crux to the left ventricular apex is decreased and the distance between the apex and the LVOT increases giving the characteristic "goose-neck" deformity. The elongation and narrowing of the LVOT in conjunction with the chordal attachment to the septum increases the risk of subaortic stenosis and coarctation of the aorta.

Clinical Pearl

Patients with AVSDs have an anterior displacement of the aorta, increasing the elongation and narrowing of the LVOT. It is important to evaluate for the presence of LVOT obstruction and subaortic stenosis by echocardiography.

What is the characteristic defect of the AVV in patients with AVSD defect?

The AVV is abnormal, with a coaptation defect frequently referred to as a cleft. The presence of a cleft results in regurgitance, occurring mainly at the left-sided AVV.

What are the cardiac surgical considerations for a patient with an AVSD?

In general, the timing of cardiac surgical intervention is dependent on the type of AVSD and patient symptomatology. The presence of congestive heart failure (CHF) and/or failure to thrive not amenable to medical management are indications for surgery. Surgery requires the use of cardiopulmonary bypass (CPB), allowing for patch closures of the atrial and ventricular level defects and repair of the AVV. The most technically challenging part of this procedure is addressing the common AVV in cases of complete ASVD. The valve is suspended and divided into right and left AV valves. Lesion-specific complications include residual atrial

or ventricular septal defects, conduction pathway anomalies, and valvular regurgitation/insufficiency.

What are the clinical implications of AVSDs?

In both partial and transitional AVSDs, medical and surgical treatment is dictated by the degree of L-to-R shunting and the presence of other cardiac anomalies. Generally, there is significant flow from the left atrium to the right atrium, but cardiac catheterization usually demonstrates RV pressures that are less than 60% of systemic pressures. Patients are often managed with diuretics and fluid restriction and typically remain asymptomatic for years. The most common scenario involves deferral of repair until the patient is older, avoiding the necessity for CPB early in development.

A subset of patients with AVSDs, especially those with complete defects, may present with early symptoms of heart failure, necessitating more urgent repair. The severity of clinical presentation depends on the size of the L-to-R shunt, the degree of regurgitant volume at the level of the AVV, and the presence of other cardiac anomalies. These patients have higher mortality after repair and generally require more reoperations on the left AVV. Patients with trisomy 21 are at particular risk for early development of pulmonary hypertension (PH) and resultant PVOD. Early surgical management may include placement of a pulmonary artery band to restrict PBF and reduce L-to-R shunting by reducing the pressure gradient between the right and left ventricles. This procedure is more likely to be performed on smaller, sicker infants as a palliative procedure until complete repair is possible.

Interestingly, the presence of syndromic associations (trisomy) is more common in patients with complete AVSDs when compared to those with partial AVSDs. The majority of AVSDs are complete (56%–75%).

Clinical Pearl

Partial and transitional AVSDs have similar physiologic implications and are often diagnosed later in life as L-to-R shunting is not as significant. Patients with complete AVSDs have more significant L-to-R shunting with more severe pulmonary overcirculation, usually necessitating earlier intervention. Patients with trisomy 21 are at particular risk for early development of PH and resultant PVOD.

What findings are commonly seen in patients with AVSDs?

In general, the presence of an isolated ostium primum ASD is discovered by auscultation of a holosystolic murmur due to high pulmonary flow, and a mid-diastolic rumble may be noted as well depending on the degree of AVV regurgitation present. Due to pulmonary overcirculation patients may appear dyspneic or tachypneic, especially with exertion or during feeding.

Electrocardiography may demonstrate a prolonged P-R interval due to the downward displacement of the conductive tissue (AV node) and the enlargement of the right atrium. A chest radiograph may show cardiomegaly with increased pulmonary markings and a characteristic "gooseneck" appearance due to the anterior displacement of the aorta.

What are the important echocardiographic and angiographic findings?

Echocardiography is the gold standard for diagnosis of AVSDs. The ASD is usually large and appreciated from the apical and subcostal four-chamber views. Despite cavity enlargement, biventricular function in these patients is generally normal. The degree of regurgitation of the AV valves should be evaluated as well as an estimate of the RV pressures from the right-sided AV valve insufficiency jet. The position, size, and degree of shunting at the ventricular level should be well characterized, and systematic evaluation of the LVOT for the detection of narrowing, obstruction, or the presence of subaortic stenosis should be well defined. Three-dimensional echocardiography may be employed to determine the mechanism of AVV lack of coaptation in order to facilitate surgical planning.

Angiography and cardiac catheterization are generally reserved for patients in whom there is a clinical or echocardiographic suspicion of PH or PVOD in order to determine the likelihood of successful closure of the septal defect.

Clinical Pearl

Echocardiography is the gold standard for diagnosis of AVSDs. Despite cavity enlargement, biventricular function in these patients is generally normal. The position, size, and degree of shunting at the ventricular level should be well characterized, and systematic evaluation of the LVOT for the detection of narrowing, obstruction, or the presence of subaortic stenosis should be well defined.

Anesthetic Implications

What are the anesthetic implications for patients with unrepaired AVSDs?

Preoperative evaluation should focus on the type of AVSD, the degree of pulmonary overcirculation, and a detailed review of echocardiographic findings. The presence of coexisting anomalies (e.g., trisomy 21) should be considered. Functional capacity should be elucidated, as it helps to understand the degree of heart failure due to pulmonary overcirculation.

Intraoperative management is also dictated by the degree of pulmonary overcirculation, biventricular function, and comorbidities. Generally, an inhalation induction of anesthesia is well tolerated in the absence of PH. In the presence of severe heart failure, an intravenous (IV) induction is preferred, with the agent of choice depending on the degree of heart failure and severity of AVV regurgitation. In the presence of normal ventricular function, anesthetic agents that reduce systemic vascular resistance (SVR), such as sevoflurane and propofol, are usually well tolerated. In the patient with a large L-to-R shunt, the use of a low inspired oxygen concentration and mild hypoventilation increases PVR and improves systemic cardiac output.

A most important consideration is the meticulous de-airing of IV lines and the use of filters, as air bubbles may enter the arterial circulation. This risk for paradoxical embolism is increased if the shunt reverses to R-to-L. Intravenous fluids should be administered judiciously to avoid pulmonary edema from increased pulmonary flow while also recognizing that many of these patients are on chronic diuretic therapy and that commonly used anesthetic agents lead to vasodilation and reduced preload. Additionally, special consideration is required during periods of desaturation as intraoperative desaturation in patients with complete AVSDs may be the result of pulmonary pressure elevation promoting R-to-L shunting. Finally, patients with large left AVV coaptation defects and significant regurgitation benefit from reduced afterload.

In general, the use of standard American Society of Anesthesiologists recommended monitoring is sufficient. Consideration may be given to the use of invasive arterial blood pressure monitoring in cases where large fluid shifts or blood loss are anticipated, and/or for patients with ventricular dysfunction.

Clinical Pearl

Intraoperative management is also dictated by the degree of pulmonary overcirculation, ventricular function, and comorbidities. Important considerations include the meticulous de-airing of IV lines to avoid the risk of air emboli.

What specific considerations exist for this patient?

This patient, having eaten immediately prior to the incident, has not met the nil per os (NPO) standard and should therefore have an IV rapid sequence induction of anesthesia. A specific and detailed examination of the child's airway and injuries is important prior to induction of anesthesia, realizing that it may be difficult to get a good mask fit due to the extent of the injuries. As the child has received morphine in the emergency department, a peripheral IV is likely already present and may be utilized to provide additional anxiolysis if necessary, at the time of parental separation.

As the echocardiogram shows preserved ventricular function, propofol could be used for induction along with either succinylcholine or rocuronium for neuromuscular blockade. A multimodal approach to analgesia would be appropriate, with the use of intravenous acetaminophen and local anesthetic by the surgeons.

Are there special considerations for postoperative care?

Following an uneventful intraoperative course, patients with unrepaired partial or transitional AVSDs without signs of CHF may recover in the post-anesthesia care unit with standard monitoring and postoperative discharge or admission. Home medications should be continued. If large fluid shifts occurred or a large volume of fluid or blood transfusion was required, cardiology consultation may be prudent.

In patients with complete and unrepaired AVSDs, or those with preoperative signs of heart failure or indicators of PVOD, admission to the intensive care unit may be warranted, particularly after major surgeries. Following prolonged surgical procedures or procedures with expected large fluid shifts, patients should be followed closely because of the risk of pulmonary volume overload and an increased likelihood of postoperative oxygen requirements in these patients.

Suggested Reading

Calkoen E. E., Hazekamp M. G., Blom N. A., et al. Atrioventricular septal defect: from embryonic development to long-term follow-up. *Int J Cardiol* 2016; **202**: 784–95.

Davey B. T. and Rychik J. The natural history of atrioventricular valve regurgitation throughout fetal life in patients with atrioventricular canal defects. *Pediatr Cardiol* 2016; **37**: 50–4.

Krupickova S., Morgan G. J., Cheang M. H., et al. Symptomatic partial and transitional atrioventricular septal defect repaired in infancy. *Heart* 2018; **104**: 1411–16.

Mery C. M., Zea-Vera R., Chacon-Portillo M. A., et al. Contemporary results after repair of partial and transitional atrioventricular septal defects. *J Thorac Cardiovasc Surg* 2019; **157**: 1117–27.

Ross F. J., Nasr V. G., Joffe D., et al. Perioperative and anesthetic considerations in atrioventricular septal defect. *Semin Cardiothorac Vasc Anesth* 2017; **21**: 221–8.

Tishler B., Gauvreau K., Colan S. D., et al. Technical performance score predicts partial/transitional atrioventricular septal defect outcomes. *Ann Thorac Surg* 2018; **105**: 1461–8.

5

Unbalanced Atrioventricular Septal Defect

Lori Q. Riegger

Case Scenario

A 1-day-old, full-term female weighing 3.1 kg with the characteristic facies of trisomy 21 vomits after her first oral feeding and an abdominal radiograph reveals duodenal atresia. She is made nil per os and a nasogastric tube is placed to aspirate secretions and gas. The patient is scheduled for repair of duodenal atresia with a laparoscopic approach.

Current vital signs are blood pressure 75/38 mm Hg, heart rate 138 beats/minute, respiratory rate 29 breaths/minute, and SpO$_2$ 98% on room air.

Transthoracic echocardiogram revealed the following:

- *Complete atrioventricular septal defect (Rastelli type A) with a common atrioventricular valve unbalanced to the right*
- *Mild hypoplasia of the transverse aortic arch and aortic isthmus with peak gradient 21 mm Hg*
- *Moderate common atrioventricular valve regurgitation*
- *Moderately dilated right ventricle with normal biventricular function*

Key Objectives

- Review the pathophysiology of a complete atrioventricular septal defect.
- Compare the anatomic and physiologic differences between balanced and unbalanced atrioventricular septal defects.
- Formulate a perioperative anesthetic plan for an infant with an unbalanced atrioventricular septal defect.
- Discuss the implications of laparoscopic insufflation for patients with unrepaired atrioventricular septal defect.

Pathophysiology

What is a complete atrioventricular septal defect?

Also known as an endocardial cushion defect, a complete atrioventricular septal defect (AVSD) is a constellation of defects at the AV junction. Instead of two separate AV

valves, mitral and tricuspid, there is a single common valve orifice serving both ventricles. The common AV valve is situated between the right and left sides of the heart and includes two leaflets that bridge the right and left sides; these are designated as the superior (anterior) bridging leaflet and the inferior (posterior) bridging leaflet. Just superior to the plane of the common AV valve is a primum atrial septal defect (ASD), and just inferior to this plane is an inlet ventricular septal defect (VSD). These defects collectively comprise a communication between the four chambers in the center of the heart. (See Figure 5.1.)

> **Clinical Pearl**
>
> *With a septum primum ASD, an inlet VSD, and a common AV valve, a complete AVSD collectively comprises a communication between the four chambers in the center of the heart.*

What are the primary physiologic issues in a patient with a complete AVSD?

The primary physiologic aberrations in patients with AVSD include:

- ***Left-to-right (L-to-R) shunting*** of blood through the ASD and VSD that can lead to congestive heart failure (CHF), increased cardiac work, and resultant ventricular hypertrophy
- ***AV valve regurgitation*** that can lead to volume overload of the ventricles and decreased cardiac output

How does L-to-R shunting occur in the context of an AVSD?

Left-to-right shunting occurs when blood moves from the left to the right side of the heart through the septal defects such that oxygenated blood meant to flow to the systemic circulation instead flows back through the right side of the heart to the lungs.

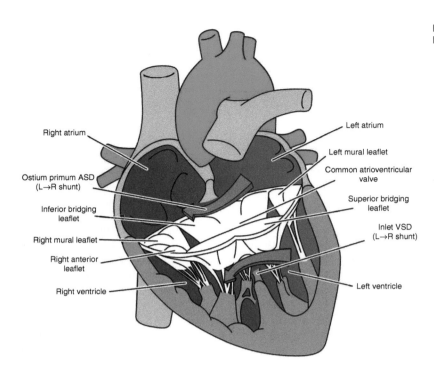

Figure 5.1 Complete atrioventricular septal defect.
Drawing by Ryan Moore, MD, and Matt Nelson.

In restrictive ASDs and VSDs, blood flows L-to-R due to the higher pressure in the LA and LV compared to the RA and RV.

With a nonrestrictive VSD, pressures are essentially equal in the LV and RV such that the direction of blood flow will proceed in the direction of lower resistance. Pulmonary vascular resistance (PVR) is usually lower than systemic vascular resistance (SVR) so blood preferentially flows away from the systemic circulation and toward the lungs. At birth, due to elevated PVR, the L-to-R shunt may not be as large, whereas several weeks later after PVR has fallen to postnatal levels the L-to-R shunt will be more significant. As PVR decreases, L-to-R shunting increases.

Clinical Pearl

With a nonrestrictive VSD, pressures are essentially equal in the LV and RV such that the direction of blood flow will proceed in the direction of lower resistance. Pulmonary vascular resistance is usually lower than SVR, so blood preferentially flows away from the systemic circulation and toward the lungs.

What is the Rastelli classification?

In 1966, Giancarlo Rastelli described a classification system to help identify different approaches for surgical repair of complete AVSD based on anatomic variation in the defects. This classification system is based on the morphology of the anterior (superior) bridging leaflet, the amount of bridging over the VSD, the location of chordal attachments, and the degree of associated hypoplasia of the tricuspid anterosuperior leaflet. Classification is not based on the inferior bridging leaflet or the posterior common leaflet.

- *Rastelli type A*: This is the most common variant, with the anterior common leaflet separated into a right and left component by extensive attachment of chordae tendineae from the superior bridging leaflet to the crest of the ventricular septum. The left superior leaflet is situated directly over the left ventricle (LV) while the right superior leaflet is directly over the RV. The superior leaflet is divided and attached to the ventricular septum.
- *Rastelli type B*: The type B atrioventricular septal defect is rare, with an anomalous papillary muscle attached to the left side of the common anterior bridging leaflet from the right side of the ventricular septum.
- *Rastelli type C*: In the type C AVSD, the ventricular septum is bridged by the anterior bridging leaflet, which is not divided and is without chordae attachments to the crest of the ventricular septum. The valve is therefore floating above the ventricular septum.

What is the relationship between trisomy 21 and an AVSD?

Trisomy 21 is the most common genetic abnormality in infants and the most frequent chromosomal anomaly associated with CHD. Forty to fifty percent of patients with trisomy 21 have CHD, which is a major cause of morbidity and mortality for these patients. For children with both trisomy 21 and CHD, 45% have some type of AVSD, of which 75% are complete AVSDs. Additionally, 50% of patients found to have an AVSD have trisomy 21. However, if repaired in the first year of life, long-term results are unchanged.

What symptoms are associated with a complete AVSD in a neonate?

A neonate with an AVSD may exhibit signs of CHF. These signs may include tachypnea, tachycardia, fatigue when feeding, sweating, and poor weight gain. In a patient with a large VSD, severe AV valve regurgitation, or other cardiac anomalies, symptoms may occur in the first week of life. In less severely affected patients, symptoms may not become evident until the postnatal PVR falls and the L-to-R shunting increases, usually within the first few months of life.

> **Clinical Pearl**
>
> *The degree of L-to-R shunting in a patient with an AVSD is a major determinant of both cardiac symptoms and the development of pulmonary hypertension.*

When anatomically describing an AVSD what does the term "unbalanced" imply?

An unbalanced AVSD occurs when the common AV valve sits disproportionately in one ventricle such that the atrioventricular junction is misaligned. The contralateral ventricle and outflow tract typically have varying degrees of hypoplasia, with the inflow to that ventricle often diminished or restricted. While only approximately 10% of AVSDs are unbalanced, this anatomic variant is more likely to be associated with poor outcomes and increased mortality [1]. (See Figure 5.2.)

> **Clinical Pearl**
>
> *An unbalanced AVSD occurs when the common AV valve sits disproportionately in one ventricle such that the atrioventricular junction is misaligned. The contralateral ventricle and outflow tract typically have varying degrees of hypoplasia, with inflow to that ventricle often diminished or restricted.*

Figure 5.2 Unbalanced atrioventricular septal defect. Drawing by Ryan Moore, MD, and Matt Nelson.

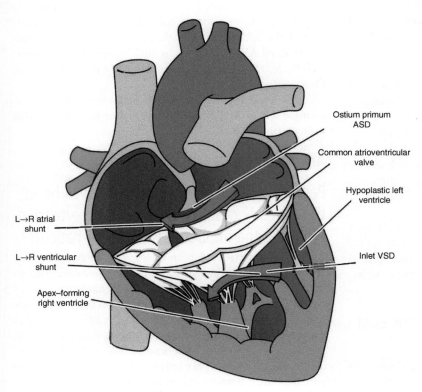

Ostium primum ASD

Common atrioventricular valve

Hypoplastic left ventricle

Inlet VSD

L→R atrial shunt

L→R ventricular shunt

Apex–forming right ventricle

In unbalanced AVSD anatomy, what is right dominance versus left dominance?

Dominance reflects the ability of blood to traverse through the valve inlet to fill the ventricle. The side contralateral to the dominant ventricle often has some degree of hypoplasia and filling may be inadequate through the diminished area of the corresponding valve leaflets. When more of the common AV valve is apportioned over the RV, this is known as *right dominance*. Those with the common AV valve distributed more over the LV have *left dominance*.

Why is it important to understand the degree to which the AVSD is unbalanced?

The degree to which the AVSD is unbalanced will guide treatment of the cardiac disease.

If common AV valve unbalance is mild, the patient may be treated similarly to a patient with a balanced AVSD, where the predominant concern is to mitigate the L-to-R shunt and decrease the risk of heart failure and pulmonary hypertension. These patients may be discharged from the hospital after birth on medical therapy (diuretics and antihypertensives) to decrease the risk of heart failure. Cardiac surgery to repair the AVSD will likely occur when the child is several months old. Early surgical intervention may be required during the neonatal period if there is significant pulmonary overcirculation or inadequate pulmonary blood flow (PBF).

If common AV valve unbalance is severe, the child generally requires single ventricle palliation as the structures on the nondominant side of the heart are hypoplastic, including the ventricle and outflow tracts.

- In a *LEFT dominant* unbalanced AVSD, the RV and outflow tract may be hypoplastic and PBF may depend on a patent ductus arteriosus (PDA), requiring a prostaglandin (PGE_1) infusion to maintain ductal patency.
- In a *RIGHT dominant* unbalanced AVSD such as this patient, the LV, left ventricular outflow tract, and aorta may be hypoplastic and therefore systemic blood flow may depend on a PDA.

The decision to repair a mildly unbalanced AVSD with a two-ventricular repair or a severely unbalanced AVSD with SV palliation may be clear. However, the optimal surgical approach for a patient with a moderately unbalanced AVSD may not always be apparent.

What cardiac surgical treatment options exist for a moderately unbalanced AVSD?

Overall, surgical options are suboptimal. In a patient with a *left dominant*, moderately unbalanced AVSD the RV is usually hypoplastic to varying degrees. Depending on the degree of hypoplasia, a two-ventricle repair may be attempted because some RV hypoplasia may be tolerated. If a two-ventricle repair is not well tolerated, a superior cavopulmonary shunt (Glenn shunt) may be added as a way to offload volume from the small RV. This anatomic configuration is referred to as a 1 ½ ventricle repair and is an option only for a left dominant unbalanced AVSD.

There is no way to offload the LV in a *right dominant* unbalanced AVSD. The options for this type of defect are dichotomous: either a two-ventricle repair or SV palliation. In this case, the patient has a gradient across the aortic arch and isthmus but has normal LV systolic function and will ultimately have a two-ventricle repair.

What is the expected long-term survival for patients with unbalanced AVSDs?

Long-term survival is dependent on the degree of AVSD imbalance and the planned surgical interventions. A patient with a mildly unbalanced AVSD who undergoes two-ventricle repair may be expected to have survival rates close to those of patients with a balanced AVSD repair. Alternatively, patients with a severely unbalanced AVSD requiring single ventricle palliation (due to one ventricle being excessively diminutive) have lower long-term survival compared to patients with two-ventricle repairs. The difference in outcome may be attributable to either coexisting congenital defects or severe dysfunction of the AV valve, or both, in a patient with severely unbalanced AVSD. There is a 30% incidence of reoperation being required to address AV valve regurgitation in these patients [2].

With regard to single-ventricle palliation, patients with a single left ventricle tend to fare better than those with a single right ventricle.

Anesthetic Implications

Patients with trisomy 21 are known to be at risk for early onset of pulmonary hypertension. What are the implications for these patients?

Rapid development of pulmonary arterial hypertension (PAH) within the first year of life has been described in trisomy 21 patients. Although the mechanisms are not clearly understood, this makes it imperative to repair lesions with large L-to-R shunts early in life before PAH can develop. Additionally, medical therapy aimed to limit the excessive PBF should be undertaken in the time preceding the cardiac surgery to lessen the risk of PAH. Some patients with trisomy 21 may not have the expected postnatal decrease in PVR seen in patients without trisomy 21. When the PVR remains high in such patients, they may not exhibit signs of CHF, since the PBF would be impeded by elevated PVR. Interestingly, patients with trisomy 21 without CHD are still at risk for developing PAH. This suggests that other pathologies such as airway obstruction (tonsillar hypertrophy or laryngotracheomalacia) may contribute to the development of PAH in these patients [2]. Because PVR is often elevated in patients with trisomy 21, single ventricle palliation is not the preferred long-term option in patients with this genetic disorder and a two-ventricle repair may be more aggressively pursued.

Should other diagnostic tests be done prior to surgery?

Preoperative laboratory studies should include hemoglobin/hematocrit, electrolyte panel, and a type and screen for blood.

A chest radiograph may show an enlarged cardiac silhouette and increased vascular markings consistent with pulmonary fluid overload. The electrocardiogram (ECG) will often show first degree AV block. Congenital heart block is also a risk in a patient with an AVSD.

Echocardiography should provide adequate information regarding cardiac anatomy and additional imaging should not be necessary prior to the abdominal surgery. Details that should be gleaned from the echocardiogram include:

- The degree of L-to-R shunting
- The degree of unbalance of the AV valve
- Is one ventricle dominant, and if so, to what degree?
- Evidence for and severity of pulmonary hypertension
- Size and function of the ventricles
- Any existence of outflow tract obstruction

What anesthetic concerns exist in a patient with trisomy 21?

Anesthetic concerns in patients with trisomy 21 focus on three main areas: risk for bradycardia, airway issues, and other comorbidities. Owing to their high vagal tone trisomy 21 patients are at increased risk for bradycardia during anesthetic induction with sevoflurane so prompt recognition and treatment – either by decrease in volatile agent concentration and/or administration of atropine – are indicated. Patients often have anatomic airway abnormalities including macroglossia, crowding of the midface, high arched palate, subglottic stenosis, wide, short neck, and adenotonsillar hypertrophy that can increase the risk of upper airway obstruction and difficult

intubation. Owing to the risk of subglottic stenosis it is often prudent to downsize the endotracheal tube. Other comorbidities frequently found in patients with trisomy 21 that should be addressed in the preoperative assessment are the potential for C1–C2 subluxation causing cervical spine instability, developmental delay, hypothyroidism, difficult intravenous (IV) access, and gastrointestinal anomalies.

Clinical Pearl

Anesthetic concerns in trisomy 21 patients include bradycardia with sevoflurane induction, airway obstruction, and cardiac disease.

What considerations exist regarding arterial and central line monitoring in this patient?

For patients with all but the most mildly unbalanced AVSD (which may effectively be treated as a large VSD or balanced AVSD) an arterial line may be useful to provide blood pressure monitoring and blood gas analysis, particularly for prolonged cases or in cases where large fluid shifts and/or blood loss are anticipated. However, it is important to realize that placement of an arterial line in infants with Down syndrome can be challenging. The patient's preoperative condition and proposed length of surgery will assist with decision making. With a laparoscopic surgical approach planned in this patient, it can also prove helpful to closely monitor the effects of insufflation on blood pressure and ventilation so that the surgical plan may be modified if necessary.

In the neonate with a severely unbalanced AVSD and significant outflow tract obstruction, a PGE_1 infusion will likely be required for maintenance of the PDA. In this situation a central line is indicated in order to administer vasoactive medications. A peripherally inserted central catheter (PICC) may have already been placed prior to surgery and can be useful for administration of PGE_1 and other vasoactive drugs. When possible, it is best to avoid placing an internal jugular vein line in a neonate who may require a future superior cavopulmonary anastomosis (Glenn procedure). Peripheral IV access will suffice for administration of anesthetic drugs and blood products if needed.

What concerns exist regarding utilizing a laparoscopic surgical approach in this particular case?

Abdominal insufflation is known to decrease cardiac output, increase SVR, increase peak inspiratory pressures, and decrease lung volumes at a given pressure. Insufflation with CO_2 may elevate right-sided pressures and increase $PaCO_2$, resulting in decreased PBF and increased R-to-L shunting. A preoperative discussion with the surgeon prior to a laparoscopic procedure in a patient with CHD should include the potential need to decrease insufflation pressure or abandon laparoscopy and open the abdomen if the patient cannot tolerate pneumoperitoneum.

Although the same study has not been repeated in children with CHD, outcome studies in patients with CHD having laparoscopic surgeries have demonstrated that as the severity of the heart disease increases, so does the morbidity and mortality.

Clinical Pearl

Laparoscopic surgery in patients with complex CHD is most successful when there is continual communication between the surgical and anesthesia teams about the effects of insufflation on the patient's hemodynamics. It may be necessary to decrease insufflation pressures or modify the original surgical plan if ventilation and hemodynamics are negatively impacted.

What medications could be used to induce and maintain anesthesia?

An IV induction is appropriate in this scenario. Care should be taken to avoid acute changes in either SVR or PVR during induction. Ketamine, etomidate, midazolam, fentanyl, and/ or dexmedetomidine along with a neuromuscular blocking agent can be utilized. Propofol, if chosen, should be given in incremental or reduced doses to avoid significant decreases in SVR.

Anesthetic maintenance may be achieved with a combination of inhalational agents and narcotics. The use of neuromuscular blocking agents is helpful during intubation and generally requested by the surgeon to achieve optimal surgical conditions. Although for most infants the goal should be to extubate the trachea at the conclusion of the procedure, consideration should be given to the length of the procedure and the infant's preoperative condition.

How should ventilation be managed in this patient?

The degree to which blood shunts and the direction in which it shunts can be heavily influenced by ventilatory techniques. Hypocarbia and the use of high inspired concentrations of oxygen can result in decreases in PVR which promote L-to-R shunting and increased PBF at the expense of systemic blood flow. These patients should be placed on low inspired oxygen concentrations and the $PaCO_2$ should be maintained near 40 mm Hg to avoid pulmonary over-circulation. However, during the period of insufflation, the increased abdominal pressure may decrease gas exchange and require increased minute ventilation and/or oxygen concentration to maintain the desired hemoglobin oxygen saturation and $ETCO_2$. Monitoring of arterial blood gases during this time may help guide ventilatory strategies as they may require frequent attention and manipulation.

Clinical Pearl

Adjusting ventilatory strategies can prove helpful in balancing cardiac shunting during abdominal insufflation.

What are the considerations for intraoperative hypotension and how should it be managed?

In addition to surgically related causes of hypotension such as bleeding and insufflation, cardiac related causes should also be considered. Intracardiac shunting can occur in either direction (L-to-R or R-to-L) and will vary throughout surgery depending on the relative systemic and pulmonary vascular resistances. Factors lowering SVR (e.g., anesthetic agents) will result in increases in systemic blood flow at the expense of PBF, and similarly factors that lower PVR and augment PBF (hypocarbia, increased FiO_2) will consequently decrease systemic blood flow. If the infant is hypotensive, it is imperative to adjust any factors which may be augmenting PBF at the expense of systemic blood flow.

In general, these patients may prove sensitive to the myocardial depressant and vasodilatory effects of inhalation and intravenous anesthetics. If an arterial line is present, an arterial blood gas should be assessed for anemia, acidosis, and calcium levels, and any abnormalities treated. Fluids should be judiciously replaced to account for blood loss and third spacing. If appropriate fluid replacement has occurred and hypotension persists, an epinephrine or dopamine infusion should be available if needed to support the patient's cardiac function. Calcium chloride 10 mg/kg or calcium gluconate 30 mg/kg can also be useful for augmenting cardiac output. Calcium gluconate is preferable for patients who have only peripheral IV access.

If laparoscopy is abandoned for laparotomy and the patient remains hypotensive, inotropic support should be instituted, and plans made to keep the infant intubated postoperatively.

What are the postoperative considerations for this patient?

If the procedure is completed via laparoscopic approach and the patient has been hemodynamically stable throughout the procedure, it may be appropriate to extubate the patient in the operating room, albeit with the usual caution utilized for a 1-day-old infant. Even so, recovery should occur in the appropriate intensive care environment, either neonatal or cardiac. In a patient with ductal-dependent physiology, recovery (with or without extubation) should preferably take place in an intensive care unit where practitioners are familiar with cardiac physiology and management (e.g., the cardiac intensive care unit). If the patient has been unstable during the procedure, it is advisable to defer extubation.

References

1. Owens G. E., Gomez-Fifer C., Gelehrter S., et al. Outcomes for patients with unbalanced atrioventricular septal defects. *Pediatr Cardiol* 2009; **30**: 431–5.

2. Craig B. Atrioventricular septal defect: from fetus to adult. *Heart* 2006; **48**: 1879–85.

Suggested Reading

Backer C. L. and Mavroudis C. Atrioventricular canal defects. In Mavroudis C., and Backer C. L., eds., *Pediatric Cardiac Surgery*. Oxford: Wiley Blackwell, 2013; 342–60.

Cetta F., Minich L. L., Maleszewski J. J., et al. Atrioventricular septal defects. In Allen H., Driscoll D. J., Shaddy R. E., et al. eds. *Moss and Adams' Heart Disease in Infants, Children and Adolescents*, 8th ed. Philadelphia: Lippincott Williams & Wilkins, 2013; 691–712.

Mitchell M. E., Litwin S. B., and Tweddell J. S. Complex atrioventricular canal. *Semin Thorac Cardiovasc Surg Pediatr Card Surg Ann* 2007; **10**: 32–41.

Nicolson S. C., Steven J. M., Diaz L. K., et al. Anesthesia for the patient with a single ventricle. In Andropoulos D. B., Stayer S., Mossad E. B. et al. eds. *Anesthesia for Congenital Heart Disease*, 3rd ed. Hoboken, NJ: John Wiley & Sons, 2015; 567–97.

Sassalos P., Si M. S., Ohye R. G., et al. Atrioventricular septal defects. In Ungerleider R. M., Meliones J. N., McMillan K. N., et al. eds. *Critical Heart Disease in Infants and Children*, 3rd ed. Philadelphia, Mosby Elsevier, 2019; 606–14.

Critical Pulmonic Stenosis

Jennie Ngai

6

Case Scenario

A 5-day-old male presents with tachypnea and poor feeding after being discharged home on day 2 of life. His mother had an uneventful pregnancy with routine prenatal care and testing and he was born via spontaneous vaginal delivery without complications. On day 4 of life his mother noted that his breathing was fast and he was not eating well and decided to seek care. At the pediatrician's office the patient was noted to have room air oxygen saturations of 75%.

Transthoracic echocardiography showed the following:

- *Critical valvular pulmonary stenosis, peak gradient 72 mm Hg*
- *Intact ventricular septum*
- *Mild right ventricular hypertrophy*
- *Normal left ventricular function*
- *Mild to moderately depressed right ventricular function*
- *Moderate tricuspid regurgitation*
- *Patent foramen ovale with bidirectional shunting*

He was admitted to the congenital cardiac intensive care unit and was started on prostaglandin E₁ and milrinone. He is scheduled for balloon valvuloplasty of the pulmonic valve in the cardiac catheterization laboratory.

Key Objectives

- Describe the role of the ductus arteriosus during fetal life.
- Discuss echocardiographic findings related to pulmonary stenosis.
- Describe perioperative management of a patient with critical pulmonary stenosis.

Pathophysiology

What is the pathophysiology of critical pulmonary stenosis?

During fetal development, little blood flows through the lungs because of high pulmonary vascular resistance (PVR). During fetal life, the majority of pulmonary artery blood flow

is directed through the ductus arteriosus (DA) to the aorta, flowing right to left (R-to-L). After birth, PVR is initially elevated and then decreases over the first few days of life. As pulmonary pressures become lower than systemic pressures, flow in the DA reverses, becoming left-to-right (L-to-R) from the aorta to the pulmonary artery.

In normal infants the DA is not needed after birth and begins to functionally close during the first 24–72 hours after birth. It is anatomically closed between the third and fourth week of life. Persistent patency of the DA can be caused by stress, hypoxia, and acidosis.

In this infant, critical PS limited the amount of antegrade pulmonary blood flow (PBF) through the pulmonary valve. Therefore, the major source of source of PBF was provided via the DA, flowing from the aorta to pulmonary artery. (See Figure 6.1.) As the DA began to close during the first few days of life, PBF was reduced. Antegrade blood flow through the critically stenosed pulmonic valve was not sufficient and the infant became hypoxemic, causing tachypnea and poor feeding. (See Figures 6.2 and 6.3.)

How is critical pulmonary valve stenosis defined?

Intervention is recommended for patients with a gradient across the pulmonary valve >50 mm Hg.

The following echocardiographic classifications are defined:

- **Mild PS**: Peak instantaneous gradient <30 mm Hg
- **Moderate PS**: Peak instantaneous gradient between 30 and 60 mm Hg
- **Severe PS**: Peak instantaneous gradient >60 mm Hg

Clinical Pearl

Echocardiographic and direct catheter measurement of PV gradients vary, as they use different measurement techniques. The peak instantaneous Doppler gradient can overestimate the catheter gradient by 20–30 mm Hg, and the mean echocardiographic gradient may underestimate the gradient compared to catheterization. During cardiac catheterization the pressures on each side of the valve are directly transduced.

33

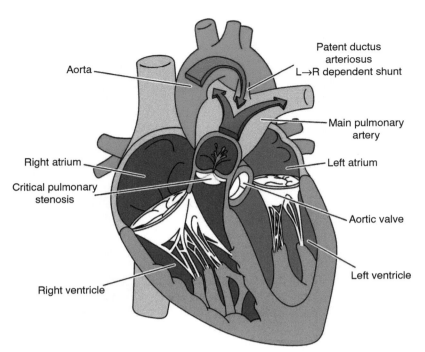

Figure 6.1 Critical pulmonic stenosis. Drawing by Ryan Moore, MD, and Matt Nelson.

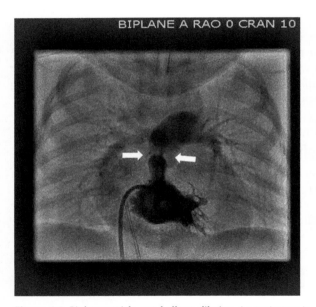

Figure 6.2 Right ventricle, pre-balloon dilation. An angiogram is performed in the right ventricle in the AP projection. The pulmonary valve is thickened and doming (arrows). Courtesy of Russel Hirsch, MD.

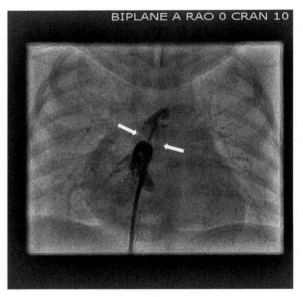

Figure 6.3 Focused injection under the pulmonary valve. A hand angiogram is performed under the pulmonary valve in the AP projection. The narrow jet of contrast flow is seen passing through the stenotic pulmonary valve and into the main pulmonary artery (arrows). Courtesy of Russel Hirsch, MD.

Is critical valvular PS associated with other lesions and syndromes?

Although PS may be an isolated abnormality, it commonly occurs in association with tricuspid atresia, tetralogy of Fallot, dextro (d)- and levo (l)-transposition of the great arteries, and double outlet right ventricle. Critical pulmonary stenosis is associated with Noonan syndrome, Alagille syndrome, Williams–Beuren syndrome, and congenital rubella syndrome.

Why was the patient started on PGE₁?

Once the DA is closed or closing, it can usually be reopened therapeutically after initiation of a PGE_1 infusion. PGE_1 relaxes ductal tissue, improving blood flow through the DA into the pulmonary circulation. The usual starting dose of PGE_1 is 0.01–0.05 mcg/kg/minute and it may be titrated up to 0.1 mcg/kg/minute. Adverse effects of PGE_1 include apnea, bradycardia, fever, flushing, and less frequently seizures, hypotension, tachycardia, sepsis, and diarrhea. Owing to these adverse effects the dose is titrated down once ductal patency has been reestablished.

Clinical Pearl

Should oxygen desaturation occur in a patient with ductal-dependent PBF, the differential includes both standard pulmonary causes of hypoxia and decreased PBF due to systemic hypotension or hypovolemia, increasing PVR, or inadequate blood flow via the DA.

What is an acceptable oxygen saturation for this patient after ductal flow is reestablished?

The effects of PGE_1 infusion can be seen within minutes. The PaO_2 can often increase as much as 20–30 mm Hg with initiation of the PGE_1 infusion. With ductal flow reestablished, the patient's oxygen saturation should be in the mid-80s. If the oxygen saturation falls below 80%, other etiologies for desaturation should be investigated and treated after assuring that the prostaglandins are being delivered. Should the oxygen saturations remain low it may be necessary to increase the PGE_1 rate. Due to the presence of the PFO, the oxygen saturation will not approach 100%, as mixing of oxygenated blood with deoxygenated blood is occurring within the heart. As the PGE_1 infusion rate is increased, the risk of apnea also increases, and endotracheal intubation may be indicated.

Clinical Pearl

Because of the presence of bidirectional shunting at the level of the PFO, the patient's systemic oxygen saturation will not approach 100%, as mixing of oxygenated blood and deoxygenated blood is occurring within the heart.

Why was the patient started on milrinone?

In this case, RV dysfunction exists due to increased right heart pressure secondary to impeded forward flow through the stenotic pulmonic valve, resulting in tricuspid regurgitation. Milrinone is both an inotrope and vasodilator for the systemic and pulmonary vasculature. It improves diastolic function, as well as myocardial contractility. As such, it is often used in patients with poor cardiac function. The usual dose of milrinone is 0.25–0.5 mcg/kg/minute. Milrinone works by decreasing the degradation of cyclic adenosine monophosphate via phosphodiesterase inhibition, with a half-life of approximately 2 hours.

What does a balloon valvuloplasty procedure entail?

Balloon pulmonary valvuloplasty is the treatment of choice for the typical dome-shaped valve characteristically seen in PS. Balloon valvuloplasty is a catheter-based procedure, performed in the cardiac catheterization suite or hybrid operating room. Vascular access is usually obtained via the femoral veins. Femoral arterial access may also be obtained for arterial pressure monitoring during the procedure. A sheath is placed in the femoral vein, with a catheter entering the right heart via the inferior vena cava, then passing through the stenotic pulmonary valve. A balloon is then inflated at the level of the pulmonic valve. (See Figures 6.4 and 6.5.) All stenosis may not be relieved, as the PV leaflets are often dysmorphic. Additionally, pulmonary insufficiency can result from balloon valvuloplasty as the thickened and calcified pulmonary valve may not coapt well after balloon dilation.

Clinical Pearl

Pulmonary insufficiency can result from balloon valvuloplasty. The thickened and calcified pulmonary valve may not coapt well after balloon dilation, and insufficiency may result.

Anesthetic Implications

What preoperative cardiac evaluation and workup is necessary?

An echocardiogram should be performed, and the following information assessed:

• Biventricular function

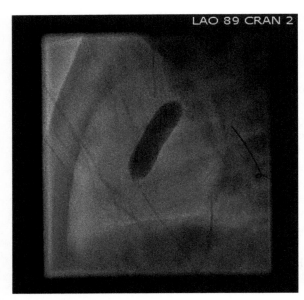

Figure 6.4 Balloon dilation of the pulmonary valve. Still frame angiogram in the lateral projection demonstrating balloon dilation across the pulmonary valve. Courtesy of Russel Hirsch, MD.

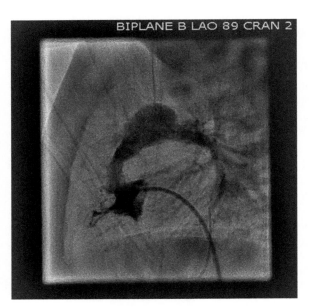

Figure 6.5 Right ventricle, post-balloon dilation. An angiogram is performed in the right ventricle in the lateral projection. Improved flow is now noted across the dilated pulmonary valve. Courtesy of Russel Hirsch, MD.

- Presence of tricuspid valve regurgitation, which can be used to estimate RV systolic pressure
- Pulmonary valve gradient to estimate severity of stenosis
- Presence of pulmonary valve insufficiency
- Any other existing valvular pathology

Echocardiographic and direct catheter measurement of PV gradients vary, as they use different measurement techniques. Echocardiography typically visualizes the PV leaflets and annulus. A peak instantaneous Doppler gradient can overestimate the catheter gradient by 20–30 mm Hg, and the mean echocardiographic gradient may underestimate the gradient compared to catheterization data. Continuous wave Doppler through the PV is used to measure the valve gradient. During cardiac catheterization the pressures on each side of the valve are directly transduced. Additionally, the physiologic state (anesthetized or awake, low or high cardiac output) will also impact gradient measurement.

What are the hemodynamic goals for patients with severe or critical PS?

RV preload: RV performance depends on adequate preload. Decreases in central venous pressure will lead to inadequate RV filling and decreased RV stroke volume.

Heart rate: Because blood flow across the stenotic pulmonary valve occurs primarily during ventricular systole, heart rate should be maintained within normal limits for age, avoiding significant bradycardia or tachycardia. Arrhythmias are an uncommon but challenging consequence of PS. Maintenance of atrial-ventricular synchrony is key to provide adequate RV filling. In severe PS, tricuspid regurgitation can develop, leading to right atrial distention and increased risk for atrial fibrillation. Additionally, in cases of severe PS severe RVH can increase the risk of subendocardial ischemia. In these cases, a slower heart rate can be considered to improve diastolic time and coronary blood flow.

Contractility: With severe or long-standing PS, RVH develops in response to the continued pressure load. Pharmacologic interventions that depress RV function should be avoided as depression of contractile state can lead to RV failure with clinical deterioration. There is particular strain on RV function during induction of anesthesia due to the transition from negative to positive intrathoracic pressure with resultant decreased RV preload and increased afterload.

Systemic vascular resistance: Afterload should be maintained to provide adequate coronary perfusion to the hypertrophied RV.

Pulmonary vascular resistance: The goals for PVR vary according to the degree of PS and the size and patency of the DA. In critical PS, the primary impedance to forward flow is the stenotic pulmonic valve, therefore reducing PVR will do little to increase blood flow to the lungs. However, in patients with mild or moderate PS, major increases in PVR and RV afterload can decrease PBF and lead to RV dysfunction.

In ductal-dependent patients, the ratio of systemic to pulmonary vascular resistance will affect PBF. Therefore, PVR should be kept in the low-to-normal range. Increases in PVR will decrease PBF and decreases in PVR may increase PBF, thereby decreasing both systemic and coronary perfusion. With ductal-dependent PBF, balancing systemic blood flow and PBF by balancing relative resistances requires constant monitoring and management.

> **Clinical Pearl**
>
> *In critical PS, the primary impedance to forward flow is the stenotic pulmonic valve; therefore, reducing PVR will do little to increase blood flow to the lungs. However, in patients with mild or moderate pulmonary stenosis, major increases in PVR and RV afterload can decrease PBF and lead to RV dysfunction.*

What is an appropriate anesthetic induction plan?

Any anesthetic that prioritizes the aforementioned hemodynamic considerations is acceptable. In patients with milder forms of PS an inhalation induction with sevoflurane and oxygen with spontaneous ventilation is an option if the patient does not have intravenous (IV) access. However, in a patient with critical (ductal dependent) PS an IV anesthetic induction is preferable. Crying and agitation during a mask induction may increase PVR, which can negatively impact PBF depending on the degree of PS. Care must be taken to maintain sufficient systemic pressure to ensure coronary perfusion, especially in the setting of RVH. Supplemental oxygen is appropriate during induction for alveolar preoxygenation and to maintain low PVR. Finally, RV workload increases after endotracheal intubation with the transition to positive pressure ventilation.

How should fluid administration be managed for this patient?

Preload should be maintained in order to optimize RV filling and stroke volume. Care should be taken not to overload the neonatal heart with excess volume.

What is the most appropriate ventilation strategy for this patient?

Children who have decreased PBF or lower SpO_2 as a result of congenital heart disease have poor tolerance for pulmonary vein desaturation due to inadequate ventilation or oxygenation. Ventilation strategies that aim for normocarbia, avoidance of $SpO_2 < 80\%$, and maintenance of functional residual capacity should optimize gas exchange and PVR.

What is an appropriate anesthetic maintenance plan?

Either inhalation or intravenous medications can be used to maintain anesthesia with attention to hemodynamic goals. Ventricular contractility should be maintained. Tachycardia should be avoided. As there is minimal postprocedural pain, opioids may be used sparingly.

What potential intraprocedural complications exist?

- *Arrhythmias* (although usually transient) can occur due to wire and catheter manipulation.
- *RV perforation* can occur, as well as damage to valve leaflets and/or chordae, from catheter manipulation.
- *Hypothermia* due to constant flushing of fluid to prevent clot in the sheaths and the cool ambient temperature necessary for the equipment.
- *Air embolism* secondary to flushing of the sheaths.
- *Accumulative blood loss* from sheath insertion site and continual aspiration of catheters.

> **Clinical Pearl**
>
> *Complications from balloon valvuloplasty are not common. However, when they occur, they can progress quickly. Prepare for emergencies by having emergency medications and a defibrillator available.*

Should this patient be extubated at the end of the procedure?

If the patient is hemodynamically stable after balloon valvuloplasty and does not require inotropic support, extubation in the procedural suite may be considered if all other extubation criteria are met. Since this infant had moderately depressed RV function requiring milrinone preprocedure, the length and success of the procedure will guide the decision to proceed toward tracheal extubation.

What is the postprocedural management for this patient?

Immediately post-procedure, bleeding at the access sites (femoral vessels) and the risk of apnea following general anesthesia in the neonate are the most common complications. Longer term, pulmonary insufficiency or residual pulmonic stenosis are frequently present. It is difficult to have a perfect result with balloon valvuloplasty, and the risk of incurring pulmonary insufficiency must be weighed against the risk of residual PS. A rare complication in severely hypertrophied ventricles is "suicide right ventricle." After obstruction is relieved, the now hyperdynamic RV may collapse inward, causing subpulmonary obstruction and decreased RV output. Avoidance of tachycardia is helpful to avoid this complication.

What criteria are used to measure the success of the intervention (balloon valvuloplasty)?

Balloon valvuloplasty for PS can either be curative or an initial intervention to improve PBF until a more definitive procedure is planned. Ideal outcomes are little or no residual obstruction in the subvalvular region or valvular level, resolution of RVH over time, decrease in the amount of tricuspid regurgitation, and no R-to-L shunting at the atrial level (PFO). For neonates who were PGE_1 dependent prior to the procedure, PGE_1 is typically stopped and the infant is monitored in hospital until the DA closes. An acceptable SpO_2 indicates that adequate antegrade blood flow through the pulmonary valve is present.

What other procedures can be done if the catheterization is not successful?

If PBF is insufficient and SpO_2 begins to fall despite balloon valvuloplasty, surgical palliation may be indicated. A modified Blalock–Taussig (mBT) shunt can be placed if oxygen saturations cannot be maintained without the DA as a source of PBF. A modified BT shunt utilizes a GORE-TEX® graft (usually 3.5 mm), to connect the right subclavian or innominate artery to the right pulmonary artery, thus providing another source of pulmonary blood flow.

For patients who have sufficient PBF but residual pulmonary valve stenosis or insufficiency, medical management is often employed in anticipation of another catheter-based or surgical procedure.

Suggested Reading

Dice J. E. and Bhatia J. Patent ductus arteriosus: an overview. *J Pediatr Pharmacol Ther* 2007; **12**: 138–46.

Gournay V. The ductus arteriosus: physiology, regulation, and functional and congenital anomalies. *Arch Cardiovasc Dis* 2011; **104**: 578–85.

Laussen P. C. and Salvin J. Diagnostic and therapeutic cardiac catheterization. In Furhman B. and Zimmerman J., eds. *Pediatric Critical Care*, 4th ed. Philadelphia, Mosby Elsevier, 2011; 266–76.

Scholz T. and Reinking B. E. Congenital heart disease. In Gleason, C. and Juul S. *Avery's Diseases of the Newborn*, 10th ed. Philadelphia: Elsevier, 2018; 801–27.

Singh Y. and Mikrou P. Use of prostaglandins in duct-dependent congenital heart conditions. *Arch Dis Child Educ Pract Ed* 2018; **103**: 137–40.

Townsley M. M. and Martin D. E. Anesthetic management for the surgical treatment of valvular heart disease. In Hensley F., Martin D., and Gravlee G. *A Practical Approach to Cardiac Anesthesia*, 5th ed. Philadelphia: Lippincott Williams & Wilkins, 2013; 319–58.

7
Tetralogy of Fallot

Matthew P. Monteleone

Case Scenario

A 6-week-old, former 32-week preterm infant weighing 3.2 kg presents with a history of vomiting and lethargy for urgent ventriculoperitoneal shunt revision. He is followed by cardiology for unrepaired tetralogy of Fallot. Noncardiac history is remarkable for a 4-week stay in the neonatal intensive care unit for respiratory and nutritional support and placement of a ventriculoperitoneal shunt to treat obstructive hydrocephalus related to a perinatal intraventricular hemorrhage. He was discharged two weeks ago on full oral feeds and no respiratory support. His only current medication is cholecalciferol.

Parents report that no hypercyanotic spells or "tet spells" have been noted at home. Elective cardiac surgical repair is planned in the next several months. The infant has not had anything by mouth in over 12 hours and is receiving maintenance fluids with dextrose through a 24-gauge peripheral intravenous line.

On physical examination vital signs are SpO$_2$ 93% on room air, heart rate 155 beats/minute, blood pressure 71/40 mm Hg, respiratory rate 38 breaths/minute, and temperature 36.8°C. The infant is sleepy but arousable and cries appropriately.

The most recent echo shows the following:

- *Severe right ventricular outflow tract obstruction, peak gradient 80 mm Hg by continuous wave Doppler; turbulence begins below the pulmonic valve with the main gradient at the valvular level*
- *Large anterior malalignment ventricular septal defect present with bidirectional shunting*
- *Patent foramen ovale with predominantly left-to-right flow*
- *Normal biventricular systolic function*

Key Objectives

- Describe the classic anatomy of tetralogy of Fallot.
- Identify typical physical examination and diagnostic test findings associated with tetralogy of Fallot.
- Understand the pathophysiology and treatment options for a hypercyanotic or "tet" spell.
- Understand considerations for the anesthetic perioperative care for the patient with uncorrected tetralogy of Fallot.

Pathophysiology

Who was Fallot and what is the history of the discovery and treatment of this lesion?

Tetralogy of Fallot (TOF) was first described in 1671 by Niels Stensen. The syndrome was eventually named for Etienne Fallot, who published the classic description in 1888 based on autopsy-confirmed diagnoses. Tetralogy of Fallot is the most common form of cyanotic heart disease and represents up to 10% of all congenital heart defects. It was first palliated surgically with a systemic-to-pulmonary artery shunt in 1944 by Blalock, Taussig, and Thomas. The first complete repair was reported by Lillehei in 1954; in the current era most cases are repaired within the first 6 months of life.

> ### Clinical Pearl
>
> *Tetralogy of Fallot is the most common form of cyanotic heart disease and represents about 10% of all congenital heart defects.*

What are the four defects present in classic TOF?

Tetralogy of Fallot with pulmonary stenosis (TOF/PS) is generally thought of as classic TOF. Although TOF is one of the most successfully repaired cardiac lesions, if left unrepaired, mortality in the first several years of life can approach 50%.

Although variants exist, classic TOF consists of a large, nonrestrictive ventricular septal defect (VSD), right ventricular outflow tract obstruction (RVOTO), an overriding

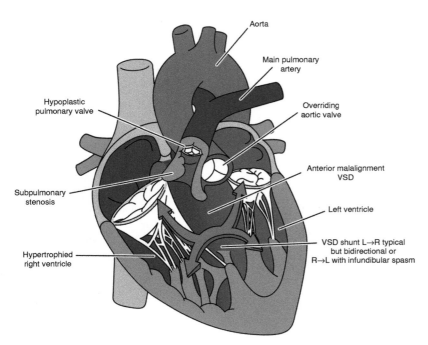

Aorta

Main pulmonary artery

Hypoplastic pulmonary valve

Overriding aortic valve

Anterior malalignment VSD

Subpulmonary stenosis

Left ventricle

VSD shunt L→R typical but bidirectional or R→L with infundibular spasm

Hypertrophied right ventricle

Figure 7.1 Tetralogy of Fallot. Drawing by Ryan Moore, MD, and Matt Nelson.

aorta, and right ventricular hypertrophy (RVH). Although named for Etienne Fallot, it was Maude Abbott in 1924 who first labeled the four classic findings as *tetralogy of Fallot.* (See Figure 7.1.)

What is meant by an "overriding aorta"?

Aortic override is created by the malalignment of the infundibular and ventricular septum. Essentially, part of the aortic valve exists on the right side of the septal plane. The aortic valve, therefore, "overrides" the interventricular septum and VSD.

What are the characteristics of the VSD in TOF?

Understanding the characteristics of the VSD in TOF is essential in order to appreciate the pathophysiology of this lesion. The VSD is large and perimembranous, often similar in diameter to the aortic annulus. This means that it is typically nonrestrictive or unrestrictive, with equal right and left ventricular pressures. The amount and direction of shunting are therefore dependent on the balance between the resistance to pulmonary blood flow, which is dependent on the degree of RVOT obstruction, and systemic vascular resistance (SVR). In contrast, a restrictive VSD is generally small and has a pressure gradient across the defect; flow is determined by the size of the VSD.

What is meant by RVOTO and what variations exist?

Right ventricular outflow tract obstruction is a key feature of TOF; the extent of obstruction can be variable, with obstruction at the valvular, subvalvular, or pulmonary artery level. The pulmonary valve is often thickened and dysplastic with some degree of hypoplasia. There is compensatory RVH as a consequence of the RVOTO. Obstruction can also exist at multiple levels and may be *fixed and/or dynamic* in nature. Fixed components occur at the valvular and supravalvular levels while dynamic components can exist due to the hypertrophied RV infundibulum and muscle bundles. Echocardiography can estimate the pressure gradient across the right ventricular outflow tract (RVOT), describe the anatomic level of obstruction and may delineate whether a dynamic obstructive component is present. Patients with a larger dynamic component of RVOTO are more likely to experience frequent tet spells during crying or agitation and may be treated with ß-blockers to decrease heart rate and contractility.

Clinical Pearl

The extent of RVOTO can be variable in TOF, with obstruction at the valvular, subvalvular, and/or pulmonary artery level that can be fixed and/or dynamic. The variable degrees of outflow tract obstruction account for the varying levels of symptomatology experienced by different patients.

Are other important cardiac lesions or abnormalities associated with TOF?

Approximately 25% of patients with TOF will also have a right-sided aortic arch (RAA) with mirror-image branching of the head and neck vessels. The origin of the subclavian artery may also be aberrant, with either the right subclavian artery arising from the descending aorta or the left subclavian artery arising from the pulmonary artery. Subclavian artery anatomy is important to consider when determining the optimal placement of an arterial line. Coronary abnormalities are also present in 5%–12% of TOF patients, with the most common anomaly being origination of the left anterior descending artery from the right coronary artery, crossing the RVOT/infundibular surface.

Patients with TOF may also have an atrial septal defect (ASD) or patent foramen ovale (PFO); when this finding is present the syndrome may be referred to as *pentalogy of Fallot*. Other associated lesions can include anomalous pulmonary venous drainage, left-sided superior vena cava, interrupted inferior vena cava, patent ductus arteriosus (PDA), a bicuspid pulmonary valve (PV), and pulmonary artery stenosis. All imaging and cardiac catheterization studies should be reviewed completely in the preanesthetic period for the presence of other associated anomalies.

Approximately 25% of patients with TOF will also have chromosomal abnormalities, most commonly trisomy 21 and chromosome 22q11.2 microdeletions. In these patient subsets the anesthesiologist must be alert for craniofacial abnormalities, immune deficiencies, hypocalcemia, and other conditions associated with genetic syndromes.

Clinical Pearl

The presence and significance of an aberrant subclavian artery should be noted, particularly when considering placement of an arterial line.

Are there other anatomic variations of TOF?

There are several important variants of TOF involving variations in pulmonary valve and pulmonary artery anatomy.

Tetralogy of Fallot/PS Stenosis of the RVOT, PV, and main pulmonary artery exists; the PV is often bicuspid and may be dysplastic.

Tetralogy of Fallot/Pulmonary Atresia (PA) Pulmonary atresia is present, along with variable hypoplasia of the main pulmonary artery. Depending on the nomenclature used, the term tetralogy of Fallot may be completely dropped and the patient's disease referred to as PA/VSD. Pulmonary artery anatomy may be complex and varies widely from patient to patient. The central pulmonary arteries may or may not be confluent, and pulmonary blood flow (PBF) may be dependent on flow supplied by a PDA. Alternatively, the patient may carry the description of TOF/PA/major aortopulmonary collateral arteries (MAPCAs); in this disease the spectrum may include a lack of central confluent pulmonary arteries and PBF may be augmented or supplied by large collaterals from the aorta. There is a wide spectrum of anatomic variants with this type of disease. (See Chapter 10.)

Tetralogy of Fallot/Absent Pulmonary Valve (APV) These patients typically have enlarged main and branch pulmonary arteries; there is often compression of the airway and resultant development of tracheobronchomalacia. The child may require mechanical ventilation, high levels of positive end expiratory pressure and even prone positioning to keep the airways open. In less severe cases, airways may remain open on moderate ventilator settings, but obstruction can occur when a transesophageal echocardiography probe or other esophageal device is placed. (See Chapter 9.)

What occurs during a "tet spell"?

A "tet" or hypercyanotic spell is a sudden and significant increase in the degree of RVOTO, with the resultant decrease in PBF resulting in a significant drop in the child's hemoglobin–oxygen saturation. The degree of RVOTO is the primary driver in determining the severity of spells. Deoxygenated systemic venous return from the body to the right side of the heart will be shunted across the VSD (R-to-L) if RVOTO significantly increases or SVR abruptly falls so that right-sided ventricular pressures are greater than left-sided pressures. While these spells may occur spontaneously, hypovolemia, acidosis, hypoxia, and/or RV infundibulum spasm with resultant increased RVOTO are among the usual contributing causes. Infundibular spasm results from increased sympathetic activity, tachycardia, and increased cardiac contractility. Agitation and pain are usual triggers. The cycle of hypoxia and acidosis can make the spell perpetuate and worsen; immediate treatment is indicated.

Clinical Pearl

The degree of RVOTO is the primary driver in determining the severity of tet spells. While these spells may occur spontaneously, hypovolemia, acidosis, hypoxia, and/or RV infundibulum spasm with resultant increased RVOTO are among the usual causes.

What is meant by a "pink tet"?

As with many congenital cardiac lesions, there is a spectrum of disease severity in TOF. A "pink tet" is a child with minimal RVOTO who generally has normal systemic oxygen saturations. The active physiology is similar to an unrestrictive VSD; they may have pulmonary overcirculation from excessive flow across the VSD and signs of congestive heart failure.

> **Clinical Pearl**
>
> *The term "pink tet" describes a child with minimal RVOTO who generally has normal systemic oxygen saturations.*

How and when is TOF with PS usually repaired?

All patients with TOF will require intervention at some time, but the optimal timing for surgery remains a matter of debate. Most centers advocate total repair in infancy unless specific anatomic features preclude this. Patients with significant RVOTO may require the placement of a systemic-to-pulmonary artery shunt prior to definitive repair. The goals of surgical repair are to close existing septal defects, to provide a patent and competent RVOT, and if necessary, to correct branch pulmonary artery stenosis. (See Figure 7.2.)

Anesthetic Implications

What diagnostic tests should be reviewed prior to anesthetizing a patient with TOF?

The *echocardiogram* is the highest-yield study. It should describe intracardiac anatomy, aortic arch pattern, presence or absence of a PDA, and relevant coronary artery anatomy. The VSD and infundibular septum can be visualized, and blood flow across the RVOT can be imaged (with Doppler) to assess the degree of RVOTO. Finally, pulmonary artery anatomy can be examined should the child have a TOF variant.

A *cardiac catheterization* report, if available, should be reviewed. However, cardiac catheterization is generally not routinely performed for TOF patients unless there is a desire for angiographic imaging or invasive assessments (e.g., the child with MAPCAs). Likewise, computed tomography and magnetic resonance imaging studies, if available, are certainly helpful in defining anatomy.

An *electrocardiogram* (*ECG*) will be consistent with the amount of RVH, showing right axis deviation and upright and peaked T waves in the right precordial leads.

Chest radiography may show the classic "boot-shaped" heart. Right ventricular hypertrophy results in an upturned cardiac apex and the shadow of the main pulmonary artery appears smaller, leading to the classic boot shape.

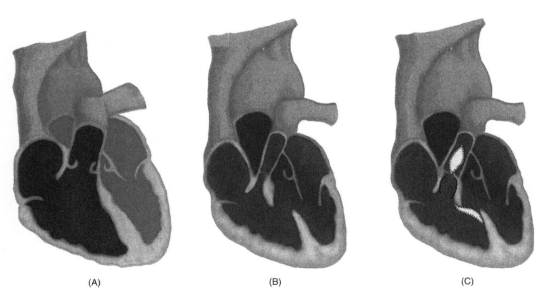

(A)   (B)   (C)

Figure 7.2 Schematic illustration of tetralogy of Fallot. (A) Normal heart. (B) Tetralogy of Fallot illustrating infundibular stenosis, ventricular septal defect (VSD), overriding aorta, and right ventricular hypertrophy. (C) Surgically repaired heart showing resection of obstructing muscle in the right ventricular outflow tract, patch closure of the VSD, and patch arterioplasty used to widen the main pulmonary artery at and/or above the pulmonary valve. From M. L. Schmitz M. L., Ullah S., Dasgupta R., et al. Anesthesia for right-sided obstructive lesions. In Andropoulos D. B., Stayer S., Mossad E. B., et al., eds. *Anesthesia for Congenital Heart Surgery*, 3rd ed. John Wiley & Sons; 2015: 516–41. With permission.

Review of a recent complete blood count with **hemoglobin and hematocrit** is useful. A higher than normal hematocrit is indicative of more frequent cyanotic spells.

> **Clinical Pearl**
>
> *A higher than normal hematocrit is indicative of more frequent cyanotic spells.*

What questions are important during the preoperative assessment?

Inquiries should be made regarding cardiac symptomatology, specifically tet spells: have they been observed by the parents, and if so, how frequently? The parents should also be asked about any ongoing issues related to prematurity, including respiratory issues, apneic events, and recent exposure to illnesses. As the infant in this case scenario has been vomiting, it would be prudent to ask about recent wet diapers and the presence of tears in order to assess the state of hydration.

What remarkable physical examination findings may be observed in a TOF patient?

A child with TOF and a stenotic RVOT will have a harsh systolic ejection murmur heard best over the left upper sternal border. In fact, if there is no murmur, there should be concern for decreased flow across the RVOT. This could occur during a tet spell or in the child with pulmonary atresia. The child with a PDA or MAPCAs may also have a continuous murmur.

> **Clinical Pearl**
>
> *A child with TOF and a stenotic RVOT generally has a harsh systolic ejection murmur; if no murmur is auscultated there should be concern for decreased flow across the RVOT.*

Should a peripheral intravenous line be placed before induction? What options are available for induction?

When planning anesthetic induction in the patient with TOF without preexisting peripheral intravenous (PIV) access one should consider the risk of decreasing SVR with inhalational agents versus the challenge and sympathetic stimulation of awake PIV placement. This risk/benefit calculation is best made in patient specific context, considering the degree of RVOTO, degree of hydration, difficulty of IV placement, and other patient or anesthetic considerations. As the spectrum of disease severity can vary widely in patients with TOF, not all unrepaired TOF patients necessarily require placement of a PIV prior to induction of anesthesia. In fact, many children with TOF will have an increase in oxygen saturation during a mask induction with sevoflurane. Even though sevoflurane reduces SVR and may cause tachycardia, anesthesia causes a significant decrease in oxygen consumption, which leads to an improvement in the mixed venous oxygen saturation.

If mask induction is chosen, plans for rapid post-induction placement of an PIV, with phenylephrine readily available if needed to increase SVR, would be prudent. It is worth noting that many infants with TOF appear robust for their age, as their parents feed them frequently to avoid agitation, which may precipitate hypercyanotic spells. Consequently, it may not always be easy to obtain PIV access and the use of ultrasound may be helpful. If the patient is actively experiencing hypercyanotic spells or is volume depleted, a PIV placement with fluid resuscitation prior to induction is prudent.

Ketamine is another induction agent that can be useful in the uncorrected TOF patient. It can be given intramuscularly if necessary. While it will increase heart rate and contractility, it will also increase SVR and may prevent a hypercyanotic spell due to the decrease in SVR which can be associated with mask induction.

In this patient, given his vomiting, a rapid sequence PIV induction with the use of neuromuscular blockade prior to intubation would be appropriate.

> **Clinical Pearl**
>
> *It is helpful to have ketamine readily available when inducing a patient with TOF as it can be given IM in patients without IV access.*

Immediately after intubation and confirmation of endotracheal tube position oxygen saturations suddenly fall to 60%. How should this be treated?

Mainstays of therapy for hypercyanotic spells fall into the following major categories:

- Increasing SVR
- Decreasing sympathetic stimulation
- Volume expansion

Inspired oxygen concentration (FiO_2) should be increased to 100%. Oxygen is a potent pulmonary vasodilator, will decrease PVR, and may serve to reduce hypoxic pulmonary vasoconstriction. Administration of phenylephrine is the initial intervention to increase SVR. Phenylephrine doses as high as 5–10 mcg/kg may be needed, though an effect may be seen initially with doses of 2–3 mcg/kg. A phenylephrine infusion may be considered if the patient requires multiple boluses.

If the patient's legs and torso are accessible, bringing the child's knees to his chest can increase SVR. Hepatic compression may also increase preload. To further increase preload, IV fluid boluses should be given to fill the right heart, dilate the RVOT, and ultimately increase cardiac output and blood pressure.

To decrease sympathetic effects, the ß-blocker esmolol can be utilized to decrease heart rate and contractility, relieving RV infundibular spasm. The appropriate dose is typically 50–250 mcg/kg/minute. Sevoflurane can also treat infundibular spasm via its action as a negative inotrope and by decreasing sympathetic stimulation via increasing anesthetic depth.

> **Clinical Pearl**
>
> *Treatments for a tet spell include administration of 100% oxygen, phenylephrine, IV fluid bolus(es), knee-to-chest position if possible, esmolol and increasing depth of anesthesia while maintaining SVR.*

What considerations exist during the maintenance of anesthesia?

Generally, anesthesia management principles for a child with TOF are similar to those for a healthy child with the added focus on avoidance of R-to-L shunting and hypercyanotic spell triggers. Hypotension and significant decreases in SVR should be avoided as they may increase the R-to-L shunting of blood across the VSD and cause systemic hypoxia. Hypovolemia will likely be poorly tolerated, so careful attention to fluid status is essential. Light anesthesia, pain, or agitation may increase catecholamines and RVOTO, causing R-to-L shunting and hypoxia. Muscle relaxation, along with a judicious amount of opioid (fentanyl) and volatile agent (sevoflurane), will provide an appropriate balanced anesthetic for this patient. Additionally, the anesthesiologist must be prepared to manage hypercyanotic spells and possible associated hemodynamic instability.

What considerations exist for postoperative care?

If the case is uneventful, extubation in the operating room and recovery in the post-anesthesia care unit is appropriate. If, on the other hand, the perioperative course is complicated by hypercyanotic spells and hemodynamic instability or continued fluid shifts are expected, the patient should be admitted to an intensive care unit postoperatively. Given this child's history of prematurity, monitoring for postoperative apnea is appropriate. A child who was previously thought to have an unobstructed RVOT who now shows signs of hypercyanotic episodes may need to be put forward for urgent surgical repair. In all perioperative patients with unrepaired congenital heart disease, cardiology consultation is suggested.

Suggested Reading

Karl T. and Stocker C. Tetralogy of Fallot and its variants. *Ped Crit Care Med* 2016; **17**: S330–6.

Rivenes S., Lewin M., Stayer S., et al. Cardiovascular effects of sevoflurane, isoflurane, halothane, and fentanyl-midazolam in children with congenital heart disease: an echocardiographic study of myocardial contractility and hemodynamics. *Anesthesiology* 2001; **94**: 223–9.

Townsley M. M., Windsor J., Briston D., et al. Tetralogy of Fallot: perioperative management and analysis of outcomes. *J Cardiothorac Vasc Anesth* 2019; **33**: 556–65.

Wise-Faberowski L., Asija R., and McElhinney D. B. Tetralogy of Fallot: everything you wanted to know but were afraid to ask. *Pediatr Anesth* 2019; **29**: 475–82.

Chapter 8

Repaired Tetralogy of Fallot

Joanna Rosing Paquin

Case Scenario

A 13-year-old boy with DiGeorge syndrome (22q11 deletion) and a history of tetralogy of Fallot repaired as an infant presents for emergency reduction of testicular torsion, orchidopexy, and possible orchiectomy. He has severe testicular pain and has been vomiting for 12 hours with minimal oral intake. He says that prior to his current illness he had occasionally become short of breath with strenuous activity and felt an occasional "funny heartbeat." His only home medication is furosemide twice daily.

He is followed yearly by his cardiologist and was last seen 11 months ago. An electrocardiogram at that time demonstrated a stable right bundle branch block.

Transthoracic echocardiography at that time showed the following:

- *A dilated right ventricle*
- *Free pulmonary insufficiency*
- *Mild to moderately diminished right ventricular function*
- *Normal left ventricular function*

Key Objectives

- Describe the anatomy of tetralogy of Fallot.
- Understand the repair of tetralogy of Fallot and its long-term implications.
- Understand the associations of DiGeorge syndrome and other genetic abnormalities.
- Describe the preoperative assessment for noncardiac surgery following repair of tetralogy of Fallot.
- Describe intraoperative management strategies.

Pathophysiology

What is tetralogy of Fallot?

Tetralogy of Fallot (TOF), more specifically tetralogy of Fallot with pulmonary stenosis (TOF/PS), describes a collection of cardiac anomalies consisting of right ventricular outflow tract obstruction (RVOTO), a ventricular septal defect (VSD), an overriding aorta, and concentric right ventricular hypertrophy (RVH). The RVOTO may involve infundibular, subvalvular, valvular, supravalvular stenosis or a combination of stenoses. These cardiac anomalies often result in cyanosis, and TOF is the most common cyanotic congenital heart disease. (See Chapter 7.)

What is the typical surgical repair for TOF?

Repair of TOF involves relieving RVOTO and closure of the VSD. The technique used will depend on the specific location of the stenoses. Relief of subvalvular obstruction is performed by resection of hypertrophied muscle bundles to open the outflow tract. This can sometimes be accomplished through the tricuspid valve but may require a right ventriculotomy and a pericardial patch. Depending on the size of the pulmonary valve annulus and the presence of any supravalvular stenosis, the pericardial patch may extend across the pulmonary valve and into the main pulmonary artery. This is commonly referred to as a transannular patch.

When possible a valve-sparing technique is performed. For a valve-sparing technique to be successful the RVOTO needs to be relieved without compromising the pulmonary valve. The intention of a valve-sparing technique is to minimize postoperative pulmonary valve incompetence while preserving RV function, minimizing conduction abnormalities, and improving exercise intolerance. When the pulmonary valve annulus is significantly hypoplastic this technique may not be possible.

While some centers may perform definitive repair of TOF in neonates, it is more common for TOF to be electively repaired between 3 and 6 months of age. Surgically created palliative systemic-to-pulmonary artery shunt procedures may be performed when necessary to augment pulmonary blood flow (PBF) during the neonatal period if anatomical complexities make elective definitive repair challenging. Another option for TOF palliation involves balloon dilation of the RVOT, with or without stent placement, or stenting of the PDA. Both of these procedures are performed in the cardiac catheterization laboratory.

What are the implications of a transannular patch in a TOF repair?

A transannular patch crosses the pulmonary valve annulus to relieve obstruction of the RVOT. However, while relieving obstruction, the patch distorts the pulmonary valve and often creates pulmonary insufficiency (PI). Over time PI can progress, ultimately compromising RV function, and leading to right ventricular dilation and failure.

> **Clinical Pearl**
>
> *A transannular patch creates free pulmonary insufficiency that in time leads to right ventricular dilation and dysfunction or failure.*

What is the implication of the ventriculotomy in TOF repair?

In neonates and small infants, a ventriculotomy is created in order to close the VSD and to aid in resection of the RVOT obstruction. This approach increases the risk of conduction system injury, causing local conduction block and predisposing patients to arrhythmias. A right bundle branch block is a common consequence of TOF repair, often seen immediately following repair. Limiting the size of the ventriculotomy can minimize the risk of arrhythmias and subsequently help to preserve RV function. Ideally, a transatrial-transpulmonary approach avoids a ventriculotomy and allows maximal preservation of the pulmonary valve, annulus, and the infundibulum. This approach is challenging and dependent on the patient's weight, and many patients may not have favorable anatomy for this repair.

What variations exist in TOF and how do they impact surgical repair?

A wide disease spectrum exists for TOF. In addition to TOF/PS, TOF can occur with pulmonary atresia (TOF/PA), with an absent pulmonary valve (TOF/APV), with major aortopulmonary collateral arteries (TOF/MAPCAs), or with an atrioventricular septal defect (TOF/AVSD). These complexities may alter the timing of repair and/or require a staged repair to establish adequate PBF and to separate pulmonary and systemic circulations. (See Chapters 7, 10, and 47).

What chronic postoperative sequelae are associated with repair of TOF?

Increased morbidity is seen as patients who have undergone TOF repair approach adulthood. Common long-term problems in patients following TOF repair are related to PI, RV dysfunction and an increasing incidence of arrhythmias over time.

Pulmonary insufficiency is initially well tolerated but places an increased volume load on the RV. Over time, long-standing severe PI leads to RV enlargement and dysfunction, heart failure, and tachyarrhythmias. Long-standing RV dysfunction can also cause LV dysfunction due to interventricular dependence. As PI is a long-standing, slowly progressive pathology in most of these patients, there is adaption over time and thus even patients with severe PI may not present with symptoms of right heart failure such as exercise intolerance and dyspnea. (See Figure 8.1.)

Atrial reentrant tachycardias and ventricular tachycardias are both possible chronic sequelae of TOF repair. These arrhythmias may result from abnormal structural conduction pathways, surgical scar tissue, and/or consequences from the chronic effects of RV dilation stretching the conduction system. These arrhythmias place patients at risk for sudden cardiac death (SCD), necessitating placement of an implantable cardioverter-defibrillator (ICD) in some patients. Monitoring for increased QRS duration will aid in identifying patients at increased risk of SCD.

Additionally, in patients who require right ventricular-pulmonary artery (RV–PA) conduits as part of their repair, the need for conduit revision due to conduit stenosis or patient growth is common. Aortic root dilation or aortic valve insufficiency may also occur as a result of the initial surgical repair. Aortic valve insufficiency may result from tension on the valve leaflets from the initial VSD repair. While it is unclear how aortic root dilation develops in patients with repaired TOF, its presence indicates a multifactorial disorder that is likely to impact long term prognosis [1].

> **Clinical Pearl**
>
> *Chronic postoperative sequelae of TOF repair include RV enlargement and dysfunction, heart failure, and tachyarrhythmias such as atrial reentrant tachycardia and ventricular tachycardia.*

When should placement of an ICD be considered?

There is an increased incidence of SCD in patients with repaired TOF, with the majority of events due to sustained

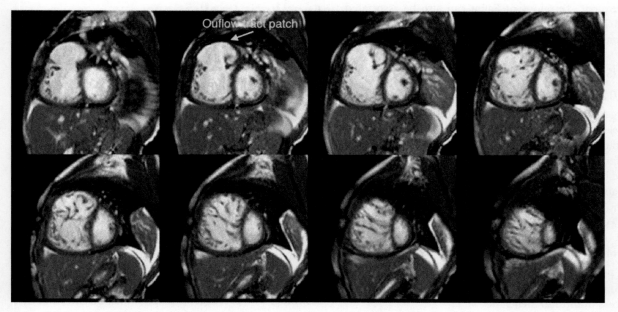

Figure 8.1 Tetralogy of Fallot. Short axis magnetic resonance imaging stack showing markedly dilated right ventricle with a dilated outflow tract patch after repair of TOF. Chronic pulmonary regurgitation results in a dilated RV and eventually leads to RV dysfunction. The RV dilation and dysfunction can lead to tricuspid regurgitation, arrhythmias and rarely sudden death. Courtesy of Michael Taylor, MD.

ventricular tachycardia (VT). These patients are typically older, over 20 years of age, and have had multiple prior cardiac operations.

Implantable cardioverter–defibrillator implantation is recommended when the following risk factors are present [2]:

- Severe PI
- Severe RV dilation
- Left ventricular dysfunction (LV end-diastolic pressure ≥12 mm Hg)
- QRS ≥180 msec on ECG
- Nonsustained VT captured on Holter monitor
- Inducible VT during an electrophysiological study

When should pulmonary valve replacement be considered?

Residual complications of TOF repair can necessitate intervention to restore pulmonary valve competence and preserve RV function before irreversible ventricular damage develops. This can be accomplished by a pulmonary valve (PV) replacement. Pulmonary valve replacement may now be performed surgically or percutaneously in the cardiac catheterization laboratory. While patients with surgically performed PV replacement have a high survival and a low rate of reintervention, transcatheter PV replacement has

a high rate of success and is a suitable, less invasive alternative for many patients that allows avoidance of surgery and cardiopulmonary bypass.

Pulmonary valve replacement is indicated when RV end-diastolic volumes are greater than 160–170 mL/m^2 or RV end-systolic volumes are greater than 80–85 mL/m^2 [3]. The presence of significant PI and/or pulmonary stenosis, RV dilation, or RV dysfunction is also considered when deciding when to proceed with PV replacement. Cardiac magnetic resonance imaging (MRI) has proven to be a valuable asset for following these patients and assessing the correct timing for valve replacement.

Following PV replacement, patients experience an improvement in symptoms, with decreased QRS time on ECG, a decrease in RV size, and decreased RV volumes. It has been noted that ejection fractions do not significantly improve following PV replacement, lending support for early intervention before severe RV dysfunction occurs [3].

Is genetic testing helpful in patients with TOF?

Genetic data can be useful to help stratify risk in patients with cardiac and noncardiac manifestations of disease. Genetic abnormalities in TOF occur equally in males and females and can be syndromic or nonsyndromic. Up to 25% of TOF patients have chromosomal abnormalities, with trisomy 21 and 22q.11.2 microdeletion being the most frequent. Tetralogy of Fallot can also be associated with *JAG1* (Alagille syndrome), *NKX2-5*, *ZFPM2*, and VEGF mutations.

What is DiGeorge syndrome and what is its relevance in TOF?

DiGeorge syndrome is the most severe form of the 22q.11.2 microdeletion and affects the development of the thymus and parathyroid glands. It includes palatal abnormalities, dysmorphic facies, learning disabilities, immune deficiencies, and hypocalcemia. Aortic arch and branching anomalies are also more common in patients with 22q11 deletion; however, they are usually not associated with a vascular ring in TOF.

The anesthetic implications of DiGeorge syndrome consist of the following:

- The potential for difficult airway management
- The need for irradiated blood products due to varying degrees of immunodeficiency
- Close monitoring for and treatment of hypocalcemia
- Increased incidence of anomalous systemic arterial or venous vessels that may impact the placement of invasive arterial or central lines

Clinical Pearl

DiGeorge syndrome is the most severe form of the 22q.11.2 microdeletion and can include palatal abnormalities, dysmorphic facies, learning disabilities, immune deficiencies, and hypocalcemia.

Are there additional genetic syndromes associated with TOF with extracardiac disease manifestations?

VACTERL (vertebral and cardiac defects, anal atresia, tracheoesophageal fistula, renal and limb abnormalities) and *CHARGE* (coloboma, heart defects, choanal atresia, genitourinary, and ear abnormalities) associations are examples of genetic syndromes in which TOF can occur along with extracardiac manifestations. Knowledge of chromosomal abnormalities and associations will guide extracardiac anesthetic management. For instance, placement of a transesophageal echocardiography probe is often contraindicated in a patient with *VACTERL* association following repair of a tracheoesophageal fistula. Patients with these syndromes and associations may more often present with challenging airway management. These patients are also more likely to present for multiple noncardiac procedures due to associated comorbidities. (See Chapter 47.)

Anesthetic Implications

What information should be gathered from these patients during a preoperative assessment?

The preoperative assessment should include a detailed history and physical exam with specific attention to the patient's functional status, cardiac anatomy and function, long-term physiologic sequelae, and a detailed review of cardiac imaging. Additional emphasis should be paid to the following:

Cardiovascular Status Evaluation of the patient's current functional status, surgical history, presence of arrhythmias, and/or pacemaker/defibrillator dependence aids in establishing the patient's baseline health. Clinical symptoms of ventricular dysfunction may include fatiguability, dyspnea, poor feeding, diaphoresis, failure to gain weight, and vomiting. The presence of palpitations, dizziness, or syncope may indicate an underlying arrhythmia.

Respiratory Status Children with previous surgery for congenital heart disease (CHD) may have a history of prolonged intubation, vocal cord paralysis, poor lung compliance, and postoperative nerve damage (i.e., phrenic and/or vagus injury). Identifying prior respiratory issues will aid in efficient intraoperative ventilation management.

Neurologic Status Children with CHD may present with a history of a neurologic insult (i.e., cerebral vascular accidents or thromboembolic events) following prior cardiothoracic surgical repairs or following low cardiac output states. Assessing patients for residual symptomatology will guide additional perioperative management.

Medications Patients with repaired TOF are frequently taking cardiac medications. While angiotensin converting enzyme inhibitors (ACEi) are not commonly used in the management of right heart failure, they are historically linked to instability on induction of anesthesia due to excessive vasodilation. The time of last preoperative administration for medications should be noted. Typically, other cardiac medications are continued without interruption prior to anesthesia; however, it is recommended to carefully examine a patient's medication list for potential interactions or complications.

Laboratory Studies Hematologic and chemical profiles as well as coagulation studies may be indicated to assess renal and hepatic function or efficacy of anticoagulation therapy.

Cardiac Imaging and Testing All pertinent imaging should be reviewed.

- *Transthoracic echocardiography (TTE)* is recommended yearly in patients with repaired TOF until 10 years of age, then once every 2 years to assess qualitative RV and LV function.
- *Yearly ECGs* are recommended to monitor the patient's rhythm and QRS duration. ECG changes, specifically a prolonged QRS (>180 msec), place a patient at an increased risk of VT and sudden cardiac death.
- *Cardiac MRI* is the preferred imaging modality in an adolescent with repaired TOF as it can assess quantitative RV and LV function, the degree of PI, presence of tricuspid valve insufficiency, and can also guide timing of PVR.

Physical Exam Each patient should be examined for cardiac-specific findings. Common concerning cardiac signs include clubbing, cyanosis, mottled skin, delayed capillary refill, lethargy, failure to thrive, murmurs, hepatomegaly, tachypnea, edema, and poor peripheral pulses.

Clinical Pearl

Patients with repaired TOF may exhibit symptoms of fatigue, dyspnea on exertion, and/or diaphoresis indicating potential ventricular dysfunction. The presence of palpitations, dizziness, or syncope may indicate an underlying arrhythmia. A QRS interval >180 msec places a patient at increased risk for sustained VT and sudden cardiac death.

What anesthetic risks should be discussed with these patients and their families?

Children with CHD experience higher perioperative morbidity and mortality; the Pediatric Perioperative Cardiac Arrest registry reported that the majority of cardiac arrests during noncardiac surgery occurred in patients with major CHD [4]. Repaired TOF with free PI is considered major CHD and places these patients at higher intraoperative risk. Once the baseline cardiac status has been evaluated additional concerns regarding potential intraoperative cardiac decompensation can be discussed with the patient and his family. Intraoperative decompensation is a risk in this patient given his significant dehydration secondary to his vomiting, prolonged fasting time, and use of diuretics.

Is additional testing indicated prior to this surgery?

Relief of a testicular torsion is a urological emergency as the survival of a torsed testicle is reported to be approximately 6–8 hours from symptom onset. If the patient's cardiac symptomatology has changed recently and resources are readily available, additional studies such as a TTE and ECG should be considered. In the event that the patient presents to a hospital other than the one where he is normally followed attempts should be made to obtain prior patient records. If records are not readily available, obtaining an emergent cardiology consult, ECG, and TTE should be considered. However, because of the urgency of this case it is important not to delay the procedure for additional imaging. In absence of complete data, treat the patient as if he has decompensated cardiac disease with necessary precautions.

Is bacterial endocarditis prophylaxis indicated?

The American Heart Association recommends subacute bacterial endocarditis (SBE) prophylaxis within the first 6 months following initial cardiac repair for patients with repaired TOF. Prophylaxis is also indicated in patients with prosthetic heart valves, when prosthetic material was used in the valve repair, or in patients with residual defects at a site adjacent to a prosthetic device or material. Complete guidelines for SBE prophylaxis can be referenced and individualized for each patient.

What premedication is appropriate?

Midazolam (oral, intravenous, or intranasal) is the most commonly used premedication. Intranasal dexmedetomidine has also proven helpful for anxiolysis. However, caution is advised with the use of dexmedetomidine in patients presenting with heart block from previous surgeries, those taking atrioventricular nodal blocking agents (such as digoxin), or in patients with heart failure who may not tolerate bradycardia. Given the nature of the surgery it is quite likely that this patient would benefit from premedication.

Should a peripheral intravenous catheter be placed prior to induction?

Placement of a peripheral intravenous (PIV) catheter is advantageous prior to induction given this patient's history of vomiting and presumed dehydration. Fluid replacement would also be indicated prior to induction, particularly as the RV is dilated and preload dependent. Additionally, an IV anesthetic induction offers more hemodynamic control than an inhalation induction and can limit the effects of potential myocardial depression due to volatile anesthetic agents when ventricular function is compromised. If placement of a preoperative IV is not successful, an IV placed with administration of nitrous oxide prior to induction is an option. It can at times be challenging to obtain PIV access in children with CHD and ultrasound guidance may be necessary.

Should additional intraoperative monitoring be considered for this procedure?

All standard American Society of Anesthesiologists (ASA) monitors should be utilized along with any additional monitoring indicated by the patient's cardiac disease and functional status. For this particular case standard ASA monitoring should suffice. A 5-lead ECG is preferred when available to monitor for cardiac arrhythmias and ischemia in all patients with CHD. Additional access and monitoring depend on the size and scope of surgery, anticipated blood loss/fluid shifts, and degree of cardiac dysfunction. An arterial line should be considered if RV function is compromised and the risk of cardiac decompensation is significant. If significant biventricular dysfunction exists, placement of a central line should be considered to infuse vasoactive drugs and monitor cardiac filling pressures. Intraoperative transesophageal echocardiography can also provide useful information in children with compromised cardiac function.

In a patient with known arrhythmias or those at high risk for arrhythmias, rapid access to a defibrillator and antiarrhythmic medications, such as adenosine, should be assured.

Clinical Pearl

Patients with repaired TOF with ventricular dysfunction or a history of arrhythmias have the potential for rapid decompensation; therefore, having safety equipment and resuscitation drugs readily available is recommended.

What type of anesthetic induction should be performed?

Patients with compromised cardiac function have the potential for rapid decompensation during induction of anesthesia due to hypotension and depressed cardiac function. A dilated, volume and pressure loaded RV with poor contractility is unlikely to be able to compensate during prolonged hypotension. In general, a slow titration of medication is the preferred means to induce anesthesia in patients with cardiac dysfunction. It is recommended for safety medications and equipment to be readily available prior to induction in the event of prolonged hypotension.

While a slow induction of anesthesia is often preferable when significant cardiac dysfunction exists, in a patient presenting with significant vomiting a rapid sequence induction (RSI) may be indicated. The risk of aspiration with titrated

induction versus hemodynamic instability with RSI should be weighed in context of the individual patient. Whatever induction method is chosen, a combination of medications should be chosen that prioritizes maintenance of cardiac function and perfusion pressure and emergency medications for resuscitation should be prepared.

What are the goals for maintenance of anesthesia in this child?

Anesthetic maintenance may be conducted with inhaled anesthetics and narcotics to achieve a balanced anesthetic. The goal is to maintain the patient's cardiac rhythm, blood pressure, and hemodynamic balance as close to baseline as possible. Decisions regarding anesthetic maintenance with inhaled anesthetics or additional intravenous drugs will also be guided by a patient's response to induction, intraoperative events, and ultimate postoperative plans. It is important to note that a stress response, such as a surgical stimulus, can be challenging in patients with little cardiac reserve; therefore, appropriate pain management is warranted. Fentanyl, a synthetic opioid, is known to blunt the surgical stress response with minimal effect on cardiac function, though it can lower the heart rate, especially in higher doses.

Clinical Pearl

Intraoperative hemodynamic goals include maintenance of adequate preload for a dilated RV, rapid detection and management of arrhythmias, and maintenance of low PVR.

What are the intraoperative fluid management goals for a child with this physiology?

Intraoperative fluid management can be challenging in patients with CHD. Ensuring adequate intravascular volume is important for maintaining cardiac output. In a patient with repaired TOF, although the RV may be dilated, it is also hypertrophic and often requires increased central venous pressures to optimize cardiac output. However, in a patient with RV dilation and dysfunction, excess fluid can lead to worsening function and decompensation. The goal of intraoperative fluid resuscitation in patients with repaired TOF is to replace the fluid deficit while being aware of potential right heart failure.

What rhythm disturbances might be anticipated?

The most common arrhythmias in patients with repaired TOF result from surgical scar tissue and structural conduction obstacles that facilitate reentrant conduction pathways. Atrial reentrant tachycardias are present in 30% of this patient population and high-grade ventricular tachycardias are observed in approximately 10% [5]. Arrhythmias may also be provoked by increasing RV strain, especially during fluid resuscitation if the RV becomes overdistended.

> **Clinical Pearl**
>
> *Atrial reentrant tachycardias are present in 30% of this patient population and high grade ventricular tachycardias are observed in approximately 10%.*

How should intraoperative arrhythmias be treated?

Pediatric Advanced Life Support algorithms should be used for management of arrhythmias, and early consultation with electrophysiology is indicated. Atrial reentrant tachycardias, typically 200 beats/minute in teenagers, consist of an accessory pathway allowing conduction through an additional circuit resulting in tachycardia. These tachycardias can be treated with vagal maneuvers (such as a Valsalva maneuver), antiarrhythmics such as adenosine, or synchronized cardioversion.

Treatment of a ventricular tachycardia will vary depending on the patient's clinical condition. If the patient is hemodynamically unstable, it is best to perform a synchronized cardioversion, with 1–2 joules/kg. If the patient is stable, intravenous lidocaine or amiodarone may be an effective alternative.

> **Clinical Pearl**
>
> *Atrial tachycardias can be treated with vagal maneuvers, antiarrhythmics such as adenosine, or cardioversion. If the patient is hemodynamically unstable, utilize synchronized cardioversion.*

Should tracheal extubation be considered in the operating room?

Tracheal extubation at the conclusion of the case is desirable and may be considered if the case is uneventful and the patient is hemodynamically stable following fluid resuscitation. Adequate reversal of neuromuscular blockade with appropriate tidal volumes should be demonstrated prior to extubation.

Where should the patient be monitored in the postoperative phase?

Following an uneventful intraoperative course, a standard post-anesthesia care unit with staff experienced in caring for children with CHD would be a reasonable location for recovery. If the case is complicated by hemodynamic instability, significant arrhythmias, or decompensated cardiac function, ongoing care in an intensive care setting is indicated.

References

1. M. Seki, S. Kuwata, C. Kurishima, et al. Mechanism of aortic root dilation and cardiovascular function in tetralogy of Fallot. *Pediatr Int* 2016; **58**: 323–30.

2. P. Khairy, L. Harris, M. J. Landzberg, et al. Implantable cardioverter-defibrillators in tetralogy of Fallot. *Circulation* 2008; **117**: 363–70.

3. T. E. Ayer Botrel, A. C. Clark, M. C. Queiroga, et al. Transcatheter pulmonary valve implantation: systemic literature review. *Rev Bras Cardiol Invasiva* 2013; **21**: 176–87.

4. C. Ramamoorthy, C. M. Haberkern, S. M. Bhananker, et al. Anesthesia-related cardiac arrest in children with heart disease: data from the Pediatric Perioperative Cardiac Arrest (POCA) Registry. *Anesth Analg* 2010; **110**: 1376–82.

5. J. Villafane, J. A. Feinstein, K. J. Jenkins, et al. Hot topics in tetralogy of Fallot. *J Am Coll Cardiol* 2013; **62**: 2155–66.

Suggested Reading

Smith C. A., McCracken C., Thomas, A. S., et al. Long-term outcomes of tetralogy of Fallot: a study from the Pediatric Cardiac Care Consortium. *JAMA Cardiol* 2019; **4**: 34–41.

Twite M. D. and Ing R. J. Tetralogy of Fallot: perioperative anesthetic management of children and adults. *Semin Cardiothorac Vasc Anesth* 2012; **16**: 97–105.

Valente A. M., Cook S., Festa, P., et al. Multimodality imaging guidelines for patients with repaired tetralogy of Fallot: a report from the American Society of Echocardiography: developed in collaboration with the Society for Cardiovascular Magnetic Resonance and the Society for Pediatric Radiology. *J Am Soc Echocardiogr* 2014; **27**: 111–41.

Wilson W., Taubert K. A., Gewitz, M., et al. Prevention of infective endocarditis: guidelines from the American Heart Association: a guideline from the American Heart Association Rheumatic Fever, Endocarditis, and Kawasaki Disease Committee, Council on Cardiovascular Disease in the Young, and the Council on Clinical Cardiology, Council on Cardiovascular Surgery and Anesthesia, and the Quality of Care and Outcomes Research Interdisciplinary Working Group. *Circulation* 2007; **116**: 1736–54.

Chapter 9

Tetralogy of Fallot with Absent Pulmonary Valve Syndrome

Andrew T. Waberski

Case Scenario

An 11-month-old boy weighing 7 kg presents for a scheduled direct laryngoscopy and bronchoscopy to evaluate moderate persistent wheezing. Pertinent medical history includes postnatal diagnosis of tetralogy of Fallot with absent pulmonary valve syndrome. He underwent cardiac repair at age 5 months, including ventricular septal defect repair, right ventricle to pulmonary artery valved conduit, and pulmonary artery plication. He is seen by a cardiologist every 6 months. He has a history of frequent respiratory infections requiring respiratory treatments, intravenous antibiotics, and admission. His current medications include albuterol, inhaled steroids, and a multivitamin.

Echocardiogram performed 3 months ago demonstrates:

- *Small atrial left-to-right shunt with 3 mm Hg gradient*
- *No residual ventricular septal defect*
- *Normal biventricular function*
- *Mild right ventricular–pulmonary artery conduit regurgitation*

Key Objectives

- Describe the anatomy of tetralogy of Fallot with absent pulmonary valve syndrome.
- Define the respiratory pathology in tetralogy of Fallot with absent pulmonary valve syndrome.
- Describe the intraoperative management for patients with repaired tetralogy of Fallot with absent pulmonary valve syndrome.
- Describe potential respiratory support in tetralogy of Fallot with absent pulmonary valve syndrome.

Pathophysiology

What are the anatomic features of tetralogy of Fallot with absent pulmonary valve?

Tetralogy of Fallot (TOF) is a spectrum, including multiple variants that differ in pulmonary artery and right ventricular

outflow tract (RVOT) characteristics. (See Chapters 7, 8, and 10.) Similar to other TOF variants, TOF with absent pulmonary valve syndrome (TOF/APVS) includes an anterior maligned ventricular septal defect (VSD), an aorta that "overrides" the septal defect, and a hypertrophied right ventricle. However, TOF/APVS is distinct in that there is an absent or rudimentary, incompetent pulmonary valve. The pulmonary valve, if present, may have some degree of stenosis but the dominant pathophysiology is pulmonary regurgitation.

Patients with TOF/APVS usually have unobstructed flow to the pulmonary arteries and therefore do not have the cyanosis or hypercyanotic "tet" spells associated with other TOF variants. The main and branch pulmonary arteries are generally dilated due to pulmonary regurgitation and excessive flow and can be large enough to cause a mass effect on surrounding structures, including the airways and lungs. (See Figures 9.1 and 9.2.)

Clinical Pearl

In TOF/APVS there is an absent or rudimentary, incompetent pulmonary valve. The pulmonary valve, if present, may have some degree of stenosis but the dominant pathophysiology is pulmonary regurgitation.

What is the respiratory pathology in TOF/APVS?

Tetralogy of Fallot/APVS commonly occurs with varying degrees of obstructive respiratory disease. Persistent pulmonary regurgitation causes abnormally large and tortuous pulmonary arteries that can cause fixed or dynamic mechanical airway obstruction, typically at the tracheobronchial level. Airway compression or collapse can cause symptoms that range from mild stridor with agitation to recurrent infections, and in severe cases, atelectasis, respiratory insufficiency, and long-term mechanical respiratory support. In the most severe cases, dilation occurs throughout the pulmonary vascular bed, impinging on gas movement within the entire respiratory tract.

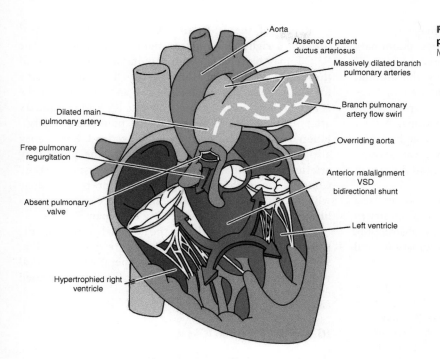

Aorta

Absence of patent
ductus arteriosus

Massively dilated branch
pulmonary arteries

Branch pulmonary
artery flow swirl

Overriding aorta

Anterior malalignment
VSD
bidirectional shunt

Left ventricle

Dilated main
pulmonary artery

Free pulmonary
regurgitation

Absent pulmonary
valve

Hypertrophied right
ventricle

Figure 9.1 Tetralogy of Fallot with absent pulmonary valve. Drawing by Ryan Moore, MD, and Matt Nelson.

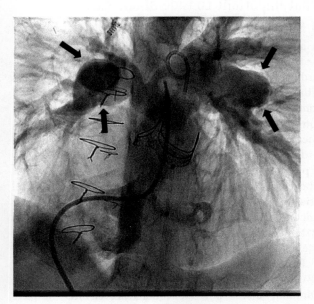

Figure 9.2 Dilated and aneurysmal branch pulmonary arteries post TOF/APVS repair. An angiogram is performed in the branch pulmonary arteries in the AP projection. The marked aneurysmal dilation of the proximal branch pulmonary arteries is noted (arrows). Courtesy of Russel Hirsch, MD.

Clinical Pearl

Airway compression or collapse can cause symptoms that range from mild stridor with agitation to recurrent infections, and in severe cases, atelectasis, respiratory insufficiency, and long-term mechanical respiratory support.

What is the role of the patent ductus arteriosus in TOF/APVS?

A patent ductus arteriosus (PDA) is typically *not* present in fetuses or neonates with TOF/APVS when significant pulmonary regurgitation is present. Absence of a PDA in TOF/APVS is associated with fetal survival.

Presence of a PDA in TOF/APVS physiology would create an unrestricted circular shunt of blood:

Aorta (via PDA) → pulmonary artery → regurgitation to RV → (via VSD) to LV → aorta

Clinical Pearl

Patients with TOF/APVS typically do not have a PDA as it would cause a circular shunt and is associated with fetal demise.

What symptomatology may be seen in unrepaired TOF/APVS?

Patients with unrepaired TOF/APVS have respiratory symptoms and cyanosis related to the degree of intracardiac shunting and airway compression. The presence of right-to-left (R-to-L) shunting at the ventricular level is dependent on relative right and left ventricular pressures and the amount of pulmonary regurgitation and stenosis (if stenosis is present). Additionally, there may be respiratory symptoms or insufficiency when large pulmonary arteries cause tracheobronchial compression.

Respiratory symptoms are dictated by the amount of airway obstruction. Mechanical obstruction of large and small bronchi may present with a pattern of obstructive airway disease, similar to asthma. Milder cases may display only tachypnea or cough, while severe obstructive pulmonary disease may cause over-inflated lung fields with limited ventilation and areas of atelectasis.

For patients with airway compression or malacia requiring treatment, prone positioning or positive airway pressure may improve symptoms of airway obstruction. However, severe cases may require intubation and mechanical ventilation.

Clinical Pearl

For infants with airway malacia due to TOF/APVS, prone positioning may reduce tracheobronchial compression and symptoms.

What chest imaging findings are commonly seen in TOF/APVS?

Chest radiography may show an enlarged cardiac silhouette related to RV hypertrophy and pulmonary artery dilation. In the presence of airway mechanical obstruction, the lungs may appear hyperinflated and/or demonstrate patchy atelectasis.

Computed tomography (CT) scan or magnetic resonance imaging (MRI) may be considered in cases where delineation of extrinsic bronchial obstruction due to compression from pulmonary arteries is necessary. For longer studies, general anesthesia is often required, which may pose additional risk for airway obstruction and difficulty with ventilation.

What are surgical repair options and considerations?

Goals for surgical repair of TOF/APVS include improvement of pulmonary blood flow (PBF) by reducing regurgitation, closure of the VSD to eliminate ventricular shunting and pulmonary arterioplasty to reduce airway compression if necessary. Timing of repair is dictated by the degree of cyanosis and effective PBF as well as the degree of respiratory obstruction. Even with adequate PBF, tachypnea and respiratory failure can cause failure to thrive prompting consideration of repair.

Repair of the VSD in TOF is typically performed through a right atriotomy or right ventriculotomy. The RVOT may be repaired with a pulmonary homograft at the level of the main pulmonary artery; the ventriculotomy for VSD repair can be used as the anchor point of the conduit. Using a *valved* conduit limits RV and pulmonary artery end-diastolic volume to reduce pulmonary regurgitation and right ventricular volume overload. Repair may also include narrowing or reduction of the pulmonary arteries by pulmonary arterioplasty or aneurysm resection. Consultation with otolaryngology and/or pulmonology with use of pre- and postoperative direct laryngoscopy/bronchoscopy may aid in directing the repair.

Low birth weight, repair in the neonatal period, and the presence of severe respiratory disease are risk factors that significantly increase mortality. Preoperative mechanical ventilation is also an independent risk factor for increased mortality following repair.

Anesthetic Implications

What important considerations exist in evaluating patients with TOF/APVS?

In addition to the routine preoperative considerations, special attention should be paid to both respiratory and cardiac systems prior to general anesthesia for patients with TOF/APVS. A focused cardiac history and physical exam should explore signs and symptoms of RV dysfunction and/or venous congestion. Dyspnea, tachypnea, wheezing, feeding difficulty, failure to gain weight, tachycardia, jugular venous distention, and liver distention may be present. Preoperative evaluation should include a recent echocardiogram to determine the presence of any residual atrial or ventricular shunts, and to evaluate ventricular function and conduit integrity. Conduit regurgitation and or stenosis may present with RV dysfunction accompanied by elevated end-diastolic pressure and volume.

Patients with a history of moderate or severe TOF/APVS may continue to experience persistent obstructive pulmonary disease and tracheomalacia even after complete repair. A small percentage of patients may require tracheostomy. Long-term respiratory pathology may include tracheo/bronchomalacia, persistent wheezing and air trapping, and recurrent pulmonary infections. Current respiratory infection secondary to ineffective clearance may require postponement of elective surgery and institution of appropriate medical therapy prior to anesthesia. Depending on symptoms, chest radiography may help assess lung fields and the degree of air trapping. Respiratory medications including bronchodilators should be continued and can be escalated in the preoperative period to support respiratory dynamics.

Although not specifically associated with TOF/APVS, patients presenting with congenital cardiac disease should be evaluated for the presence of genetic or dysmorphic syndromes. Current genetic studies estimate between 20% and 30% of congenital cardiac disease can be attributed to genetic or environmental factors. Further genetic diagnosis may have implications on anesthetic management including airway pathology and metabolic requirements.

> **Clinical Pearl**
>
> *Patients with a history of moderate or severe TOF/APVS may continue to experience persistent obstructive pulmonary disease even after complete repair.*

What induction techniques could be considered for this procedure?

The proposed anesthetic plan should consider both the degree of residual cardiac disease and/or dysfunction and the degree of existing respiratory pathology. When cardiac function is preserved, induction may be achieved through either inhalation or intravenous routes. Spontaneous ventilation for the patient undergoing direct laryngoscopy in this instance is nearly always desired to allow for in situ assessment of tracheobronchial tree anatomy and airway dynamics, including the degree of tracheobronchomalacia. Intravenous medications such as propofol or dexmedetomidine can be titrated to maintain spontaneous ventilation and limit operating room pollution of inhaled gases during direct laryngoscopy. The use of aerosolized lidocaine by the proceduralist will aid in decreasing airway irritability. Oxygen may be insufflated via an endotracheal tube placed in the side of the mouth during the procedure to assist in maintaining adequate saturations. Monitoring of adequacy of ventilation with chest excursion, tidal volumes, and capnography must be used in combination to continually evaluate the patient's respiratory status. Patients with significant respiratory disease will experience profound airway collapse without the support of positive airway pressure.

In patients with long-standing cardiac disease and poor RV function, changes in intrathoracic pressure related to mechanical ventilation, positive end-expiratory pressure and/or airway obstruction during spontaneous ventilation may precipitate worsening RV performance and impair cardiac output via increased intrathoracic pressure and RV afterload. Particular attention to cardiac output is warranted in these patients, and the anesthetic plan may

include intravenous induction and availability or administration of vasoactive medications to support cardiac function. However, in most patients with TOF/APVS the respiratory pathology after repair is more significant than the degree of residual cardiac pathology.

During inhalational induction the patient develops significant retractions with limited chest excursion: what should be done?

These symptoms are generally indicative of lower airway obstruction related to bronchomalacia. They are frequently accompanied by decreased capnography waveform and tidal volume. Standard upper airway manipulations of jaw thrust, chin lift, and oral airway should be tried but frequently do not relieve the obstruction as it is distal and not related to the upper airway. Without resolution, air trapping may occur and the patient may desaturate and become hypercarbic.

The use of positive pressure usually aids in relieving the distal airway obstruction. Titrating the adjustable pressure-limiting valve with mask ventilation to achieve adequate tidal volumes will determine the amount of positive end-expiratory pressure required to maintain lower airway patency. A balance should be considered between maintaining expiratory airway pressure to prevent lower airway obstruction and minimizing end-expiratory pressure to allow for complete exhalation. If end-expiratory pressure is ineffective, pressure support or mechanical ventilation may be beneficial.

Neuromuscular blockade may provide better conditions for controlled ventilation but may not resolve airway collapse in the setting of mechanical intrathoracic obstruction from large pulmonary arteries.

> **Clinical Pearl**
>
> *Neuromuscular blockade may provide better conditions for controlled ventilation but may not resolve airway collapse in the setting of mechanical intrathoracic obstruction from large pulmonary arteries.*

What ventilation strategies could be utilized during laryngoscopy and bronchoscopy?

During bronchoscopy, use of a supraglottic airway device or endotracheal tube can maintain upper airway patency and allow for titration of inhaled anesthetics. However, positive end-expiratory pressure may be required to support tracheobronchial integrity if significant malacia is present.

The approach to positive pressure ventilation in patients with TOF/APVS should always consider the likelihood of significant tracheobronchomalacia in this patient population. Spontaneous ventilation, if tolerated, or moderate end-expiratory pressure may be good choices to support airway patency. Adequate ventilation and oxygenation with spontaneous ventilation and sufficient depth of anesthesia to tolerate bronchoscopy may be difficult to achieve. Periods of apnea during laryngoscopy may be tolerated in combination with periods of intermittent mask ventilation.

Whatever technique is chosen, meticulous monitoring for signs of airway collapse or obstruction, along with $ETCO_2$, chest rise, exhaled tidal volumes, and SpO_2 is necessary. Constant communication between the otolaryngologist and anesthesiologist before and during the procedure is vital to patient safety and procedural efficiency.

What postoperative issues can arise?

Patients who have undergone TOF/APVS repair are at ongoing risk for bronchomalacia and airway clearance challenges; these risks are increased both intraoperatively and postoperatively. Management should include measures to decrease airway resistance and improve airflow throughout the upper and lower airways. Perioperative steroids and postoperative racemic epinephrine may decrease swelling and airway resistance from laryngoscopy and bronchoscopy.

For patients with severe bronchomalacia, postoperative continuous positive airway pressure via mask or high flow nasal cannula may provide airway support and may be necessary until residual anesthetic effects have dissipated. For acute, short-term reduction in airway resistance and turbulent flow, helium and oxygen may be administered through a nasal cannula or mask. Patients requiring continuous positive pressure or helium should be closely monitored in an intensive care setting following diagnostic or interventional laryngoscopy and bronchoscopy.

Suggested Reading

Cowan J. R. and Ware S. M. Genetics and genetic testing in congenital heart disease. *Clin Perinatol* 2015; **42**: 373–93.

Dorobantu D. M., Stoicescu C., Tulloh R. M., et al. Surgical repair of tetralogy of Fallot with absent pulmonary valve: favorable long-term results. *Semin Thorac Cardiovasc Surg* 2019; **31**: 847–9.

Hew C. C., Daebritz S. H., Zurakowski D., et al. Valved homograft replacement of aneurysmal pulmonary arteries for severely symptomatic absent pulmonary valve syndrome. *Ann Thorac Surg* 2002; **73**: 1778–85.

Rabinovitch M., Rabinovitch S., David I., et al. Compression of intrapulmonary bronchi by abnormally branching pulmonary arteries associated with absent pulmonary valves. *Am J Cardiol* 1982; **50**: 804–13.

Yeager S. B., Van D. V., Waters B. L., et al. Prenatal role of the ductus arteriosus in absent pulmonary valve syndrome. *Echocardiography* 2002; **19**: 489–493.

Zach M., Beitzke A., Singer H., et al. The syndrome of absent pulmonary valve and ventricular septal defect–anatomical features and embryological implications. *Basic Res Cardiol* **74**: 54–68.

Chapter 10

Tetralogy of Fallot, Pulmonary Atresia, and Aortopulmonary Collaterals

Mikel Gorbea and Lisa Wise-Faberowski

Case Scenario

A 2-year-old child weighing 11.5 kg with a history significant for tetralogy of Fallot, pulmonary atresia, multiple aortopulmonary collaterals, and DiGeorge syndrome presents for thyroglossal duct cyst excision under general anesthesia. He had a prenatal diagnosis of tetralogy of Fallot and pulmonary atresia, and at age 4 months underwent unifocalization of his left- and right-sided aortopulmonary collaterals via thoracotomies, along with placement of a 4 mm central shunt from the aorta to the unifocalized neopulmonary artery. The ventricular septal defect remains open. He has had multiple cardiac catheterizations for balloon dilation of pulmonary arteries and sees his cardiologist regularly.

Physical exam is notable for dysmorphic facies, slight clubbing, and bilateral thoracotomy incision scars. A holosystolic murmur is auscultated at the left sternal border. Lungs are clear and liver edge is 2 cm below the right costal margin. The hemoglobin count is 15 and hematocrit 44%, with all other laboratory results within normal limits. Current vital signs are heart rate 111 beats/minute, blood pressure 90/50 mm Hg, respiratory rate 25 breaths/minute, and SpO$_2$ 82% on room air.

Recent transthoracic echocardiography shows the following:

- *Atretic pulmonic valve*
- *Large ventricular septal defect with bidirectional flow*
- *Patent central shunt to small neopulmonary arteries with diastolic flow reversal in the descending aorta*
- *Low-normal right ventricular function*
- *Normal left ventricular function*

Key Objectives

- Describe key anatomic and physiologic features of tetralogy of Fallot, pulmonary atresia, and multiple aortopulmonary collaterals.
- Discuss current surgical palliations in this patient population and their impact on subsequent perioperative anesthetic management.
- List hemodynamic and physiologic considerations in perioperative care for a patient with tetralogy of Fallot, pulmonary atresia, and multiple aortopulmonary collaterals.

Pathophysiology

What are key anatomic characteristics of tetralogy of Fallot with pulmonary atresia and aortopulmonary collaterals?

Tetralogy of Fallot with pulmonary atresia (PA) and multiple aortopulmonary collaterals (MAPCAs) represents an extreme variation of tetralogy physiology with an incidence of 0.7 per 10,000 live births. While TOF/PA includes the basic findings of TOF, including an aorta that "overrides" an unrestrictive ventricular septal defect (VSD) and right ventricular hypertrophy (RVH), instead of pulmonary stenosis (PS) there is complete atresia of the pulmonary valve and right ventricular outflow tract. There is variable hypoplasia of the main pulmonary artery, and in severe cases the right and left pulmonary arteries are not confluent.

When complete pulmonary atresia is present, no blood flow path exists from the right ventricle (RV) into the pulmonary arteries. In addition, native pulmonary vasculature is typically hypoplastic, stenotic, or atretic. In TOF/PA/MAPCAs, pulmonary blood flow (PBF) occurs via MAPCAs. Multiple aortopulmonary collaterals are vessels that arise from the descending thoracic aorta or any of its branches (subclavian, bronchial, celiac, or intercostal), often anastomosing proximal to branch pulmonary arteries. Pulmonary blood flow via MAPCAs is variable and nonuniform. Bronchopulmonary segments can have multiple vascular contributions arising from one or more vascular sources, and PBF may vary between segments.

57

What is the path of blood flow at birth in this patient?

- Systemic venous blood returns via the inferior vena cava (IVC) and the superior vena cava (SVC) to the right atrium (RA).
- Blood passes via the nonrestrictive VSD from the RV to the LV, mixing deoxygenated systemic venous return with oxygenated pulmonary venous blood return.
- Blood exits via the LV outflow tract.
- Pulmonary blood flow is provided via a PDA (if present) or via MAPCAs from the aorta.

How do patients with TOF/PA/MAPCAS receive pulmonary blood flow?

In TOF with PS some of the systemic venous blood passes through the RV outflow tract to the PAs. In contrast, *in TOF/PA ALL pulmonary blood flow is from the aorta*: either via flow from a patent ductus arteriosus (PDA), MAPCAs, or a combination of the two.

In more than half of cases the native central pulmonary arteries are well developed and supplied by the PDA. Confluence between the right and left pulmonary arteries is a key differentiator in disease spectrum severity. Confluent branch pulmonary arteries occur in the majority (85%) of patients. In the absence of pulmonary artery (PA) confluence, MAPCAs are always present and lung segments are perfused via individual MAPCAs as well as the nonconfluent PAs.

In TOF/PA, in the absence of a path from the RV to the pulmonary vasculature, presence of a VSD is vital for establishing a path that allows systemic venous return to enter the LV, aorta, and subsequently MAPCAs.

How do MAPCAs provide pulmonary blood flow?

There is variation in PBF in patients with TOF/PA/MAPCAs due to variability of MAPCA size, origin, and connection to the lungs. Collateral arteries may be classified as *direct* when arising from the aorta and *indirect* when originating from the brachiocephalic (25%) or coronary arteries (7%). Total number of MAPCAs usually range from two to six with indirect collaterals being less numerous when compared to direct collaterals. Collaterals may course directly into the pulmonary parenchyma to supply a discrete bronchopulmonary segment or toward the lung hilum with direct anastomosis to branches of the pericardial pulmonary arteries at extrapulmonary, hilar, lobar, or segmental levels. Bronchopulmonary segments can contain a dual supply of blood from both intrapericardial pulmonary and systemic-to-pulmonary collaterals in 4%–14% of patients.

What is the physiologic impact of MAPCAs and what are their characteristics?

Multiple aortopulmonary collaterals may induce anatomic and physiologic changes in pulmonary vessels due to chronic endothelial exposure to systemic arterial pressures. They may also induce arterialization of distal low pressure pulmonary arterial tributaries, and the resultant increased pressure and volume burden results in discrete dilations within vascular branch points distal to their respective MAPCA insertions. Long-standing elevated pressures in pulmonary vessels often induce vascular endothelial muscular changes and increased vascular reactivity.

In addition to abnormal PBF, lung parenchymal development is also impacted in TOF/PA/MAPCAs. In utero, diminished PBF contributes to decreased distal pulmonary vessel arborization. As a result of compromised perfusion, lungs may be hypoplastic. Importantly, MAPCAs anastomotic sites may become stenotic over time, negatively impacting PBF.

What cardiac surgical palliative or repair pathways are available for these patients?

The ultimate surgical treatment goal, if possible, is restoration of two discrete and non-mixing systemic and pulmonary circulations. Complete separation of the systemic and

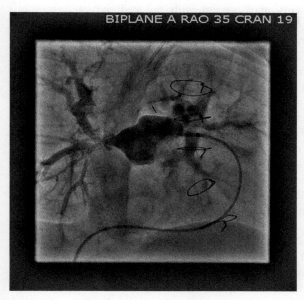

Figure 10.1 Unifocalized right pulmonary artery. An angiogram is performed in the right pulmonary artery in the AP projection. The dilated proximal conduit extending into the proximal right pulmonary artery is noted, with the stenotic, unifocalized right pulmonary artery branches extending distally. Courtesy of Russel Hirsch, MD.

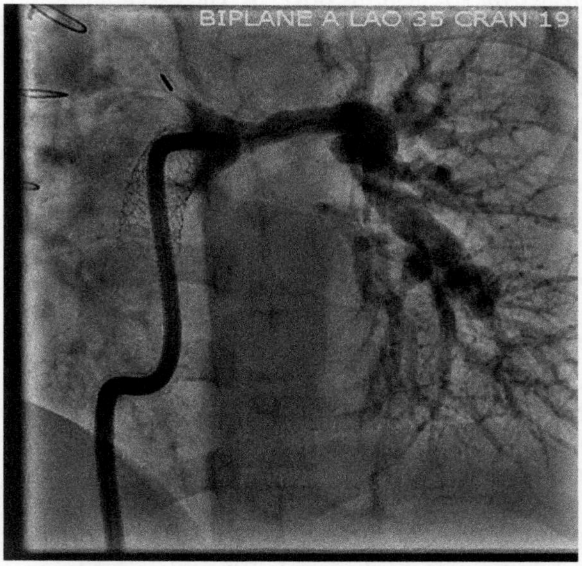

Figure 10.2 Unifocalized left pulmonary artery. An angiogram is performed in the left pulmonary artery in the AP projection. The long segment stenotic proximal conduit is noted with the small unifocalized left pulmonary artery branches extending distally. Courtesy of Russel Hirsch, MD.

pulmonary circuits with the lowest possible RV pressure is the ultimate goal. Because of anatomic complexity in TOF/PA/MAPCAs, single step complete repair may not be achievable, and a staged approach or palliation may be utilized. The feasibility of complete repair is heavily dependent on the arborization of the pulmonary bed, the size and morphology of the pulmonary arteries and MAPCAs, and the amount of PBF.

Complete repair includes the following:

- Collateral pulmonary arteries are "unifocalized" into a neopulmonary artery confluence. (See Figures 10.1 and 10.2.) Aortopulmonary collaterals and pulmonary arteries supplying bronchopulmonary segments are combined into a single source via an augmented and reconstructed PA.
- Right ventricular outflow tract obstruction is corrected and a valved conduit connecting the RV to the PA confluence is placed.
- Intraventricular/atrial connections are closed.

A staged or palliated approach is common in TOF/PA/MAPCAs.

- Complex anatomy may require unifocalization in stages and a surgically created central (aortopulmonary) shunt may be placed. The centrally created shunt or conduit is connected to the small but

functional unfocalized neopulmonary arteries to provide a source of PBF and support pulmonary arterial vascular growth.

- A right ventricular to pulmonary artery conduit to the neopulmonary confluence can be placed.
- It may not be possible to close the VSD if the pulmonary arteries and the pulmonary vascular bed are not of sufficient caliber (<50%–75% of normal) to handle the entire cardiac output from the RV. The VSD is left open and acts as a "pop off" to allow for some blood flow from the RV to LV; mixing at the ventricular level of deoxygenated and oxygenated blood means that child will remain cyanotic. When the VSD is closed before the pulmonary vascular bed is able to handle the entire RV cardiac output, the child will exhibit signs and symptoms of RV hypertension and RV failure.

Some institutions utilize a staged procedure via thoracotomy, unifocalizing the pulmonary arterial supply to a single lung, either the left or right lung. The pulmonary blood supply to the contralateral lung is unifocalized at a later date. Correction of the VSD can occur after the complete restoration of pulmonary arterial supply to both lungs during the final staged correction.

Regardless of anatomy, evidence suggests that single stage complete correction may offer advantages and improved outcomes compared to staged unifocalization in greater than four-fifths of cases. The exception to this rule is noted when confluent central PAs with normal arborization share dual blood supply with MAPCAs and present with cyanosis. Patients undergoing complete unifocalization with intracardiac repair, however, are at risk of developing prolonged postoperative respiratory failure. In either staged or complete repair, pulmonary arteries are often hypoplastic and stenosis occurs over time. Frequent interventional catheterizations for balloon angioplasty and/or stenting are common.

Clinical Pearl

In either staged or complete repair, pulmonary arteries are often hypoplastic and stenosis occurs over time. Frequent interventional catheterizations for balloon angioplasty and/ or stenting are common.

What is the physiology of PBF supplied by MAPCAs?

At birth, anatomic variations in MAPCAs, lung development and PVR determine the severity of cyanosis. In patients with TOF/PA/MAPCAs, PBF is often limited by abnormal, hypoplastic pulmonary vessel anatomy and neonatal pulmonary vascular elevation; $Q_p{:}Q_s$ may be low-normal or low, resulting in low oxygen saturations.

Assessing the importance of the contribution of the PDA to overall PBF is a key in the perinatal period. The PDA may be a significant source of PBF via either MAPCAs or hypoplastic native pulmonary arteries. If saturations fall to unacceptable levels with PDA closure, prostaglandins are utilized to reopen the PDA and the patient will require neonatal intervention to maintain ductal patency. This can be accomplished either via an interventional cardiac catheterization with stenting of the PDA or placement of a surgical aortopulmonary shunt in the cardiac operating room. In the less common setting of abundant or unrestricted MAPCAs, PBF increases as PVR falls after birth resulting in pulmonary overcirculation and congestion.

After the neonatal period, dominant physiology and hemodynamic expectations depend on anatomy of the MAPCAs, $Q_p{:}Q_s$, potential lung disease, and pulmonary vascular reactivity.

What are the expectations for oxygen saturation, $Q_p{:}Q_s$, and hemodynamics?

Patients whose lesions are completely repaired and who no longer have interventricular or atrial connections should have normal oxygen saturations. Palliated and unoperated patients may present with reduced oxygen saturations depending on the palliation, degree of residual collaterals, intracardiac shunting, and PVR.

Because of the variation in PBF and resultant oxygen saturations that can exist in patients with unrepaired or palliated TOF/PA/MAPCAs, a thorough understanding of each patient's current anatomy and palliative stage is essential in order to determine appropriate hemodynamic and saturation goals. Baseline oxygen saturations should be noted at both rest and with exertion (elevated RV pressure) in order to better define current physiology. In order to minimize over-circulation of both pulmonary and systemic arterial systems, an optimal oxygen saturation should ideally reflect a balanced $Q_p{:}Q_s$ on room air, resulting in oxygen saturations of 75%–85%. The combination of abnormal pulmonary vessel anatomy, hypoplastic lungs, and variable pulmonary vascular reactivity often creates a resultant physiology that typically has low or low-normal $Q_p{:}Q_s$ and may present challenges with oxygenation and ventilation. Oxygen saturations may be 70%–80% with physical and physiologic sequelae of chronic hypoxemia such as clubbing and polycythemia. Patients with elevated pulmonary vascular reactivity may be chronically taking pulmonary vasodilators.

Clinical Pearl

A thorough preoperative assessment and cardiology consultation is recommended for understanding of the individual child's dominant physiology, as a wide spectrum of variation can exist in PBF and resultant oxygen saturations in patients with TOF/PA/MAPCAs.

What long-term complications may occur with TOF/PA/MAPCAs?

After repair or palliation, patients with TOF/PA/MAPCAs can suffer from short- and long-term respiratory insufficiency. Immediate postoperative respiratory complications following complete repair with unifocalization are common. Prolonged postprocedural intubation, longer exposure to anesthetics, intricate surgical dissection, vascular reconstruction, and extensive suture lines contribute to increased postoperative respiratory compromise. Prolonged intubation may result in tracheal mucosal and/or vocal cord injury as well as worsen preexisting or new bronchomalacia. Dissection within the thorax may increase the risk of iatrogenic unilateral or bilateral recurrent laryngeal nerve damage resulting in postoperative stridor, airway obstruction, and potential respiratory failure.

Airway obstruction or malacia due to changing intrathoracic anatomy is possible. Left and right reconstructed pulmonary arteries may cause compression of posterior airway structures including the bronchi. Intrathoracic obstruction secondary to compression of bronchi may go unnoticed in these patients until chest closure is attempted, resulting in the need for anastomosis revision, intraoperative bronchoscopy, or surgical fixation of structures anterior to the site of compression to the chest wall to relieve the obstruction.

Clinical Pearl

Airway obstruction or malacia due to changing intrathoracic anatomy is possible. Left and right reconstructed pulmonary arteries may cause compression of posterior airway structures including the bronchi.

Although most collateral arteries are present at birth, evidence suggests that more collaterals may develop postnatally and post-palliation resulting in "acquired" or unmasked collateral arteries. Origins for these acquired collateral arteries include intercostal, bronchial, or systemic arteries. "Aggravated" acquired collateral arteries develop after a surgically created systemic-to-pulmonary shunt. Residual MAPCAs can be unmasked following complete repair when initial anatomic location or vessel size prevented discovery at the time of repair. Increased collateral flow or persistent MAPCAs can contribute to pulmonary congestion, systemic hypoperfusion, and gradually increased PVR over time due to collateral flow.

Patients with TOF/PA/MAPCAs often require repeated diagnostic and interventional cardiac catheterization procedures. Stenosis of the newly reconstructed pulmonary vasculature after complete repair may require reintervention in up to one-third of patients in order to maintain the lowest possible systolic PA pressures. Diagnostic pressure measurements and coiling of persistent MAPCAs or newly developed collaterals may be indicated.

Heterografts, homografts, and synthetic conduits are often used in palliation or complete repair of TOF/PA/MAPCAs. Right ventricle-to-pulmonary artery (RV-PA) conduits are subject to the development of progressive stenosis, regurgitation, and calcification. Homograft deterioration is progressive, with only 30% being intact at 15 years. Prolonged conduit regurgitation and/or stenosis increases RV strain, resulting in ventricular fibrosis, restriction, dilation, and increased risk for arrhythmias and failure. Additionally, conduits are nonnative and do not grow with the pediatric patient. Therefore, conduits need periodic catheter-based reintervention or surgical replacement.

Clinical Pearl

Follow-up recommendations following partial or complete repair include routine catheterization 1 year after repair. It is not uncommon for balloon angioplasty to be performed at that time, even for minor stenoses, in an effort to maintain the lowest total resistance to pulmonary flow possible. Surgical reintervention on the pulmonary arteries is not uncommon and generally occurs at the time of conduit replacement.

Anesthetic Implications

Are there associated genetic syndromes to consider? Would they affect the perioperative plan?

Multiple syndromes can be associated with TOF/PA/MAPCAs including chromosome 22q11 microdeletion (DiGeorge syndrome) and Alagille syndrome. Between 17% and 40% of patients with TOF/PA/MAPCAS have chromosome 22q11 microdeletion. In affected patients a 14% incidence of airway abnormalities including laryngeal web, subglottic stenosis, and laryngomalacia has been noted. In these instances, direct laryngoscopy can provide upper airway evaluation but chest computed tomography (CT) and bronchoscopy may be necessary to provide lower airway evaluation. Preoperative genetic testing and counseling are helpful as these syndromes have associated noncardiac manifestations that can impact anesthetic planning. Issues may include potential difficult airway management, immunodeficiency, hypocalcemia, and liver dysfunction.

Clinical Pearl

Between 17% and 40% of patients with TOF/PA/MAPCAS have chromosome 22q11 microdeletion. In affected patients a 14% incidence of airway abnormalities including laryngeal web, subglottic stenosis, and laryngomalacia has been noted.

What imaging modalities may be utilized to guide surgical intervention and outcomes in patients with TOF/PA/MAPCAs?

Annual transthoracic echocardiography should be performed with a focus on both size and function of the right and left ventricles, including pressure gradient estimates through the right ventricular outflow tract that may rule out or diagnose new or worsening obstruction. The presence of aortic valvulopathies or history of previous aortic balloon dilation places patients at risk of developing progressive aortic insufficiency. Poor visualization of pulmonary arteries within the adult population relative to their pediatric counterparts can hinder adequate echocardiographic assessment of these vessels.

Computed tomography and angiography (CTA) may be utilized when detailed interrogation of the complex pulmonary circulation is needed. Improved spatial resolution enhances visualization of preexisting stents and the extent of collateralization with the added benefit of assessment of ventricular function via cine viewing. Computed tomography/angiography is also useful in identifying the proximity of conduit location relative to the sternum that may warrant peripheral cannulation in patients that have undergone multiple sternotomies. Unfortunately, the use of CT presents patients with the risks of both radiation and contrast exposure. Patients with abnormal CT scans should reflexively undergo catheterization for hemodynamic quantification and potential intervention to correct any newly discovered lesions.

What priorities exist for preoperative assessment of a patient with TOF/PA/MAPCAs?

The initial preanesthetic evaluation should elicit a complete history including original cardiac anatomy and current palliation stage. Detailed surgical palliative histories including both surgical and anesthetic courses should be reviewed. Recent echocardiographic and catheterization reports for patients undergoing noncardiac surgery should be reviewed. Consultation with cardiology preoperatively is recommended.

Exercise tolerance should be queried, and the most recent echocardiogram and imaging studies reviewed. Airway assessment including any history of prior prolonged intubations, tracheostomy, presence and severity of bronchomalacia, mass effect of the vasculature on airway segments, vocal cord integrity, and recurrent nerve injury is paramount for these patients.

Physical examination may be significant for systolic ejection murmurs with a loud palpable S2 component secondary to preexisting conduits. "To and fro" murmurs over a preexisting conduit location may indicate prominent conduit regurgitation. Classic diastolic murmurs indicating aortic regurgitation are not uncommon. Persistent, continuous murmurs noted laterally or around the posterior thorax may raise concern for the presence of new or persistent MAPCAs or previous surgical shunts that should be clinically correlated. The liver should be palpated to assess for congestion because of increased

right heart pressure. A superficial examination of the skin may be notable for previous posterolateral thoracotomy scars on the trunk from prior systemic-to-pulmonary artery shunt procedures.

Preoperative instructions for cyanotic patients should emphasize the importance of minimizing fasting time. American Society of Anesthesiologists fasting guidelines should be followed, and clear liquid intake should be encouraged until 2 hours prior to surgery. If the patient is not the first case of the day, consideration should be given to starting an intravenous (IV) line with administration of maintenance fluids until the start of surgery. The patient's level of preoperative anxiety should be assessed as well; the use of distraction techniques, child life preparation, or oral premedication may all be considered if needed to allay anxiety.

What considerations are important during induction and maintenance of anesthesia?

Anesthetic induction and maintenance management goals for patients with TOF/PA/MAPCAs center on two goals:

- *Balancing Q_p:Q_s in palliated patients* can be achieved by knowing the patient's baseline oxygen saturation at rest, utilizing fraction of inspired oxygen concentration (FiO_2) during the procedure to maintain saturations in this range, and avoiding triggers that may increase PVR.
- *Decreasing the hemodynamic burden experienced by the RV* associated with changes in preload and afterload; a knowledge of baseline RV function and maintenance of adequate preload are useful for accomplishing this goal.

The choice of IV or inhalational induction and maintenance should be made based on the patient's previous palliation(s), current physiology, and degree of RV dysfunction. Palliated patients presenting without overt signs of severe congestive heart failure or cyanosis may undergo inhalational induction with sevoflurane with titration of the FiO_2 based on the patient's Q_p:Q_s. In this patient, with baseline oxygen saturations of 82% and low-normal RV function, an inhalation induction of anesthesia could be performed, or if the patient had undergone a prolonged period of fasting, placement of an IV preinduction would allow for a more controlled induction of anesthesia.

During induction and intubation an increased FiO_2 is often utilized and then adjusted once the patient is intubated. Ideally, the FiO_2 is adjusted to maintain an oxygen saturation between 75% and 85% to reflect a balanced Q_p:Q_s. Depending on the number and size of MAPCAs, changes in PVR may have significant impact on systemic and pulmonary flow. Decreasing PVR may cause considerable runoff from the systemic system into the lower pressure pulmonary arterial system and may result in systemic hypoperfusion and subsequent acidosis. Similarly, children with TOF/PA/MAPCAs are at risk for increased pulmonary vascular reactivity and may experience decreased PBF if PVR is acutely increased.

Patients with TOF/PA/MAPCAs are at risk for RV dysfunction. Right ventricular pressure overload may result from stenosis within the conduit, branch pulmonary arteries, previously unifocalized MAPCAs, hypoplastic pulmonary arteries, or other vascular arborization anomalies within the pulmonary system that may increase afterload experienced by the RV. In the setting of prolonged RV pressure overload, the right heart may dilate with subsequent development of tricuspid regurgitation, causing a volume and pressure loaded failing ventricle. Inhalational induction of anesthesia and the increased RV afterload associated with positive pressure ventilation (PPV) may cause worsening RV function or failure.

As volatile anesthetics decrease mean arterial blood pressure (MAP), systemic vascular resistance (SVR), and cardiac output (CO) in a dose-dependent manner, it may be prudent to limit the total dose of inhalational anesthetic or consider a total intravenous anesthetic for patients with severe RV dysfunction. Combinations of fentanyl and dexmedetomidine infusions may be used along with a long-acting nondepolarizing neuromuscular blocker if needed. Prior studies demonstrated hemodynamic stability when using high-dose fentanyl, either in bolus dosing or as a continuous infusion. Fentanyl in combination with midazolam leads to a decrease in MAP and CO but an increase in heart rate and SVR. Dexmedetomidine is an α_2-agonist with sedative properties; when used in combination with fentanyl, it minimally decreases heart rate and MAP, while potentiating the analgesic properties of fentanyl.

In older patients with long-standing severe disease, biventricular heart dysfunction and arrhythmias may be present. Left heart failure resulting from the presence of residual MAPCAs may lead to aortic insufficiency from progressive root dilation. Supraventricular arrhythmias (atrial fibrillation, atrial flutter, or atrial tachycardia) related to progressive pathology of the right heart and previous surgical insult to myocardial conduction tissue may be present. Patients can be at increased risk for ventricular arrhythmias due to prior ventriculostomies, abnormalities of the native myocardium, or progressive ventricular dilation and dysfunction.

Clinical Pearl

Anesthetic induction and maintenance management goals for patients with TOF/PA/MAPCAs center on the goals of balancing $Q_P:Q_S$ in palliated patients and decreasing the hemodynamic burden experienced by the RV.

What is the appropriate postoperative disposition for this patient undergoing elective surgery?

Patients with complex congenital heart disease presenting for noncardiac surgery are at high risk for complications in the perioperative period. Postoperative observation in an intensive care unit may be warranted to permit rapid assessment and treatment of potentially fatal complications inherent to this unique subset of patients after complex surgeries. Depending on the complexity of surgical procedure and degree of preoperative morbidity, perioperative complications can include arrhythmias, cardiac ischemia or failure, and acute respiratory compromise. Assuming a stable intraoperative course this patient should be able to recover in the post-anesthesia care unit followed by overnight observation with monitoring of pulse oximetry. As with all patients, adequate pain relief, control of nausea and vomiting, maintenance of normothermia, and adequate volume status are essential for a stable postoperative recovery.

Suggested Reading

Ho S. Y., Catani G., and Seo J. W. Arterial supply to the lungs in tetralogy of Fallot with pulmonary atresia or critical pulmonary stenosis. *Cardiol Young* 1992; **2**: 65–72.

Huntington G. S. The morphology of the pulmonary artery in the mammalia. *Anat Rec* 1919; **17**: 164–201.

Jefferson K., Rees S., and Somerville J. Systemic arterial supply to the lungs in pulmonary atresia and its relation to pulmonary artery development. *Br Heart J* 1972; **34**: 418.

Mainwaring R. D., Reddy V. M., Peng L., et al. Hemodynamic assessment after complete repair of pulmonary atresia with major aortopulmonary collaterals. *Ann Thorac Surg* 2013; **95**: 1397–402.

Quinonez Z. A., Downey L., Abbasi R. K., et al. Anesthetic management during surgery for tetralogy of Fallot with pulmonary atresia and major aortopulmonary collateral arteries. *World J Pediatr Congenit Heart Surg* 2018; **9**: 236–41.

Rossi R. N., Hislop A., Anderson B. H., et al. Systemic-to-pulmonary blood supply in tetralogy of Fallot with pulmonary atresia. *Cardiol Young* 2002; **12**: 373–88.

Webb G., Mulder B. J., Aboulhosn J., et al. The care of adults with congenital heart disease across the globe: current assessment and future perspective: a position statement from the International Society for Adult Congenital Heart Disease (ISACHD). *Int J Cardiol* 2015; **195**: 326–33.

Chapter

11

Pentalogy of Cantrell

Jennifer E. Lam

Case Scenario

A 2-week-old neonate with unrepaired, prenatally diagnosed pentalogy of Cantrell presents to the general operating room for an omphalocele repair. She was born via cesarean section at 38 weeks weighing 2.9 kg, with Apgar scores of 6 and 8. She initially required continuous positive airway pressure support, but quickly weaned to nasal cannula. The omphalocele is large and contains mostly bowel but also parts of the stomach and liver. The umbilical sac is intact and covered by sterile gauze. The patient currently has one 24-gauge peripheral intravenous line and a nasogastric tube in place. She is on 1 L of oxygen per nasal cannula. On examination, she is noted to be tachypneic with paradoxical respiratory motion, and a pulsatile mass is seen under her skin just superior to the omphalocele sac.

Echocardiography reveals the following:

- *Moderately sized perimembranous ventricular septal defect with left-to-right shunting*
- *Elevated right ventricular pressures*
- *Preserved biventricular function*

Key Objectives

- Describe the five congenital defects that comprise pentalogy of Cantrell.
- Understand the surgical options, timing, and staging of repairs for this patient.
- Describe the preoperative assessment and studies necessary before surgery.
- Describe intraoperative concerns and management strategies.
- Describe postoperative destination and concerns.

Pathophysiology

What five congenital defects comprise pentalogy of Cantrell?

Pentalogy of Cantrell (POC) was first described in 1958 by James Cantrell and consists of the following findings:

1. A midline, supraumbilical abdominal wall defect

2. A congenital heart defect (CHD)
3. A lower sternal defect
4. An anterior diaphragmatic defect
5. A diaphragmatic pericardial defect [1]

William Toyama further classified the syndrome into three subcategories:

- **Class I** is considered definite, with all five defects as described by Cantrell.
- **Class II** is probable but incomplete, with four of five defects present, which must include both congenital heart and abdominal wall defects.
- **Class III** is incomplete phenotypic expression with various combinations of defects that must include a sternal malformation [2].

Various other malformations have been associated with POC, including craniofacial (cleft lip/palate), central nervous system (meningocele/hydrocephalus), limb (club feet), thoracic (lung atresia), and abdominal defects (pyloric stenosis/colon malrotation/cryptorchidism) [3].

What is the prevalence, epidemiology, and embryology of POC?

Pentalogy of Cantrell is a rare defect with reported incidences between 1/65,000 and 1/200,000 live births. The male/female ratio is approximately 2:1, and females tend to be more severely affected. Most cases are sporadic, although associations have been reported with trisomies 13, 18, and 21 and Turner syndrome, and some familial, X-linked cases have been reported. Pentalogy of Cantrell occurs between days 14 and 18 of embryonic life around the time of differentiation of the primitive mesoderm into the splanchnic and somatic layers, which give rise to the pericardium, myocardium, abdominal wall, diaphragm, and sternum. It is the abnormal differentiation, migration, and fusion of the mesoderm at this time that leads to the defects seen in POC [3, 4].

What types of abdominal wall defects are seen in POC?

Most patients with POC have an omphalocele, a ventral wall defect of the umbilical ring with herniation of the abdominal viscera covered by the umbilical sac. Other possible defects in the abdominal wall include wide diastasis of the abdominal muscles (diastasis recti), epigastric hernia, umbilical hernia, and gastroschisis (protrusion of the abdominal viscera through the defect to the side of the umbilical cord).

What are the various congenital heart defects seen with POC?

The most common intracardiac defects seen in POC are ventricular septal defect (72%–100%), atrial septal defect (53%), pulmonary stenosis (33%), tetralogy of Fallot (20%), and left ventricular (LV) diverticulum (20%). Complex congenital heart defects are present in 51% and include partial anomalous pulmonary venous return, transposition of the great arteries, truncus arteriosus, hypoplastic left heart syndrome, complete atrioventricular canal, and double outlet right ventricle. Other findings can include bilateral superior vena cava, single coronary anatomy, dextrocardia, and dextroversion. The most common pericardial defect is an absent pericardium, with the minority of patients having only a ventral defect [1, 3].

What is an LV diverticulum?

An LV diverticulum is either a muscular or fibrous appendix arising from the LV apex that extends beyond the myocardial border. The muscular type is associated with POC. It results in a narrow connection to the LV cavity (versus a wide connection in the fibrous type) that contracts synchronously with the true LV, although it is usually thin walled and hypokinetic. It often appears as a pulsating umbilical mass under the skin. The risks associated with LV diverticulum include spontaneous rupture, thrombus formation, and ventricular tachyarrhythmias. The left anterior descending coronary artery may also course through the diverticulum and put the patient at risk for LV failure after repair. Surgical intervention is indicated for those at high risk for rupture (dyssynchronous contraction), severe tachyarrhythmias, or progressive congestive heart failure (CHF) [5].

Clinical Pearl

Risks associated with LV diverticulum include spontaneous rupture, thrombus formation, and ventricular tachyarrhythmias. The left anterior descending coronary artery may also course through the diverticulum and put the patient at risk for LV failure after repair.

What sternal malformations are associated with POC?

Sternal malformations occur due to failed fusion of the mesenchymal plate during embryonic development and vary in significance from absence of the tip of the sternum (short sternum) to complete sternal absence. They are categorized according to location of the defect: (1) cervical, (2) thoracic, (3) thoracoabdominal, and (4) cleft or bifid sternum. Patients with sternal clefts have normal heart position and skin coverage and intact pericardium, and these malformations are typically more benign in nature, whereas those in the first three categories are associated with ectopia cordis [6].

Sternal instability may result in severe paradoxical movement of the mediastinum with respirations, leading to dyspnea, hypoxemia, and ventilatory failure in infants. In addition, sternal malformations leave the patient susceptible to respiratory infections and blunt or piercing trauma to the heart.

What is ectopia cordis?

Ectopia cordis (EC) occurs when the heart lies outside the thoracic cavity due to sternal, pericardial, diaphragmatic, and/or abdominal wall defects. It can lie partially or completely outside the chest and may also be deficient in both pericardial and skin coverings ("naked heart"). The apex of the heart is usually anterior and cephalad in both cervical and thoracic EC, both of which are nearly universally fatal [6]. Pentalogy of Cantrell is associated with thoracoabdominal EC, which often has a thin membrane/skin covering and the apex is typically not as rotated. In addition to being susceptible to infection and trauma, complete EC results in the development of a small chest cavity with associated lung hypoplasia. (See Figures 11.1 and 11.2.)

Clinical Pearl

In addition to susceptibility to infection and trauma, complete ectopia cordis results in the development of a small chest cavity with associated lung hypoplasia.

Are these patients at risk for pulmonary hypertension?

Patients with POC often have some degree of pulmonary hypoplasia and up to 55% present with pulmonary hypertension (PH) [7]. After birth they may require pulmonary vasodilators (inhaled nitric oxide [iNO], sildenafil) or respiratory assistance, including high-frequency oscillatory ventilation. Pulmonary hypoplasia may be attributed

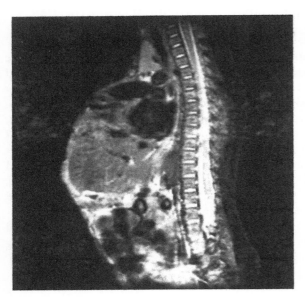

Figure 11.1 MRI, sagittal scan. The heart is located outside the thorax.

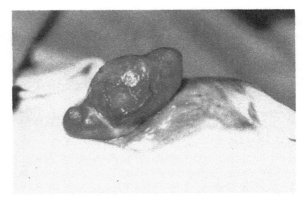

Figure 11.2 Cantrell's pentalogy (thoracoabdominal ectopia cordis). The heart is protruding from the thoracic cavity above an omphalocele. From Engum S. Embryology, sternal clefts, ectopia cordis, and Cantrell's pentalogy. *Semin Ped Surg* 2008; **17**: 154–60. With permission.

to the markedly decreased chest capacity but also to abnormal postnatal pulmonary growth. Pulmonary hypertension is more likely to occur with giant omphaloceles or when the liver is located inside the omphalocele sac. Pulmonary hypertension may also result from CHD due to cyanotic lesions resulting in hypoxia-induced tension on arterial smooth muscle and vascular remodeling, severe left-sided obstructive lesions, or lesions with significant left-to-right shunting. Pulmonary hypertension in POC has also been attributed to a possible genetic component, as it has been known to exist without the aforementioned comorbidities.

What surgical options and strategies should be considered in POC?

General Considerations The biggest challenge in caring for a patient with POC lies in consideration of the wide spectrum of anomalies with various complexities that complicate surgical planning. Planning dictates a multidisciplinary approach involving neonatology, cardiology, cardiac surgery, general surgery, anesthesiology, and pertinent subspecialties to determine the best course of action. Generally, corrective strategies include separation of the peritoneal and pericardial cavities with coverage of midline defects, omphalocele correction, repair of intracardiac lesions, and restoration of the heart into the thoracic cavity, all while preserving/establishing musculoskeletal structural integrity and hemodynamic stability. Early staged approaches

are reserved for the most severe cases, while postponing surgery until after the more vulnerable neonatal period is advocated for less severe cases. In general, surgical mortality rates are higher in patients requiring early intervention. Alternative options include supportive/symptomatic care and comfort care/withdrawal.

Omphalocele An intact and well-epithelialized omphalocele does not necessarily need to be repaired immediately after birth, but early intervention is surgically easier. Smaller defects (<5 cm) can be repaired earlier by primary closure or with a synthetic mesh. Larger, more complex omphaloceles will require a staged approach with gradual reduction into the abdominal cavity to allow for growth within the cavity and to minimize the effects of increased intraabdominal pressure, especially in patients with significant cardiac malformations. Conservative management is preferred, if possible, for larger lesions to allow for epithelialization of the omphalocele sac and maturation of the lungs. This includes prophylactic antibiotics and coverage of the omphalocele to protect it from injury and desiccation.

Intracardiac Repair Unstable, hemodynamically significant intracardiac defects demand early intervention, which may include definitive surgical correction or surgical palliation. If possible, repair is delayed until there is sufficient growth of both the thoracic cavity and the lungs.

Left Ventricular Diverticulum Because of the risk of rupture and lethal arrhythmias, LV diverticula are repaired early. Repair of an LV diverticulum can be done concomitantly with EC and/or cardiac repair in less complex cases [5].

Ectopia Cordis The main goal in repairing EC is to provide coverage to the heart and return it to the thoracic cavity to prevent fluid losses, desiccation, and trauma. This can be accomplished initially by primary closure for smaller defects or with the use of skin grafts or prosthetic material. Returning the heart into the thorax can cause compression or kinking of the great arteries and may have to be done in stages to allow for growth of the smaller thoracic cavity. The timing of intracardiac repairs in relation to reduction of the heart into the chest depends on the cardiac defect. Smaller, less significant lesions (such as an atrial or ventricular septal defect) may be repaired at the same time but more complex lesions may be delayed until the child is older and the thoracic cavity is large enough to accommodate the heart [4].

Sternal Malformations Repair of sternal malformations in the neonatal period is preferred because the compliant chest wall becomes more rigid by the age of 3 months, making surgery more complicated. Simple malformations can be repaired by primary closure, but complex lesions may require a staged approach because of the risk of cardiac compression/decompensation secondary to the limited size of the small chest cavity. Various techniques such as the use of autologous tissue (rib, costal cartilage, clavicle), sliding/rotating chondrotomies, and pectoralis major myoplasty may be used [4].

> **Clinical Pearl**
>
> *Pentalogy of Cantrell has a wide spectrum of anomalies with various complexities; therefore surgical planning dictates a multidisciplinary approach.*

Anesthetic Implications

What preoperative information is necessary before surgery?

A preoperative evaluation for a patient with POC must include a multidisciplinary discussion prior to surgery. Imaging including echocardiogram, cardiac catheterization, computed tomography/magnetic resonance imaging studies, and ultrasound to assess cardiac/sternal/abdominal defects will help with anesthetic planning. The child's cardiorespiratory status should be evaluated for signs of compromise including shunting, arrhythmias, congestive heart failure (CHF), low cardiac output, aspiration, respiratory failure, and PH, as early and aggressive support may be necessary. Patients may require mechanical ventilation at birth, as well as inotropic support, the use of iNO, and systemic pulmonary vasodilators. Patients are also at risk for sepsis, dehydration, hypothermia, and renal failure.

> **Clinical Pearl**
>
> *A thorough preoperative investigation of available imaging to ascertain the presence and severity of associated anomalies is paramount. The cardiorespiratory status should be evaluated for signs of compromise, as early and aggressive support may be necessary.*

What are the intraoperative concerns regarding omphalocele repair in a patient with POC?

The main concern with an omphalocele repair in a patient with POC is the effect of increased intraabdominal pressure (and translated increase in intrathoracic pressure) on reduction of viscera into the abdominal cavity. This increase in abdominal pressure and physical presence of additional viscera in the abdomen may compress the exposed heart and lungs, compromise alveolar ventilation, induce arrhythmias, and reduce venous return to the heart. This, in turn, may worsen right-to-left shunting (or reverse left-to-right shunting), induce a PH crisis, decrease cardiac output, or hinder the ability to ventilate effectively. The potential for severe cardiac compromise is magnified in patients with EC and LV diverticula, who may not tolerate even mild increases in intraabdominal pressure or direct compression.

> **Clinical Pearl**
>
> *The increase in intraabdominal pressure and physical presence of additional viscera in the abdomen may compress the exposed heart and lungs, compromise alveolar ventilation, induce arrhythmias, and reduce venous return to the heart.*

What are the intraoperative concerns regarding sternal malformation repair?

Large sternal malformation repair, especially in patients with EC, significant CHD, or LV diverticulum, may lead to rapid blood loss, arrhythmias, impaired cardiac function, and pneumothorax. Internalization of an EC or further reduction of the heart into the thoracic cavity may increase intrathoracic pressure enough to impair ventilation and reduce venous return to the heart or may twist or kink the great vessels. Intraoperative echocardiography may be necessary to assess cardiac function.

The operating room setup should consist of a typical setup for a neonatal omphalocele repair. The room should be warmed, blood should be available, and dextrose-containing intravenous fluids should be administered.

A naso- or orogastric tube is necessary to decompress the stomach. In patients with significant CHD/PH, it is wise to have vasoactive drugs available (epinephrine, milrinone, vasopressin, phenylephrine, and calcium chloride) both in bolus form and as infusions. Nitric oxide should also be readily available. In patients with an LV diverticulum who are at risk for arrhythmias, antiarrhythmic drugs such as adenosine and amiodarone should be available and defibrillation pads should be placed. Ventilation can prove challenging and it may be necessary to use an intensive care unit (ICU) ventilator intraoperatively.

What types of vascular access and monitoring are necessary intraoperatively?

The type of vascular access and monitoring necessary will be determined by the severity of the cardiac lesion(s) and the size of the abdominal wall defect. Anesthesia for repair of a small omphalocele with a simple cardiac defect and no significant hemodynamic compromise or shunting (such as a small atrial or ventricular septal defect) can be accomplished with one or two peripheral intravenous (IV) lines and standard American Society of Anesthesiologists monitoring. However, placement of arterial and central venous access is warranted for either primary closure of a large omphalocele with reduction into the abdominal cavity or in the presence of complex, hemodynamically significant cardiac lesions as the potential for cardiac compromise, arrhythmias, need for vasoactive medications, fluid shifts, and concerns for respiratory compromise and PH crisis exist. It should also be noted that an electrocardiogram (ECG) tracing in patients with EC (especially when the heart is completely outside the chest) may not be possible. Heart rate and rhythm may have to be assessed through direct visualization.

What are the anesthetic induction and intubation considerations for this patient?

An IV induction is warranted when an omphalocele is present because of possible delayed gastric emptying and risk for aspiration. Induction goals for these patients should be tailored toward the specific cardiac lesion. Epinephrine should be drawn up and immediately available in the event of cardiovascular collapse on induction of anesthesia. The abdomen must be decompressed to minimize aspiration risk and bowel distension. Care must be taken to ensure the omphalocele sac and exposed heart are covered and not compressed during mask ventilation and intubation. Intubation may be difficult in patients with severe EC due to the heart sitting on the chest and the

anterior/cephalad direction of the heart. There may be little to no room for the laryngoscope handle to be placed while manipulating the blade into the oropharynx. When appropriate, a difficult airway cart with fiberoptic intubating equipment should be present.

Clinical Pearl

Intubation may be difficult in patients with severe EC due to the heart sitting on the chest and the anterior/cephalad direction of the heart. There may be little to no room for the laryngoscope handle to be placed while manipulating the blade into the oropharynx.

What ventilatory strategies should be planned for this patient?

These patients are already at risk for ventilatory failure, as they often have pulmonary hypoplasia and some degree of PH, a deficient anterior chest wall, and a diaphragmatic malformation. Significant left-to-right shunting with fluid overload and CHF further compromise ventilation. Cardiopulmonary compromise is made worse with the reduction of the omphalocele into the abdominal cavity. Even slight pressure on the lower sternum or abdomen during positioning can impair ventilation. Permissive hypercapnia with a higher respiratory rate and lower tidal volumes and peak inspiratory pressures may be indicated to minimize reduced venous return to the heart as well as pulmonary hyperinflation and lung injury. Caution should be exercised, however, in patients with PH, as hypercapnia may lead to an increase in pulmonary vascular resistance and a pulmonary hypertensive crisis may ensue. It may be necessary to use an ICU ventilator during the procedure.

Clinical Pearl

Permissive hypercapnia with a higher respiratory rate and lower tidal volumes and peak inspiratory pressures may be indicated to minimize reduced venous return to the heart as well as pulmonary hyperinflation and lung injury.

What is abdominal compartment syndrome?

During an omphalocele repair an increase in abdominal pressure >20 mm Hg and/or an increase in central venous pressure (CVP) >4 mm Hg places the patient at risk for abdominal compartment syndrome (ACS). Abdominal compartment syndrome occurs when an increase in intraabdominal pressure results in hypoperfusion to the splanchnic circulation leading to lactic acidosis, renal failure, intestinal ischemia, reduced cardiac output, and impaired ventilation. Signs of intraoperative ACS include difficulty with ventilation, lower extremity edema or duskiness in color, failure of the SpO_2 monitor in the lower extremities, oliguria, decreased femoral pulses, and differences in upper versus lower extremity blood pressures. Close monitoring of intraabdominal pressure and/or CVP is helpful in guiding surgical repair in patients who are at higher risk for ACS.

What are the postoperative concerns for this patient?

Postoperative concerns include ACS, low cardiac output syndrome, CHF, arrhythmias, LV diverticulum rupture, respiratory failure, PH/pulmonary hypertensive crisis, hypoxemia, infection/sepsis, small bowel obstruction, feeding difficulties/parenteral nutrition dependence, fluid and electrolyte abnormalities, and hypothermia. Because of the significant postoperative concerns, most infants remain intubated and recover in the intensive care unit after surgery.

What is the prognosis for patients with POC?

Owing to the low incidence and extreme heterogeneity of POC, it is difficult to approximate the prognosis, but it is generally poor. Recent data state a survival rate between 37% and 61%, depending on the type and severity of associated malformations and intracardiac defects. Risk factors for high mortality include Class I POC, younger age at first operation, respiratory failure exceeding 100 days, hypoxia, complex CDH, and complete EC. The causes of death are cardiac failure, tachyarrhythmias, ruptured LV diverticulum, CHF, respiratory failure, and sepsis [3, 8].

References

1. J. R. Cantrell, J. A. Haller, and M. M. Ravitch. A syndrome of congenital defects involving the abdominal wall, sternum, diaphragm, pericardium, and heart. *Surg Gynecol Obstet* 1958; **107**(5): 602–14.

2. W. Toyama. Combined congenital defects of the anterior abdominal wall, sternum, diaphragm, pericardium, and heart: a case report and review of the syndrome. *Pediatrics* 1972; **50**(5): 778–92.

3. J. F. Vazquez-Jimenez, E. G. Meuhler, S. Daebritz, et al. Cantrell's syndrome: a challenge to the surgeon. *Ann Thorac Surg* 1998; **65**: 1178–85.

4. S. A. Engum. Embryology, sternal clefts, ectopia cordis, and Cantrell's pentalogy. *Semin Pediatr Surg* 2008; **17**: 154–60.

5. H. Kawata, H. Kishimoto, T. Ueno, et al. Repair of left ventricular diverticulum with ventricular bigeminy in an infant. *Ann Thorac Surg* 1998; **66**: 1421–3.

6. R. C. Shamberger and K. J. Welch. Sternal defects. *Pediatr Surg Int* 1990; **5**: 156–64.

7. E. Duggan and P. S. Puligandla. Respiratory disorders in patients with omphalocele. *Semin Pediatr Surg* 2019; **28**: 115–17.

8. C. S. O'Gorman, T. A. Tortoriello, and C. J. McMahon. Outcome of children with pentalogy of Cantrell following cardiac surgery. *Pediatr Cardiol* 2009; **30**: 426–30.

Suggested Reading

Balderrabano-Saucedo N., Vizcaino-Alarcon A., Sandoval-Serrano E., et al. Pentalogy of Cantrell: forty-two years of experience in the hospital infantile de Mexico Federico Gomez. *World J Pediatr Congenit Heart Surg* 2011; **2**: 211–18.

Cantrell J. R., Haller J. A., and Ravitch M. M. A syndrome of congenital defects involving the abdominal wall, sternum, diaphragm, pericardium, and heart. *Surg Gynecol Obstet* 1958; **107**: 602–14.

Duggan E. and Puligandla P. S. Respiratory disorders in patients with omphalocele. *Semin Pediatr Surg* 2019; **28**: 115–17.

Laloyaux P., Veyckemans F., and Van Dyck M. Anaesthetic management of a prematurely born infant with Cantrell's pentalogy. *Pediatr Anesth* 1998; **8**: 163–66.

Nicols J. H. and Nasr V. G. Sternal malformations and anesthetic management. *Pediatr Anesth* 2017; **27**: 1084–90.

Williams A. P., Marayati R., and Beierle E. A. Pentalogy of Cantrell. *Semin Pediatr Surg* 2019; **28**: 106–10.

Ebstein Anomaly

Chapter 12

Joseph McSoley and Joseph P. Previte

Case Scenario

A 4-year-old boy weighing 16 kg with known Ebstein anomaly presents from the emergency department for urgent upper endoscopy and foreign body removal. His mother found him choking and coughing at home several hours ago and chest radiography reveals a radiopaque toy in the lower esophagus.

The mother states that the child has a "heart problem" and that he sees a cardiologist. She also adds that he often seems more easily tired than his siblings. The most recent clinic note from nearly a year ago states that the patient has Ebstein anomaly. He has not had any previous surgeries, and the cardiologist recommended yearly follow-up and imaging.

Currently the child looks uncomfortable and is drooling, but he is without any respiratory distress. His vital signs are blood pressure 85/52, heart rate 94 beats/minute, respiratory rate 22 breaths/minute, room air SpO$_2$ 94%, and temperature 36.8°C. A right-sided cardiac murmur and mild liver enlargement are noted.

The most recent echocardiogram from 11 months ago demonstrated:

- *An inferiorly displaced tricuspid valve with mild-to-moderate tricuspid regurgitation*
- *Mildly reduced right ventricular cavity size*
- *Mildly diminished right ventricular function*
- *Normal left ventricular function*
- *Presence of an atrial connection with bidirectional flow*

Key Objectives

- Describe the anatomy and spectrum of disease in Ebstein anomaly.
- Define the term "atrialized ventricle."
- Describe perioperative management considerations for a patient with Ebstein anomaly.

Pathophysiology

What is Ebstein anomaly?

Ebstein anomaly (EA) is a rare heart defect affecting the tricuspid valve (TV) and right ventricle (RV). The TV is dysplastic, with downward displacement of the septal and posterior leaflets inferiorly into the RV. The anterior leaflet is elongated and frequently has fenestrations and abnormal chordal attachments. As a result, there is dilation of the TV annulus resulting in tricuspid regurgitation (TR) and, depending on the degree of TV displacement, loss of RV cavity volume. (See Figure 12.1.) Right atrial enlargement frequently exists, and arrhythmias may occur related to right atrial dilation and abnormalities of the conduction system. Ebstein anomaly represents a wide spectrum of anatomic and clinical presentations, ranging from minimally symptomatic disease presenting in late childhood or early adolescence that requires medical management over time to critical disease requiring neonatal surgical intervention.

While the mildest forms of EA include minimal TV regurgitation and TV displacement, more severely affected patients will have greater TV displacement with resultant loss of RV volume and RV dysfunction. Varying degrees of

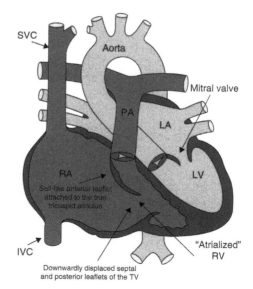

Figure 12.1 Ebstein anomaly of the tricuspid valve. Ao, aorta; LA, left atria; LV, left ventricle; PA, pulmonary artery; RA, right atria; RV, right ventricle; TV, tricuspid valve. From Nasr V. G. and DiNardo J. A. *The Pediatric Cardiac Anesthesia Handbook*, 1st ed. John Wiley & Sons, 2017; 239–42. With permission.

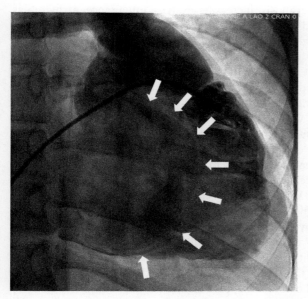

Figure 12.2 Right ventricular injection. An angiogram is performed in the right ventricle in the AP projection. The displacement of the tricuspid valve leaflets into the right ventricular cavity is indicated by the arrows. Courtesy of Russel Hirsch, MD.

cyanosis via right-to-left (R-to-L) shunting at the atrial level via either an atrial septal defect (ASD) or patent foramen ovale (PFO) can occur. The most severely affected patients may require single ventricle palliation, as the RV is diminutive and insufficient to support adequate antegrade pulmonary blood flow (PBF). (See Figure 12.2.)

Clinical Pearl

Ebstein anomaly represents a wide spectrum of anatomic and clinical presentations, ranging from minimally symptomatic disease that requires medical management over time to critically ill neonates with severe disease requiring neonatal surgical intervention.

How common is Ebstein anomaly?

While EA is the most common congenital malformation of the TV (1 in 20,000 live births), it is extremely rare, accounting for fewer than 1% of congenital cardiac defects. The true cause of EA is unknown but there are associations with usage of benzodiazepines in the first trimester of pregnancy and lithium usage.

What are the key anatomic characteristics of Ebstein anomaly?

Ebstein anomaly includes abnormalities of the TV and the RV. The hinge points of the septal and posterior leaflets of the TV are downwardly displaced from the atrioventricular junction into the RV itself, while the anterior leaflet is elongated with a hinge point at the true TV annulus. Depending on the severity of the TV abnormalities the resultant degree of "atrialization" of the RV varies, and in the most severe forms of EA the RV may have only trabecular and outflow portions. The atrialized portion of the RV is thin and dilated; it has ventricular morphology but functionally serves as part of the right atrium. An atrial level communication, either ASD or PFO, also exists in nearly all patients. In more severely affected patients R-to-L shunting at the atrial level results in varying degrees of cyanosis.

What are typical symptoms of Ebstein anomaly?

Ebstein anomaly has a wide spectrum of presentations. The clinical presentation will depend on the extent of TV displacement, RV size and function, right atrial pressure, and the degree of R-to-L shunting. Patients with EA are at particular risk for arrhythmias related to abnormal conduction patterns in the atrialized RV and right atrial dilation due to TR. Many patients with EA display findings on electrocardiogram (ECG) of preexcitation and/or Wolff–Parkinson–White syndrome (WPW).

Mildly affected patients may display mild exercise intolerance and there may initially be minimal symptomatology. The diagnosis may not be established until early adolescence or adulthood with the advent of diminished RV function and/or atrial arrhythmias.

Moderately affected patients may have cyanosis related to inadequate RV size, moderate TV malformation, TR, and atrial level R-to-L shunting. Symptoms may be exacerbated by exercise. There may be progressive dilation and dysfunction of the RV related to the degree of TR.

The most *severely affected patients* are often recognized in utero or present early in the neonatal period with refractory cyanosis (due to obligatory R-to-L shunting at the atrial level), extreme cardiomegaly, and arrhythmias. Inadequate blood flow through the pulmonary valve can result in functional or anatomic pulmonary stenosis or atresia. Infants with less severe forms of EA may be mildly cyanotic and will continue to improve as pulmonary vascular resistance (PVR) falls after birth, allowing increased antegrade PBF. Neonates with severe TR and a diminutive, poorly contractile RV with little to no antegrade PBF may be dependent on a prostaglandin E_1 infusion to maintain ductal patency and assure adequate PBF until palliative surgery can take place.

What are surgical options for EA and when would they be considered?

Surgical intervention for EA is prompted by severity of symptomatology, with multiple options existing depending on the patient's specific anatomy and physiology. The morphology and size of the RV are important in determining the patient's suitability for either a two-ventricle, one-and-a-half-ventricle, or single-ventricle approach.

- A two-ventricle repair, with TV repair and plication of the atrialized portion of the RV, is proposed for patients with an adequate RV and antegrade PBF. Several methods of TV repair have been described. An annuloplasty ring may be added if necessary. In patients with compromised RV function a small atrial fenestration may be left to augment cardiac output. Although a last resort in children, TV replacement may be required in adults.
- A one-and-a-half-ventricle palliation can be considered for patients with insufficient RV size or function. This operation consists of TV repair, a superior cavopulmonary anastomosis (bidirectional Glenn), and a fenestrated ASD. In this scenario blood from the inferior vena cava would traverse the TV and RV while blood from the superior vena cava would passively flow directly to the pulmonary vascular bed.
- In the most severe cases of EA, when anatomic pulmonary atresia exists as a result of right ventricular outflow tract obstruction, a Starnes procedure can be performed, consisting of oversewing or pericardial patch closure of the TV, an atrial septectomy, and construction of a modified Blalock–Taussig (mBT) shunt to provide PBF. If significant pulmonary insufficiency exists, the pulmonary valve may be oversewn and the main pulmonary artery divided. Typically, patients who have undergone the Starnes procedure will then proceed with single-ventricle palliative procedures (bidirectional Glenn followed by completion Fontan). (See Chapters 10, 27–30.)

Anesthetic Implications

What findings should be considered in the preoperative evaluation of a patient with unrepaired EA?

In addition to a comprehensive preoperative history and physical, special considerations for patients with EA include an understanding of the patient-specific anatomy, physiology, and rhythm. The history should include a review of symptoms, with special attention to any history of cyanosis, increasing exercise intolerance, arrhythmias, and/or failure to thrive. Consultation with the patient's cardiologist may be beneficial if there has been a significant change in his cardiac symptoms since the last office visit. If available, findings from the most recent cardiology visit, echocardiogram, and ECG should be reviewed.

Other concerns include any history of a recent upper respiratory infection or other recent illnesses that might adversely affect PVR. Information should be sought regarding the patient's last oral intake and whether he has taken anything by mouth since the ingestion.

While a patient with only mild TR may present with no signs or symptoms, those with more significant pathology may present with signs and symptoms related to TR and/or RV dysfunction. Cardiac auscultation may reveal a widely split first heart sound and a soft pansystolic murmur of TR. In the presence of significant RV dysfunction, a cardiac gallop may be appreciated.

In this patient, the preoperative hemoglobin–oxygen saturation of 94% on room air that was noted in the emergency department is significant. If possible, it would be useful to find previous measurements from cardiology office visits to determine whether a saturation of 94% is chronically seen in this patient (due to shunting at the atrial level) or whether it is due in part to the current foreign body ingestion.

> **Clinical Pearl**
>
> *In patients with EA, exercise tolerance is an indicator of the severity of the disease and ability to tolerate the stress of anesthesia.*

Is review of imaging necessary in a patient with unrepaired EA?

Echocardiography is used to assess size of the tricuspid annulus and severity of TR, the size of the RV, and degree of pulmonary stenosis and RV dysfunction. In addition, echocardiography may reveal other associated defects; although rare, they can include ventricular septal defects, congenitally corrected transposition of the great arteries, and atrioventricular canal defects. Atrial septal defects are nearly always present, allowing R-to-L shunting to occur when right atrial pressures are high, contributing to cyanosis. Additionally, left heart function can be compromised due to abnormal positioning of the interventricular septum and decreased left ventricular chamber size.

Cardiac magnetic resonance imaging (MRI) is also useful for ongoing assessment of patients with Ebstein anomaly. Recent studies have shown this imaging modality to be useful for defining the volume of RV atrialization and ratio of right to left cardiac volumes, providing information about exercise capacity and heart failure in patients with Ebstein anomaly.

Preoperative imaging choices should be made with consideration of the history and physical examination findings and the urgency of the planned procedure. Echocardiography is generally most accessible and provides useful information. When the most recent echocardiographic findings are not available or it is not feasible to obtain an echocardiogram due to procedural urgency, physical examination and history may provide clues to right heart function and degree of TR. Recent changes in exercise capacity should be noted with concern. Without recent echocardiographic data, it is wise to proceed with caution and have emergency plans and resuscitation medications available.

Is premedication appropriate for this patient?

Midazolam is one of the most common preoperative sedatives used to ease separation anxiety. Though frequently used as an oral premedication, in this case administration of an oral sedative to a patient with an esophageal foreign body would not be advisable. Because this is an urgent procedure, an intravenous line should be placed prior to the procedure, if not already done in the emergency department. Depending on the child's level of anxiety and symptomatology administration of a small dose of midazolam via IV could be considered prior to separation and would likely prove beneficial in decreasing agitation and anxiety.

What are the predominant concerns during induction of anesthesia?

In this case predominant concerns involve the presence of an esophageal foreign body in a patient with preexisting TR and mildly depressed RV function. Patients with esophageal foreign bodies often have hypersalivation, pooled secretions, and difficulty swallowing. This patient has had difficulty managing secretions since the aspiration event and is at risk for aspiration during induction due to his lack of fasting as well as his ingestion of a foreign body. Additionally, foreign body migration from the esophagus to airway during induction is a concern. If not already present, IV access should be placed prior to a planned intravenous rapid sequence induction and intubation.

In this patient with mildly depressed RV function, IV induction of anesthesia may be achieved with either propofol (1–2 mg/kg) or ketamine (2–4 mg/kg) depending on

the child's functional status. Etomidate can be utilized for patients with severe RV dysfunction. Patients with Ebstein anomaly are dependent on preload and will respond poorly to anesthetic-induced vasodilation, therefore IV fluid replacement may be necessary.

The potential impact of anesthetic agents and positive pressure ventilation (PPV) on RV performance should be considered, and peak airway pressures minimized. Appropriate steps should also be taken to keep PVR normal, with avoidance of hypercarbia, hypoxemia, acidosis, and hypothermia. Owing to the propensity for atrial arrhythmias close attention should be paid to the underlying rhythm and any changes that occur intraoperatively.

In patients with significant RV dysfunction, RV failure may present with hypotension, hypoxemia, and bradycardia. When an intraatrial connection is present, hypoxia may be prominent while hemodynamics are preserved as elevated right atrial pressures exceed left atrial pressures, causing R-to-L shunting. Left ventricular preload is preserved by systemic venous return shunted from the right to left atrium.

> **Clinical Pearl**
>
> *Induction of anesthesia and the transition from negative to positive pressure ventilation increases demand on the RV.*

In addition to standard monitoring, is an arterial line indicated?

Standard monitoring as recommended by the American Society of Anesthesiologists should be utilized for this procedure. If possible, a 5-lead ECG should be employed, as patients with EA are at increased risk for atrial arrhythmias. The planned case will have minimal blood loss and fluid shifts and therefore arterial line placement would not be warranted in this case. The risk for hemodynamic instability for this patient is likely greatest during induction of anesthesia.

What are the major considerations in patients with EA who require mechanical ventilation?

The main consideration in mechanical ventilation of the patient with EA and presumed RV dysfunction is minimizing RV afterload. This is achieved through careful ventilation strategies and avoidance of increases in PVR.

As increases in intrathoracic pressure result in increased RV afterload, ventilation utilizing minimal mean airway pressures is advisable. A low tidal volume and high respiratory rate strategy will achieve adequate ventilation while maintaining low mean airway pressures.

As increases in PVR will increase RV work and perhaps decrease PBF, care should be taken to avoid those factors that can result in increasing PVR such as hypercarbia, hypoxemia, acidosis, and hypothermia. Atelectasis also increases PVR; a successful ventilation strategy should balance the need to minimize mean airway pressure with maintaining functional residual capacity.

What are the anesthetic management considerations for patients with EA?

Tricuspid regurgitation causes RV volume and pressure overload and may contribute to RV dysfunction. Intraoperative management of TR involves reducing RV afterload to encourage forward flow and maintenance of RV function. A normal or slightly elevated heart rate may be required to support RV forward flow to the pulmonary circulation. Bradycardia in patients with EA and TR may not be well tolerated due to an increase in regurgitation with longer diastolic times and decrease in cardiac output. Vasoactive infusions or inhaled nitric oxide may be required to support RV function in severe cases.

The nurse in the post-anesthesia care unit is concerned about a sudden change in the ECG tracing. What specific concerns exist for this patient?

An abnormal ECG in a patient with EA is not uncommon. If a 12-lead ECG was obtained prior to the case, it may have identified baseline abnormalities. An elevation in P wave morphology is often seen due to right atrial enlargement. Other baseline findings may include right-sided bundle branch block or first-degree heart block.

Patients with EA are also at particular risk for arrhythmias. Up to 20% of patients will have an accessory conduction pathway, most often recognized as Wolff–Parkinson–White (WPW). Characteristic ECG findings in WPW include a short PR interval, a wide QRS complex, and a delta wave. Right atrial enlargement predisposes the patient to atrial fibrillation and atrial flutter. Atrialization of the RV can also create a dysynchrony between the left and right sides of the heart, increasing the likelihood of ventricular arrhythmias.

Atrial and ventricular arrhythmias should be triaged and treated as per American Heart Association Pediatric Advanced Life Support Guidelines. Atrial arrhythmias are most common, including supraventricular tachycardia (SVT) due to WPW, atrial flutter, and atrial fibrillation. If the patient is unstable as a result of the arrhythmia, rapid treatment may be indicated. Urgent SVT treatment may include vasovagal maneuvers (if hemodynamically stable), adenosine, or cardioversion. Given the patient's underlying diagnosis of EA, management of atrial arrhythmias is best done in consultation with a pediatric cardiologist.

Clinical Pearl

Patients with EA are at risk for arrhythmias, particularly if they have had a history of arrhythmias in the past. The preoperative history should include any history of arrhythmias and a baseline ECG to assist with perioperative ECG interpretation.

Should the patient be admitted after the procedure?

The decision whether to admit the patient for overnight observation depends on the child's baseline disease and perioperative course. In patients with minimal cardiac symptoms and uneventful perioperative course, discharge after extended post-anesthesia care unit stay can be considered. If the child has significant cardiac symptoms or a complicated operative course, consultation with pediatric cardiology and admission may be indicated.

Suggested Reading

Jaquiss R. D. and Imamura M. Management of Ebstein's anomaly and pure tricuspid insufficiency in the neonate. *Semin Thorac Cardiovasc Surg* 2007; **19**: 258–63.

Morray B. Preoperative physiology, imaging, and management of Ebstein's anomaly of the tricuspid valve. *Semin Cardiothorac Vasc Anesth* 2016; **20**: 74–81.

Ross F. J., Latham G. J., Richards M., et al. Perioperative and anesthetic considerations in Ebstein's anomaly. *Semin Cardiothorac Vasc Anesth* 2016; **20**: 82–92.

Rutz T. and Kühn A. The challenge of risk stratification in Ebstein's anomaly. *Int J Cardiol* 2019; **278**: 89–90.

Chapter 13

Ebstein Anomaly, Palliated

David Faraoni

Case Scenario

A 2-year-old boy, weighing 11.5 kg, is seen in the preoperative clinic prior to planned outpatient ptosis repair. He is currently growing and developing well despite a complex cardiac history. The patient was born at 32 weeks gestational age with an antenatal diagnosis of severe Ebstein anomaly. He was intubated shortly after birth for hypoxia and required an emergent Starnes procedure (oversewing of the tricuspid valve and placement of a systemic-to-pulmonary artery shunt) at day 2 of life. His postoperative course was complicated by cardiac dysfunction and need for extracorporeal membrane oxygenation for 3 days. He remained stable following decannulation and was discharged home at 6 weeks of age. At age 5 months he underwent an uneventful bidirectional Glenn shunt (superior vena cava to right pulmonary artery anastomosis) and ligation of previous systemic-to-pulmonary artery shunt. His only current medication is aspirin.

Key Objectives

- Describe the presentation, anatomy, and decision making for newborns with severe Ebstein anomaly.
- Describe cardiac surgical options for patients with severe Ebstein anomaly.
- Describe pulmonary blood flow in patients after bidirectional Glenn procedure and expected hemoglobin–oxygen saturations.
- Discuss anesthetic management for patients having noncardiac surgery after bidirectional Glenn procedure, including perioperative risk stratification and planning.

Pathophysiology

What is Ebstein anomaly?

Ebstein anomaly is a rare and highly variable congenital abnormality, comprising fewer than 1% of all congenital heart disease (CHD), affecting the tricuspid valve (TV) and adjacent right ventricular myocardium. The TV is dysplastic and displaced inferiorly into the RV. Valve leaflets may be larger or smaller than normal, resulting in failure of coaptation with resultant tricuspid regurgitation (TR) of varying degrees. Depending on the degree of apical TV displacement, there is loss of effective right ventricular volume and size, with "atrialization" of the right ventricle (RV). Right ventricular outflow tract obstruction can exist, limiting functional ejection and resulting in decreased pulmonary blood flow (PBF). Ebstein anomaly represents a wide spectrum of anatomic and clinical presentations, ranging from minimally symptomatic patients who require medical management over time to critically ill neonates with severe cyanosis who require intensive medical and surgical intervention. (See Chapter 12 and Figures 13.1 and 13.2.)

Clinical Pearl

Ebstein anomaly is a highly variable lesion in which forward flow through the right heart can be limited because of an apically displaced, dysplastic, and incompetent TV with resultant functional impairment of the "atrialized" RV.

What are the anatomic characteristics of Ebstein anomaly?

Newborns with severe Ebstein anomaly present with significant apical displacement of the TV, leading to severe TR and an ineffective RV. Nearly all patients have an atrial communication [either an atrial septal defect (ASD) or patent foramen ovale (PFO)], and they are therefore cyanotic, as most systemic venous return is shunted right-to-left (R-to-L) across the atrial communication. There is often insufficient antegrade flow through the RV to the pulmonary circulation, resulting in inadequate PBF. Particularly in the neonatal period, pulmonary vascular resistance (PVR) is a major determinant of RV antegrade flow.

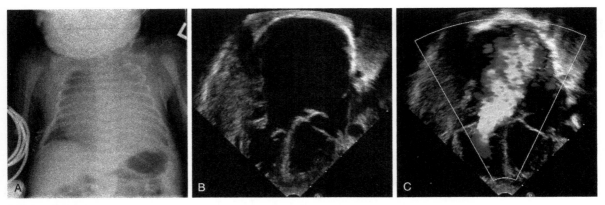

Figure 13.1 Ebstein anomaly in a neonate. (A) Chest plain film showing marked cardiomegaly. (B, C) Echocardiogram four-chamber view showing a severely dilated right atrium, a secundum atrial septal defect, and severe tricuspid regurgitation. From Kussman B., et al. Congenital cardiac anesthesia. Non bypass procedures. In Davis P. J. and Cladis F. P., eds. *Smith's Anesthesia for Infants and Children*, 9th ed. Elsevier; 2017: 699–743. With permission.

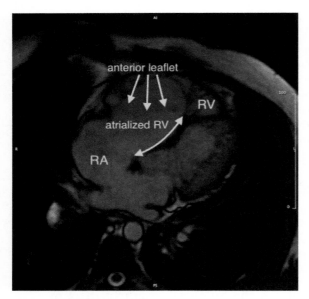

Figure 13.2 Ebstein anomaly. Four-chamber magnetic resonance imaging of severe Ebstein anomaly. There is marked apical displacement of the tricuspid septal leaflet creating a very small right ventricle and a large atrialized right ventricle. Courtesy of Michael Taylor, MD.

In the presence of anatomic RV outflow tract obstruction (RVOTO) or pathophysiologic pulmonary atresia, PBF is dependent on left-to-right (L-to-R) flow via a patent ductus arteriosus (PDA) from the aorta to the pulmonary artery. When the disease is less severe, the natural progressive reduction in PVR will improve RV to pulmonary artery antegrade flow, leading to clinical improvement.

Severe cardiomegaly is also present in Ebstein anomaly, typically due to the dilated right atrium. The right atrial dilation and stretch on the conduction system makes these patients prone to atrial tachyarrhythmias.

> **Clinical Pearl**
>
> *Newborns with severe Ebstein anomaly present with significant apical displacement of the TV, leading to severe TR and an ineffective RV. As nearly all patients have an atrial communication, they are cyanotic, as most systemic venous return is shunted right-to-left across the atrial communication.*

Is the left ventricle affected in Ebstein anomaly?

In the presence of right atrial and RV enlargement, the ventricular septum may bulge to the left, reducing the size of the left ventricle (LV). When severe, this may reduce LV filling and ability to generate appropriate cardiac output. The LV myocardium may also show variable degrees of fibrosis, usually beyond childhood.

What is the natural course and survival of patients with Ebstein anomaly?

In neonates with severe TR or cardiomegaly who are otherwise asymptomatic and who do not have medical or surgical intervention the associated mortality rate is 45% within the first year of life. In the presence of severe and symptomatic Ebstein anomaly, nearly all neonates will die without surgical intervention. However, patients who survive early childhood can expect reasonable longevity, while those undergoing single-ventricle palliation will have survival rates comparable to other single-ventricle patients.

What is the medical management and decision making for a newborn with severe Ebstein anomaly?

Initial management of the newborn with severe Ebstein anomaly is focused on maintaining effective PBF and oxygen saturation. Tricuspid valve and RV anatomy and amount of antegrade PBF are assessed at birth via echocardiography, oxygen saturation, and physical examination. Neonates who are stable are treated with supplemental oxygen and prostaglandin E_1 (PGE_1) to maintain PBF through the PDA.

Daily echocardiograms are obtained to assess antegrade PBF via the native RV outflow tract while the patient is slowly weaned off PGE_1, the PDA closes, and PVR decreases. Approximately 50% of neonates with severe Ebstein anomaly will stabilize, with sufficient antegrade PBF to maintain oxygen saturations of >75%–80%, while the other 50% will require neonatal surgical intervention.

Patients are closely monitored in an intensive care setting during this time to allow rapid assessment and treatment of decreases in cardiac output or oxygen desaturations. Therapy may include restarting or increasing PGE_1 to reopen the PDA, and, if the neonate is unstable, intubation, sedation, and paralysis may be required. Once the patient is intubated, high tidal volumes (10–12 mL/kg) may be needed due to the deleterious effect of cardiomegaly on lung expansion. Initiation of inotropic support may be necessary, including epinephrine, milrinone, and calcium infusions.

Clinical Pearl

In neonates with severe Ebstein anomaly, early decision making about surgical intervention is dependent on the amount of effective PBF as PVR falls and the PDA closes.

When would a patient require a surgical intervention?

Neonates with persistent deterioration (oxygen saturation <75%) despite adequate medical management or who are unable to wean from PGE_1 will require surgical intervention. Additionally, patients who successfully wean from PGE_1 but cannot tolerate feeding or fail to thrive may also require early intervention.

What are the major pathways for a patient with severe Ebstein anomaly requiring surgical intervention?

Surgical intervention depends on the individual patient's anatomic and pathophysiologic characteristics.

Initial decision making depends on the amount of antegrade PBF and oxygen saturation. Longer term surgical decision making is directed toward either a single-ventricle palliation pathway, a one-and-a-half ventricle repair, or a two-ventricle repair, based on the size and function of the RV. When the size and function of the TV and RV are adequate, a two-ventricle repair with creation of an RV-pulmonary artery conduit (if needed) may be performed.

Clinical Pearl

Depending on the individual patient's anatomy and pathophysiology, either a single-ventricle palliative pathway or a two-ventricle repair may be chosen.

What are the surgical options for a patient who cannot be weaned from PGE_1?

For the neonate with inadequate antegrade PBF who is unable to be weaned from PGE_1, the initial surgical procedure will include creation of a modified Blalock–Taussig (mBT) shunt, typically a GORE-TEX® shunt from the subclavian or innominate artery to the pulmonary artery, to establish another source of PBF. Determining whether the infant's pulmonary atresia is anatomic or functional will determine the surgical approach taken in addition to the mBT shunt. (See Figure 13.3.)

Anatomic Pulmonary Atresia with Moderate to Severe TR The Starnes procedure may be utilized for anatomic pulmonary atresia with moderate to severe TR. As the Starnes procedure excludes the RV, this plan most often commits the patient to the single-ventricle palliation pathway, including a bidirectional Glenn procedure and, eventually, Fontan completion.

The Starnes procedure consists of the following:
- Oversewing/pericardial patch closure of the TV
- Atrial septectomy (allowing mixing of systemic and pulmonary venous return)
- Creation of a mBT shunt for pulmonary blood flow

Systemic venous return now flows to the common atrium, through the mitral valve to the left ventricle, and exits via the aorta. Pulmonary blood flow is provided via the mBT shunt.

Functional Pulmonary Atresia The size of the RV and severity of the TR will determine the most appropriate surgical option. If the RV is adequately sized or may grow to allow for two-ventricle repair and the TV function is

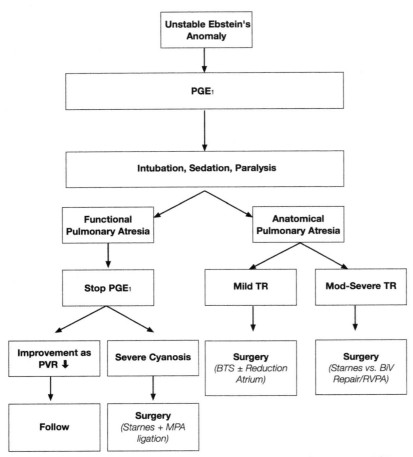

Figure 13.3 Simplified algorithm for neonatal decision making in severe Ebstein anomaly.

Starnes, Starnes Procedure; BiV, Biventricular; PVR, pulmonary vascular resistance; PGE1, Prostaglandin E1; BTS, Blalock-Taussig Shunt; RVPA, Right Ventricle to Pulmonary Artery Shunt)

sufficient, the initial surgical approach will be directed at establishing PBF, perhaps through a mBT shunt, while maintaining RV antegrade flow. This approach leaves the option for either one- or two-ventricle surgical pathways in the future. When the size and function of the TV and RV are adequate, a two-ventricle repair with creation of an RV–pulmonary artery conduit (if needed) may be performed.

Clinical Pearl

Initial decision making depends on the amount of antegrade PBF and oxygen saturations. Longer term surgical decision making is directed toward either a single-ventricle palliation or a two-ventricle repair, based on the size and function of the RV.

What is the Starnes procedure and what is the long-term strategy for patients in this pathway?

In 1991, Starnes et al. reported a single-ventricle palliation for critically ill neonates with Ebstein anomaly. He described a procedure including a pericardial patch closure of the TV orifice, atrial septectomy, and creation of an mBT shunt. To address the issue of pulmonary regurgitation, ligation of the main pulmonary artery may also be performed. Starnes et al. later described two important modifications to their technique: coronary sinus retained in the right atrial side of the TV patch to prevent drainage into the excluded RV and fenestration of the TV patch with a 4 mm opening to prevent RV distension.

Patients who undergo the Starnes palliation are generally obligated to the single-ventricle palliative pathway and will require a Glenn procedure at the age of 3–9 months and Fontan completion around the age of 2–4 years.

Clinical Pearl

Patients who undergo the Starnes procedure are generally obligated to the single-ventricle palliative pathway and will require a Glenn procedure at the age of 3–9 months, and Fontan completion around the age of 2–4 years.

What is a bidirectional Glenn procedure?

The bidirectional Glenn (BDG) procedure is frequently performed as part of staged surgical palliation of single-ventricle patients, including severe Ebstein anomaly. The BDG shunt procedure involves rerouting upper body systemic venous return directly to the lungs by anastomosing the superior vena cava (SVC) to the right pulmonary artery. This anastomosis provides a source of PBF and reduces ventricular work, as upper body systemic venous return does not return to the heart. Blood flows passively from the SVC to the pulmonary artery, without a pump. As originally described, the Glenn procedure provided blood flow to one lung only; modern modification has blood flowing from the SVC into both right and left lungs, thus the term *bidirectional* Glenn shunt or procedure. (See Chapter 27.)

What are the sources of PBF and venous return to the single ventricle after BDG?

Pulmonary blood flow in a BDG shunt is dependent on SVC flow. Superior vena cava flow accounts for approximately 50% of cardiac output in newborn infants, reaching a maximum of 55% at 2.5 years old and then gradually decreasing to the adult value of 35% by 6 years of age.

After BDG, blood enters the single ventricle from two sources: oxygenated blood enters the heart from the pulmonary veins and deoxygenated blood from the lower body enters via the inferior vena cava (IVC). Because patients have had a complete atrial septectomy as part of their first-stage procedure, flow from the IVC mixes with flow from the pulmonary veins in the atrium and then proceeds to the single ventricle before being ejected into the systemic circulation. Due to this mixing, expected oxygen saturations in patients with BDG physiology are 75%–85%.

Anesthetic Implications

What preoperative assessment should be done in a patient with a BDG?

Prior to providing an elective anesthetic in a patient with a BDG, a complete preoperative assessment should include a review of the most recent cardiology visit, including echocardiographic, catheterization, and recent laboratory data. Information regarding current ventricular function, the presence of valvular regurgitation, PVR, ventricular end-diastolic pressure, and the presence of any collateral circulation should be reviewed. Questions during the preoperative interview should be directed at eliciting information regarding exercise tolerance, syncope or other symptoms of arrhythmias, and growth and development. Symptoms of ventricular dysfunction, severe valvular regurgitation, and/or a history concerning for heart failure or arrhythmias may prompt further discussion and optimization. Laboratory tests such as complete blood count, electrolytes, urea nitrogen, creatinine, coagulation profile, and liver function may be considered depending on the patient's history, medication profile, and scope of the anticipated procedure.

What should the parents be told regarding anesthetic and surgical risk in this patient?

Children with congenital heart disease (CHD) undergoing noncardiac surgery are known to be at higher risk for morbidity and mortality than patients without cardiac disease. Among patients with CHD, those with single-ventricle physiology or ventricular dysfunction are at particular risk. The patient's functional capacity should be carefully reviewed. Recent studies support a lack of correlation between intrinsic surgical risk and the risk of complications in children with CHD undergoing noncardiac surgery, suggesting that the severity of the cardiac lesion and the patient's functional status are more important in risk assessment.

What are the guidelines for endocarditis antibiotic prophylaxis?

Preoperative antibiotic prophylaxis is necessary for all procedures likely to produce bacteremia (e.g., dental extraction) in patients with unrepaired CHD, including palliative shunts and conduits such as the BDG. In this particular case, no endocarditis prophylaxis would be required.

What are the key points regarding BDG physiology?

Bidirectional Glenn flow is passive; there is no pump between the SVC and the pulmonary artery. Pulmonary blood flow is therefore dependent on SVC pressure, pulmonary artery pressure/PVR, intrathoracic pressure, and volume status. Reductions in PBF with resultant oxygen desaturation can occur with increased PVR, hypovolemia, or increased intrathoracic pressure due to coughing, laryngospasm, excessive positive pressure ventilation (PPV), or breath holding. Desaturations due to reduced PBF in BDG physiology can be significant, but saturations will typically return to baseline when the cause is addressed.

Clinical Pearl

Pulmonary blood flow in BDG physiology is passive as there is no ventricular pump. Pulmonary blood flow will decrease with increases in either intrathoracic pressure (due to coughing, laryngospasm, or positive pressure ventilation) or increases in pulmonary vascular resistance, resulting in hypoxemia.

With Glenn physiology, hemodynamic performance tends to be resilient because the single ventricle is less volume loaded than it was prior to BDG, when the presence of parallel circulations required the single ventricle to handle both pulmonary and systemic volumes. Cardiac output after BDG is not entirely dependent on PBF because the IVC remains directly connected to the heart, providing venous return even when pulmonary blood flow is decreased. Therefore, should PBF be compromised by an increase in PVR or intrathoracic pressure, cardiac output can be maintained via IVC flow.

Clinical Pearl

Cardiac output after a Glenn shunt is not entirely dependent on PBF because the IVC remains directly connected to the heart, providing venous return even when PBF is decreased. Therefore, should PBF be compromised by an increase in PVR or intrathoracic pressure, cardiac output can be maintained via IVC flow.

What oxygen saturations are expected for a child with a BDG?

Due to intracardiac mixing in the common atrium of deoxygenated blood (from the IVC) with oxygenated blood (following the path from the SVC/Glenn anastomosis → pulmonary arteries → lungs → pulmonary veins), the typical oxygen saturations for a patient with Glenn physiology are between 75% and 85% on room air.

Clinical Pearl

After a BDG, mixing in the common atrium of deoxygenated blood from the IVC with oxygenated blood from the pulmonary veins means that typical oxygen saturations for a patient with Glenn physiology are between 75% and 85% on room air.

What considerations exist for a BDG patient with a recent or current respiratory infection?

Recent respiratory illness or recent changes in oxygen saturation merit careful consideration in patients with Glenn physiology. In addition to the increased risk of pulmonary complications following recent infection that is common to all patients, the increased PVR and airway hyperreactivity that can accompany respiratory infections may result in increased cyanosis and hypoxemia in patients with passive PBF. Therefore, the risk–benefit analysis of anesthesia for BDG patients in the presence of a recent or current respiratory tract infection should be carefully assessed.

What are the anesthetic considerations for a BDG patient presenting for noncardiac surgery?

In patients with Glenn physiology and preserved ventricular function, the mild to moderate fluid or pressure shifts associated with surgery and general anesthesia are typically well tolerated. Inhalation induction may take slightly longer than in a patient with biventricular physiology because of the decreased ratio between pulmonary and systemic blood flow. Anesthetic induction can also be associated with peripheral vasodilatation, which may require volume administration and sometimes vasoconstrictor agents such as phenylephrine to maintain mean arterial pressure. Anesthetic management is directed to preserving cardiac output by supporting ventricular function and promoting PBF. Hypovolemia is disadvantageous because it significantly reduces PBF, ventricular preload, and output. The most appropriate ventilation strategy should be considered in the context of the planned procedure with the understanding that positive pressure ventilation (PPV) may negatively impact PBF.

> **Clinical Pearl**
>
> *Inhalation induction may take slightly longer than in a patient with biventricular physiology because of the decreased ratio between pulmonary and systemic blood flow. Anesthetic management is directed to preserving cardiac output by supporting ventricular function and promoting PBF.*

What ventilation strategy is most appropriate?

Ventilatory management should aim to promote PBF by minimizing mean airway pressure. Maintenance of low to baseline PVR is essential and can be accomplished by a ventilation strategy that maintains adequate tidal volume and utilizes a short inspiratory time, minimizing mean airway pressure. While significant hypercarbia increases PVR, mild hypercarbia may improve PBF and oxygen saturations by increasing cerebral blood flow and SVC flow to the pulmonary bed. Hyperventilation should be avoided due to its association with a decrease in cerebral blood flow and consequently PBF. Although the use of a laryngeal mask airway may be preferred over intubation when possible, as it encourages the use of spontaneous ventilation and lower mean airway pressures, securing the airway with an endotracheal tube may be preferable based on patient or procedural considerations.

> **Clinical Pearl**
>
> *While significant hypercarbia increases PVR, mild hypercarbia may improve PBF and oxygen saturations by increasing cerebral blood flow and SVC flow to the pulmonary bed.*

What fluid management and transfusion strategy should be applied?

Patients with BDG physiology require adequate fluid status (normovolemia) to maintain passive PBF while avoiding fluid overload for the single ventricle. Crystalloid fluids may be utilized to account for fasting deficits and any decrease in SVR associated with general anesthesia. A bolus of 5–10 mL/kg is sometimes useful during or immediately following induction if desaturation or hypotension due to PPV and decreased PBF occurs. However, fluid management should be carefully weighed in patients with decreased cardiac function. Although the surgical procedure planned in this scenario presents a relatively low bleeding risk, patients with single-ventricle physiology are at risk for increased bleeding due to therapeutic use of anticoagulant medications and intrinsic coagulopathy. Patients with cyanotic heart disease require a higher hemoglobin for improved oxygen delivery; the preoperative hemoglobin should therefore be assessed, and patient contextualized transfusion triggers considered. At a minimum, an appropriate hemoglobin level of 9–10 g/dL or higher should be targeted; most practitioners advocate a hemoglobin level of 13–15 for a patient with single-ventricle physiology.

Is a patient with severe Ebstein anomaly at increased risk for arrhythmias?

Conduction system abnormalities may be present in children with Ebstein anomaly. The right bundle may be fibrotic and, occasionally, accessory pathways have been noted with pre-excitation syndrome. Supraventricular tachycardias due to right atrial dilation are challenging and sometimes refractory to therapy in patients with Ebstein anomaly. Care of patients with Ebstein anomaly who have a history of arrhythmias should be coordinated in consultation with cardiologists and electrophysiologists to assist in perioperative medication administration and planning for potential intraoperative rhythm disturbances.

What are the major anesthesia concerns during emergence and the postoperative period?

As PBF is passive in BDG patients, avoiding significant increases in PVR or intrathoracic pressure should be the goal during emergence and postoperatively. Adequate pain control is necessary. Dexmedetomidine is useful to decrease the incidence of postoperative agitation and coughing without adversely affecting spontaneous respiratory drive. Antiemesis prophylaxis is also recommended, as vomiting may cause dehydration and impair respiratory mechanics, leading to cyanosis.

Where should this patient recover?

Clear guidelines regarding postoperative destination do not exist for patients with BDG physiology. However, the decision to recover the patient in the postoperative anesthesia care unit versus intensive care unit should be based on the patient's functional status and perioperative hemodynamic stability as well as local practice patterns. If the patient has good functional status, is well palliated, and the case is uneventful, post-anesthesia care unit recovery may be appropriate. Patients with single-ventricle physiology should be recovered in an environment where nurses and physicians are familiar and comfortable with the pathophysiology.

Can this procedure be performed on an outpatient basis?

Single-ventricle patients may not be suitable candidates for surgery in centers that do not have a cardiac program and cardiac-trained anesthesiologists. However, patients with good functional status for low-risk procedures may be treated in a same-day surgery unit of a tertiary care hospital following the collaborative decision-making of cardiologist, surgeon, and anesthesiologist.

Suggested Reading

Holst K. A., Dearani J. A., Said S. M., et al. Surgical management and outcomes of Ebstein anomaly in neonates and infants: a Society of Thoracic Surgeons Congenital Heart Surgery Database Analysis. *Ann Thorac Surg* 2018; **106**: 785–91.

Kumar S. R., Kung G., Noh N., et al. Single-ventricle outcomes after neonatal palliation of severe Ebstein anomaly with modified Starnes procedure. *Circulation* 2016; **134**: 1257–64.

Kumar T. K. S., Boston U. S., and Knott-Craig C. J. Neonatal Ebstein anomaly. *Semin Thorac Cardiovasc Surg* 2017; **29**: 331–7.

Leyvi G. and Wasnick J. D. Single-ventricle patient: pathophysiology and anesthetic management. *J Cardiothorac Vasc Anesth* 2010; **24**: 121–30.

Luxford J. C., Arora N., Ayer J. G., et al. Neonatal Ebstein anomaly: a 30-year institutional review. *Semin Thorac Cardiovasc Surg* 2017; **29**: 206–12.

Chapter

14

Critical Aortic Stenosis

Vannessa Chin

Case Scenario

A 2-day-old male neonate, diagnosed with critical aortic stenosis, is scheduled for emergent balloon valvuloplasty in the cardiac catherization laboratory. He was born at 38 weeks gestational age via spontaneous vaginal delivery. His Apgar scores were 9 at 1 and 5 minutes, and he was admitted to the neonatal intensive care unit due to mild tachypnea and a murmur on auscultation. No obvious dysmorphic features were noted. On day 2 of life he was noted to be more tachypneic and tachycardic, with diminished pulses, cool extremities, and poor capillary refill. A chest radiograph revealed cardiomegaly and pulmonary edema.

Venous lactate is 4 with a blood pH of 7.1.
A prostaglandin E_1 infusion and low-dose inotropic support were started.

Transthoracic echocardiogram was remarkable for the following:

- A dysplastic aortic valve with a mean gradient of 45 mm Hg
- A dilated, thick left ventricle with qualitatively moderately reduced function
- No patent ductus arteriosus

Key Objectives

- Define critical aortic stenosis.
- Discuss the options for treatment of a patient with ductal-dependent aortic stenosis.
- Describe the preoperative assessment and intraoperative management of this patient.
- Discuss the potential complications and expected outcomes of balloon valvuloplasty.
- Discuss the postprocedural management and disposition.

Pathophysiology

What is critical aortic stenosis?

Critical aortic stenosis (AS) is defined as the presence of severe aortic valve stenosis with systemic perfusion that is dependent on right ventricular (RV) output through a patent ductus arteriosus (PDA). Mean gradients of >40 mm Hg or peak-to-peak gradients >50 mm Hg are usually reported. As the PDA begins to close, left ventricular function deteriorates, with signs of decreased perfusion to end organs such as the kidneys, gastrointestinal tract, and brain, manifesting as renal failure, necrotizing enterocolitis, and intracerebral bleeds, respectively. Critical AS is not defined by an absolute valve area or gradient because in patients with ventricular dysfunction (either systolic or diastolic) critical AS may exist with larger valve areas and gradients may be underestimated. (See Figure 14.1.)

Clinical Pearl

Critical AS is not defined by an absolute valve area or gradient because in patients with ventricular dysfunction (either systolic or diastolic) critical AS may exist with larger valve areas and gradients may be underestimated.

What is the pathophysiology of AS in a neonate?

Aortic stenosis in older infants, children and adults leads to left ventricular (LV) pressure overload and progressive LV concentric hypertrophy and failure, with resultant elevation in end-diastolic pressure and pulmonary edema. The hypertrophied LV thus becomes susceptible to subendocardial hypoperfusion and ischemia.

In neonates with critical AS, a PDA provides systemic cardiac output via flow from the RV to the descending aorta via right-to-left (R-to-L) shunting, and thus systemic perfusion is preserved. The degree of LV hypertrophy in these neonates, though not as severe, still exists, and the ventricle may be dilated and poorly contractile. This heart failure is associated with increases in heart rate and LV end-diastolic pressure which can lead to inadequate coronary blood flow and the risk of ischemia. The elevated left atrial (LA) pressure leads to pulmonary edema and pulmonary hypertension with dilation of the RV; in addition,

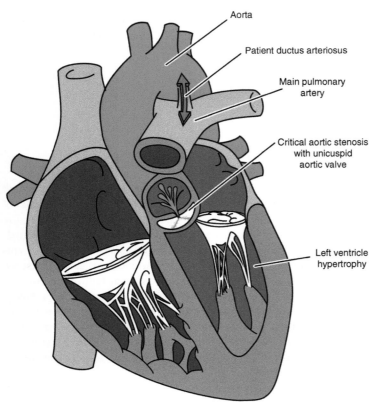

Aorta

Patient ductus arteriosus

Main pulmonary artery

Critical aortic stenosis with unicuspid aortic valve

Left ventricle hypertrophy

Figure 14.1 Critical aortic stenosis. Drawing by Ryan Moore, MD, and Matt Nelson.

LA hypertension leads to stretching of the foramen ovale and left-to-right (L-to-R) shunting at the atrial level.

What are the options for treatment of a patient with ductal-dependent AS?

The immediate treatment of patients presenting with critical AS is to ensure systemic output and perfusion by maintaining a PDA or reopening a closed ductus. A prostaglandin E_1 (PGE_1) infusion is immediately initiated at birth in patients with a prenatal diagnosis or when critical AS is suspected postnatally. Additional details for medical management are discussed later in this chapter.

Once PGE_1 is initiated and the patient stabilized, then the intervention to relieve the outflow obstruction can be planned. This intervention can be either catheter or surgically based. The decision is based on other associated cardiac factors such as hypoplasia of the LV, mitral valve, or aortic arch.

First, it must be determined whether a biventricular repair is feasible; the question of whether or not the left heart structures are of adequate size to sustain the systemic circulation needs to be answered.

Echocardiography is used to assess all the left-sided structures, namely:

- The size and function of the LV
- The extent of endocardial fibroelastosis
- The size of the aortic annulus and the morphology of the aortic valve
- The size and function of the mitral valve
- The presence of coarctation of the aorta

Once it is determined that a biventricular repair can be undertaken, the next step involves deciding what intervention will be the most beneficial for the individual neonate: surgical aortic valvotomy (SAV) versus balloon aortic valvuloplasty (BAV) in the cardiac catheterization laboratory. Results from the most recent meta-analysis showed that although the rate of reintervention following BAV is higher than following SAV, the survival rates, need for aortic valve replacement, and development of late aortic insufficiency (AI) are equivalent [1]. The final decision will often depend on the patient's weight and clinical condition, local experience, the skills and preference of the surgical and interventional cardiology teams, and overall center outcomes.

How is SAV performed?

Surgical aortic valvotomy can be done either using a transventricular approach without cardiopulmonary bypass (CPB), or more commonly, via open valvotomy utilizing CPB. In the former approach, after a thoracotomy or sternotomy, the valve is accessed through the LV apex and is serially dilated with balloons or Hegar dilators. Open valvotomy is achieved via sternotomy and may involve just detaching commissures from the aortic wall to reduce doming of the valve (commissurotomy), or a two-stage process. The two-stage process involves thinning the leaflets to improve mobility, followed by commissurotomy.

How is BAV performed?

Balloon aortic valvuloplasty can be approached either from a retrograde or antegrade direction. (See Figure 14.2A and B.) Using a retrograde approach, the balloon sheath is most commonly advanced from the femoral artery, and less commonly from the umbilical artery or carotid artery (usually after surgical cutdown). For the antegrade approach the femoral vein or umbilical vein is cannulated and the catheter advanced through the foramen ovale into the left atrium and ventricle; this approach is easier if the LV is somewhat dilated.

Critical information to be obtained includes:

- Mixed venous saturation
- Aortic valve gradient
- Left ventricular end diastolic pressure (LVEDP)
- Angiograms demonstrating the annulus size; valve anatomy; degree of AI; and LV anatomy, size, and function

The aim of BAV is to adequately relieve the LV outflow tract obstruction (as demonstrated by a reduction in the gradient and/or LA pressure) without causing significant AI, allowing recovery of LV function. The intention is not to dilate the valve annulus but rather to tear the valve leaflets, which are often partially fused, ideally along the fused commissure.

With poor LV function and stable wire position in the aorta, balloon dilatation can be undertaken with minimal chance of the balloon being ejected from the aortic position by a forceful ventricular contraction against the balloon-occluded outflow. If there is adequate LV function, either rapid overdrive pacing or a bolus of adenosine or esmolol, followed by an esmolol infusion, may be administered prior to dilating the valve, to transiently lower cardiac output.

The valve is dilated until the largest reasonable balloon has been inflated across the valve with minimal AI; that is, a balloon usually not exceeding the diameter of the aortic root or a balloon to annulus ratio <0.9. A reduction in the gradient by approximately 50% or to <30 mm Hg is deemed a success. (See Figure 14.3.) If LV function is poor and the gradient is low at baseline, the gradient may

(a)

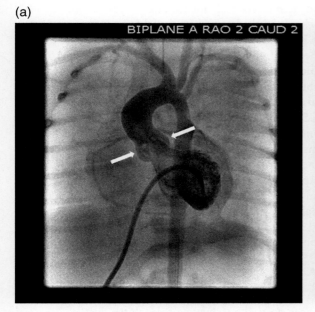

(b)

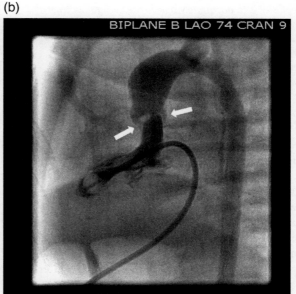

Figure 14.2 Doming aortic valve. An angiogram is performed in the left ventricle in the AP (A) and lateral (B) projections. The thickened and doming aortic valve is noted (arrows). Courtesy of Russel Hirsch, MD.

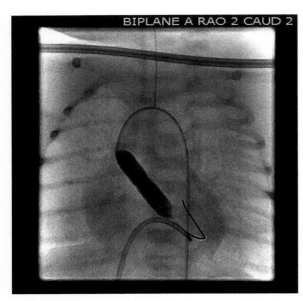

Figure 14.3 Balloon inflation across the aortic valve. Still frame angiogram in the AP projection demonstrates the balloon inflated across the aortic valve. Courtesy of Russel Hirsch, MD.

remain the same after a successful dilation, and it may actually increase days after the procedure once the LV function begins to improve.

> **Clinical Pearl**
>
> *The aim of BAV is to adequately relieve the LV outflow tract obstruction (as demonstrated by a reduction in the gradient and/or LA pressure) without causing significant AI, allowing recovery of LV function. The intention is not to dilate the valve annulus but rather to tear the valve leaflets, which are often partially fused, ideally along the fused commissure.*

What are the advantages of SAV versus BAV?

Open valvotomy carries the advantage that the surgeon directly visualizes and probes the valve before performing a defined, anatomically sound valvotomy with potentially less resultant AI. However, because this approach requires CPB it carries a greater potential risk to the neonate. Balloon aortic valvuloplasty avoids the need for CPB and sternotomy but may lead to potentially higher rates of cusp disruption with resulting AI that may progress over time, ultimately requiring a surgical repair. However, it is interesting to note that while the development of AI often occurs secondary to BAV, Ewert et al. reported a 49% incidence of AI in patients with untreated AS, suggesting a natural course toward insufficiency [2].

Anesthetic Implications

What key information should be obtained in the preoperative cardiac assessment of a neonate with critical AS?

The aim is to establish whether the neonate has been optimized for the catheterization laboratory: determining what treatment has been implemented, its effectiveness, and any need for further interventions prior to transfer to the catheterization laboratory. A neonate with critical AS and a closed PDA is a medical emergency. Medical management involves establishing intravenous (IV) access and administering PGE_1 to reopen the ductus arteriosus, and utilizing inotropic therapy if necessary to improve LV dysfunction. There should be signs of improvement in systemic perfusion usually within 4 hours. These would include improvements in tachycardia, capillary refill and pulses, decreasing lactate levels, resolution of acidosis, and increased urine output. A preductal/postductal oxygen saturation gradient (SpO_2) suggests R-to-L shunting is occurring through the PDA and is also reassuring. All existing lines should be evaluated for functionality and to confirm that infusions are being delivered to the patient. Dextrose-containing IV fluids should be infusing for this 2-day-old neonate; some centers add calcium gluconate as well. In critically ill infants in whom the duct has closed and remains closed despite PGE_1, surgical and extracorporeal membrane oxygenation (ECMO) backup should be readily available.

Respiratory status should be assessed to decide whether tracheal intubation and ventilatory support, which would decrease the work of breathing and contribute to the overall stabilization of the patient, is warranted prior to transfer to the lab. Often patients on PGE_1 are intubated due to the occurrence of frequent apneic episodes caused by administration of prostaglandins, rather than because of deteriorating pulmonary function. In addition, findings from the chest radiograph, electrocardiogram (ECG), echocardiography, and the most recent lab results should be evaluated. It is also important to ensure the availability of packed red blood cells during procedures in the catheterization laboratory.

> **Clinical Pearl**
>
> *A preductal/postductal SpO_2 gradient suggests an open duct; R-to-L shunting through the duct is reassuring.*

What useful information can be ascertained from the chest radiograph, ECG, and echocardiogram?

Chest Radiograph Heart size, the presence or absence of pulmonary edema, appropriate endotracheal tube position, and, if in situ, appropriate positioning of umbilical vein catheter (UVC) and umbilical artery catheter (UAC) should be evaluated. The UVC and UAC should both be above the level of the diaphragm; the UAC should be between thoracic vertebrae 6 and 9 and UVC should be in the inferior vena cava as it enters the right atrium.

Electrocardiogram Right axis deviation and RV hypertrophy (RVH) should be within normal limits for age. In some infants, significant RVH is noted, with tall right precordial R waves and upright T waves in the right precordial leads.

Echocardiogram The following should be assessed: location and nature of the left ventricular outflow tract obstruction (valvular, subvalvular, supravalvular); assessment of the severity of obstruction (peak/mean gradients (PG/MGs); LV wall thickness and chamber size; LV function; patency of the ductus arteriosus and flow through it, atrial level L-to-R shunting through the foramen ovale; and the presence of associated cardiac lesions.

When is an echocardiographic gradient not accurate?

These conditions will result in an inaccurate estimation of the gradient across the aortic valve:

- Presence of a PDA that provides flow from the RV to the descending aorta
- Presence of other obstructive lesions, particularly mitral valve stenosis and coarctation of the aorta
- Depressed LV function

Clinical Pearl

Depressed LV function results in underestimation of the degree of severity of AS.

What should parents be told about anesthetic risk?

Though several scoring systems have been developed to predict the risk of serious adverse events during cardiac catheterization, none specifically address the anesthetic risk. An adverse event is defined as any event leading to mortality, permanent morbidity, need for further interventions, or extended length of hospital stay. The Catheterization Risk Score for Pediatrics (CRISP), created from information obtained from 20 international centers [3], allows points to be assigned according to the patient's age, weight, level of inotropic support/need for extracorporeal membrane oxygenation, systemic illness/organ failure, physiologic status, pre-catheterization diagnosis, procedure type, and the procedure performed. Patients are then placed into one of five CRISP categories and assigned their individual risk for serious adverse events. This risk ranges from a 1% risk for serious adverse events in a CRISP 1 patient to a 36.8% risk for a CRISP 5 patient. Based on a CRISP risk category of 4, this patient would be quoted an incidence of serious adverse events of 14.4%. In considering the risks of general anesthesia, younger age, higher American Society of Anesthesiologists (ASA) status, and emergency procedures have all been reported as risk factors for cardiac arrest during pediatric procedures [4]. Specific to catheterization procedures, infants requiring interventional procedures are at a higher risk for adverse events and hence this patient would fall into the high-risk category. Recent expert consensus statement recommendations have stated that these patients should ideally be managed by a pediatric cardiac anesthesiologist [5]; at a minimum, care should be provided by a pediatric practitioner familiar with the cardiac anatomy and physiology along with the catheterization laboratory environment.

What are the special considerations involved in providing care in the cardiac catheterization laboratory?

The following considerations make the cardiac catheterization laboratory a challenging environment:

- Satellite location, often located away from operating room and intensive care environments
- Suboptimal lighting
- Limited space due to equipment, leading to limited patient access
- Ionizing radiation exposure
- Difficulty with direct communication with other team members
- Increased patient risk for pressure injuries or nerve traction injuries (such as brachial plexus injuries) due to the requirement for arms to be above the head in order to facilitate imaging; meticulous positioning and padding are important
- Difficulty maintaining normothermia in neonates due to both low room temperature (to prevent overheating of cameras) and frequent flushing of catheters and sheaths

- Volume overload, also due to frequent flushing of catheters and sheaths

What are the anesthetic management goals for this patient?

Anesthetic management is directed toward meeting the increased oxygen requirement of the hypertrophied LV myocardium and optimizing cardiac output.

The goals of management include:

- *Maintain preload*: A thick LV requires adequate volume loading. However, in the setting of reduced systolic function +/− LV dilation, coupled with preexisting diastolic dysfunction, fluid administration should be judicious.
- *Maintain afterload*: A thickened LV requires adequate perfusion pressures to minimize sub/ endocardial ischemia; vasoconstrictors such as phenylephrine will help with a fall in systemic vascular resistance.
- *Maintain contractility*: If systolic function becomes reduced, inotropes may become necessary, but should be used judiciously given their propensity to increase heart rate and thus myocardial oxygen requirements.
- *Maintain heart rate and sinus rhythm*: Avoid bradycardia as neonatal cardiac output is dependent on heart rate given their fixed stroke volume, even in the absence of AS. It should be noted that most infants are tachycardic at baseline, but increases in tachycardia should be avoided, as these will increase oxygen demand and increase ischemic risk in a thick, failing LV.

What are the monitoring requirements for this case?

Standard ASA monitoring is required, but with a few special considerations. As for all catheterization cases where the groin is being accessed, monitoring and vascular access should be on the upper limbs where possible. A preductal SpO_2 monitor will accurately reflect changes in ventilation and respiratory status. Noninvasive blood pressure measurements from a cuff on an arm elevated above the head may underestimate the actual reading and should be correlated with the direct femoral artery pressures that the interventionist can intermittently transduce. End-tidal CO_2 ($ETCO_2$) is a useful surrogate for pulmonary artery blood flow and cardiac output; an abrupt decrease in $ETCO_2$ may be the first indication of a decrease in cardiac output and/or pending disaster.

Clinical Pearl

End-tidal CO_2 is a useful surrogate for pulmonary artery blood flow and cardiac output; it may be the first indication of a decrease in cardiac output and/or pending disaster.

What are special steps in preparation for the case?

In addition to induction drugs and intubation equipment, the following are necessary:

- *Upper limb IV access* for volume resuscitation; if the groin is accessed, the interventionist's catheter may obstruct the vessel or the IV may be distal to potential vessel injury.
- *Blood product* availability.
- *Resuscitation drugs* such as epinephrine, phenylephrine, and calcium gluconate/chloride. Start with low doses as boluses, for example 1 mcg/kg of epinephrine or 1–2 mcg/kg of phenylephrine and repeat as necessary. Calcium gluconate may be used in a bolus of 25 mg/kg. A norepinephrine infusion may become necessary, commencing at 0.02 mcg/kg/minute and titrated to effect.
- *Defibrillator* with appropriate size pads/paddle.

What are the most critical points during this case?

As some life-threatening events are preventable, the importance of preparation, anticipation, prevention, and communication has to be emphasized at every step.

Anesthetic induction: An opioid-based anesthetic plus the use of neuromuscular blockade with intubation and mechanical ventilation is generally well tolerated. Regardless of the choice of drug, a slow titration of the induction agent is important given the depressed LV function.

As the catheter courses through the heart, dysrhythmias can frequently occur, including ventricular fibrillation.

Balloon inflation obstructs antegrade blood flow and leads to a drop in cardiac output and blood pressure with a fall in $ETCO_2$. These effects may be less significant if some cardiac output or pulmonary blood flow is maintained via a PDA. However, significant hypotension and bradycardia may be commonly seen at this time. The patient may or may not require pharmacologic intervention to recover.

What are the possible procedural complications?

- Blood loss during vessel cannulation by the interventional team
- Dysrhythmias
- Valve or heart perforation
- Cardiac arrest from decreased cardiac output during balloon dilatation
- Stroke
- Air embolism
- Acute severe AI (leaflet avulsion, cusp prolapse, disruption of the annulus) requiring urgent surgical valve repair or replacement
- Femoral vein or artery thrombus; heparin should be considered early for lower extremities that show signs of compromised perfusion
- Endocarditis

What are the results of BAV?

Balloon aortic valvuloplasty has been shown to decrease the gradient of AS by 50% but at the expense of a 15% incidence of AI. In the meta-analysis recently published [1], mortality rates following BAV were 11% (95% CI: 8–14). Reintervention following an initial BAV procedure for treatment of AS was 37% (95% CI: 30%–44%) with a mean time to reintervention of 2.7 years (95% CI: 1.4–4.1). This is probably a reflection of the growing preference for a graduated approach to relief of AS, and a trend toward leaving a higher degree of residual stenosis to reduce the risk of significant AI. The incidence of aortic valve replacement following BAV was 20% (95% CI: 17–23). Long-term and mid-term follow-up showed moderate to severe AI was present in 28% of patients (95% CI: 20–37).

Where should the patient be transferred following the procedure?

The patient should be transferred to the appropriate intensive care unit (ICU) for postprocedural monitoring. If stable post-dilatation with normal lactate levels and mixed venous saturations, extubation may be considered. Frequently, however, the patient is transferred to the ICU sedated, intubated, and ventilated. The cardiologist usually decides if PGE_1 can be discontinued in the catheterization laboratory or later during recovery in the ICU, with the decision usually based on how confident he or she is that there will be adequate forward flow through the balloon dilated aortic valve. Post-catheterization chest radiograph and echocardiogram are routinely obtained. Groin access is observed, with a low threshold to start a heparin infusion if no distal pulses are palpable even after the bandage is loosened.

In conclusion, the neonate with critical AS is dependent on a PDA for maintenance of systemic cardiac output, and PGE_1 should be initiated while the management decision regarding catheter versus surgical intervention is being discussed.

References

1. M. T. Saung, C. McCracken, R. Sachdeva, et al. Outcomes following balloon aortic valvuloplasty vs surgical valvotomy in congenital aortic valve stenosis: a meta-analysis. *J Invasive Cardiol* 2019; **31**: E133–44.

2. P. Ewert, H. Bertram, J. Breuer, et al. Balloon valvuloplasty in the treatment of congenital aortic valve stenosis: a retrospective multicenter survey of more than 1000 patients. *Int J Cardiol* 2011; **149**: 182–185.

3. D. G. Nykanen, T. J. Forbes, W. Du, et al. CRISP: catheterization risk score for pediatrics: a report from the congenital cardiac interventional study consortium (CCISC). *Catheter Cardio Inte* 2016; **87**: 302–9.

4. C. Ramamoorthy, C. M. Haberkern, S. M. Bhananker, et al. Anesthesia-related cardiac arrest in children with heart disease: data from the pediatric perioperative cardiac arrest (POCA) registry. *Anesth Analg* 2010; **110**: 1376–82.

5. K. C. Odegard, R. Vincent, R. Baijal, et al. SCAI/CCAS/SPA expert consensus statement for anesthesia and sedation practice: recommendations for patients undergoing diagnostic and therapeutic procedures in the pediatric and congenital cardiac catheterization laboratory. *Catheter Cardio Inte* 2016; **88**: 912–22.

Suggested Reading

Daaboul D. G., Dinardo J. A., and Nasr V. G. Anesthesia for high-risk procedures in the catheterization laboratory. *Pediatric Anesthesia* 2019; **29**: 491–8.

Odegard K. C., Bergersen L., Thiagarajan R., et al. The frequency of cardiac arrests in patients with congenital heart disease undergoing cardiac catheterization. *Anesth Analg* 2014; **118**: 175–82.

Vergnat M., Asfour B., Arenz C., et al. Aortic stenosis of the neonate: a single-center experience. *J Thorac and Cardiovasc Surg* 2019; **157**: 318–26.

Chapter 15

Aortic Stenosis

Deborah A. Romeo

Case Scenario

A 13-year-old male with new-onset headaches and right-sided weakness presents for craniotomy and resection of an intracranial mass. He has a past medical history of well-controlled asthma, taking albuterol as needed. His past surgical history includes a Ross procedure performed at age 5 years for congenital aortic stenosis. He reports playing basketball daily with his friends and denies cardiac symptoms of exertional dyspnea, chest pain, or syncope. He currently takes no medications. Preoperative vital signs are heart rate 73 beats/minute, blood pressure 110/69 mm Hg, respiratory rate 18 breaths/minute, and SpO$_2$ 97% on room air. A II/VI high-pitched diastolic murmur can be heard on auscultation of the right upper sternal border. Laboratory values are all within normal limits.

His last cardiology visit was 3 months ago, at which time the cardiologist was pleased with his progress and reported to the boy's mother that his echo looked "fine."

Key Objectives

- Understand the criteria for observation versus intervention on a stenotic aortic valve.
- Discuss potential cardiac surgical interventions for aortic stenosis.
- Understand the difference between the Ross procedure and the Ross–Konno procedure.
- Discuss preoperative assessment of this patient.
- Discuss intraoperative management for this patient.
- Discuss postoperative care and airway management strategies.

Pathophysiology

What is aortic stenosis?

Aortic stenosis (AS) is one of the most common congenital cardiac defects, with a bicuspid aortic valve occurring in approximately 2% of the population. Stenosis can occur anywhere along the left ventricular outflow tract (LVOT) and can be classified as subvalvular, valvular, or supravalvular. (See Figure 15.1.) Nearly two-thirds of stenotic LVOT lesions occur at the level of the aortic valve. Congenital valvular AS occurs in approximately 3%–5% of patients with congenital heart disease (CHD) with a male predominance of 3:1. Evidence suggests that the development of AS is influenced by both genetic and environmental factors [1].

What is the anatomy of valvular AS?

Aortic valve stenosis results from narrowing of the orifice size. While a normal aortic valve is tricuspid, an aberrant aortic valve can be unicuspid, bicuspid, or quadricuspid. The unicuspid valve has a single, thickened leaflet resulting in either an eccentric slit-like orifice or a pinhole central orifice, severely limiting flow through the valve during systole. A bicuspid aortic valve occurs from fusion of two of the three aortic valve cusps. With time these cusps undergo myxomatous changes that result in thickened, fibrous leaflets that further contribute to worsening stenosis. The quadricuspid aortic valve is the most rarely seen and is thought to be due to abnormal division of the developing aortic valve leaflets. This lesion is more often associated with aortic regurgitation than with AS. Symptoms associated with a quadricuspid aortic valve generally do not present until adulthood.

A stenotic aortic valve can be associated with other cardiac lesions including patent ductus arteriosus, coarctation of the aorta, and ventricular septal defects. Aortic root dilation frequently occurs with bicuspid aortic valves, even in the absence of clinical stenosis.

What is the physiology of critical valvular AS in the neonate?

At birth, when the low-resistance placenta is removed from circulation, the left ventricle (LV) experiences an increase in afterload. As ventilation begins and the neonate's lungs expand, pulmonary vascular resistance (PVR) decreases,

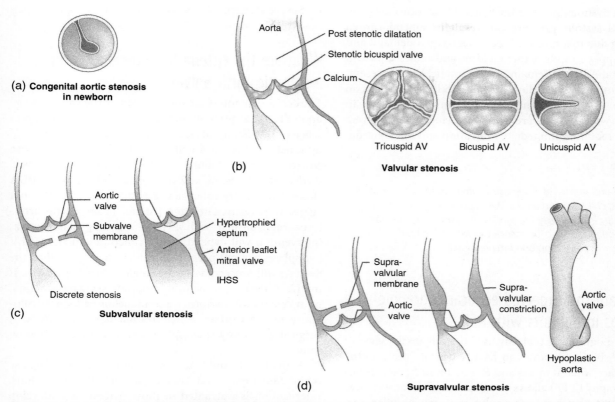

Figure 15.1 Types of aortic stenosis. (a) Congenital aortic stenosis in the newborn, characterized by hypoplastic aortic valve annulus and malformed unicuspid, unicommissural aortic valve with keyhole appearance to narrow orifice. **(b) Valvular aortic stenosis**, characterized by abnormal number of valve cusps or three-cuspid valve. **(c) Subvalvular aortic stenosis**, characterized by a thickened ring or collar of dense endocardial fibrous tissue below the level of the valve cusps causing narrowing in the outflow tract from the left ventricle. **(d) Supravalvular aortic stenosis**, characterized by narrowing of the ascending aorta just above the aortic valve. From Ottaviani G. and Buja L. M. Congenital heart disease: pathology, natural history, and interventions. In Buja L. M. and Butany J., eds. *Cardiovascular Pathology*, 4th ed. Elsevier, 2015; 611–47. With permission.

resulting in an increase in pulmonary blood flow and increased volume return, or preload, to the left heart. In critical AS, the right ventricle (RV) can generally compensate for compromised LV output in the presence of a patent foramen ovale and patent ductus arteriosus (PDA). Compromised LV output through the stenotic aortic valve is augmented by right to left (R-to-L) shunting through the PDA. As the PDA closes over the first 2–4 days of life the LV is then unable to provide adequate systemic circulation and signs of inadequate systemic circulation and congestive heart failure ensue. The initiation of prostaglandin E_1 (PGE$_1$) is required for neonates with critical AS to maintain ductal patency, thereby ensuring adequate flow to the systemic circulation. Aortic perfusion distal to the PDA is then largely derived from systemic venous blood, resulting in **differential cyanosis**, or lower oxygen saturations in the lower extremities compared to the upper extremities. (See Chapter 14.)

Clinical Pearl

While patients with mild AS often remain asymptomatic, newborns with critical AS will become severely ill and present in cardiogenic shock when the PDA closes, requiring immediate intervention. These patients require urgent resuscitation, PGE$_1$ infusion to maintain the PDA, and intervention to relieve AS.

What is the physiology of valvular AS in children and adolescents?

The obstruction caused by the stenotic aortic valve results in an increase in LV systolic pressure followed by the development of LV wall hypertrophy. This concentric hypertrophy preserves wall stress such that heart rate, stroke volume, and cardiac output are maintained in a normal range. With time, progressive AS will result in diastolic dysfunction. The thickened LV myocardium and increased systolic pressure can result in subendocardial ischemia due to a mismatch between oxygen demand and blood supply. In spite of this, children and adolescents with congenital AS often remain asymptomatic. When present, symptoms generally include easy fatigability or dyspnea on exertion. Chest pain and syncope can also be seen in patients with AS and are ominous symptoms of severe stenosis requiring immediate evaluation and intervention.

Clinical Pearl

Congenital aortic valve stenosis is often asymptomatic in infants, children, and adults. When present, symptoms generally include easy fatigability or dyspnea on exertion. Chest pain and syncope associated with AS require immediate evaluation and intervention.

What are the expected echocardiographic findings in patients with AS?

Echocardiography is typically used to evaluate the severity of AS. A bicuspid valve can have a typical "fish mouth" appearance when it opens and closes. Transthoracic echocardiography (TTE) allows visualization of the aortic valve in different planes to assess valve anatomy, annular size, aortic root diameter, and LV function. The anatomy of the ascending aorta, aortic arch, and any other associated cardiac anomalies may also be evaluated.

Measurement of the peak-to-peak transvalvular pressure gradient during cardiac catheterization has historically been used to quantify the degree of aortic valvular stenosis to aid in determining the need for intervention. However, there can be a significant discrepancy between the peak instantaneous Doppler echocardiographic gradient and the peak-to-peak pressure gradient obtained by cardiac catheterization; as peak instantaneous Doppler gradients can overestimate the transvalvular gradient, most clinicians prefer to use continuous wave mean Doppler gradient to guide timing of intervention on a stenotic valve. The mean pressure gradient is relatively consistent between Doppler and catheterization measurements. The following are the guidelines for Stages of Valvular AS from the 2014 American Heart Association/American College of Cardiology Guidelines for the Management of Patients with Valvular Heart Disease [2].

- **Mild stenosis**: Mean gradient <20 mm Hg or aortic V_{max} 2.0–2.9 m/s
- **Moderate stenosis**: Mean gradient 20–39 mm Hg or aortic V_{max} 3.0–3.9 m/s
- **Severe stenosis**: Mean gradient >40 mm Hg or aortic V_{max} >4.0 m/s

What are the criteria for intervention on a stenotic aortic valve?

The decision to intervene on a stenotic aortic valve is based upon the age at presentation, severity of the stenosis, presence of coexisting cardiac lesion(s) and the degree of LV dysfunction. Neonates with critical AS will present with congestive heart failure, respiratory distress, hypoxia, inadequate perfusion, and metabolic acidosis as the PDA closes. Circulatory collapse will ensue if the patient is not aggressively resuscitated and patency of the ductus arteriosus reestablished with PGE_1. Following stabilization, intervention will depend on LV function and size. If LV hypoplasia will not permit a biventricular repair, then the neonate will proceed down the single-ventricle pathway. If the LV is deemed to be of appropriate size and function, most centers will perform a percutaneous balloon valvuloplasty in the cardiac catheterization laboratory, though surgical valvotomy is an option that may be preferred by some.

Patients with mild AS can be monitored with regular echocardiography and require no activity restrictions. Intervention is warranted in those patients who develop either a peak-to-peak gradient >50 mm Hg accompanied by symptoms or electrocardiogram (ECG) changes, or an isolated peak-to-peak gradient >70 mm Hg [3].

Clinical Pearl

Neonates with critical AS can present in cardiogenic shock with metabolic acidosis, respiratory distress, and poor systemic perfusion. These patients require urgent resuscitation, PGE_1 infusion to maintain ductal patency, and intervention to relieve AS.

How is balloon valvuloplasty performed in neonates with critical AS?

The neonate is brought to the cardiac catheterization laboratory and vascular access is obtained. The anterograde approach involves gaining access via the femoral or umbilical veins and then advancing the catheter into the left atrium via the foramen ovale. Alternatively, a retrograde approach can be utilized by cannulating the umbilical, femoral or carotid artery and advancing the catheter to the left side of the heart. The catheter is then positioned across the aortic valve and the balloon inflated, causing disruption of the fused aortic valve leaflets. The goal is to relieve stenosis while inflicting minimal aortic insufficiency (AI) from the balloon valvuloplasty. This procedure is palliative, and patients will require intervention later in life for either restenosis of the aortic valve or for AI.

What cardiac surgical options exist for patients with AS?

- *Repair of the aortic valve* is the first option. In some centers this is the preferred approach for management of the neonate with critical AS instead of balloon valvuloplasty in the cardiac catheterization laboratory. When possible, surgical repair offers certain advantages. It allows growth, delays aortic valve replacement, and avoids anticoagulation with its associated morbidity. Disadvantages include the need for cardiopulmonary bypass (CPB), potentially at a very early age. Surgical repair may also be complex if associated congenital cardiac abnormalities exist. Studies have demonstrated excellent long-term survival exceeding 95% at 10 years. However, a surgical procedure does not obviate the need for reintervention, with freedom from a second procedure on the aortic valve ranging from 50% to 80% at 10 years [4].
- The *Ross procedure* for AS was first described in 1967 by Donald Ross. Described in further detail in the text that follows, the Ross procedure is favored in children and adolescents due to the advantages of potential for growth, freedom from anticoagulation and durability when compared to placement of an aortic homograft. Disadvantages include the fact that the previously healthy right ventricular outflow tract (RVOT) will now have a pulmonary homograft, which is at risk for becoming incompetent and requiring intervention as the patient ages. Additional disadvantages include high early mortality for the Ross procedure when performed on neonates and infants and the high rate of second intervention when performed on young children.
- *Aortic valve replacement with a mechanical valve* is the least preferred surgical technique to address AS in pediatric patients. Though this technique carries low early mortality, it is associated with significant morbidity. A mechanical valve requires life-long anticoagulation requiring medication compliance. Patients on anticoagulation cannot participate in contact sports and should avoid becoming pregnant because of teratogenic effects to the fetus. Risks of thromboembolic events and endocarditis exist. Mechanical valves also carry a risk of requiring

replacement as children age because the valve does not provide for any growth potential.

What is the Ross procedure?

The Ross procedure involves resecting the stenotic aortic valve and replacing it with the patient's own pulmonary valve (pulmonary autograft). A valved pulmonary homograft is then placed between the RV and pulmonary artery.

After CPB is commenced the diseased aortic valve is removed and coronary buttons dissected. Depending on the comparative sizes of the aortic annulus and the pulmonary autograft the resection can also involve a portion of the aortic valve annulus. This will allow expansion of the annulus to accommodate a larger pulmonary autograft. The pulmonary autograft is then sutured into the LVOT and the coronary buttons are attached. A pulmonary homograft is constructed and placed in the RVOT. (See Figure 15.2.)

What is the Konno procedure?

The Konno operation was described by Konno in 1975 and serves to alleviate LVOT obstruction at the subvalvular, valvular, and supravalvular levels. This is a desirable option when the aortic annulus is very small. Here the incision is made from above the level of the aortic commissures to the aortic annulus and through the RVOT. Another incision is then made across the annulus and extended into the LVOT via the interventricular septum, taking care to avoid the conduction system. A mechanical or bioprosthetic aortic valve is placed in the LVOT, which has been expanded to adequately accommodate the new valve. Both the RV and LV outflow tracts are then augmented with patch closures.

What is the Ross–Konno procedure?

The Konno procedure by itself is rarely utilized but has been combined with the Ross operation to perform a shortened incision through the interventricular septum. The initial dissection of the aortic valve, pulmonary autograft, and coronary buttons are carried out as discussed earlier for the Ross procedure. Again, a portion of the aortic annulus is resected, and an incision made in the interventricular septum. This allows a smaller aortic annulus to accommodate a larger pulmonary autograft. A shorter incision in the interventricular septum than

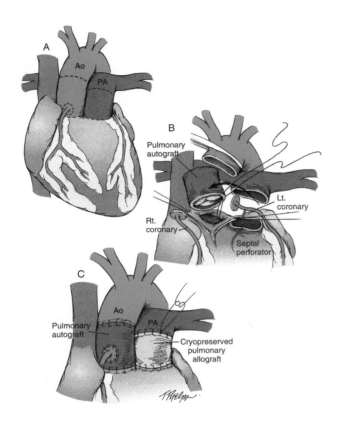

Figure 15.2 Ross procedure. (A) Great arteries are transected, aortic sinuses are excised, and coronary arteries are mobilized. **(B)** Pulmonary autograft is excised from the right ventricular outflow tract. The proximal end of the autograft is anastomosed to the annulus. **(C)** The coronary arteries are anastomosed to the pulmonary autograft. Autograft-to-aorta anastomosis is completed and the right ventricular outflow tract is reconstructed usually with a cryopreserved pulmonary allograft. From Alsoufi R., Aljiffry A., and Ungerleider R. M. Left ventricular outflow tract obstruction. In Undgerleider R. M., Meliones J. N., McMillan K. N., et al., eds. *Critical Heart Disease in Infants and Children*, 3rd ed. Elsevier, 2019; 615–31. With permission.

that performed in the classic Konno operation decreases the risk for injury to the conduction system. Coronary buttons are implanted, and a pulmonary homograft placed in the RVOT to complete the Ross–Konno procedure. (See Figure 15.3.)

What are outcomes for patients undergoing the Ross or Ross–Konno procedures?

An analysis of the Society of Thoracic Surgery, Congenital Heart Surgery Database from 2000 to 2009 evaluating outcomes in neonates and infants undergoing aortic valve replacement by the Ross or Ross–Konno procedures found in-hospital mortality to be 40% [5]. This is likely because neonates present with more complex left-sided structural abnormalities and significant LV dysfunction. Long term outcomes in older patients have been favorable, with >75% freedom from re-operation at 10 years. One study also associated the type of surgical reintervention with age at the time of the Ross/Ross–Konno intervention, with infants more likely needing later surgery on the RVOT and children and adolescents needing subsequent reintervention on their LVOT [6].

Anesthetic Implications

What valvular disease might be anticipated in this patient?

After the Ross procedure patients can develop AI. The exact physiology is unclear, but it is thought to be due to either dilation of the neoaortic root or degeneration of the pulmonary cusps of the autograft. Despite concerns about the Ross procedure creating two diseased valves from one dysfunctional valve, observational data do not support this. Pulmonary homograft dysfunction is much less common than AI after the Ross procedure.

What are the physical findings of AS? AI?

Vital signs are generally normal in patients with AS. The classic murmur associated with AS is a systolic crescendo–decrescendo murmur heard best at the right upper sternal border, though in younger children it can be auscultated at the left upper sternal border. The murmur will often radiate to the bilateral carotid arteries.

The murmur of AI is classically a diastolic high-pitched, decrescendo murmur heard best at the right upper sternal

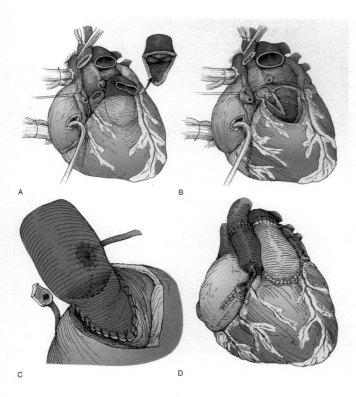

Figure 15.3 Ross–Konno procedure. (A) The pulmonary valve is harvested after the aorta has been divided and the coronary arteries removed as buttons. **(B)** An incision is made across the infundibular septum. **(C)** The pulmonary autograft is anastomosed to the aortic root using the infundibular muscle to repair the interventricular septal defect. The coronary arteries are placed into the neoaorta. **(D)** The procedure is completed with a pulmonary homograft to repair the right ventricular outflow tract. From Alsoufi R., Aljiffry A., and Ungerleider R. M. Left ventricular outflow tract obstruction. In Undgerleider R. M., Meliones J. N., McMillan K. N., et al., eds. *Critical Heart Disease in Infants and Children*, 3rd ed. Elsevier, 2019; 615–31. With permission.

border. Severe aortic regurgitation can cause a mid-to-late diastolic rumbling murmur heard best at the apex of the heart. This lesion is also associated with wide pulse pressures and bounding pulses when chronic in nature.

Clinical Pearl

The murmur of AS is a systolic crescendo–decrescendo murmur radiating to the carotids while that of aortic regurgitation is a diastolic high-pitched, decrescendo murmur.

How should this patient be evaluated preoperatively?

A thorough history and physical exam will need to be performed before his craniotomy. While discussing his history, particular attention should be paid to his functional status, activity level, and the presence and/or nature of cardiac symptoms such as shortness of breath, chest pain, or syncope. His medication list should be reviewed and medication compliance confirmed. Current vital signs and laboratory values, particularly his hematocrit, should be assessed.

As part of the preoperative evaluation the most recent pediatric cardiology consultation should be reviewed, and the cardiologist made aware of the impending surgery. A recent ECG and echocardiogram should also be reviewed. When evaluating the echocardiogram, it is important to note the status of the neoaortic valve, noting any significant regurgitation or restenosis. The RVOT should also be evaluated for any pulmonary homograft dysfunction.

The preoperative evaluation should include a discussion about fasting status. If restenosis of the neoaortic valve has occurred, particular care should be taken to avoid prolonged fasting and perioperative hypovolemia. In general patients should be encouraged to eat solid food up until 8 hours before their scheduled procedure and to drink clear liquids up until 2 hours before their procedure. Patients with pre-existing intravenous (IV) access may receive maintenance fluids until the time of surgery.

Clinical Pearl

The most recent pediatric cardiology consultation should be reviewed, and the cardiologist made aware of the impending surgery. Results of the last echocardiographic exam should be thoroughly reviewed, with attention to the status of the RVOT and the pulmonary homograft as well as the neoaortic valve, noting significant regurgitation or restenosis.

Is there a need for invasive monitoring during the craniotomy?

Craniotomies require close blood pressure monitoring due to the potential for volume shifts with the administration of mannitol. Given this, and the patient's history of palliative cardiac surgery, invasive arterial pressure monitoring would be appropriate during this procedure. A central line allows monitoring of central venous pressure and administration of inotropes if needed. In this patient, the placement of a central line would be best in the subclavian or femoral veins because of the nature of the surgical procedure. However, in the absence of a central line, volume status can also be accurately measured by monitoring urine output, closely following vital signs trends and evaluating arterial blood gas values for base deficits.

What perioperative management concerns exist for this patient?

Placement of a preoperative IV catheter, if not already present, would be appropriate for this patient. In the setting of a neoaortic valve with restenosis, goals of an anesthetic IV induction include avoidance of tachycardia and maintenance of appropriate preload and afterload. Similarly, intraoperative anesthetic goals should include maintenance of appropriate preload, afterload, and contractility while avoiding tachycardia and arrhythmias. In the presence of aortic regurgitation, a higher heart rate is better tolerated. A total IV anesthetic with propofol and narcotic infusions would allow for hemodynamic stability and optimize cerebral oxygen supply and demand. Euvolemia should be maintained and volume replacement should be guided by urine output and arterial blood gas measurements of base deficit. The patient should be monitored closely for anemia; if necessary, packed red blood cells should be available for transfusion.

Clinical Pearl

Anesthetic goals in patients with AS include maintenance of preload, afterload, and contractility with avoidance of tachycardia, arrhythmias, and hypovolemia.

What are the postoperative management considerations for this patient?

In the absence of significant respiratory disease or intraoperative complications, extubation should be considered in the operating room environment. It is important to avoid significant tachycardia on emergence and to ensure adequate analgesia. Postoperative care should take place in an intensive care unit.

References

1. G. K. Singh. Congenital aortic valve stenosis. *Children* 2019; **6**: 1–12.

2. A. P. Vlahos, G. R. Marx, D. McElhinney, et al. Clinical utility of Doppler echocardiography in assessing aortic stenosis severity and predicting need for intervention in children. *Pediatr Cardiol* 2008; **29**: 507–14.

3. P. S. Rao. Management of congenital heart disease: state of the art; Part I – ACYANOTIC heart defects. *Children* 2019; **6**: 1–27.

4. I. Bouhout, P. Salmane, I. El-Hamamsy, et al. Aortic valve interventions in pediatric patients. *Semin Thorac Cardiovasc Surg* 2018; **31**: 277–87.

5. R. K. Woods, S. K. Pasquali, M. L. Jacobs, et al. Aortic valve replacement in neonates and infants: an analysis of the Society of Thoracic Surgeons Congenital Heart Surgery Database. *J Thorac Cardiovasc Surg* 2012; **144**: 1084–90.

6. J. S. Nelson, S. K. Pasquali, C. N. Pratt, et al. Long-term survival and reintervention after the Ross procedure across the pediatric age spectrum. *Ann Thorac Surg* 2015; **99**: 2086–95.

Suggested Reading

Gottlieb E. A. and Andropoulos D. B. Anesthesia for the patient with congenital heart disease presenting for noncardiac surgery. *Curr Opin Anaesthesiol* 2013; **26**: 318–26.

Mavroudis C., Mavroudis C. D., and Jacobs J. P. The Ross, Konno, and Ross-Konno operations for congenital left ventricular outflow tract abnormalities. *Cardiol Young* 2014; **24**: 1121–33.

Stulak J. M., Burkhart H. M., Sundt T. M., et al. Spectrum and outcome of reoperations after the Ross procedure. *Circulation* 2010; **122**: 1153–58.

Subvalvular Aortic Stenosis

16

Rahul G. Baijal

Case Scenario

A 5-year-old male, who was a restrained rear-seat passenger, presents to the emergency department following a T-bone motor vehicle accident. The child's medical history is significant for repaired subvalvular aortic stenosis at age 3. The child is able to keep up with his older siblings and classmates without difficulty.

Primary assessment reveals a nonobstructive respiratory rate of 12 breaths/minute, SpO_2 99% on room air, heart rate of 140 beats/minute, and a Glasgow Coma Scale score of 14. Secondary assessment reveals a distended, tender abdomen along with bruising and tenderness over the right femur. Radiographic assessment confirms a right femur fracture while computed tomography of the abdomen reveals potential intraperitoneal air. The child is scheduled for an emergent exploratory laparotomy along with placement of an intramedullary nail in the right femur. Transthoracic echocardiography 6 months previously showed the following:

- Moderate to severe subvalvular aortic stenosis with a peak velocity of 3.9 m/s
- 40 mm Hg mean gradient across the aortic valve
- Normal ejection fraction (55%) with qualitatively normal diastolic function
- Moderate left ventricular hypertrophy

Key Objectives

- Understand the pathophysiology of subvalvular aortic stenosis.
- Describe the natural progression of subvalvular aortic stenosis.
- Describe appropriate intervention(s) for subvalvular aortic stenosis.
- Understand echocardiographic findings in subvalvular aortic stenosis.
- Construct a perioperative plan for the patient with subvalvular aortic stenosis.

Pathophysiology

What is the epidemiology of subvalvular aortic stenosis?

Fixed subvalvular aortic stenosis (AS) is the second most common type of left ventricular outflow tract obstruction (LVOTO) following valvular AS, accounting for approximately 15% of all cases. Subvalvular AS has a male predominance with a ratio of approximately 1.5–2.5:1.

What is the pathology of subvalvular AS?

- *Membranous subvalvular AS* is the most common type, accounting for approximately 70%–80% of all cases of subvalvular pathology. (See Figure 16.1.) A thin, fibrous, circumferential membrane, often with attachments to the anterior mitral valve leaflet, is typically located 1–2 mm inferior to the aortic valve.

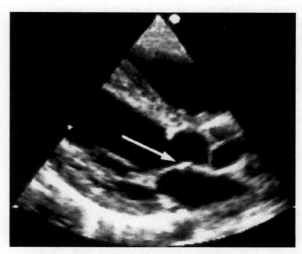

Figure 16.1 Parasternal long axis view of subvalvular aortic stenosis with membrane.

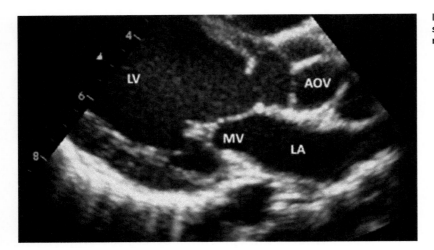

Figure 16.2 Parasternal long axis view of subvalvular aortic stenosis with fibromuscular ridge.

- A *fibromuscular ridge*, located slightly more inferior to the aortic valve than the membrane, is the second most common type of subvalvular AS. (See Figure 16.2.)

Both types are acquired conditions. Turbulent flow and shear stresses within the left ventricular outflow tract (LVOT), producing endothelial damage, cellular proliferation, and collagen deposition, are theorized as the etiologies for the formation of both membranous and fibromuscular ridge subvalvular AS. The turbulent flow and the increased shear stresses are postulated to result from an abnormally shaped LVOT, where the angle between the long axis of the left ventricle (LV) and aorta is more acute than normal. The endothelial damage, cellular proliferation, and collagen deposition result in LVOTO, producing further turbulent flow and abnormal shear stresses. (See Figure 16.3.)

- *Tunnel-type subvalvular AS*, extending for several centimeters below the aortic valve, is the most severe type of subaortic stenosis. (See Figure 16.4.) Tunnel-type obstruction is also acquired, typically following previous repair of congenital heart defects, including double outlet right ventricle, interrupted aortic arch, and Shone's complex. (See Chapter 20.) Turbulent flow and shear stresses caused by residual postoperative obstruction are again postulated as the etiology for tunnel-type obstruction.
- *Other etiologies of subvalvular AS include*:
  - Abnormal attachment of the anterior mitral valve leaflet or accessory atrioventricular valve tissue, as seen in cleft mitral valve or complete atrioventricular septal defect

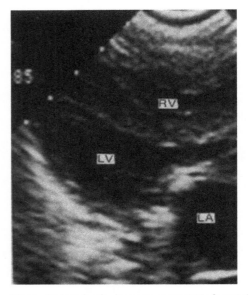

Figure 16.3 Subvalvular aortic stenosis: Left ventricular injection. An angiogram is performed in the left ventricle in the AP projection. The subaortic stenosis immediately below the valve is noted (arrows). Courtesy of Russel Hirsch, MD.

  - Conal septal projection into the LVOT with a posterior malaligned ventricular septal defect (VSD)
  - Asymmetric septal hypertrophic cardiomyopathy

Aortic insufficiency (AI) develops in approximately 70% of children with subvalvular AS. (See Figure 16.5.) Aortic insufficiency develops secondary to long-standing damage to the aortic valve from the increased turbulent

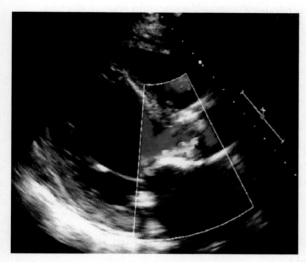

Figure 16.4 Parasternal long axis view of subvalvular aortic stenosis tunnel type.

Table 16.1 Lesions Associated with Subvalvular Aortic Stenosis

Lesion	%
Bicuspid aortic valve	40
Valvular aortic stenosis	28
Ventricular septal defect	24
Coarctation of the aorta	12
Patent ductus arteriosus	12
Atrial septal defect	4

flow and shear stresses. The thickening and distortion of the valve leaflets result in failure of leaflet coaptation or prolapse, producing AI. The peak echocardiographic Doppler gradient is the strongest predictor for AI in children with subvalvular AS.

> **Clinical Pearl**
>
> *The peak echocardiographic Doppler gradient is the strongest predictor for AI in children with subvalvular AS.*

What lesions may be associated with subvalvular AS?

See Table 16.1 for lesions associated with subvalvular AS.

What are the physiologic considerations with subvalvular AS?

Left ventricular outflow tract obstruction is the primary physiologic derangement in subvalvular AS, increasing LV systolic pressure and wall stress, which is directly proportional to LV pressure and indirectly proportional to LV wall thickness. Left ventricular wall hypertrophy is a compensatory mechanism that increases LV wall thickness to maintain constant LV wall stress in the setting of increasing LV systolic pressure.

$$T = Pr/2h,$$

where T = LV wall stress, P = LV systolic pressure, r = ventricular radius, and h = LV wall thickness.

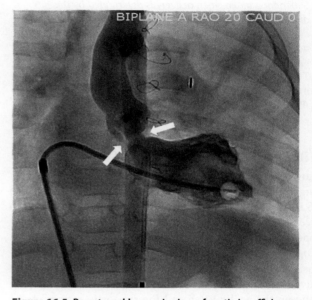

Figure 16.5 Parasternal long axis view of aortic insufficiency.

Left ventricular wall stress normalization initially maintains normal systolic and diastolic function despite an increased impedance to ejection. However, long-standing pressure overload to the LV results in ventricular remodeling with both diastolic and systolic dysfunction and subsequent clinical heart failure.

Subendocardial ischemia may also result from high intracardiac compressive forces that limit systolic coronary artery flow. Oxygen delivery to the subendomyocardium occurs during diastole, driven by the gradient between aortic diastolic pressure and left ventricular end-diastolic pressure (LVEDP). Increased myocardial oxygen demand is typically compensated for by increased oxygen delivery through coronary vasodilation. Further subendocardial coronary vasodilation in children with subvalvular AS during periods of stress is limited by the high intracardiac compressive forces. Subsequently, subendocardial oxygen delivery is determined by the duration of diastole and the gradient between aortic diastolic pressure and LVEDP. This diastolic gradient is additionally reduced from increased LVEDP secondary to decreased LV compliance due to compensatory hypertrophy. Hemodynamic data from a cohort of 80 children with AS demonstrated that myocardial oxygen delivery is determined by aortic valve area, diastolic function, and heart rate. All patients with severe AS with a heart rate <100 beats/minute demonstrated adequate oxygen delivery.

Clinical Pearl

Subendocardial oxygen delivery is determined by the duration of diastole and the gradient between aortic diastolic pressure and LVEDP. This diastolic gradient is additionally reduced from increased LVEDP secondary to decreased LV compliance due to compensatory hypertrophy. Tachycardia, particularly a heart rate >100 beats/minute, may be poorly tolerated in children with severe subvalvular AS.

What is the natural history of subvalvular AS?

Subvalvular AS is an acquired progressive disease, producing symptoms late in the disease course. Mild or moderate AS is typically asymptomatic. Symptoms with moderate to severe AS include dyspnea on exertion, angina, presyncope, syncope, and fatigue. Although the rate of disease progression may be variable, an increased gradient at diagnosis, attachment of the subaortic membrane to the mitral valve, aortic valve thickening, and decreased distance between the aortic valve and the subaortic membrane or fibromuscular ridge are risk factors for disease progression. Additionally, an increased mean gradient at diagnosis and increased time since diagnosis are risk factors for progression of AI.

What physical examination findings might be expected in subvalvular AS?

In children with moderate to severe subvalvular AS, the LV impulse will be displaced further laterally, and a systolic thrill may be appreciated over the base of the heart. The first heart sound is normal, and the second heart sound may be narrow, secondary to delayed aortic valve closure.

- A physiologically split S2 is the most reliable physical examination finding to *exclude* severe stenosis.
- S3 and S4 gallops are also present in children with LVOTO but do not correlate with the degree of stenosis in children <12 years of age. An S4 gallop in children >12 years of age may indicate severe stenosis and left ventricular diastolic dysfunction.

- A harsh crescendo–decrescendo systolic ejection murmur, loudest at the left mid-sternal border and radiating to the carotid arteries, is heard in subvalvular AS. The intensity of the murmur correlates with the severity of the obstruction. An early diastolic decrescendo murmur at the left lower sternal border may also be heard if AI is present.

Clinical Pearl

*A physiologically split S2 is the most reliable physical examination finding to **exclude** severe stenosis. The intensity of the harsh crescendo–decrescendo systolic ejection murmur correlates with the severity of the obstruction.*

Is electrocardiography a useful diagnostic tool?

Electrocardiographic findings are neither highly sensitive nor specific for severe stenosis. Only 74% and 70% of children with moderate or severe AS display LVH and strain, respectively, on ECG, whereas 24% and 10% of children with mild AS display LVH and strain, respectively.

What echocardiographic parameters are important in subvalvular AS?

Echocardiography is the only class I recommendation by the American Heart Association/American College of Cardiology (AHA/ACC) for the diagnostic evaluation of suspected AS and the monitoring of disease progression. An echocardiogram may determine not only the location and severity of the obstruction, but also the LV response to the obstruction, including hypertrophy and systolic and diastolic function. Doppler interrogation of the aortic valve accurately estimates disease severity and predicts the need for intervention in children.

The mean echocardiographic Doppler velocity more closely approximates the peak-to-peak pressure gradient obtained in the cardiac catheterization laboratory as an accurate reflection of disease severity, whereas the peak instantaneous echocardiogram Doppler velocity may overestimate the catheter-derived gradient.

Doppler interrogation may underestimate disease severity in the setting of severe myocardial dysfunction, multiple levels of obstruction, or the presence of a pop-off (e.g., an atrial or ventricular septal defect).

Preferred echocardiographic views are as follows:

- *Parasternal long axis*: Aortic valve annulus and aortic root dimensions
- *Parasternal short axis*: Aortic valve assessment

Aortic valve gradient may be estimated by the Doppler velocity through the modified Bernoulli equation:

$$\Delta P = 4\ v^2,$$

where ΔP is the calculated gradient and v is either the interrogated mean or peak velocity.

Severe aortic stenosis is defined as a peak velocity >4.0 m/s across the aortic valve or a mean gradient of 40 mm Hg across the valve. An aortic valve area ≤ 1.0 cm^2 or an indexed valve area of ≤0.6 cm^2/m^2 in the setting of severe myocardial dysfunction is consistent with severe stenosis.

Moderate aortic stenosis is defined as a peak velocity of 3.0–3.9 m/s or a mean gradient between 20 and 39 mm Hg.

Mild stenosis is defined as a peak velocity between 2.0 and 2.9 m/s or a mean gradient ≤20 mm Hg.

Clinical Pearl

Doppler interrogation of the aortic valve accurately estimates disease severity and predicts the need for intervention in children, but Doppler interrogation may underestimate disease severity in the setting of severe myocardial dysfunction, multiple levels of obstruction, or the presence of a pop-off (e.g., an atrial or ventricular septal defect).

How is subvalvular AS medically managed?

There is a limited role for medical management of LVOTO. Guidelines from the ACC/AHA recommend interval transthoracic echocardiography (TTE) to assess disease progression. A TTE is recommended every 6 months to 1 year in children with asymptomatic severe stenosis, every 1–2 years in asymptomatic moderate stenosis, and every 3–5 years in asymptomatic mild stenosis. Symptomatic patients require urgent evaluation. Asymptomatic children with mild stenosis may participate in all sports without restriction whereas all competitive sports should be avoided in patients with severe stenosis. Children with moderate stenosis without moderate or greater LVH on echocardiography, a normal stress test, and no strain on a baseline ECG may participate in sports with a low static component and low to moderate dynamic component.

Is there a role for interventional cardiac catheterization in subvalvular AS?

There is limited evidence that balloon aortic valvuloplasty is effective for subvalvular AS.

What is the surgical management in subvalvular AS?

The surgical approach to subvalvular AS repair depends on the type of obstruction. Although resection of the thin, fibrous membrane or fibromuscular ridge is a relatively straightforward procedure, indications for the procedure are unclear. Since the stenosis is progressive, some studies suggest early repair with a peak gradient as low as 20 mm Hg. Reoperation rates range between 0.6% and 1.8% per year, with risk factors for reoperation including an increased peak gradient at the time of diagnosis >40 mm Hg, early age at diagnosis, distance of <5 mm between the aortic valve and the membrane or fibromuscular ridge, and immediate postoperative LVOT peak pressure gradient >10 mm Hg. (See Figure 16.5.)

Tunnel type obstruction requires either a Konno or Ross–Konno operation (see Chapter 15) with resection of the conal septum, or revision of previously placed LV-to-aorta baffle. Reoperation rates in tunnel-type obstruction range from 15% to 50%. Overall recurrence rate is 20% and higher in children <10 years of age. New-onset AI is an indication for surgical repair. Some centers prefer to defer surgery in children with gradients <40–50 mm Hg without AI, or in children <5–10 years of age, given the high recurrence rate in patients <10 years of age.

Anesthetic Implications

What preoperative workup is appropriate for a child with subvalvular AS presenting for emergent surgery?

A history and physical examination may help elucidate the severity of the LVOTO. The patient/family should be interrogated for any symptoms of dyspnea on exertion, angina, presyncope, syncope, or fatigue. On physical examination, the quality and intensity of the murmur and any new findings are assessed and compared to previous examinations if possible. Previous echocardiographic data should be reviewed for Doppler interrogation of the aortic valve and the degree of stenosis, along with the presence of AI, LVH, and degree of myocardial systolic and diastolic dysfunction. Symptomatic patients require urgent reevaluation with an echocardiogram preoperatively. A limited point of care ultrasound via TTE allows rapid assessment of the degree of subvalvular AS and myocardial dysfunction if there is limited time for a more thorough examination before an emergent procedure.

What are the fasting considerations for patients with subvalvular AS?

The American Society of Anesthesiologists (ASA) nil per os (NPO) guidelines are 8 hours for heavy meals, 6 hours for light meals, 6 hours for formula, and 2 hours for clear liquids for elective procedures. Excessive fasting should be limited in children with LVOTO, including subvalvular AS. Clear liquids should be administered liberally until 2 hours prior to surgery in children presenting for elective procedures. Extended periods without fluid intake or maintenance intravenous (IV) fluid hydration can significantly decrease preload or afterload, increasing the risk of hypotension resulting in decreased aortic diastolic blood pressure and subsequent myocardial ischemia. These NPO guidelines, however, do not apply for children presenting for emergent procedures. Children presenting for emergent procedures may be hypovolemic secondary to previous fasting or fluid or hemorrhagic losses. These losses may need to be replaced with fluid boluses or blood transfusion therapy preoperatively prior to the induction of anesthesia.

What are the primary anesthetic considerations in subvalvular AS?

Perioperative goals should entail reducing the physiologic trespass of surgery and anesthesia. Concentric LVH due to chronic pressure overload, a preload-dependent LV with poor myocardial compliance, and poor coronary artery reserve secondary to fixed LVOTO impede appropriate hemodynamic responses during surgery and anesthesia. Extended periods without fluid intake or maintenance IV

fluid hydration can significantly decrease preload, increasing the risk of hypotension with decreased aortic diastolic blood pressure and subsequent myocardial ischemia.

Anesthetic goals include the following:

- *Maintenance of adequate preload and systemic vascular resistance (SVR)*, or afterload, to ensure an appropriate aortic diastolic pressure for an adequate pressure gradient during diastole for coronary blood flow, and maintenance of myocardial contractility with a normal-to-low heart rate.
- *Avoidance of decreases in SVR* due to anesthetic agents as exaggerated hypotension may be seen secondary to a compromised compensatory increase in cardiac output from the fixed outflow tract obstruction.
- *Avoidance of increased contractility with associated tachycardia*: Inadequate anesthetic depth may cause subendocardial ischemia from already maximally dilated subendocardial coronary arteries due to high intracardiac compressive forces. Tachycardia also prevents adequate early-diastolic filling of the LV that already has impaired relaxation necessary for early-diastolic filling, further reducing cardiac output.

Is premedication appropriate in this child?

This child is tachycardic: possible etiologies include pain, anxiety, hypovolemia, or a combination thereof. Premedication with IV, intranasal or oral agents, including midazolam, ketamine, opioids, or dexmedetomidine may reduce preoperative anxiety and decrease the risk of subsequent subendocardial ischemia secondary to tachycardia.

What induction technique is most appropriate for this child?

Although induction of anesthesia may be achieved with either inhalational agents, IV agents, or a combination of both, the method chosen should allow preservation of preload, afterload, and contractility with a normal-to-low heart rate. Hypotension, myocardial ischemia, and subsequent cardiac arrest may occur even with low incremental dosing of inhalational agents. A titrated IV induction offers optimal control of hemodynamics. Options for a titrated IV induction include etomidate, fentanyl, midazolam, dexmedetomidine, and ketamine. In this case, with an emergent surgery due to trauma, a rapid sequence induction utilizing narcotic along with etomidate and a rapid-onset neuromuscular blocking agent would be most appropriate. The use of vecuronium may be preferable due to the sympathomimetic effects of rocuronium. Administration of a preinduction IV fluid bolus of 20 mL/kg isotonic crystalloid, guided by heart rate response, pulse pressure variability on the pulse oximeter, or inferior vena cava collapsibility on point of care ultrasound, should be considered prior to induction to maintain normovolemia and prevent exaggerated effects on SVR. Up to three 20 mL/kg fluid boluses may be administered prior to vasopressor initiation.

A balanced anesthetic technique combining volatile anesthetic and IV agents for maintenance of anesthesia is appropriate as long as SVR is maintained and tachycardia is prevented. ST changes on ECG may herald subendocardial ischemia, and afterload should be increased with agents that increase SVR such as phenylephrine or vasopressin. Infusions may be utilized if necessary to maintain SVR. Phenylephrine may be the vasopressor of choice, as it not only improves coronary perfusion by increasing SVR but also improves LV filling dynamics by possibly increasing left atrial pressure through reflex bradycardia. Tachycardia without hypotension should also be treated aggressively to improve early-diastolic filling of the left ventricle, ideally with short-acting β_1 agents.

What additional monitoring may be necessary? Is a preinduction arterial line appropriate prior to emergent surgery?

This child has moderate-to-severe AS with a peak velocity of 3.9 m/s and a mean gradient of 40 mm Hg with preserved myocardial function. This child is also presenting for two invasive procedures that may both have a propensity for significant blood loss and fluid shifts: an exploratory laparotomy and an intramedullary pinning of a femur fracture. Invasive monitoring, including an arterial line for hemodynamic monitoring and volume assessment via pulse pressure variation will be necessary not only for the procedure but also for appropriate monitoring of moderate-to-severe AS. Although a preinduction arterial line may be ideal to monitor hypotension during induction of anesthesia, placement of an awake arterial line (even with local anesthetic infiltration, anxiolytic, and ultrasound guidance) may elicit a detrimental tachycardic response in a child who is already tachycardic. A central venous line should be placed to monitor fluid status with central venous pressure trends and for vasopressor administration, given the

expected blood loss and fluid shifts with the planned procedures. Although transesophageal echocardiography is an invaluable tool to monitor wall motion abnormalities, intracardiac volume, valvular and myocardial function, the limited experience of many providers may limit this modality intraoperatively. However, limited point of care ultrasound with TTE may allow rapid assessment of intracardiac volume and myocardial function with myocardial collapse.

What perioperative pain management strategies are appropriate?

Perioperative pain management is not only critically important for functional recovery, but also to alleviate pain-associated tachycardia that is detrimental to LV early-diastolic filling in patients with AS. Although neuraxial anesthesia may provide both sensory and motor blockade for this child for both the exploratory laparotomy and the intramedullary rod placement, it should be used judiciously in a child with moderate-to-severe AS. Several case reports describe the successful use of neuraxial anesthesia in patients with AS, however sympathetic blockade decreasing SVR may produce exaggerated hypotension secondary to a compromised compensatory increase in cardiac output from the fixed outflow tract obstruction, resulting in subsequent myocardial ischemia. A peripheral nerve block for perioperative pain may offer less risk of hypotension, particularly for surgical procedures where expected blood loss and fluid shifts are expected. A truncal nerve block with an indwelling catheter, such as a quadratus lumborum or transversus abdominal block, along with a femoral nerve block and an indwelling catheter would provide coverage perioperatively for the exploratory laparotomy and the femoral intramedullary rod pinning. Postoperative mechanical ventilation should be considered in children who require significant intraoperative cardiopulmonary support, including significant changes in positive pressure ventilation, vasopressor support, or ongoing fluid or blood product resuscitation. In this instance IV analgesia with opioids, α-agonists, or ketamine would be appropriate.

What is the appropriate venue for postoperative recovery?

Decisions regarding postoperative extubation will depend on the length of surgery, blood loss and intraoperative fluid shifts, and hemodynamic stability during the procedure. If vasopressor support has been required during surgery, postoperative care in an intensive care unit should be considered and arranged. Assuming the child is at cardiopulmonary baseline, consideration can be given to extubation in the operating room with postoperative care in the post-anesthesia care unit.

Suggested Reading

Bengur A. R., Snider A. R., Serwer G. A., et al. Usefulness of the Doppler mean gradient in evaluation of children with aortic valve stenosis and comparison to gradient at catheterization. *Am J Cardiol* 1989; **64**: 756–61.

Braunwald E., Goldblatt A., Aygen M. M., et al. Congenital aortic stenosis. I. Clinical and hemodynamic findings in 100 patients. II Surgical treatment and the results of operation. *Circulation* 1963; **27**: 426–62.

Lopes R., Lourenço P., Gonçalves A., et al. The natural history of congenital subaortic stenosis. *Congenit Heart Di* 2011; **6**: 417–23.

Nishimura R. A., Otto C. M., Bobo R. O., et al. 2014 AHA/ACC guidelines for the management of patients with valvular heart disease: a report of the American College of Cardiology/ American Heart Association Task Force on Practice Guidelines. *J Am Coll Cardiol* 2014; **63**: e57-e185.

Pickard S. S., Geva A., Gauvreau K., et al. Long-term outcomes and risk factors for aortic regurgitation after discrete subvalvular aortic stenosis resection in children. *Heart* 2015; **101**: 1547–53.

Talwar S., Anand A., Gupta S. K., et al. Resection of subaortic membrane for discrete subaortic stenosis. *J Card Surg* 2017; **32**: 430–35.

Uysal F., Bostan O. M., Signak I. S., et al. Evaluation of subvalvular aortic stenosis in children: a 16-year single-center experience. *Pediatr Cardiol* 2013; **34**: 1409–14.

Vincent W. R., Buckberg G. D., and Hoffman J. I. Left ventricular subendocardial ischemia in severe valvar and supravalvar aortic stenosis: a common mechanism. *Circulation* 1974; **49**: 326–33.

Vlahos A. P., Marx G. R., McElhinney D., et al. Clinical utility of Doppler echocardiography in assessing aortic stenosis severity and predicting need for intervention in children. *Pediatr Cardiol* 2008; **29**: 507–14.

Supravalvular Aortic Stenosis

Stephanie N. Grant and Bruce E. Miller

Case Scenario

A 2 ½-year-old male with Williams syndrome is evaluated preoperatively prior to dental rehabilitation. He presented last week to the preoperative clinic for evaluation prior to repair of his supravalvular aortic stenosis; however, on examination he was found to have multiple dental caries and his cardiac surgery was rescheduled to first optimize his dental health. Current vital signs are heart rate 105 beats/minute, respiratory rate 22 breaths/minute, SpO_2 98% on room air, and blood pressure 120/60 mm Hg. He is very friendly but appears anxious while his vital signs are being checked.

A transthoracic echocardiogram obtained last week showed the following:

- *Supravalvular aortic stenosis gradient of 65 mm Hg*
- *Mild peripheral pulmonary artery stenosis*
- *Mild right ventricular hypertrophy*
- *Moderate left ventricular hypertrophy*
- *Normal biventricular function*
- *Coronary arteries could not be visualized*

Key Objectives

- Describe the characteristic phenotype of Williams syndrome.
- Understand the cardiac anomalies common in patients with Williams syndrome.
- Understand why Williams syndrome patients are at high risk for cardiac events during sedation and general anesthesia.
- Describe the preoperative planning necessary for patients with Williams syndrome.
- Describe perioperative hemodynamic goals for patients with supravalvular aortic stenosis.

Pathophysiology

What is Williams syndrome?

Williams syndrome (WS), also known as Williams–Beuren syndrome, was first reported in 1961 by Williams and subsequently in 1962 by Beuren; each described four children with similar phenotypes consisting of supravalvular aortic stenosis (SVAS), characteristic facial features, and developmental delay [1, 2]. The incidence of WS is 1 in 7500 to 10,000, with an equal distribution among males and females [3].

The syndrome is a multisystem disorder with a variable clinical presentation resulting from a microdeletion on chromosome 7q11.23 encompassing 27 genes including the *ELN* gene that codes for the protein elastin [3]. The microdeletion is usually sporadic but can be familial [4]. Other genes that are deleted within the region of the microdeletion are responsible for the other features commonly associated with WS. The systems most affected in WS include cardiovascular, renal, endocrine, and psychiatric. Patients with WS have a high risk of cardiac events and sudden death, especially during sedation and general anesthesia [5].

What is the significance of the elastin deficiency in WS patients?

The elastin deficiency is caused by deletion of one elastin allele, resulting in a significant reduction in the quantity of elastin produced by affected patients. Consequently, an elastin arteriopathy develops as the elastin in arterial walls is replaced by a proliferation of smooth muscle cells in the vascular media that causes obstructive, hyperplastic intimal lesions of medium and large arteries. Abnormal circumferential growth of arteries also contributes to luminal narrowing. Elastin deficiency is responsible for many of the cardiovascular abnormalities associated with WS [6]. The aorta and coronary, carotid, renal, and pulmonary arteries can be affected [7]. Stenosis occurs most commonly at the sinotubular junction of the aorta, causing SVAS.

What cardiac abnormalities are associated with WS?

Eighty percent of patients with WS have cardiovascular abnormalities, which are the leading cause of morbidity and mortality [8]. The most common cardiac malformation is SVAS, occurring in 45%–70% of patients with WS. Supravalvular aortic stenosis occurs at the sinotubular junction of the aorta due to a circumferential ridge of tissue that causes luminal narrowing [4]. (See Figure 17.1A and B.) Other cardiovascular abnormalities associated with WS patients include supravalvular pulmonary artery stenosis (SVPS), peripheral pulmonary artery stenosis, coronary artery obstructions, aortic valve defects, hypoplasia of the aorta, coarctation of the aorta, and renal artery stenosis [8]. Forty to fifty percent of patients have systemic hypertension, which may be caused by renal artery stenosis [4].

The etiology of coronary artery obstructions includes not only medial hypertrophy but also narrowing of the ostia by a thickened aortic wall, ostial obstruction due to superior displacement of the ostia to just below the sinotubular ridge of the aorta, fusion of the free edges of the coronary cusps to the site of SVAS, and accelerated atherosclerotic lesions and aneurysm formations due to exposure to high pressures in the presence of SVAS [9]. The degree of SVAS is not correlated to the degree of coronary artery involvement [10].

Clinical Pearl

Supravalvular aortic stenosis is the most common lesion in WS and occurs at the sinotubular junction. The degree of SVAS does not correlate with the degree of coronary involvement.

What abnormality of the electrical conduction system is common in WS patients?

Prolongation of the corrected QT (QTc) interval occurs in 13.6% of patients with WS [11]. Prolonged QTc may deteriorate into malignant ventricular arrhythmias, such as torsades de pointe or ventricular fibrillation, and may contribute to an increased risk of periprocedural morbidity and mortality. It is important to perform an electrocardiogram (ECG) on all patients with WS prior to an anesthetic to screen for evidence of QTc prolongation.

Clinical Pearl

It is important to perform an electrocardiogram on all patients with WS prior to an anesthetic to screen for evidence of QTc prolongation.

Does SVAS occur in patients without WS?

Supravalvular aortic stenosis can occur in patients without WS and is often due to point mutations in the *ELN* gene. Patients with nonsyndromic elastin arteriopathy can have the same cardiovascular manifestations as patients with WS but have a reduced incidence of prolonged QT interval [12].

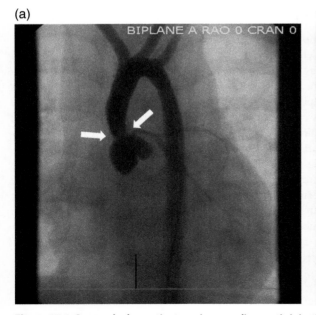
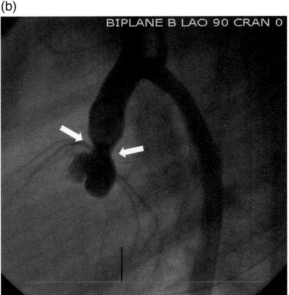

Figure 17.1 Supravalvular aortic stenosis: ascending aortic injection. An angiogram is performed in the ascending aorta in the AP (A) and lateral (B) projection. The arrows indicate the area of stenosis at the sinotubular junction. Courtesy of Russel Hirsch, MD.

What are the risk factors for cardiac arrest in WS?

Patients with WS have a 25- to 100-fold higher risk of sudden death compared to an age-matched normal population [13]. The risk of sudden death and major adverse cardiac events (MACE) – including cardiac arrest, need for postoperative mechanical circulatory support, and in-hospital mortality – are high during the perioperative period in patients with WS [5, 12]. An analysis of the Society of Thoracic Surgeons Congenital Heart Surgery Database in 2015 by Hornik et al. reported that 9% of WS patients undergoing cardiac surgery had MACE in the perioperative period with an in-hospital mortality rate of 5% [14]. Latham et al. reported cardiac arrest in 5% of WS patients undergoing an anesthetic [12].

The two conditions associated with a high risk of cardiac arrest are biventricular outflow tract obstructions and coronary artery obstruction by ostial or intraluminal stenosis [15]. Age <3 years and prolongation of the QTc interval have also been identified as risk factors for cardiac arrest. Biventricular outflow tract obstruction with right ventricular (RV) and left ventricular (LV) gradients >20 mm Hg increases the risk of cardiac arrest. The rate of cardiac arrest increases as the gradients of the biventricular outflow tract obstruction increase, with the highest risk with gradients >50 mm Hg [12].

Clinical Pearl

Risk factors for cardiac arrest in the perioperative period are biventricular outflow tract obstruction and coronary artery obstruction by ostial or intraluminal stenosis. The risk increases as the gradients of the biventricular outflow tract obstruction increase.

When is cardiac surgery indicated for patients with SVAS?

Supravalvular aortic stenosis repair is indicated when the patient develops symptoms related to the obstruction, there is a documented gradient >50 mm Hg, or there is evidence of coronary obstruction [16]. Approximately 30% of patients with WS who have SVAS will require surgical repair [4].

Anesthetic Implications

Why are patients with WS at high risk for cardiac arrest when undergoing anesthesia?

The balance between myocardial oxygen supply and demand may be in a continually precarious state in patients with WS, as the cardiovascular abnormalities associated with WS and their pathophysiologic consequences predispose patients to myocardial ischemia.

Factors that can negatively impact myocardial oxygen supply and demand in WS include the following:

- *Reduced coronary blood flow* can decrease myocardial oxygen supply. Stenotic lesions may be present within the coronary artery and at the ostium. Restriction of blood flow into the sinus of Valsalva can occur secondary to adhesion of aortic leaflets to the sinotubular junction.

- *Ventricular hypertrophy* secondary to ventricular outflow tract obstruction(s) can result in both decreases in coronary perfusion AND increases in oxygen demand. Decreases in subendocardial perfusion can occur due to increased left ventricular end-diastolic pressure (LVEDP) in the setting of decreased coronary perfusion pressure. Increased myocardial oxygen consumption leading to increased myocardial oxygen demand results from the increased muscle mass of ventricular hypertrophy.

Patients with WS are at high risk for cardiac arrest when undergoing anesthesia due to a further imbalance in myocardial oxygen supply and demand induced by anesthetic medications that alter hemodynamics. Several commonly utilized anesthetic medications may decrease systemic vascular resistance (SVR) and thus decrease coronary blood flow and myocardial oxygen delivery. Other anesthetic agents may increase heart rate and thus increase myocardial oxygen demand [9]. Changes in preload, afterload, contractility, and heart rate that occur during anesthesia may lead to myocardial ischemia and subsequent cardiovascular collapse in children with WS [12]. When hemodynamic instability occurs during anesthesia it progresses rapidly from initial hypotension and bradycardia to cardiac arrest that many times fails to respond to aggressive resuscitation measures [12, 15].

Clinical Pearl

Patients with WS are at high risk for cardiac arrest when undergoing sedation or general anesthesia due to an imbalance in myocardial oxygen supply and demand that can be further accentuated by anesthetic medications.

What physical characteristics are consistent with WS?

Patients with WS have distinct facial features, neurodevelopmental findings, and personalities, although considerable phenotypic variability exists. The facial features consistent with WS include a broad forehead, wide-set eyes, flat nasal bridge, short nose with a bulbous nasal tip, long philtrum, wide mouth with a thick vermillion of the lips, heavy cheeks, and a pointed chin [1, 17]. Children are often described as having pixie-like or elfin-like facial features. Many patients have a developmental delay, with an average IQ of 50–60; however, there are some patients who have IQs of 100 [17]. Patients have a distinct "cocktail party" personality, meaning that they do not display social anxiety and are very friendly. Despite this personality, patients often experience significant periprocedural anxiety that can evolve quickly into agitation in the setting of medical procedures. Most patients with WS have a normal airway exam; however, in some patients difficulty with mask ventilation and tracheal intubation may be noted secondary to a flattened midface, mild micrognathia, small teeth, and malocclusion [18].

What preoperative laboratory abnormalities might be expected?

Endocrine abnormalities frequently associated with WS include hypercalcemia, hypothyroidism, and diabetes mellitus type 2. Hypercalcemia is generally mild but can be severe during infancy. Subclinical hypothyroidism occurs in 15%–30% of patients with WS. Patients are often asymptomatic but general anesthesia may precipitate unwanted symptoms, including depression of myocardial function, poor temperature regulation, and impaired hepatic drug metabolism [17, 18]. Diabetes mellitus type 2 is more common in adults with WS than in children. A thyroid function panel and calcium and glucose levels should be checked at appropriate age intervals according to the American Academy of Pediatrics (AAP) guideline for patients with WS [19]. Additionally, these laboratory results should be checked preoperatively if there is clinical suspicion of an endocrinopathy or if they have not been recently measured.

What preoperative diagnostic studies should be reviewed?

Prior to an anesthetic, all available cardiac diagnostic studies should be reviewed, and a determination should be made as to whether additional studies need to be performed. At a minimum, an ECG and a transthoracic echocardiogram (TTE) should be performed.

- *The electrocardiogram* should be analyzed for changes indicative of prolonged QTc interval, evidence of ventricular hypertrophy suggestive of outflow tract obstructions, and changes indicative of myocardial ischemia, such as ST segment abnormalities.
- *Transthoracic echocardiography* should be reviewed and assessed for any degree of biventricular outflow

tract obstruction caused by SVAS and/or SVPS. While the contribution of peripheral pulmonary artery stenosis to RV outflow tract obstruction may be more difficult to assess with echocardiography, a finding of RVH in the absence of obvious SVPS may prove insightful. *Coronary artery obstructions are also difficult to assess by echocardiography, but ventricular wall motion abnormalities may be suggestive of coronary lesions.* Echocardiography can also be used to assess cardiac function.

- *Cardiac catheterization* with coronary and aortic angiography is the gold standard for assessing coronary arterial anatomy but carries risk. Catheter manipulations during cardiac catheterization may further compromise myocardial oxygen supply and demand balance by blocking coronary blood flow, inducing valvular regurgitation, producing dysrhythmias, or acutely increasing ventricular outflow tract obstruction(s). Contrast injection into a stenotic coronary artery may cause acute myocardial ischemia secondary to the lack of oxygen carrying capacity in contrast.
- *Cardiac magnetic resonance imaging* (MRI) and *computed tomography* (CT) scans also provide valuable data on cardiovascular anatomy.

Patients often require sedation or general anesthesia when diagnostic studies are performed. Therefore, the anesthesia team may be required to proceed with limited and incomplete data. An anesthetic must be planned as if the child's coronary blood flow and myocardial oxygen balance exist in a tenuous state.

Clinical Pearl

An anesthetic must be planned as if the child's coronary blood flow and myocardial oxygen balance exist in a tenuous state.

Where should this procedure be performed?

All patients with WS are at high risk for major adverse cardiac events during the perioperative period. Morbidity and mortality may occur in patients with WS despite the most cautious anesthetic care [12]. Elective procedures requiring anesthesia should be planned only after consideration by all participants of the balance between the benefits of the procedure and the potential adverse events of anesthetizing patients with WS. All elective procedures requiring sedation or general anesthesia should be performed at a medical center with pediatric cardiac care subspecialists who are available for immediate consultation [4]. The facility must be equipped to handle unexpected cardiac emergencies, initiate extracorporeal membrane oxygenation (ECMO) immediately, and adequately monitor the patient post-procedure.

> **Clinical Pearl**
>
> *Administration of sedation or general anesthesia for elective procedures should be performed at a medical center with immediate access to cardiac multidisciplinary specialists and the capability to provide ECMO support.*

What preoperative preparations are necessary for patients with WS?

Thorough preoperative preparations should take place before every elective procedure in patients with WS [4]. Brown et al. reported a low rate of cardiac events in 75 patients with WS who each had a preanesthetic evaluation. The authors of this review concluded that high anesthetic risk can be mitigated with appropriate planning and adherence to hemodynamic goals [20]. Patients with WS should attend a preoperative anesthetic clinic at least 1–2 weeks before scheduled procedures. The preanesthetic evaluation should include the following:

- *History and physical* should be conducted with attention to any new symptoms or signs of cardiac disease progression.
- *Cardiology consultation* and new imaging studies should be completed if necessary due to the progressive nature of cardiac lesions. Recently obtained diagnostic studies, such as an ECG, echocardiogram, or cardiac catheterization report, should be reviewed. An updated ECG and TTE within the previous 6 months prior to an anesthetic should be available.
- *Preoperative laboratory results* should be reviewed and ordered according to the AAP guidelines to evaluate for hypercalcemia, hypothyroidism, and hyperglycemia [19].
- *Fasting guidelines* should include continuing hydration with clear fluids until 2 hours before the procedure to preserve myocardial preload. The procedure should be scheduled as a first start case to avoid unexpected delays that would increase fasting times and to ensure adequate personnel resources are available for assistance if needed. If there are any delays, an intravenous (IV) line should be placed preoperatively for fluid administration.
- *The ECMO support team* should be notified about patients with severe SVAS gradients or known involvement of the coronary arteries.

- *Postoperative recovery location* and intensive care unit availability should be discussed prior to all procedures requiring sedation or general anesthesia.

If appropriate, a *child life* specialist should explain perioperative events to the patient.

> **Clinical Pearl**
>
> *The risk of perioperative cardiovascular events can likely be mitigated by proper planning, preparation, and coordination of resources. Ideally WS patients should attend a preoperative anesthetic clinic at least 1–2 weeks prior to the procedure.*

What risks should be discussed with the patient's parents before the case?

The anesthetic plan, along with the risks and benefits of anesthesia, should be discussed with the patient's family before the case. The significant potential for cardiac arrest and the possibility of ECMO support should be discussed before the procedure. Many parents of patients with WS are well aware of the risks while undergoing anesthesia and should be given the proper time to ask questions.

What are the perioperative hemodynamic goals for patients with WS?

For patients with WS, the perioperative goal is to decrease the incidence of myocardial ischemia by maximizing the oxygen supply and minimizing the myocardial oxygen demand. The hemodynamic goals are to maintain an age-appropriate heart rate, sinus rhythm, adequate preload, contractility, and SVR. It is important to avoid tachycardia, hypotension, and increases in pulmonary vascular resistance (PVR). Tachycardia increases myocardial oxygen consumption and decreases diastolic perfusion time. A decrease in coronary perfusion pressure resulting from hypotension will be especially hazardous when coronary artery lesions are present or when myocardial hypertrophy has developed. Changes in the hemodynamic status of patients should be treated quickly to avoid deterioration that may lead to myocardial ischemia and cardiac arrest.

> **Clinical Pearl**
>
> *The perioperative goal is to decrease the incidence of myocardial ischemia by maximizing the oxygen supply and minimizing the myocardial oxygen demand. Hemodynamic goals include maintaining an age-appropriate heart rate, sinus rhythm, preload, contractility, and SVR. Tachycardia and hypotension should be avoided.*

Does this patient need premedication for anxiolysis?

Despite the "cocktail party" personality of patients with WS, many patients have significant periprocedural anxiety and will require premedication for anxiolysis. It is important to avoid tachycardia related to anxiety because this increases myocardial oxygen demand, decreases the time needed for coronary perfusion in diastole, and may contribute to potential hemodynamic instability caused by anesthetic medications [4]. It is important for the anesthesiologist to develop rapport with the patient and family to establish trust. A calm environment should be created and maintained in the preoperative area. Many children with WS have hyperacusis and therefore loud noises should be avoided. Patients with WS have a near universal enjoyment of music, which can serve as a distraction [17]. Child life specialists can work with patients to create additional distractions. In addition to nonpharmacologic methods of anxiolysis, medications are often needed. Midazolam and dexmedetomidine are well tolerated and do not induce tachycardia.

What type of anesthetic should be performed — sedation, monitored anesthesia care, or general anesthesia?

Both patient and procedural factors should guide the depth of sedation and anesthesia [4]. Many patients with WS will require sedation or general anesthesia for noninvasive diagnostic studies. General anesthesia is the best plan for dental rehabilitation in this patient due to his age and likely inability to cooperate with the duration and discomfort of the procedure.

How should anesthetic induction be conducted for this patient?

Following premedication, establishment of a peripheral IV prior to induction of anesthesia not only allows for the careful titration of induction medications but also secures a route for the immediate treatment of any potentially adverse hemodynamic changes that may occur during induction. Thus, *an intravenous induction is strongly preferred over an inhalational induction* [21]. Topical local anesthetics or needleless local anesthetic applications can be used to minimize pain during placement of an awake IV line. Prior to induction, American Society of Anesthesiologists (ASA) standard monitors should be placed on the patient to provide continuous monitoring during induction. The ECG should be carefully monitored

for any changes in the appearance of the ST segments. During induction of anesthesia a balanced technique should be used in which small incremental doses of a combination of medications are given until the desired plane of sedation or anesthesia is reached. Anesthetic medications should be selected that avoid tachycardia, hypotension, and myocardial depression to minimize the risk of myocardial ischemia. Narcotics, such as fentanyl, have been successfully used for induction. Ketamine maintains SVR and contractility but when used in larger doses may increase the heart rate. Nevertheless, ketamine has been used successfully for induction of patients with WS. In this case the use of neuromuscular blockade would be useful to facilitate placement of a nasal endotracheal tube for a dental procedure. Care should be taken to achieve an adequate anesthetic depth prior to intubation to avoid undue tachycardia.

If a patient is uncooperative and an IV is unable to be placed prior to induction, an inhalational induction is possible; however, a greater chance for hemodynamic instability exists. Inhalational anesthetics cause a decrease in the SVR and subsequent hypotension. Propofol should also be avoided for this reason. If an inhalational induction is necessary, additional anesthesia providers should be readily available to assist if needed. If a patient decompensates with loss of a perfusing heart rhythm during induction or any time during the perioperative period, Pediatric Advanced Life Support protocols should be initiated, advancing to ECMO if necessary.

> **Clinical Pearl**
>
> *Careful intravenous titration of small incremental doses of a combination of medications seems to be the safest technique for induction of general anesthesia. The ECG should be carefully monitored for any changes in the appearance of the ST segments.*

In addition to standard ASA monitoring, what other monitors should be available for this patient?

Depending on the degree of ventricular outflow tract obstruction(s) and coronary artery involvement, additional monitoring may be needed. A 5-lead continuous ECG should be used for all patients with WS and ST segments monitored closely for any change. External defibrillation pads should be available. Placement of an arterial line should be considered for all patients with WS, with the decision for placement based on the severity of cardiac disease, hemodynamic status during induction, and procedure to be performed. Placement of an arterial line prior to induction may be considered in patients with severe biventricular outflow tract obstructions and coronary artery stenosis. This should be placed after an IV line has been established, and sedation may be given for its placement. The patient in this case is at high risk for cardiac arrest because his SVAS gradient is >50 mm Hg, and therefore placement of an arterial line before induction would not be unreasonable, if feasible.

How should anesthetic maintenance be conducted for this patient?

After a hemodynamically stable induction, low concentrations of volatile anesthetics can be used for maintenance as part of a balanced anesthetic technique. If hypotension develops, phenylephrine, norepinephrine, and vasopressin infusions or boluses can be used to improve blood pressure without increasing the heart rate. Medications that prolong the QT interval, such as ondansetron, should be avoided in patients with prolonged QTc to prevent further deterioration into malignant ventricular arrhythmias. (See Chapter 49.) Narcotic medications should be titrated to blunt painful procedural stimuli to prevent tachycardia. Regional anesthesia techniques should be considered for postoperative pain management for appropriate procedure. A multimodal approach to analgesia is also helpful, utilizing IV acetaminophen and other nonnarcotic modalities.

Where should this patient recover after the procedure? Can this case be performed as an outpatient?

Regardless of the type of procedure performed, WS patients may need to be admitted for postoperative monitoring depending on the severity of cardiac involvement and any intraoperative events. Patients with WS should have continuous monitoring with ECG, pulse oximetry, and blood pressure until the patient recovers their baseline level of cognition [21]. Parental presence in the postanesthesia care unit may help to relieve anxiety. Patients with known risk factors for perioperative cardiac arrest – biventricular outflow tract obstructions and/or coronary artery stenosis – should be admitted for postoperative monitoring in a unit with continuous telemetry. Patients with severe biventricular outflow tract obstruction and coronary artery stenosis should be admitted to an intensive care unit for monitoring. Patients without significant cardiac involvement may be discharged after low-risk procedures, such as dental rehabilitation or an esophago-duodenoscopy, after return to baseline.

If a patient has had previous uneventful anesthetics, does this impact the approach to anesthetic care?

All patients with WS are considered high-risk for cardiac events during sedation or general anesthesia regardless of past anesthetic history. The natural history of cardiac lesions in WS includes progression of SVAS lesions and possible spontaneous resolution of branch or peripheral pulmonary artery stenosis lesions [8]. Cardiac lesions may have worsened since the last anesthetic placing the patient at higher risk for myocardial ischemia. *Therefore, the same resources should be available for all patients with WS during every anesthetic.*

Clinical Pearl

All patients with WS are considered high risk for cardiac events during sedation or general anesthesia regardless of past anesthetic history. The natural history of cardiac lesions in WS includes progression of SVAS lesions.

What if the child has had prior cardiac surgery and the coronaries are "fixed"?

If a child has had an anatomic repair of known coronary defects, a recent CT or MRI may provide reassurance; however, it is important to remain vigilant. Patients with WS may have occult coronary artery abnormalities even with the absence of echocardiographic or angiographic evidence [12]. All patients with WS have the possibility of undiagnosed coronary artery disease.

Is it acceptable to perform a subsequent procedure at a community hospital?

All patients with WS are at high risk for major adverse cardiac events while undergoing a general anesthetic [12, 20]. Since cardiac morbidity and mortality may occur despite careful planning and the most cautious vigilant care, patients with WS should receive anesthetic care at tertiary care medical centers where immediate access to cardiac multidisciplinary specialists and the capability to provide ECMO support exists[12].

References

1. J. C. P. Williams, B. G. Barratt-Boyes, and J. B. Lowe. Supravalvular aortic stenosis. *Circulation* 1961; 24: 1311–18.

2. A. J. Beuren, J. Apitz, and D. Harmjanz. Supravalvular aortic stenosis in association with mental retardation and a certain facial appearance. *Circulation* 1962; 26: 1235–40.

3. P. Stromme, P. G. Bjornstad, and K. Ramstad. Prevalence estimation of Williams syndrome. *J Child Neurol* 2002; **17**: 269–71.

4. M. D. Twite, S. Stenquist, and R. J. Ing. Williams syndrome. *Pediatr Anesth* 2019; **29**: 483–90.

5. D. Taylor and W. Habre. Risk associated with anesthesia for noncardiac surgery in children with congenital heart disease. *Pediatr Anesth* 2019; **29**: 426–34.

6. A. K. Ewart, C. A. Morris, D. Atkinson, et al. Hemizygosity at the elastin locus in a developmental disorder, Williams syndrome. *Nat Genet* 1993; **5**: 11–16.

7. Z. Urbán, J. Zhang, E. C. Davis, et al. Supravalvular aortic stenosis: genetic and molecular dissection of a complex mutation in the elastin gene. *Hum Genet* 2001; **109**: 512–20.

8. R. T. Collins, P. Kaplan, G. W. Somes, et al. Long-term outcomes of patients with cardiovascular abnormalities and Williams syndrome. *Am J Cardiol* 2010; **105**: 874–8.

9. P. E. Horowitz, S. Akhtar, J. A. Wulff, et al. Coronary artery disease and anesthesia-related death in children with Williams syndrome. *J Cardiothorac Vasc Anesth* 2002; **16**: 739–41.

10. V. C. Baum and J. E. O'Flaherty. *Anesthesia for Genetic, Metabolic, and Dysmorphic Syndromes of Childhood*. 3rd ed. Philadelphia: Wolters Kluwer 2015; 475–6.

11. R. T. Collins, P. F. Aziz, M. M. Gleason, et al. Abnormalities of cardiac repolarization in Williams syndrome. *Am J Cardiol* 2010; **106**: 1029–33.

12. G. J. Latham, F. J. Ross, M. J. Eisses, et al. Perioperative morbidity in children with elastin arteriopathy. *Pediatr Anesth* 2016; **26**: 926–35.

13. A. Wessel, V. Gravenhorst, R. Buchhorn, et al. Risk of sudden death in the Williams-Beuren syndrome. *Am J Med Genet* 2004; **127A**: 234–7.

14. C. P. Hornik, R. T. Collins, R. D. B. Jaquiss, et al. Adverse cardiac events in children with Williams syndrome undergoing cardiovascular surgery: an analysis of the Society of Thoracic Surgeons Congenital Heart Surgery Database. *J Thorac Cardiovasc Surg* 2015; **149**: 1516–22.

15. L. M. Bird, G. F. Billman, R. V. Lacro, et al. Sudden death in Williams syndrome: report of ten cases. *J Pediatr* 1996; **129**: 926–31.

16. A. R. Castañeda, R. A. Jonas, J. E. Mayer, et al. *Cardiac Surgery of the Neonate and Infant*. 1st ed. Philadelphia: W.B. Saunders, 1994; 327–32.

17. B. R. Pober. Williams-Beuren syndrome. *N Engl J Med* 2010; **362**: 239–52.

18. J. Medley, P. Russo, and J. D. Tobias. Perioperative care of the patient with Williams syndrome. *Pediatr Anesth* 2005; **15**: 243–7.

19. Committee on Genetics. American Academy of Pediatrics: healthcare supervision for children with Williams syndrome. *Pediatrics* 2001; **107**: 1192–204.

20. M. L. Brown, V. G. Nasr, R. Toohey, et al. Williams syndrome and anesthesia for non-cardiac surgery: high risk can be mitigated with appropriate planning. *Pediatr Cardiol* 2018; **39**: 1123–8.

21. R. T. Collins, M. G. Collins, M. L. Schmitz, et al. Peri-procedural risk stratification and management of patients with Williams syndrome. *Congenit Heart Dis* 2017; **12**: 133–42.

Suggested Reading

Brown M. L., Nasr V. G., Toohey R., et al. Williams syndrome and anesthesia for non-cardiac surgery: high risk can be mitigated with appropriate planning. *Pediatr Cardiol* 2018; **39**: 1123–28.

Burch T. M., McGowan F. X., Kussman B. D., et al. Congenital supravalvular aortic stenosis and sudden death associated with anesthesia: what's the mystery? *Anesth Analg* 2008; **107**: 1848–54.

Collins R. T., Collins M. G., Schmitz M. L., et al. Peri-procedural risk stratification and management of patients with Williams syndrome. *Congenit Heart Dis* 2017; **12**: 133–42.

Latham G. J., Ross F. J., Eisses M. J., et al. Perioperative morbidity in children with elastin arteriopathy. *Pediatr Anesth* 2016; **26**: 926–35.

Matisoff A. J., Olivieri L., Schwartz J. M., et al. Risk assessment and anesthetic management of patients with Williams syndrome: a comprehensive review. *Pediatr Anesth* 2015; **25**: 1207–15.

Pober B. R. Williams-Beuren syndrome. *N Engl J Med* 2010; **362**: 239–52.

Twite M. D., Stenquist S., and Ing R. J. Williams syndrome. *Pediatr Anesth* 2019; **29**: 483–90.

Hypertrophic Cardiomyopathy

Chapter 18

Bridget Pearce

Case Scenario

A 5-year-old boy with a history of hypertrophic cardiomyopathy is booked for an emergency post-tonsillectomy bleed after he presents to the emergency department spitting out blood. Five days ago, he underwent an elective tonsillectomy and adenoidectomy and preoperative evaluation at that time included an electrocardiogram that showed normal sinus rhythm and biventricular hypertrophy.

Following the adenotonsillectomy and an uneventful postoperative recovery, he was discharged home. This morning he woke up and started vomiting blood. He is awake and alert but anxious. His current blood pressure is 80/40 mm Hg, heart rate is 145 beats/minute, and hemoglobin is 10 g/dL. He takes metoprolol daily but did not take his medication this morning.

Transthoracic echocardiography prior to adenotonsillectomy demonstrated:

- *Severe hypertrophic cardiomyopathy with hyperdynamic left ventricular systolic function*
- *Mildly impaired left ventricular relaxation*
- *Severe asymmetric septal hypertrophy*
- *Left ventricular outflow gradient 40 mm Hg at rest and 60 mm Hg with Valsalva*

Key Objectives

- Describe the genetics and pathophysiology of hypertrophic cardiomyopathy.
- Identify the clinical symptoms and diagnosis of hypertrophic cardiomyopathy.
- Discuss an appropriate preoperative evaluation of patients with hypertrophic cardiomyopathy.
- Describe anesthetic considerations for elective or emergent procedures in patients with hypertrophic cardiomyopathy.

Pathophysiology

What is hypertrophic cardiomyopathy?

Hypertrophic cardiomyopathy (HCM) is the most common autosomal dominant cardiac disease and is characterized by asymmetric septal hypertrophy. It is a genetically heterogeneous disease characterized by myocyte disarray, intermittent left ventricular outflow obstruction (LVOTO), diastolic dysfunction, and sudden cardiac death (SCD) [1].

What are the genetics of HCM?

Hypertrophic cardiomyopathy is genetically heterogeneous due to incomplete penetrance and variable expressivity. It is estimated that as many as 1 in 200 people may carry the gene but only 1 in 500 develop the disease [2]. Along with incomplete penetrance, HCM has variable expressivity. For example, some patients with HCM can have septal hypertrophy but no left ventricular (LV) outflow gradient and normal sinus rhythm, while others have near complete outflow tract obstruction or life-threatening arrhythmias.

The genetic heterogeneity leads to a variable clinical presentation and many people remain asymptomatic and undiagnosed. It is estimated that 750,000 people in the United States have HCM but only 100,000 have been diagnosed. However, lack of symptomatology does not imply benign expression of this disease. Sudden cardiac death (SCD) has occurred when neither the patient nor the provider was aware of the diagnosis. In fact, HCM is the leading cause of SCD in young athletes and the diagnosis is typically established postmortem. A thorough understanding of the pathophysiology is needed to safely care for a patient with HCM.

Clinical Pearl

Asymptomatic and undiagnosed patients with HCM may present for an anesthetic, but lack of symptomatology does not imply benign expression of the disease.

113

What genes are involved?

Mutations in at least 11 genes that encode proteins of the cardiac sarcomere are responsible for HCM [3]. The majority of mutations are missense with a single amino acid substitution, but there are also insertions, deletions, and splice mutations that result in abnormal proteins being incorporated into the cardiomyocyte contractile apparatus. Both actin and myosin filaments of the sarcomere may be involved. Most frequently, the mutation involves the β-myosin heavy chain but there are as many as 1400 variants and every part of the contractile apparatus can be abnormal. The myriad of sarcomere proteins involved contributes to the heterogeneity of clinical expression.

What are the effects on the myocardium?

Abnormal sarcomere proteins can alter actin–myosin crossbridge cycling, potentially affecting both contraction and relaxation. These altered physical and functional properties of the sarcomeres cause abnormal growth, disorganized architectural patterns, and myocyte disarray [4]. Abnormal growth leads to septal hypertrophy, the hallmark of the disease. Disturbed cardiomyocyte architecture may result in rhythm disturbances and the abnormal sarcomere function can result in decreased cardiac relaxation.

What is the pathophysiology of HCM?

Hypertrophic cardiomyopathy is predominantly an obstructive disease. Obstruction occurs when there is mechanical impedance to outflow of blood from the LV, produced by the hypertrophied septum and systolic anterior motion (SAM) of the mitral valve. The mechanism of SAM is multifactorial and includes decreased LV diameter, Venturi effect, and twisting mechanism of the ventricle during systole. The enlarged septum and dysfunctional mitral valve result in distortion of the LV cavitary anatomy, which impedes blood flow from the ventricle. In addition, the mitral leaflets may fail to coapt in a normal fashion, causing regurgitation. (See Figure 18.1.)

What are the symptoms of HCM?

Symptoms of the disease may include dyspnea, angina, syncope, and palpitations. Children may present with asthma-like symptoms and fail to keep up with their peers. Infants may present with failure to thrive, tachypnea, and diaphoresis with feeding.

Why do these patients have dyspnea?

In patients with HCM, diastolic dysfunction and/or mitral regurgitation may lead to increased left atrial pressure

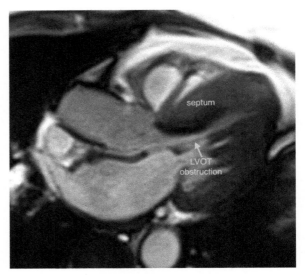

Figure 18.1 Hypertrophic cardiomyopathy. Magnetic resonance imaging of severe hypertrophic cardiomyopathy resulting in left ventricular outflow tract obstruction. Courtesy of Michael Taylor, MD.

(LAP). Dyspnea occurs when the elevated LAP impedes pulmonary venous outflow leading to congestion of the lungs. Higher pulmonary capillary pressure drives fluid into the interstitium, impeding diffusion of oxygen and resulting in symptomatic shortness of breath.

Why do patients with HCM experience angina?

The etiology of angina in HCM is subendocardial ischemia from an imbalance of myocardial oxygen supply and demand. Oxygen demand is increased due to the myocardial hypertrophy; more muscle mass requires additional oxygen for actin–myosin crossbridge cycling. Even though myocardial oxygen demand is higher, capillary density is 33% lower compared to the normal heart, and this too results in lower oxygen delivery [5]. In addition, when LV end-diastolic pressure is elevated due to diastolic dysfunction, the pressure gradient driving coronary flow is diminished, and flow through the coronary arteries decreases, thereby further reducing oxygen supply. The result of the supply/demand imbalance is subendocardial ischemia, experienced subjectively as angina.

Why do HCM patients have syncope?

Syncope is due to inadequate cerebral perfusion. With HCM, decreased cardiac output (CO) and insufficient cerebral perfusion can occur from either increased LVOTO or dysrhythmias.

What is the etiology of palpitations in HCM patients?

Rhythm disturbances are frequently observed with HCM, including sinus pauses, intermittent atrioventricular (AV) block, premature atrial and ventricular contractions, atrial fibrillation and flutter, and supraventricular and ventricular tachycardia. Sudden cardiac death is predominantly caused by ventricular fibrillation during intense physical exertion or stress despite a normal sinus rhythm at baseline.

How is HCM diagnosed?

Transthoracic echocardiography (TTE) is the gold standard for diagnosis of HCM. Asymmetric septal hypertrophy is the hallmark and LV function is typically preserved.

- *For adults*, septal wall thickness of >15 mm in the absence of abnormal loading conditions is a diagnostic criterion [1].
- *For children*, the criterion is a maximal LV wall thickness with a Z score >2 (greater than 2 standard deviations above average, corrected for body surface area) [6].

Pertinent features of the history include the patient's symptoms and any family history of HCM. Additionally, patients suspected to have HCM should undergo an electrocardiogram (ECG) to rule out dysrhythmias.

Cardiac magnetic resonance imaging (MRI) has been utilized to aid in the diagnosis of patients where TTE has yielded equivocal results due to poor acoustic windows or hypertrophy localized to regions not well visualized by TTE. Late gadolinium enhancement on MRI is indicative of myocardial fibrosis, which likely represents areas subjected to poor perfusion and subendocardial ischemia [7].

Genetic testing is an option, but the heterogeneity of the disease and variable penetrance make interpretation of the results difficult. In addition, recent studies indicate that identifying a particular sarcomere abnormality does not predict prognosis and cannot be used to guide treatment [8].

Clinical Pearl

Transthoracic echocardiography is the gold standard for diagnosis of HCM. Asymmetric septal hypertrophy is the hallmark and LV function is typically preserved.

What is the difference between HCM and HOCM?

Hypertrophic cardiomyopathy and hypertrophic obstructive cardiomyopathy (HOCM) are different expressions of the same disease. In a resting state, a ventricle may have asymmetric hypertrophy without obstruction defined as HCM; but obstruction can be provoked by different physiologic states and hence become HOCM. Tachycardia, hypovolemia, and hypotension may all cause outlet obstruction in these patients. With outlet obstruction, CO is impaired, leading to a downward spiral of hypotension, inadequate perfusion of the cerebral and cardiac vessels, syncope, ischemia, dysrhythmias, and death.

Clinical Pearl

In a resting state, a ventricle may have asymmetric hypertrophy without obstruction defined as HCM; obstruction can be provoked by different physiologic states and hence become HOCM. Tachycardia, hypovolemia, and hypotension may all cause LVOT obstruction in these patients.

What happens when a patient with HCM becomes tachycardic?

Increased heart rate is deleterious in a patient with HCM for a number of reasons.

- Diastolic time decreases, allowing less time for isovolumetric LV filling. Ventricular diameter decreases and LVOTO is provoked.
- Shortened ventricular relaxation time impairs oxygen delivery because coronary perfusion occurs during diastole.
- Finally, tachycardia increases workload because the myocardium develops tension more frequently each minute, thereby increasing oxygen demand. The net result is a supply/demand imbalance that increases the risk for subendocardial ischemia.

What happens when these patients become hypovolemic?

If a patient has a decrease in intravascular volume, preload diminishes, and consequently both LV filling and diameter decrease, causing LVOTO. Impaired venous return will elicit reflex mechanisms to maintain CO, resulting in tachycardia that further exacerbates the situation.

How does a HCM patient decompensate when he or she becomes hypotensive?

The decrease in both systolic and diastolic blood pressures is problematic. Elevated afterload mechanically stents open the outflow tract, helping to maintain ventricular geometry. Lower systolic blood pressures can result in outflow tract collapse, provoking or worsening the obstruction. Lower diastolic pressure decreases coronary perfusion, limiting oxygen delivery to the myocardium.

How is HCM medically treated?

The main goal of treatment is to decrease or prevent outlet obstruction. Medical aims are as follows:

- *Maintain low-normal heart rate* to allow for a longer ventricular filling time and hence improved coronary perfusion.
- *Avoid increases in sympathetic stimulation* to decrease and/or prevent obstruction during ejection.
- *Prevent dysrhythmias.*
- *Decrease diastolic dysfunction.*

β-Adrenergic receptor blockade for negative inotropy and chronotropy has been the mainstay of pharmacologic treatment. Virtually all patients diagnosed with HCM will take ß-blockers unless there is a contraindication. Calcium channel blockers are used with caution. Their negative inotropic and lusitropic properties are helpful, but they both vasodilate and venodilate, decreasing both preload and afterload. Disopyramide is sometimes used as an anti-arrhythmic and to decrease contractility. Amiodarone may also be used to suppress dysrhythmias.

Lifestyle modification is part of the treatment plan. Avoidance of dehydration, caffeine, and competitive sports is advisable. Both genetic and family counseling is helpful for patients and families with the diagnosis.

Clinical Pearl

The main goal of treatment for HCM patients is to decrease or prevent LVOT obstruction.

Are there surgical therapies to address HCM?

Surgical myectomy can be performed, in which a portion of the hypertrophied muscle is excised from the ventricular septum, enlarging the outflow tract. It is the primary therapeutic option for patients who are refractory to pharmacologic intervention and have a LVOT gradient >50 mm Hg at rest or with provocation [9]. An additional benefit with myectomy is that the mitral apparatus may function in a more normal fashion if SAM and mitral regurgitation are improved.

Catheter-based alcohol ablation performed in the cardiac catheterization laboratory is a potential alternative to surgical myectomy. Alcohol is injected into an artery supplying the septum, causing transmural myocardial infarction, reducing septal wall thickness, and enlarging the

LVOT diameter. Patients can avoid cardiopulmonary bypass with this technique, but potential side effects of alcohol treatment include increased conduction abnormalities and residual LVOT gradient.

Automatic implantable cardioversion devices (AICDs) have been used prophylactically to prevent SCD. Indications for AICD placement include a family history of SCD, unexplained syncope, repetitive episodes of nonsustained ventricular tachycardia, massive left ventricular hypertrophy (LVH), and extensive late gadolinium enhancement on MRI or fibrosis. Patients with systolic or diastolic heart failure who are refractory to pharmacologic and surgical treatment may require implantation of a left ventricular assist device (LVAD) or cardiac transplantation.

Anesthetic Implications

What are the potential anesthetic complications in a patient with HCM?

Anesthesia and surgery can cause catecholamine surges resulting in tachycardia, hypotension, and hypovolemia, all of which may exacerbate LVOTO. Adverse perioperative outcomes for HCM patients can include congestive heart failure, myocardial ischemia, systemic hypotension, dysrhythmias, and death [10]. Adverse events in children are more likely to occur in the setting of LVH, LVOTO, diastolic dysfunction, and a history of ventricular arrhythmias [11]. In an adult study, patients with HCM and a LVOTO gradient >30 mm Hg at rest and intraoperative hypotension had a higher rate of adverse events [12].

What preoperative evaluation is necessary for a 5-year-old patient with HCM presenting for elective adenotonsillectomy?

Identification of high-risk patients can help guide clinical management and ensure adequate allocation of resources. Evaluation includes a thorough family history to rule out familial SCD, patient history to ascertain symptomatology, and an ECG to rule out rhythm disturbances. In addition, a chest radiograph may show pulmonary edema or an enlarged cardiac silhouette due to LVH and/or left atrial enlargement. An echocardiogram or cardiac MRI is mandatory to determine if the patient has outflow obstruction at rest or with provocation, the latter typically elicited with a Valsalva maneuver to decrease venous return. Preoperative instructions should include short nil per os (NPO) times to minimize hypovolemia and maintain preload, and continuation of pharmacologic management such as ß-blockers to blunt the sympathetic nervous system (SNS) response to anesthesia and surgical stress.

The surgeon would like to perform the adenotonsillectomy at an outpatient facility. What is the most appropriate venue?

Caution should be exercised regarding location of surgery. Due to the increased risk of adverse events and death when patients with HCM are anesthetized, it is not advisable to anesthetize a patient with HCM in a free-standing ambulatory setting [12]. It is recommended to proceed in a specialized center with pediatric anesthesiologists, cardiologists and intensivists that are experienced in managing a child with HCM.

If a patient with HCM has an AICD, how should it be managed in the perioperative period?

The decision to disable an AICD is made by an electrophysiologist. The Heart Rhythm Society/American Society of Anesthesiologists (ASA) Expert Consensus Statement recommends that the decision be individualized for each patient and the decision made by the physician who monitors the patient's AICD function [13]. If the device is reprogrammed or deactivated, the Class I recommendation is for continuous cardiac monitoring during the entire time of deactivation and immediate availability of an automatic external defibrillator. The AICD should be reprogrammed in the immediate postoperative period. Prophylactic cutaneous defibrillator pads for cardioversion of a dysrhythmia is advisable if the patient's AICD has been disabled or if the patient does not have an AICD.

The patient has normal LV function with an LVOTO gradient of 40 mm Hg at rest and mild diastolic dysfunction. He is asymptomatic and ECG shows normal sinus rhythm. What perioperative monitoring would be appropriate?

Decisions regarding intraoperative monitoring are made according to the severity of HCM and nature of the operative procedure. For a minor procedure in a patient with insignificant LVOTO, standard ASA monitors with 5-lead ECG would suffice.

What are anesthetic management goals for a patient with HCM?

The primary anesthetic goal is to prevent LVOTO by avoiding tachycardia, hypotension and hypovolemia. This is achieved by reducing SNS activity as well as maintaining normal sinus rhythm, left ventricular filling and systemic vascular resistance. Fluid strategy is tailored to euvolemia, which will help maintain preload and afterload. Excessive fluid administration in the setting of a stiff ventricle with diastolic dysfunction can cause pulmonary edema.

How should anesthesia be induced in this patient for an *elective* case?

There is no single best agent for induction of anesthesia. The aim is to keep the hemodynamic goals in mind and titrate anesthetic agents accordingly. Although inhalation induction with sevoflurane might be an option in the patient with a mild form of HCM, it is important to recognize that an inhalational induction with sevoflurane can cause significant increases in heart rate and a reduction in SVR, both of which may place the patient at risk for cardiac ischemia. In addition, without intravenous (IV) access it will not be possible to rapidly treat hypotension or rhythm abnormalities. If the child has IV access, small doses of propofol slowly titrated to maintain stable hemodynamics may be an option. However, a large bolus dose of propofol is not advisable as venodilation and vasodilation can decrease preload and afterload. If SVR drops, small doses of phenylephrine (0.5–1 mcg/kg) can be used. Etomidate is a safe choice because it has a stable cardiovascular profile, but it should be administered with another anesthetic agent such as fentanyl to aid in blunting the sympathetic response to endotracheal intubation.

Prior to direct laryngoscopy, the SNS can be attenuated with a short-acting ß-blocker (e.g., esmolol) or short-acting opioid such as remifentanil. In most cases, if muscle relaxation is required, a nondepolarizing agent such as vecuronium or rocuronium can be used, but caution is advised with agents such as atracurium that cause histamine release and hypotension. If a rapid-acting agent is needed, succinylcholine is an option, but it may cause bradycardia or asystole. If the fall in heart rate is hemodynamically significant, glycopyrrolate or atropine can be administered. The use of glycopyrrolate may be preferable to atropine as it can accomplish the goal of treating bradycardia while minimizing the risk of incurring tachycardia. It is also important to recognize that atropine causes a greater reduction in diastolic time than other ß-adrenergic agents. Ephedrine can be used to increase heart rate without compromising diastolic time.

What agents can be used for maintenance of anesthesia?

Maintenance of anesthesia may be accomplished with volatile agents. Sevoflurane has minimal effects on the cardiovascular system and may be preferable to isoflurane which has negative inotropic and vasodilatory properties. If volatile agents are not tolerated, IV adjuncts can be used to maintain the depth of anesthesia necessary for the operative procedure. Benzodiazepines are desirable given their anxiolytic and amnestic properties. Dexmedetomidine infusion can be useful because it blocks sympathetic stimulation and decreases heart rate, but bolus dosing can cause hypotension. In longer cases maintenance of muscle relaxation may be necessary, especially if the patient is unstable.

What are the goals during emergence from anesthesia?

An important goal during anesthetic emergence is to attenuate the SNS response as the child awakens. Titration of fentanyl or morphine, and administration of nonopioid analgesics such as IV acetaminophen or administration of dexmedetomidine, 0.5–1 mcg/kg, can ameliorate the catecholamine surge with emergence.

If the perioperative course is uneventful, how should postoperative disposition be determined?

Postoperative recovery of HCM patients depends on the severity of the disease, the type of procedure, and intraoperative course. Disposition to the post-anesthesia care unit is appropriate for patients with benign expressions of HCM undergoing minor surgery who have an uneventful anesthetic. For patients with more severe symptoms, major surgery and/or perioperative cardiovascular instability, the intensive care unit (ICU) is more appropriate. Many patients fall within that spectrum and the decision should

be made following a multidisciplinary discussion with the anesthesiologist, surgeon, and cardiologist/intensivist if available.

Postoperatively the patient is agitated and crying: what are the considerations and how should they be addressed?

Pain will increase catecholamines, contractility and heart rate so it is important to intervene in a timely fashion to avoid increased LVOTO. Opioid analgesics, benzodiazepines, and dexmedetomidine, alone or in combination, will help lower SNS activity. If the patient remains hyperdynamic and tachycardic despite adequate analgesia and anxiolysis, then a fast-acting ß-blocker (e.g., esmolol) can be given.

What are the anesthetic considerations in a HCM patient presenting with a post-tonsillectomy hemorrhage?

A HCM patient who has been hemorrhaging is likely to be hypovolemic and may be hemodynamically unstable with outlet tract obstruction and impending cardiovascular collapse. Hence, immediate preoperative fluid resuscitation is a must. Intravenous access should be placed, and a fluid bolus given, if necessary, prior to induction of anesthesia. In addition to being hypovolemic, the patient may also be anemic with decreased oxygen carrying capacity, which increases the risk of myocardial ischemia. Obtaining a hematocrit and blood typing and cross match should be done as soon as possible. Minimizing anxiety to prevent a SNS surge is important and may be accomplished with benzodiazepines or by utilizing support from child life specialists or distractions such as video games and movies. The parents should also be asked about compliance with cardiac medications.

If the patient has an AICD but cardiologists are not immediately available to reprogram the device, how should you proceed?

There is a risk of AICD malfunction when using monopolar electrocautery. The device may be inhibited by the monopolar electrocautery and fail to defibrillate when needed or may fire inappropriately when electromagnetic interference causes false detection of arrhythmias [14]. In an emergent situation, bipolar electrocautery should then be used, since it uses less current and will not interfere with the AICD unless directly applied to it.

What perioperative monitors should be used for this patient?

Standard ASA monitoring with 5-lead ECG should be placed prior to induction. Although an arterial line is useful for hemodynamic monitoring in a potentially unstable child, placement of an arterial line in an awake child can be challenging and cause further anxiety and catecholamine release. Additionally, with an emergent post-tonsillectomy bleed the priority is achieving control of bleeding. If arterial line placement is warranted, it should take place while surgical control of bleeding is occurring. Although transesophageal echocardiography is helpful to determine volume status as well as dynamic outflow obstruction, it is not feasible given the surgical site for this patient. Transthoracic echocardiography could be utilized instead if needed. Adequate peripheral venous access for volume resuscitation should be obtained as well. Decisions should be individualized based on the clinical and hemodynamic assessment of the patient.

What are the anesthetic goals?

The primary anesthetic goal is to prevent increases in LVOTO. Although the patient did not have symptomatic LVOTO before he started bleeding, the possibility that obstruction may have been provoked by hypovolemia, tachycardia, and hypotension must always be considered. Anemia exacerbates the situation by further increasing heart rate. The goal is to reduce SNS activity while maintaining normal sinus rhythm, left ventricular filling, and systemic vascular resistance. In addition, treating intravascular depletion and restoring hematocrit to normal levels should be undertaken.

What is an anesthetic induction strategy for this patient with post-tonsillectomy hemorrhage?

A rapid sequence induction is indicated to secure an airway with ongoing pharyngeal bleeding and a full stomach from swallowed blood. Etomidate is a safe choice for an IV induction agent. Propofol in this clinical scenario would not be advisable because it may not be safely titrated in a timely fashion. Bolus dosing of propofol in the hypovolemic patient with HCM may precipitate outflow obstruction that could lead to ventricular fibrillation. For muscle relaxation, succinylcholine or rocuronium can be used. It is important to keep in mind that succinylcholine can lead to significant bradycardia. To blunt the SNS response to airway instrumentation, judicious use of opioid analgesia may be used. Esmolol could be used (standard dosing at 0.5 mg/kg bolus with infusions of 50–300 mcg/kg/minute) to attenuate the SNS response to intubation but hypotension may occur with coexisting intravascular volume depletion.

The patient becomes hypotensive after induction: What are the concerns and possible actions?

Post-induction hypotension can precipitate outlet obstruction, decrease coronary perfusion, and evoke ventricular fibrillation. Timely treatment with a vasoconstrictor is essential to maintain afterload and coronary perfusion pressure. To increase SVR, the preferred agent is the α_1-adrenergic agonist phenylephrine, with a bolus dose of 1–2 mcg/kg and/or infusion of 0.1mcg/kg/minute. The use of inotropes such as epinephrine is inadvisable in HCM patients as epinephrine will increase contractility and heart rate and may precipitate cardiovascular collapse [1]. Caution should also be used with other ß-adrenergic agonists such as dopamine, dobutamine, ephedrine, and isoproterenol. If the response to phenylephrine is inadequate, vasopressin, a potent vasoconstrictor, is another option. An added benefit with direct vasoconstrictors is the reflex bradycardia elicited by the increase in blood pressure, which is beneficial with HCM physiology.

Post-induction hypotension can also be minimized by decreasing the concentration of volatile anesthetic agent. Giving a fluid bolus of crystalloid or packed red blood cells will expand intravascular volume and increase preload and afterload.

What is an appropriate ventilation strategy for this patient?

High inspiratory airway pressures during positive pressure ventilation will decrease venous return, and the effect is exaggerated with hypovolemia. This can be achieved by avoiding high positive end-expiratory pressure, maintaining physiologic ventilation and allowing resumption of spontaneous ventilation as soon as safely possible.

The patient becomes hypertensive when the mouth gag is placed: How might this be treated?

Caution should be used with direct vasodilators as they can worsen LVOTO and precipitate cardiovascular collapse. Vasodilators such as hydralazine and nitroprusside should be avoided. In addition to provoking outlet obstruction, they can also induce ischemia by lowering diastolic pressure. A safer approach to lowering blood pressure is to decrease SNS stimulation with higher volatile agent concentrations and opioid analgesics. After ensuring adequate anesthesia and analgesia, if the patient remains hyperdynamic, consider ß-blockers to lower blood pressure into the desired range.

Clinical Pearl

Caution is indicated with direct vasodilators because they can worsen LVOTO and precipitate cardiovascular collapse.

On arrival in the ICU the patient's ECG rhythm changes to atrial fibrillation with a heart rate of 140. What is the most appropriate therapeutic action?

Patients with HCM are dependent on active ejection of blood from the atria into the LV for adequate filling. Loss of coordinated atrial systole with atrial fibrillation can be catastrophic and the recommendation is immediate direct cardioversion to restore sinus rhythm [1]. Pharmacologic restoration to sinus rhythm does not have a favorable time course and is a second line of therapy.

References

1. L. C. Poliac, M. E. Barron, and B. J. Maron. Hypertrophic cardiomyopathy. *Anesthesiology* 2006; **104**: 183–92.
2. R. M. Cooper, C. E. Raphael, M. Liebregts, et al. New developments in hypertrophic cardiomyopathy. *Can J Cardiol* 2017; **33**: 1254–65.
3. B. J. Maron, M. S. Maron, and C. Semsarian. Genetics of hypertrophic cardiomyopathy after 20 years: clinical perspectives. *J Am Coll Cardiol* 2012; **60**: 705–15.
4. A. M. Varnava, P. M. Elliott, N. Mahon, et al. Relation between myocyte disarray and outcome in hypertrophic cardiomyopathy. *Am J Cardiol* 2001; **88**: 275–79.
5. B. Johansson, S. Morner, A. Waldenstrom, et al. Myocardial capillary supply is limited in hypertrophic cardiomyopathy: a morphological analysis. *Int J Cardiol* 2008; **126**: 252–7.
6. S. D. Colan, S. E. Lipshultz, A. M. Lowe, et al. Epidemiology and cause-specific outcome of cardiomyopathy in children. Findings from the Pediatric Cardiomyopathy Registry. *Circulation* 2007; **115**: 773–81.
7. M. S. Maron, B. J. Maron, C. Harrigan, et al. Hypertrophic cardiomyopathy phenotype revisited after 50 years with cardiovascular magnetic resonance. *J Am Coll Cardiol* 2009; **54**: 220–8.
8. B. J. Maron and M. S. Maron. Hypertrophic cardiomyopathy. *Lancet* 2013; **381**: 242–55.
9. B. J. Gersh, B. J. Maron, J. A. Dearani, et al. 2011 ACCF/AHA guideline for the diagnosis and treatment of hypertrophic cardiomyopathy: Executive Summary, a Report of the American College of Cardiology Foundation/American Heart Association Task Force on Practice Guidelines. *J Am Coll Cardio* 2011; **58**: 2703–38.
10. H. Hreybe, M. Zahid, A. Sonel, et al. Noncardiac surgery and the risk of death and other cardiovascular events in patients with hypertrophic cardiomyopathy. *Clin Cardiol* 2006; **29**: 65–8.
11. B. Norrish, N. Forshaw, C. Woo, et al. Outcomes following general anesthesia in children with hypertrophic cardiomyopathy. *Arch Dis Child* 2019; **104**: 471–5.
12. A. Dhillon, A. Khanna, M. S. Randhawa, et al. Perioperative outcomes of patients with hypertrophic cardiomyopathy undergoing non-cardiac surgery. *Heart* 2016; **102**: 1627–32.
13. G. H. Crossley, J. E. Poole, M. A. Rozner, et al. The Heart Rhythm Society (HRS)/American Society of Anesthesiologists (ASA) Expert Consensus Statement on the perioperative management of patients with implantable defibrillators, pacemakers and arrhythmia monitors. *Heart Rhythm* 2011; **8**: 1114–54.
14. J. D. Madigan, A. F. Choudhri, J. Chen, et al. C. Surgical management of the patient with an implanted cardiac device *Ann Surg* 1999; **230**: 639–47.

Suggested Reading

Dhillon A., Khanna A., Randhawa M. S., et al. Perioperative outcomes of patients with hypertrophic cardiomyopathy undergoing non-cardiac surgery. *Heart* 2016; **102**: 1627–32.

Norrish B., Forshaw N., Woo C., et al. Outcomes following general anesthesia in children with hypertrophic cardiomyopathy. *Arch Dis Child* 2019; **104**: 471–75.

Coarctation of the Aorta

Nicholette Kasman

Case Scenario

A 9-month-old former full-term male presents for repair of nonsyndromic craniosynostosis. He was diagnosed via fetal ultrasound with a discrete coarctation of the aorta and underwent complete surgical repair with end-to-end anastomosis on day 10 of life. Postoperative transthoracic echocardiogram prior to discharge showed no residual gradient. His mother states that he has been feeding and growing well but she did not keep his 6-month cardiology follow up appointment. Current vital signs are heart rate 140 beats/minute, respiratory rate 25 breaths/minute, and SpO$_2$ 97% on room air. The heart beat is regular with no perceptible murmur; the lungs are clear, and the abdomen is soft. He was seen in cardiology clinic today, and right upper extremity blood pressure was 105/70 mm Hg whereas blood pressure in the lower extremity was 70/40 mm Hg.

Transthoracic echocardiography revealed the following:

- *Mild aortic valve regurgitation*
- *Mildly decreased left ventricular systolic function with mild hypertrophy*
- *Turbulent flow below the subclavian artery origin; estimated peak systolic pressure gradient 27 mm Hg*

Key Objectives

- Understand the anatomy and physiology of coarctation of the aorta.
- Understand the natural history of coarctation of the aorta.
- Understand echocardiographic and catheterization data for evaluation of a coarctation gradient.
- Describe preoperative assessment and intraoperative management for this patient.
- Understand major concerns for craniosynostosis repair and how residual coarctation can affect anesthetic management.

Pathophysiology

What is the anatomy and physiology of coarctation of the aorta?

Coarctation of the aorta is defined as any form of narrowing of the aorta, but it is often a discrete narrowing of the aorta distal to the left subclavian artery, just past the point of insertion of the ductus arteriosus. It can occur in isolation or as part of a long segment of aortic arch hypoplasia, which can sometimes involve the transverse aortic arch. It is one of the most common forms of congenital heart disease, representing 4%–7% of cases [1]. If left untreated, aortic coarctation leads to chronic hypertension of the upper extremities, left ventricular (LV) pressure overload, LV hypertrophy, pulmonary edema, and the development of aortic collaterals. (See Figure 19.1A and B.)

What other cardiac defects can be associated with coarctation of the aorta?

The spectrum of clinical manifestations is highly variable and depends upon the presence of other associated lesions as well as the degree of obstruction at the level of the coarctation. In a series of severely symptomatic neonates isolated coarctation was seen in 40%, an associated ventricular septal defect (VSD) in 36%, and the remainder had more complex anomalies including atrioventricular septal defect, transposition of the great arteries, a hypoplastic ventricle, or double outlet right ventricle. Coarctation presenting in a child or an adult can occur either in isolation or with any other left-sided obstructive lesion such as bicuspid aortic valve, aortic valve stenosis, subaortic or supravalvular aortic stenosis. It can also be seen in patients with Turner syndrome or Shone complex. [1–3]. (See Chapter 20.)

(a)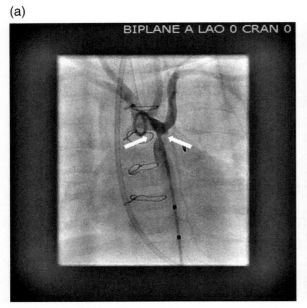

(b)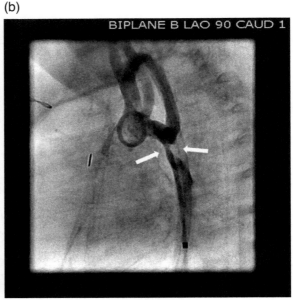

Figure 19.1 (A, B) Aortic coarctation: transverse aortic injection. An angiogram is performed in the AP and lateral projection. The arrows demonstrate the region of the recurrent coarctation at the aortic isthmus, distal to the origin of the left subclavian artery. Courtesy of Russel Hirsch, MD.

How is the diagnosis of coarctation of the aorta made?

The hallmark of coarctation of the aorta is upper extremity hypertension characterized by a differential gradient of at least 20 mm Hg between the systolic blood pressures of the upper and lower extremities. A neonate with coarctation may remain asymptomatic as long as the ductus arteriosus remains open; some neonates present in cardiogenic shock when the ductus closes. A delay in femoral pulses or auscultation of a cardiac murmur or click due to an associated defect may help the practitioner identify the coarctation. Patients may present with symptoms of left-sided heart failure including tachypnea, diaphoresis with feeds, hypotension, tachycardia, and hepatomegaly.

In children and adults aortic coarctation generally presents as hypertension. Murmurs from associated collateral vessels or other defects may be auscultated. Despite the differences in regional blood flow adequate perfusion is generally maintained due to the development of collateral circulation and by autoregulatory vasoconstriction in hypertensive areas and vasodilation in hypotensive areas. Most older patients are asymptomatic, but symptoms related to untreated hypertension such as headache, epistaxis and claudication can occur. If left untreated, the natural history involves the development of accelerated coronary artery disease, stroke, heart failure, and/or aortic dissection. The average survival age for people with untreated aortic coarctation is 35 years of age, with a 75% mortality rate by 46 years of age [4–5].

What echocardiographic and catheterization data can aid in evaluating the severity of coarctation?

Transthoracic echocardiography can establish the diagnosis of coarctation of the aorta by revealing areas of aortic narrowing and turbulent flow seen via color flow Doppler. Using continuous color flow Doppler, the maximum flow velocity and the pressure gradient across the narrowed area can be calculated. The presence of collateral vessels may be detected as well as associated cardiac anomalies. Pressure criteria for diagnosis include a trans-coarctation gradient >20 mm Hg or a gradient <20 mm Hg in the presence of collaterals or reduced cardiac output. Cardiac catheterization is considered the gold standard for diagnosis, with clinically significant aortic coarctation defined as a peak-to-peak pressure gradient difference ≥20 mm Hg. Given the invasive nature of catheterization, however, it is no longer indicated for diagnosis unless warranted for evaluation of associated defects. Although echocardiography is generally adequate for diagnosis in children, cardiac magnetic resonance imaging (MRI) or computed tomography (CT) imaging may be used as adjuncts in the evaluation of older children and adults as they not only clearly delineate the area and severity of coarctation but also describe associated collateral vessels [4, 5].

> **Clinical Pearl**
>
> *Cardiac catheterization is considered the gold standard for diagnosis, defining clinically significant aortic coarctation as a peak-to-peak pressure gradient difference ≥ 20 mm Hg. Given the invasive nature of catheterization, however, it is no longer indicated for diagnosis unless evaluation of associated defects warrants it.*

What is "critical" coarctation? When should coarctation of the aorta be repaired?

Newborns born with critical aortic coarctation (Figure 19.2) are dependent on blood flow through a patent ductus arteriosus (PDA) to provide systemic blood flow to the distal aorta. Because maintaining ductal patency is essential, prostaglandin (PGE₁) infusion is continued until the time of repair. As they lack significant collaterals, neonates and infants are at risk for depressed ventricular function caused by high LV afterload when the PDA closes. If a critical coarctation goes undiagnosed, the patient may present in cardiogenic shock when the PDA closes.

Children and adults meeting the following criteria are considered to have disease significant enough to warrant repair:

- Gradient between upper extremity and lower extremity systolic blood pressure >20 mm Hg or mean Doppler gradient >20 mm Hg
- Upper extremity to lower extremity gradient or mean Doppler gradient >10 mm Hg with either:
    ○ Decreased LV systolic function or aortic valve regurgitation
    ○ Collateral flow

Early intervention is thought to decrease the risk of developing long-standing hypertension and its associated sequelae [5].

> **Clinical Pearl**
>
> *A gradient between the upper and lower extremity systolic blood pressure or a peak-to-peak Doppler gradient of >20 mm Hg is the hallmark of aortic coarctation. However, a blood pressure gradient may not exist in the setting of collateral flow, aortic valve regurgitation, or decreased left ventricular systolic function.*

How is the decision made between a surgical or cardiac catheterization approach to treating aortic coarctation?

The treatment of choice for neonatal coarctation is surgical repair. Compared to balloon angioplasty, surgical repair is

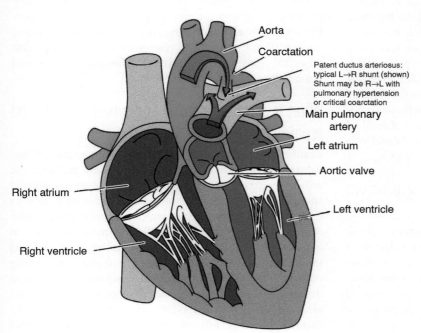

Figure 19.2 Coarctation of the aorta. Drawing by Ryan Moore, MD, and Matt Nelson.

Aorta

Coarctation

Patent ductus arteriosus: typical L→R shunt (shown) Shunt may be R→L with pulmonary hypertension or critical coarctation

Main pulmonary artery

Left atrium

Aortic valve

Left ventricle

Right atrium

Right ventricle

associated with fewer reinterventions, improved aortic arch growth, and a decreased risk of aneurysm formation and need for antihypertensive medication. While balloon angioplasty can be done in infants, it is essentially a palliative procedure in small, critically ill neonates with associated medical conditions that render them poor surgical candidates [1, 7]. Coarctation repair is generally performed via a left thoracotomy unless other associated cardiac defects will be simultaneously repaired on cardiopulmonary bypass via a median sternotomy. A variety of options for surgical repair exist including subclavian flap aortoplasty, aortic arch advancement with end-to-end or end-to-side reconstruction, tube graft interposition, and a resection of the coarctation with end-to-end anastomosis. Of these the latter is most commonly performed [7].

In older children the decision to treat aortic coarctation surgically versus catheterization lab intervention is more complex. Balloon angioplasty was introduced in the 1980s but was associated with a higher rate of recoarctation, aneurysm formation and aortic dissection. In the 1990s endovascular balloon-expandable stents were introduced in place of balloon dilation and have been associated with lower rates of recoarctation and aneurysm formation. An adult-sized stent can be placed in patients weighing >25 kg, and the stent can be redilated multiple times, eventually reaching adult size. This is not possible in neonates and infants, and simple balloon angioplasty remains the main transcatheter option for these patients [1, 3].

In patients >4 months of age but weighing <25 kg the decision to perform balloon angioplasty versus surgery depends upon the anatomy of the lesion and the expertise of the institution. Balloon angioplasty alone is associated with a higher rate of intimal tears and aneurysm formation compared with stent placement; however, in a patient with a discrete coarctation without evidence of arch hypoplasia it may be preferable to perform balloon angioplasty rather than a surgical approach via thoracotomy. Balloon angioplasty is, however, the first choice for treatment of residual or recurrent coarctation after surgical repair. Worldwide the preferred approach continues to be surgery [3, 5].

Does repair of aortic coarctation fix the problem or do residual concerns exist?

Despite successful surgical repair or transcatheter intervention, hypertension often persists. Hypertension is the most common sequela of coarctation, whether repaired or unrepaired. Systemic hypertension may not be consistently identifiable at rest and ambulatory blood pressure monitoring can be useful in identifying patients with a hypertensive response to exercise. Up to 80% of patients with prior coarctation intervention manifest an abnormally elevated upper extremity exercise blood pressure response and peak blood pressure is correlated with increased LV mass [4, 5].

Restenosis of the previously repaired or stented regions also occurs. In a retrospective comparison between balloon angioplasty and surgery for the treatment of neonatal coarctation in patients <4 months, 18% of patients who underwent surgery had recurrence of stenosis requiring follow-up angioplasty. Nevertheless, freedom from any intervention was significantly greater in the surgically treated cohort as opposed to the angioplasty cohort and the rate of complication was significantly lower [5, 6]. Among adult patients successfully treated for coarctation, long-term follow-up with MRI or CTA reveals that approximately 11% of patients may require reintervention for restenosis [4, 5].

In patients with a history of balloon angioplasty, aneurysms often occur in the ascending aorta. Patients who have undergone coarctation repair can develop aneurysms in the descending thoracic aorta or arch. Dissection can occur, presumably more likely in the setting of uncontrolled hypertension [5]. Multiple studies have demonstrated an increased frequency of intracranial aneurysm in adults with coarctation of the aorta as well. Approximately 10% of adult patients with coarctation of the aorta have intracranial aneurysms identified by MR angiography or CT angiography. Whether this is a byproduct of the coarctation itself or other factors such as hypertension is unclear [5].

What is evident is that lifelong follow up is needed not only for the prompt recognition and treatment of hypertension, cardiovascular disease, and postprocedural complications, but also for recurring or residual coarctation. Even with an excellent surgical repair or catheter-based intervention, hypertension remains common and predisposes the patient to myocardial infarction, stroke, and heart failure.

What is craniosynostosis and when should it be repaired?

Craniosynostosis is a condition in which one or more of the sutures in an infant's skull fuse prematurely and alter the growth pattern of the skull. It can occur as an isolated sporadic event or as part of a larger syndrome such as Crouzon or Apert syndromes which also involve hypoplasia of the mid-face, skull base and limb abnormalities. These associated problems can lead to issues such as elevated intracranial pressure (ICP), airway obstruction, and feeding difficulties as well as abnormal behavioral and psychological development. The most significant surgical risks are blood loss and venous air embolism. The repair is not merely cosmetic and is performed at an early age to allow normal brain growth and cognitive development [7, 8].

Anesthetic Implications

What preoperative evaluation is appropriate for this patient?

Preoperative evaluation should include a thorough assessment of preexisting medical conditions, medications, allergies, previous anesthetic or airway issues, relevant family history, and physical examination. Given this patient's prior coarctation repair and the existing noninvasive blood pressure (NIBP) gradient between upper and lower extremities, it is essential that during his cardiology visit an electrocardiogram, chest radiograph and transthoracic echocardiogram be obtained and reviewed.

With regard to the patient's craniosynostosis it is appropriate to look for clinical signs of increased ICP such as visual difficulties, nausea, vomiting, or somnolence. Although problems with increased ICP are unusual in infants with craniosynostosis, it can occur in older children or when fusion of multiple sutures exists. [7]

Preoperative laboratory evaluation should include a complete blood count and coagulation studies as well as a type and cross for packed red blood cells. Availability of blood should be confirmed prior to the start of the procedure and blood should be present in the operating room environment.

Does the restenosis of the coarctation need to be addressed prior to the craniotomy?

Given the patient's mildly diminished LV function and gradient between upper and lower extremity blood pressures, the results of the cardiology visit may prompt communication between physicians from neurosurgery, cardiology, and cardiac surgery regarding the appropriate sequence of interventions for this patient as he may need to undergo balloon angioplasty of the recoarctation in the cardiac catheterization laboratory prior to craniosynostosis repair. The existing upper extremity hypertension and relative hypotension below the level of the coarctation puts the patient at greater risk for perioperative complications during the craniosynostosis repair.

For a surgery involving significant blood loss, techniques such as permissive hypotension and acute normovolemic hemodilution have been employed in some centers. Neither has been found to be helpful in the setting of craniosynostosis repair mostly due to the small size of the patient, the increased risk of hemodynamic instability and the increased risk of venous air embolism. While neither permissive hypotension nor acute normovolemic hemodilution has gained widespread acceptance, hypertension should be avoided in the face of ongoing blood loss. In the presence of an aortic coarctation it will be important to maintain normal blood pressures above the coarctation and to avoid hypotension which would place the patient at risk for hypoperfusion of the kidneys, gastrointestinal tract, and spinal cord.

The general hemodynamic goals for craniosynostosis repair involve mild hypotension and euvolemia, attempting to decrease blood loss while maintaining adequate perfusion and minimal risk of venous air embolism. In this patient, however, the presence of the unrepaired recoarctation places the patient at risk for hypoperfusion to organs supplied by arteries distal to the recoarctation, thus an anesthetic strategy allowing mild hypotension may not be in the patient's best interest.

Clinical Pearl

The anesthetic goals for craniosynostosis repair include mild hypotension and euvolemia. The aim is to decrease blood loss while maintaining adequate perfusion and minimal risk of venous air embolism. The hemodynamic effects of the unrepaired recoarctation already put the patient at risk for hypoperfusion of the gastrointestinal tract, kidneys, and spinal cord and thus the use of deliberate mild hypotension may not be in the patient's best interest.

Are there special concerns that need to be communicated to the parents in the preoperative area?

On the day of surgery it should be confirmed that the patient is appropriately nil per os (NPO) and without recent signs of upper or lower respiratory infections or fevers. The patient's level of stranger anxiety should be assessed and if helpful an oral premedication such as midazolam may be administered. As with any preoperative evaluation, adequate time should be spent addressing any questions or concerns the parents have. Parents should be fully informed of the likelihood of transfusion. Although the child has already been through a major surgery and follow up visit to the catheterization lab, most likely without transfusion, there is a very high probability that during craniosynostosis repair he will require transfusion. The need for transfusion and potential development of coagulopathy may affect the ability to extubate the child at the end of the case.

What are the most significant concerns during a craniosynostosis repair?

The surgical approach to craniosynostosis repair depends not only upon which sutures are fused but also institutional experience. All approaches involve elevation of the vascular periosteum. Once the osteotomy is performed, blood loss is usually slow and continuous. Dural sinuses are another potential source of blood loss. Bleeding from the sinuses can be dramatic and require an immediate response. Given their small size at time of repair it is not unusual for a patient to lose 25%–50% of their blood volume during repair, sometimes more [7, 8].

The patient's small size increases the impact of blood loss as well as the metabolic effects of transfusion. Cardiovascular function in infants is more sensitive to calcium homeostasis as well as acidosis. With a smaller and relatively less compliant heart than an older child or adult an infant has less cardiovascular reserve so the relative impact of a potassium load from older blood that has been in storage has greater consequence.

The most significant intraoperative concerns for an infant undergoing craniosynostosis repair include blood loss, coagulopathy, hemodynamic instability, and venous air embolism. Other important issues in small children include glucose regulation, acidosis, calcium homeostasis, hemodilution, and temperature regulation.

Clinical Pearl

During surgical repair of craniosynostosis the most important risks are blood loss and venous air embolism. It is imperative to plan for significant blood loss and to have packed red blood cells readily available in the operating room environment.

What drugs could be utilized for induction and maintenance of anesthesia?

An inhalation induction of anesthesia followed by placement of a peripheral intravenous (IV) line is generally well tolerated. A balanced anesthetic including volatile agents, opioids and muscle relaxant can be used throughout the case. Neuromonitoring is not employed for these cases and the use of total intravenous anesthesia is usually unnecessary. The goal is a readily titratable anesthetic that can be altered to accommodate varying levels of surgical stimulation and changing hemodynamic conditions.

What monitoring would be appropriate?

Monitoring should include American Society of Anesthesiologists standard monitoring along with placement of an arterial line. Although the coarctation has been repaired the preference for a right radial arterial line over a left-sided arterial line still exists.

An NIBP cuff can be placed on the left arm or a lower extremity as well. Other indicators of adequate perfusion such as upper and lower extremity pulse oximeters would also be useful. Central venous pressure monitoring is not routine, but adequate access should be ensured for volume resuscitation, necessitating two peripheral IV lines at a minimum.

Although venous air embolism is a reported complication of craniosynostosis repair, the incidence of hemodynamically significant air embolism is rare. The patient should be carefully positioned, and table controls checked ahead of time so that the table can be put into Trendelenburg position quickly if necessary. Emergency drugs such as epinephrine diluted to 10 mcg/mL should be readily available. Sterile saline should be at hand for the surgeon to flood the field as necessary. Constant monitoring of end-tidal CO_2 is necessary and changes in end-tidal CO_2 or other signs of hemodynamic instability should be communicated to the surgeon immediately.

Although placement of a central venous line is not necessary for the repair, the evaluation of volume status should be a constant process via other mechanisms. Pulse pressure variation noted via the pulse oximeter and/or arterial line, maintenance of appropriate urine output and the development of a base deficit or lactic acidosis should be monitored and adequate volume resuscitation maintained. Regular arterial blood gases should be checked during the portion of the procedure involving significant blood loss. The hemoglobin and hematocrit may be deceptive in an underresuscitated child. It is not until one is already behind with volume resuscitation that a base deficit or lactic acidosis is observed. Although it is not possible to monitor cerebral near-infrared spectroscopy during a craniosynostosis repair, it may be helpful to place a sensor over the flank in an effort to optimize monitoring of lower extremity perfusion.

How does residual coarctation affect induction and management strategies?

If a blood pressure gradient exists between upper and lower extremities, it is important to know the patient's underlying baseline pressure both above and below the coarctation with the goal being to "keep him where he lives." Under such circumstances the surgery would be performed at a higher cerebral pressure than might be favored by the surgeon, but the potential need for additional blood transfusion and ideal surgical conditions is offset by the necessity of maintaining adequate kidney, spine, and gastrointestinal perfusion. Under such circumstances, regular monitoring of arterial blood gases becomes even more critical.

What inotropic or vasoactive infusions might be helpful?

Antifibrinolytics such as tranexamic acid have been shown to reduce blood loss and the need for transfusion in some studies. The loading dose of tranexamic acid varies between 10 and 100 mg/kg, followed by an infusion of 5–10 mg/kg/hour for the duration of the surgery. Although the use of a nicardipine infusion for potential control of residual upper extremity hypertension could be considered, an appropriate level of hemodynamic control can generally be achieved with a combination of inhaled anesthetic and narcotic [8].

Are there transfusion issues that are unique to infants?

Transfusion guidelines are similar in children and adults. Unless a child suffers from complex cyanotic heart disease, is premature, or requires invasive respiratory or hemodynamic support, transfusion for a hemoglobin level >10 g/dL is usually unnecessary. Transfusion for a hemoglobin level of 6 g/dL or below is indicated. In the setting of ongoing surgical blood loss, regular arterial blood gases along with other sources of clinical information help to guide transfusion. In small children it is helpful to calculate the estimated maximum allowable blood loss to utilize as a guideline along with regular arterial blood gases.

$$\text{Allowable blood loss} = [EBV \times (H_i - H_f)]/H_i,$$

where

H_i = initial hemoglobin and H_f = final hemoglobin
EBV = estimated blood volume.

All blood used in young children should be leukocyte-depleted, cytomegalovirus negative, and washed or stored less than 2–3 weeks. It should be warmed and filtered prior to administration to the patient.

If the apparent blood loss exceeds half of the patient's EBV, a new set of baseline labs should be sent *STAT* and the provider should consider ordering platelets or fresh frozen plasma (FFP). Although the need for red blood cell transfusion is common, the need for transfusion of platelets, FFP or cryoprecipitate occurs less frequently.

Nevertheless, platelet transfusion is appropriate if the blood loss approaches the patient's blood volume or if the platelet count is known to be <50,000. The usual therapeutic dose of platelets in children under 10 kg is 10 mL/kg. When INR is >1.5 times normal, effective hemostasis can generally be achieved with a minimum of 30% of the normal level of factor concentration. Administration of 10 mL/kg FFP is generally appropriate in small children. If fibrinogen levels drop below 80 mg/dL, one unit of cryoprecipitate per 10 kg of body weight or 0.1 unit/kg can be administered and should correct fibrinogen concentration by approximately 50 mg/dL [7].

Where should the patient recover after surgery and what concerns might the managing team have?

Patients are generally extubated after craniosynostosis repair. Factors that can delay extubation include large volume fluid shifts due to transfusion, facial swelling due to patient positioning or underlying airway obstruction concerns due to associated airway defects such as midface hypoplasia. Even if extubated, the patient should still be transferred to a unit with a high level of care. Postoperative coagulopathy is an ongoing concern. Children with a coarctation are at risk for hypertension even after repair, which may complicate postoperative hemostasis. Dramatically elevated levels of norepinephrine have been noted following coarctation repair and are thought to be due to baroreceptor adaptation. The use of nonsteroidal antiinflammatory drugs should be avoided. Attention should be paid to postoperative electrolyte disturbances; hyponatremia can result from intraoperative crystalloid infusions as well as syndrome of inappropriate antidiuretic hormone [4, 7].

References

1. E. B. Fox, G. J. Latham, F. J. Ross, et al. Perioperative and anesthetic management of coarctation of the aorta. *Semin Cardiothorac Vasc Anesth* 2019; **23**: 221–4.

2. J. R. Boris. Primary-care management of patients with coarctation of the aorta. *Cardiol Young* 2016; **26**: 1537–42.

3. L. M. S. Padua, L. C. Garcia, C. J. Rubira, et al. Stent placement versus surgery for coarctation of the thoracic aorta (review). *Cochrane Database Syst Rev* 2012; **5**: 1–18.

4. M. Astengo, C. Berntsson, A. A. Johnsson, et al. Ability of noninvasive criteria to predict hemodynamically significant aortic obstruction in adults with coarctation of the aorta. *Congenit Heart Dis* 2017; **12**: 174–80.

5. K. K. Stout, C. J. Daniels, J. A. Aboulhosn, et al. 2018 AHA/ACC Guideline for the management of adults with congenital heart disease. *J Am Coll Cardiol* 2019; **73**: e81–192.

6. A. C. Fiore, L. K. Fischer, T. Schwartz, et al. Comparison of angioplasty and surgery for neonatal aortic coarctation. *Ann Thorac Surg* 2005; **80**: 1659–65.

7. J. L. Koh and H. Gries. Perioperative management of pediatric patients with craniosynostosis. *Anesthesiol Clin* 2007; **25**: 465–81.

8. A. Pearson and C. T. Matava. Anaesthetic management for craniosynostosis repair in children. *BJA Educ* 2016; **16**: 410–16.

Suggested Reading

Fox E. B., Latham G. J., Ross F. J., et al. Perioperative and anesthetic management of coarctation of the aorta. *Semin Cardiothorac Vasc Anesth* 2019; **23**: 221–4.

Koh J. L. and Gries H. Perioperative management of pediatric patients with craniosynostosis. *Anesthesiol Clin* 2007; **25**: 465–81.

Pearson A. and Matava C. T. Anaesthetic management for craniosynostosis repair in children. *BJA Educ* 2016; **16**: 410–16.

Chapter 20

Shone Complex

Nicole Dobija

Case Scenario

A 4-year-old female with a history of Shone complex is scheduled for an umbilical hernia repair. She has a twin sister and is a bit slower and smaller than her twin, requiring more frequent breaks while playing. She has no other medical conditions or comorbidities. Her only previous surgery was a repair of coarctation of the aorta during infancy and she experienced no anesthetic issues. The patient's mother is very concerned about separation anxiety and the effects of anesthesia on her daughter's heart.

On physical exam she appears anxious, hiding in her mother's arms and making no eye contact with healthcare providers. Lungs are clear to auscultation and a 2/6 systolic ejection murmur is appreciated, which is unchanged from prior exams. Vital signs include a heart rate of 98 beats/minute, lower extremity noninvasive blood pressure reading 88/60 mm Hg, respiratory rate 26 breaths/minute, and SpO$_2$ 99% on room air. She appears healthy, with no pallor, cyanosis, or diaphoresis.

Two months earlier, echocardiography showed the following:

- *Parachute mitral valve with mild stenosis, mean gradient 5 mm Hg*
- *Bicuspid aortic valve with moderate stenosis, mean gradient 30 mm Hg*
- *Mild to moderate gradient (10 mm Hg) across the area of aortic coarctation repair*
- *Normal left ventricular function with mild hypertrophy*
- *Normal right-sided structures and function*

Key Objectives

- Describe the characteristic cardiac anomalies of Shone complex.
- Understand treatment options for patients with Shone complex.
- Describe preoperative planning for patients with Shone complex.
- Describe perioperative management for the various cardiac anomalies associated with Shone complex.
- Understand concerns for postoperative pain control and disposition in the Shone complex patient.

Pathophysiology

What is Shone complex?

Shone complex is a group of typically obstructive left-sided lesions of the heart, also referred to as Shone syndrome, disorder, or anomaly. It is a rare congenital cardiac disease, occurring in fewer than 1% of patients with congenital heart disease (CHD). Shone complex was first described by John D. Shone et al. in 1963 as four left-sided heart lesions consisting of a supravalvular ring of the left atrium, a "parachute" mitral valve, muscular or membranous subaortic stenosis, and coarctation of the aorta [1]. (See Figure 20.1.) These anomalies cause a progressive problem with inflow into the left ventricle (LV) and outflow obstruction from the LV and aorta. There is also an association with smaller LV size and decreased LV function. Lesions may progressively worsen over time, causing significant heart failure symptoms, pulmonary hypertension, and arrhythmias [2]. (See Figure 20.2.)

Partial Shone complex comprises two or three of the described four lesions [3]. There may be up to eight lesions (all involving the left side of the heart) and patients may have a combination of several of the lesions. The patient's symptoms are typically related to the lesion that is most severe, with mitral valve stenosis commonly being most symptomatic.

Is there a surgery or technique to correct Shone complex?

The treatment of Shone complex is based on the presence of the lesions and their severity. Each lesion brings a different and distinct set of physiological aberrations. These may act together to cause a series of obstructions that may magnify a single lesion. Each cardiac lesion

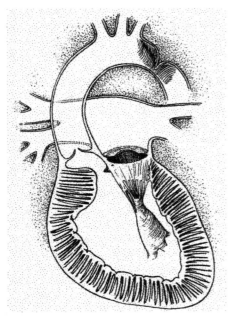

Figure 20.1 Shone complex. Diagrammatic representation of the four obstructive anomalies forming the complex: supravalvular ring of the left atrium, parachute mitral valve, subaortic stenosis, and coarctation of aorta, in that order, according to the direction of blood flow. From Shone J., et al. The developmental complex of "parachute mitral valve," supravalvular ring of left atrium, subaortic stenosis, and coarctation of aorta. *Am J Cardiol* 1963; **11**: 714–25. With permission.

must be evaluated individually and then reexamined as part of the whole cardiac complex to understand the pathophysiology and determine management. Each patient with Shone complex has a range in the variety and severity of left-sided lesions and must be evaluated individually: no two patients with Shone complex are the same. There is not a single surgical procedure to correct Shone complex. Surgical intervention may range from a single intervention such as aortic arch repair to a combination of multiple procedures such as repair of aortic coarctation along with mitral valve repair and aortic valvotomy. In severe cases patients may require multiple surgeries for recurrent left-sided obstructive lesions, including mitral and/or aortic valve replacements. (See Figure 20.3.)

Clinical Pearl

No two patients with Shone complex have exactly the same cardiac abnormalities. It is imperative to evaluate and understand each patient's pathophysiology. Surgical intervention may range from a single intervention such as aortic arch repair to a combination of multiple procedures such as repair of aortic coarctation along with mitral valve repair and aortic valvotomy.

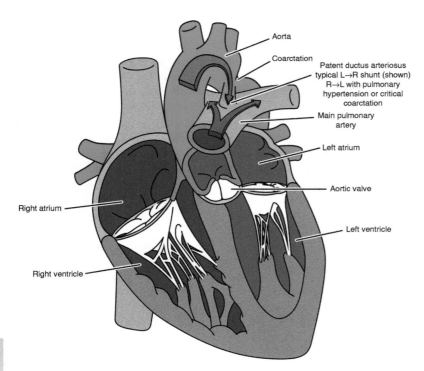

Figure 20.2 Shone complex. Drawing by Ryan Moore, MD, and Matt Nelson.

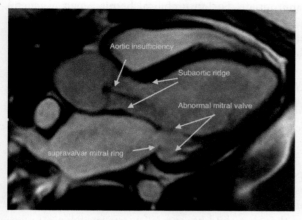

Figure 20.3 Multiple left-sided lesions. Three-chamber magnetic resonance imaging showing supravalvular mitral ring, hypoplastic mitral valve annulus, abnormal mitral valve, small subaortic ridge, and aortic regurgitation. Courtesy of Michael Taylor, MD.

What is a parachute mitral valve?

A normal mitral valve has two leaflets and two papillary muscles; the chordae from each leaflet each insert into a separate papillary muscle. A parachute mitral valve is an abnormality in the mitral valve apparatus in which the chordae of the mitral valve insert into a single papillary muscle [4]. During the first trimester of development, a disruption in embryonic formation of the papillary muscles leads to a single papillary muscle being formed [5]. The chordae in a parachute mitral valve become shorter and thicker, resulting in limited opening of the valve and functional mitral stenosis (MS) [1].

Mitral stenosis, or any LV inflow obstruction, should be evaluated for its etiology and severity. Moderate to severe MS due to a parachute mitral valve may necessitate valve repair or a valve replacement depending on the severity of the stenosis. Congenital MS due to a parachute mitral valve historically has carried a poor surgical prognosis [6]. A supravalvular membrane causing mitral (MS) or aortic stenosis (AS) may require resection depending on how much inflow and outflow obstruction it causes.

Some patients with mitral and aortic stenosis may also have an underdeveloped or hypoplastic LV. The degree of this hypoplasia, LV function, and the ability of the LV to produce adequate cardiac output may all impact surgical planning. A severely hypoplastic LV with a stenotic aortic valve may require single-ventricle palliation. This decision would be made in a multidisciplinary session including cardiologists and cardiac surgeons.

Clinical Pearl

The severity of MS is directly related to the morbidity and mortality of patients with Shone complex. Patients with severe MS are the most symptomatic and have the highest morbidity with surgery.

Why should coarctation of the aorta be corrected?

Coarctation of the aorta causes an increase in LV afterload, hypertension in the head vessels and upper extremities, and hypotension with decreased perfusion to the remainder of the body distal to the narrowing. Without repair, over time, the LV will become hypertrophied and there is an increased risk of coronary artery disease and stroke [7].

What are the surgical approaches to correction of aortic coarctation?

A coarctation repair is generally performed during infancy via a thoracotomy. There are many different approaches to surgical repair such as an end-to-end anastomosis (with a possible extended resection), a subclavian flap angioplasty, and an interposition graft repair. With a subclavian flap angioplasty repair, the subclavian artery becomes discontinuous with the aorta, and consequently blood pressure monitoring on the left upper extremity may not be indicative of the true blood pressure.

Coarctation relief may also be attempted in the cardiac catheterization laboratory via an endovascular approach. Arterial access is obtained through the femoral artery. In infants and small children, angioplasty is typically performed with balloon dilation of the stenosis. In older patients and for re-coarctation of the aorta, angioplasty with stent placement may be performed. Long-term surveillance is required following coarctation repair to evaluate for recurrent coarctation and aneurysm formation. If there is a longer segment of arch hypoplasia, an aortic arch reconstruction may have to be performed via a median sternotomy and utilizing cardiopulmonary bypass.

Clinical Pearl

If the technique previously employed for coarctation repair is unknown, place the blood pressure cuff on the right upper extremity, as this will provide a reliable blood pressure for coronary artery and cerebral perfusion.

Are Shone complex patients prone to respiratory involvement?

Patients with left-sided obstructive lesions may have increased pulmonary pressures from increased left atrial pressures. Not surprisingly, pulmonary hypertension causes long-term increases in morbidity and mortality in patients with Shone complex [8]. These patients may experience shortness of breath from pulmonary edema. They may also experience an exacerbation of respiratory symptoms with a concomitant respiratory infection.

Clinical Pearl

Patients with Shone complex who have developed pulmonary hypertension have increased anesthetic risk.

Anesthetic Implications

Is a visit to the cardiologist needed prior to elective surgery?

Since the manifestations of Shone complex are so variable, knowing the individual patient's cardiac pathophysiology is of utmost importance. Results of a recent visit to his or her cardiologist should be documented along with an echocardiogram and electrocardiogram (ECG) to delineate disease progression. A discussion with the cardiologist may be beneficial to understand which lesions are causing the most influence on cardiac output and how changes in preload or afterload would affect the patient's hemodynamics. The cardiologist can also help determine if the patient is optimized for an elective surgery.

Once the cardiac pathophysiology is confirmed, an understanding of the patient's functional status and symptomatology is important. Symptoms may occur at rest or with activity. The most commonly elicited symptom is shortness of breath with exertion. Patients with moderate to severe obstructive lesions may have chest pain, dizziness, or even syncope from decreased cardiac output.

How should the type of anesthetic be determined and how should parental concerns about the effect of anesthesia be addressed?

Children with CHD have a disproportionately high risk of perioperative cardiac arrest and anesthetic morbidity [9]. The type of surgery will dictate the anesthetic requirements. For instance, if this patient were to undergo a diagnostic procedure such as magnetic resonance imaging (MRI), sedation or monitored anesthesia care might

be appropriate. For an umbilical hernia repair a general anesthetic is required. Maintenance of adequate preload, afterload, and contractility is of utmost importance, along with judicious titration of anesthetic medications.

How could the mother's concerns about her daughter's anxiety be addressed?

Preoperative management is similar to the management of any pediatric patient who will undergo general anesthesia for an umbilical hernia repair. The goal is to minimize the stress response associated with the anxiety of undergoing anesthesia and a surgical procedure. Multiple methods can be used, such as behavioral management techniques facilitated though a child life specialist, pharmacological management with medications such as oral midazolam, and involving a parent in the induction of anesthesia to avoid separation anxiety. The technique or combination of techniques utilized will be determined by the anesthesia team, with the aim of reducing the child's stress while introducing the lowest possible risk. A stress response will elicit tachycardia, which in a patient with Shone complex may cause a reduction in cardiac output and poor perfusion and should be avoided. Child Life specialists, if available, should be utilized early in the preoperative process. Some institutions have a separate preoperative appointment with the Child Life team. Having the child comfortable in his or her surroundings prior to the presence of medical personnel will help reduce the anxiety of a new environment. The use of premedication and/or parental presence depends on the anesthesiologist's comfort with having a parent in the operating room during induction as well as the institutional policy. The safety of the child during anesthetic induction is of utmost importance independent of which modality is utilized to relieve preoperative anxiety.

Should an intravenous catheter be placed preoperatively?

Depending on the severity of the patient's individual pathophysiology induction of general anesthesia may occur either via inhalational mask induction or intravenous (IV) induction. Most patients with mild to moderate MS or AS will be able to tolerate an inhalational induction with vigilant hemodynamic monitoring. Patients with regurgitant lesions will generally tolerate a gentle inhalational induction. This patient has left-sided outflow tract gradients at the mitral and aortic level, as well as a residual gradient at the site of the coarctation repair. Although none of the gradients are severe individually, they should be considered cumulatively and thus a cautious approach to anesthetic induction is warranted. In the patient with severe stenosis, it may be prudent to place an IV prior to induction of anesthesia and slowly induce anesthesia with precise hemodynamic monitoring. The specific pharmacologic agents chosen may vary as long as meticulous care is taken to maintaining preload, contractility, and afterload while avoiding the development of significant tachycardia.

Clinical Pearl

This patient has left-sided outflow tract gradients at the mitral and aortic level, as well as a residual gradient at the site of the coarctation repair. Although none of the gradients are severe individually, they should be considered cumulatively and thus a cautious approach to anesthetic induction is warranted. In the patient with severe stenosis, it may be prudent to place an IV prior to induction of anesthesia and slowly induce anesthesia with precise hemodynamic monitoring.

What intraoperative considerations exist with umbilical hernia closure?

Most small umbilical hernias close spontaneously, prior to the child's third or fourth birthday. When the defect has failed to close on its own, is large, or the bowel is at risk for strangulation, the patient will be scheduled for surgical closure. Typically, repair involves a periumbilical incision with primary suture closure of the hernia defect. Unlike the adult population, mesh and laparoscopy is rarely utilized. Depending on the size of the umbilical hernia and the surgeons' approach to the repair, the airway may be secured with either an endotracheal tube or a supraglottic airway device such as a laryngeal mask airway. Some surgeons may also prefer the use of neuromuscular blockade depending on the size of the defect. Spontaneous ventilation, if possible, offers the benefit of having less effect on preload. However, care should be taken to avoid the potentially negative effects of hypercarbia on the pulmonary vascular bed.

How should adequate preload be ensured and monitored perioperatively?

An initial assessment should be made to evaluate the patient's baseline hydration/preload status. Ensure that the patient is appropriately fasted per the American Society of Anesthesiologists (ASA) guidelines but avoid extended periods of fasting that can cause decreased preload. These patients should be scheduled early in the day and should be encouraged to drink clear fluids until 2 hours prior to the procedure. Dehydration should be avoided. If the patient appears dehydrated, has decreased

urine output, a lack of wet diapers, or decreased capillary refill, the patient may need to receive IV fluids prior to the induction of anesthesia. Monitoring of preload for a hernia repair is usually not done invasively through a central venous line but is based on clinical signs and symptoms.

Both inhaled and IV anesthetic agents can decrease preload. While one specific anesthetic agent is not preferred over another, the judicious and careful titration of anesthetic agents to the desired effect is recommended.

Management of positive pressure ventilation can also influence preload. While one particular ventilation strategy is not favored over another, maintaining thoracic volumes that allow for optimal venous return to the right side of the heart is important.

The surgical approach can also influence preload. An open repair may manually compress a discrete area of the abdomen whereas a laparoscopic approach may cause unintended compression of small vessels, thus causing decreases in preload and cardiac output. Insufflation pressures can also lead to increased abdominal pressure, resulting in increased intrathoracic pressures and hence an increase in afterload. Maintaining lower insufflation pressures may be necessary when utilizing a laparoscopic approach.

Clinical Pearl

Preload may be affected by hydration status, anesthetic agents, ventilation strategy, and surgical technique.

How should adequate afterload be monitored and ensured?

Afterload is commonly defined as the pressure the LV must produce to pump the volume out of its chamber. It is influenced by the volume in the LV, wall thickness of the ventricle, and systemic vascular resistance (SVR). Patients with Shone complex can have perturbations in all three of these categories.

For the patient with MS, obstruction of blood flow into the LV exists, thus decreasing the volume within the chamber. The LV volume may also be influenced by the patient's heart rate, which relates to the length of time in the cardiac cycle for diastole, or cardiac filling.

Aortic stenosis causes afterload obstruction for the LV. Over time, this increased afterload may result in left ventricular hypertrophy (LVH). An increase in wall thickness may lead to increased LV pressures and decreased or dyskinetic LV function. Maintaining adequate coronary perfusion is critical for a thickened ventricle. Decreases in afterload, commonly seen with induction of anesthesia, can lead to decreased diastolic flow to the coronary arteries and myocardium, thus causing ischemia.

From an anesthesia perspective, SVR is the afterload that the LV must pump against. Most anesthetic agents cause a decrease in SVR. Patients with Shone complex may have other perturbations in anatomy that influence SVR such as a coarctation of the aorta and/or AS. Depending on the location of the lesion, there may be an area of "fixed" or relatively high SVR proximal to the lesion and an area of decreased SVR distal to the lesion. The patient with moderate AS has a fixed lesion that is not influenced by the choice of anesthetic. With induction of anesthesia, the LV continues to pump against the same afterload, the stenotic aortic valve. Distal to the aortic valve, if anesthetic agents have caused SVR to decrease, consequently blood pressure and the amount of blood flow to the coronary arteries are decreased. This decrease in coronary perfusion leads to myocardial ischemia, as the LV is required to do the same amount of work to eject blood across the stenotic aortic valve. In the patient with aortic coarctation, the aortic pressure proximal to the coarctation (from the heart to the coarctation, typically around the level of the left subclavian artery) will be higher than the pressure distal to this lesion. This would clinically manifest as a higher noninvasive blood pressure (NIBP) measurement on the right upper extremity compared to the lower extremity.

How should adequate contractility be monitored and ensured?

Contractility is described as systolic function. Echocardiography is typically used to measure systolic function. Being familiar with the results of previous transthoracic echocardiograms and knowing the patient's heart rate and blood pressure during those studies is important. Anesthetic agents typically cause a decrease in preload secondary to vasodilatation, thus reducing cardiac output. With escalating doses of anesthetic medications, a reduction in contractility may be observed. Decreased cardiac output may also lead to decreased contractility because of poor coronary perfusion. Arrhythmias may develop from myocardial ischemia, compromising filling time for the LV, and thus leading to further reductions in cardiac output. A stable sinus rhythm is essential for the maintenance of adequate cardiac output.

Typical intraoperative monitoring for this patient would include an NIBP cuff and heart rate monitoring via a 5-lead ECG. Knowing the preoperative baseline vital signs is important in this patient population. During the perioperative period, including recovery, it is imperative to keep the patient near their baseline parameters. Tachycardia in particular is not well tolerated, as it decreases the filling and

ejection time of the LV, thus causing decreased cardiac output. Slight hypertension is better tolerated than hypotension, as hypotension can lead to decreased coronary perfusion in an already stressed myocardium and a subsequent reduction in cardiac function.

Clinical Pearl

Tachycardia in particular is not well tolerated, as it decreases the filling and ejection time of the LV, thus causing decreased cardiac output. Slight hypertension is better tolerated than hypotension.

Is there a preferred method for postoperative pain control?

Intraoperative and postoperative pain control is of paramount importance. Inadequate pain control causes sympathetic stimulation that can increase heart rate, leading to decreased cardiac output and coronary ischemia in a patient with LV outflow tract obstruction. The specific surgical approach as well as individual patient factors will help determine which pain modalities are optimal. A multimodal approach to pain management may be achieved with a combination of preoperative oral medications, IV medications, and regional or local anesthesia. Intraoperative pain control for an umbilical hernia may be achieved with inhalational agents, IV agents such as opioids and nonsteroidal medications (ketorolac), and preoperative oral or IV acetaminophen. Regional anesthesia can also be utilized and modalities such as infiltration of local anesthesia at the surgical site by the surgeons, rectus sheath blocks, or caudal anesthesia have all been shown to be equally efficacious [10]. With umbilical hernia repair, one should aim to reduce postoperative nausea and/or retching. A reduction in the amount of opioid or an opioid-free approach may aid in decreasing this adverse event.

Can a patient with Shone complex be discharged home following hernia repair?

The appropriate postoperative disposition of congenital cardiac patients undergoing noncardiac surgery is institution, provider, and patient dependent. An umbilical hernia repair can be scheduled and safely performed as an outpatient procedure in most instances. However, in this scenario this surgery would rarely be performed at a freestanding ambulatory surgical center due to the patient's comorbidities. A preoperative discussion with the family to ensure that they are comfortable managing postoperative care and maintaining adequate pain control and hydration is important. This asymptomatic patient with mild to moderate obstruction, once adequately recovered from anesthesia, tolerating oral intake without difficulties and with adequate pain control, may be discharged home with parents or guardians. However, if there is concern for decreased cardiac output, hypoperfusion, or respiratory insufficiency postoperatively, the anesthesiologist and cardiologist should discuss the symptoms and an overnight stay may be warranted.

References

1. J. D. Shone, R. D. Sellers, R. C. Anderson, et al. The developmental complex of "parachute mitral valve," supravalvular ring of left atrium, subaortic stenosis, and coarctation of aorta. *Am J Cardiol* 1963; **11**: 714–25.

2. C. M. Ikemba, B. W. Eidem, J. K. Fraley, et al. Mitral valve morphology and morbidity/mortality in Shone's complex. *Am J Cardiol* 2005; **95**: 541–3.

3. A. Grimaldi, A. C. Vermi, S. Y. Ho, et al. Surgical outcome of partial Shone complex. *Interact Cardiovasc Thorac Surg* 2012; **14**: 440–4.

4. B. S. Marino, L. E. Kruge, C. J. Cho, et al. Parachute mitral valve: morphologic descriptors, associated lesions, and outcomes after biventricular repair. *J Thorac Cardiovasc Surg* 2009; **137**: 385–93.

5. P. W. Oosthoek, A. C. Wenink, L. J. Wisse, et al. Development of the papillary muscles of the mitral valve: morphogenetic background of parachute-like asymmetric mitral valves and other mitral valve anomalies. *J Thorac Cardiovasc Surg* 1998; **116**: 36–46.

6. R. A. Brauner, H. Laks, D. C. Drinkwater, et al. Multiple left heart obstructions (Shone's anomaly) with mitral valve involvement: long-term surgical outcome. *Ann Thorac Surg* 1997; **64**: 721–9.

7. N. P. Jenkins and C. Ward. Coarctation of the aorta: natural history and outcome after surgical treatment. *QJM* 1999; **92**: 365–71.

8. G. T. Nicholson, M. S. Kelleman, C. M. De la Uz, et al. Late outcomes in children with Shone's complex: a single-centre, 20-year experience. *Cardiol Young* 2017; **27**: 697–705.

9. C. Ramamoorthy, C. M. Haberkern, and S. M. Bhananker. Anesthesia-related cardiac arrest in children with heart disease: data from the Pediatric Perioperative Cardiac Arrest (POCA) registry. *Anesth Analg* 2010; **110**: 1376–82.

10. L. M. Relland, J. D. Tobias, D. Martin, et al. Ultrasound-guided rectus sheath block, caudal analgesia, or surgical site infiltration for pediatric umbilical herniorrhaphy: a prospective, double-blinded, randomized comparison of three regional anesthetic techniques. *J Pain Res* 2017; **10**: 2629–34.

Suggested Reading

Atkinson T. M., Giraud G. D., Togioka B. M., et al. Cardiovascular and ventilatory consequences of laparoscopic surgery. *Circulation* 2017; **135**: 700–10.

Friesen R. H. Anesthetic drugs in congenital heart disease. *Semin Cardiothorac Vasc Anesth* 2014; **18**: 363–70.

Schimke A., Majithia A., Baumgartner R., et al. Intervention and management of congenital left heart obstructive lesions. *Curr Treat Options Cardiovasc Med* 2013; **15**: 632–45.

Shone J. D., Sellers R. D., Anderson R. C., et al. The developmental complex of "parachute mitral valve," supravalvular ring of left atrium, subaortic stenosis, and coarctation of aorta. *Am J Cardiol* 1963; **11**: 714–25.

Spaeth J. P. and Loepke A. W. Anesthesia for left-sided obstructive lesions. In Andropoulos D. B., Stayer S., Mossad E. B., et al., eds. *Anesthesia for Congenital Heart Disease*, 3rd ed. Hoboken, NJ: John Wiley & Sons, 2015; 497–515.

Chapter

21

D-Transposition of the Great Arteries (Arterial Switch)

Leah Landsem and Gregory J. Latham

Case Scenario

A 10-year-old male presents for elective upper endoscopy and colonoscopy. He has a 2-week history of persistent vomiting and weight loss with new-onset diarrhea. He has a history of dextro-transposition of the great arteries and underwent an arterial switch operation shortly after birth. He has been followed since by his cardiologist for residual pulmonic stenosis. He and his family report he is able to participate in sports but has begun to tire more quickly than his peers; he has felt considerably more fatigued since the start of the vomiting and diarrhea. His current vital signs include heart rate 100 beats/minute, respiratory rate 18 breaths/minute, and SpO_2 99% on room air. His abdomen is soft, mildly distended, and nontender to palpation. He has mild eczema on his extremities.

Transthoracic echocardiography 1 week earlier showed the following:

- *Peak velocity of 3.5 m/s and peak gradient of 50 mm Hg across the pulmonary valve*
- *Right ventricular hypertrophy*
- *Qualitatively normal biventricular function*

Key Objectives

- Understand the anatomy of dextro-transposition of the great arteries.
- Describe the arterial switch operation and identify potential sequelae.
- Describe the preoperative assessment and anesthetic management of a patient with repaired dextro-transposition.
- Understand considerations regarding performing procedures in remote or offsite locations in patients with repaired congenital heart disease.

Pathophysiology

What is transposition of the great arteries?

Transposition of the great arteries (TGA) is most accurately an umbrella term for all congenital cardiac lesions whereby the aorta arises from the right ventricle (RV) and the pulmonary artery (PA) arises from the left ventricle (LV). This is termed ventriculoarterial discordance. Most typically the term TGA is used to denote dextro (d)-TGA, whereas other forms of TGA are called by their specific names, as discussed in the text that follows.

What is d-TGA?

D-transposition of the great arteries is one of the most common cyanotic congenital heart lesions, characterized by ***ventriculoarterial discordance***, the origination of the great vessels from the incorrect ventricles, in a heart with otherwise normal connections. Deoxygenated systemic blood flows from the vena cavae to the right atrium (RA), on to the RV, and then to the aorta. Oxygenated pulmonary venous blood enters the left atrium (LA), flows to the LV, and exits the PA. This anatomy results in a parallel circulation. (See Figure 21.1.) Fetal shunts between the parallel circulations, including a patent foramen ovale (PFO) and patent ductus arteriosus (PDA), are required to provide mixing between the separate circulations and thus some degree of oxygen delivery to the tissues. Without intervention, d-TGA is uniformly fatal in infancy, with a 30% mortality in the first week of life and 50% in the first month. Transposition represents 5% of all congenital heart lesions (32 per 100,000 live births) with a 2:1 predilection for males.

What are other types of TGA and how are they distinct from d-TGA?

D-transposition is a morphologically distinct entity wherein the "d" denotes dextroposition of the bulboventricular loop embryologically, resulting in atrioventricular concordance, ventriculoarterial discordance, and a typically anterior and rightward position of the aortic valve.

Congenitally corrected, or levo-TGA (l-TGA), is also characterized by ventriculoarterial discordance; however, the addition of atrioventricular discordance results in a series circulation, with the left-sided morphologic RV responsible for systemic blood flow. (See Chapter 23.) Because l-TGA results in a series blood flow, it is a separate entity both anatomically and physiologically, as well as embryologically. Other congenital cardiac lesions that also have transposed great vessels include those with associated mitral or tricuspid atresia, double inlet left or right ventricle, and some forms of double outlet RV.

What is the newborn physiology of d-TGA?

D-transposition is characterized by a parallel circulation. There are three primary d-TGA subtypes that influence a newborn's clinical presentation. (See Table 21.1.)

In infants with **TGA-IVS**, after birth the preexisting fetal shunts (PDA and PFO) become critical sources for mixing of oxygenated and deoxygenated blood between the separate circulations. (See Figure 21.2.) The ductus arteriosus is almost always patent immediately after birth, and intravenous prostaglandin E_1 (PGE_1) infusion is immediately initiated to maintain ductal patency. The PDA alone is unable to provide sufficient mixing, which requires robust bidirectional flow. As a result, patency at the atrial level (ASD and/or PFO) is necessary to provide countercurrent flow in equal volume to the flow across the PDA. A countercurrent flow across two shunts allows the possibility of sufficient mixing in the short term. Although the foramen ovale typically remains open due to higher pressures in the RA, it can be closed or restrictive. In these cases, emergent balloon atrial septostomy (BAS) is undertaken, generally in the cardiac catheterization laboratory, to enlarge the communication between the atria and allow adequate mixing. (See Figure 21.3.)

Table 21.1 d-TGA Subtypes and Incidences

Subtype	Incidence
d-TGA with intact ventricular septum (TGA-IVS)	60%–70%
d-TGA with ventricular septal defect (TGA-VSD)	25%–45%
d-TGA with VSD and left ventricular outflow tract obstruction (TGA-LVOTO)	5%–25%

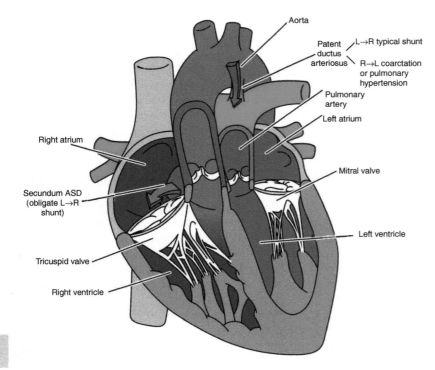

Figure 21.1 Unrepaired d-TGA with intact ventricular septum. Drawing by Ryan Moore, MD, and Matt Nelson.

Aorta

Patent ductus arteriosus — L→R typical shunt
R→L coarctation or pulmonary hypertension

Pulmonary artery

Left atrium

Right atrium

Mitral valve

Secundum ASD (obligate L→R shunt)

Left ventricle

Tricuspid valve

Right ventricle

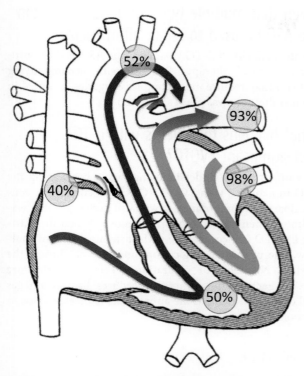

Figure 21.2 d-TGA with intact ventricular septum. The ductus arteriosus and foramen ovale are restrictive, leading to poor mixing and severe hypoxemia. Courtesy of Greg Latham, MD.

Figure 21.3 d-TGA-IVS with improved mixing after initiation of PGE₁ and a balloon atrial septostomy. Courtesy of Greg Latham, MD.

Clinical Pearl

The most common form of d-TGA, TGA-IVS, relies on shunting at the ductal and atrial level to adequately mix the parallel circulations. A prostaglandin E₁ infusion is usually required to maintain ductal patency, and a BAS may be required to create or maintain an atrial shunt.

In patients with **TGA-VSD**, there are usually, but not always, ample saturations due to robust mixing at three levels: arterial (PDA), atrial (PFO), and ventricular (VSD). Therefore, these children may not be cyanotic at birth. In these cases, a trial of discontinuing PGE₁ is warranted to reduce the risk of excessive pulmonary blood flow (PBF) as pulmonary vascular resistance (PVR) decreases, therefore reducing the risk of heart failure.

Neonates with **TGA-LVOTO** may have adequate mixing from the VSD; however, the amount of PBF will be dependent on the degree of subpulmonic LVOTO, which may range from a mild to severe reduction in PBF, thus resulting in variable degrees of hypoxemia.

As PVR decreases after birth, children with either TGA-IVS or TGA-VSD will experience a gradual increase

in blood flow into the pulmonary side of the parallel circulation (pulmonary veins to LA, to LV, to PA, and back to pulmonary veins), which can lead to pulmonary congestion and heart failure.

Clinical Pearl

D-transposition relies on adequate mixing to prevent severe hypoxemia after birth. This generally requires patency of two out of three possible cardiac shunts (arterial level: PDA, atrial level: PFO, ventricular level: VSD) to allow circular mixing between the parallel circulations. Regardless, adequate oxygenation and perfusion may be tenuous prior to surgery.

What other anomalies are associated with d-TGA?

Regardless of the subtype, d-TGA may also be associated with aberrant coronary anatomy and/or ostial abnormalities, as well as accompanying aortic arch hypoplasia, coarctation, or interruption. Unlike most other complex congenital heart lesions, d-TGA usually appears in isolation without extracardiac anomalies or genetic syndromes.

How and when is d-TGA repaired?

Because transposition physiology has been demonstrated to cause variable degrees of brain matter changes, early surgical repair is preferred. Days 3–5 of life are considered ideal, which strikes an appropriate balance, allowing reduction of postnatal PVR but occurring prior to the deconditioning of the LV that occurs as a result of the decreased afterload on the LV as it perfuses the pulmonary circulation.

Surgical management of d-TGA has changed over the past 40 years. Initially, d-TGA was repaired via a Mustard or Senning atrial switch operation. (See Chapter 22.) Today, the arterial switch operation (ASO) has become the mainstay of modern surgical management due to excellent outcomes, with more than 90%–95% of patients living into adulthood. The ASO results in anatomic correction (see Figure 21.4), whereby the great arteries are switched to create ventriculoarterial concordance, with reanastomosis of the coronary arteries to the neo-aorta. The ductus arteriosus, if patent, and any other residual septal shunts are closed.

> **Clinical Pearl**
>
> *The arterial switch operation is the preferred repair for d-TGA and is appropriate in the majority of patients, with excellent surgical outcomes and more than 90% of patients surviving into adulthood.*

Given that multiple types of d-TGA exist, can the ASO be used to repair all of them?

For the majority of d-TGA patients, the ASO is the appropriate surgical therapy. Patients with accompanying LVOTO may require more complex surgeries, as noted in the text that follows. (See Table 21.2.)

What happens to patients with d-TGA and significant LVOTO?

It is important to understand that while performing the ASO in neonates with TGA-LVOTO will correct the ventriculoarterial discordance, it will also exchange what was pulmonic stenosis for neoaortic stenosis. When the existing LVOTO is incompatible with sustaining systemic outflow, one of several surgical options may be chosen: the Rastelli, Nikaidoh, or réparation á l'étage ventriculaire (REV). Each of these three procedures has advantages and disadvantages, and the appropriate choice depends in part on the specific anatomy.

> **Clinical Pearl**
>
> *It is important to understand that while performing the ASO in neonates with TGA-LVOTO will correct the ventriculoarterial discordance, it will also exchange what was pulmonic stenosis for neoaortic stenosis.*

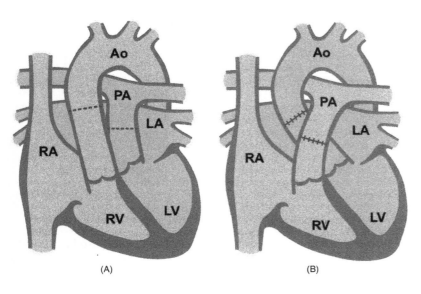

(A) (B)

Figure 21.4 The arterial switch operation (ASO). Schematic representation of d-transposition of the great arteries anatomy before (A) and after (B) the ASO. AO, aorta; LA, left atrium; LV, left ventricle; PA, pulmonary artery; RA, right atrium; RV, right ventricle. From McEwan A. and Manolis M. Anesthesia for transposition of the great arteries. In Andropoulos D. B., Stayer S., Mossad E. B., et al., eds. *Anesthesia for Congenital Heart Surgery*, 3rd ed. John Wiley & Sons, 2015: 542–66. With permission.

Table 21.2 Surgical Repairs for d-TGA Variants

Lesion	Surgical Repair
d-TGA with intact ventricular septum	ASO
d-TGA with intact ventricular septum and interrupted arch or coarctation	ASO with arch/coarctation repair
d-TGA with VSD	ASO with VSD closure
d-TGA with VSD and significant PS	Rastelli, REV, or Nikaidoh procedure

ASO, arterial switch operation; PS, pulmonary stenosis; VSD, ventricular septal defect.

The *Rastelli procedure* leaves the great vessels and semilunar valves in place and a VSD patch is used as a baffle to direct LV output across the VSD and to the anterior-rightward aortic valve that overlies the RV. Because the Rastelli baffle invades the RV outflow tract and precludes RV outflow to the leftward PA, the pulmonary valve is over-sewn, and an external valved RV-to-PA conduit is placed. A disadvantage is that the synthetic external conduit obligates future reinterventions, including surgical conduit changes, percutaneous stenting of the conduit, and/or percutaneous transcatheter pulmonary valve replacements. Recurrent LVOTO is also a risk with the long LV outflow baffle.

The *REV procedure* is very similar to the Rastelli procedure but includes resection of the conal septum and directly connects the native PA to the RV, allowing for growth and eliminating the need for a prosthetic conduit. However, obligate pulmonary regurgitation will also eventually require reinterventions.

The *Nikaidoh procedure* is characterized by translocation of not only the great vessels but the aortic valve as well. The aortic root is harvested from the RV, and the LVOTO is relieved by dividing the posteriorly positioned pulmonary valve and outlet septum. The aortic valve, aorta, and coronary arteries are reimplanted above the reconstructed LV outflow tract, and the VSD and outlet septum are closed. Anastomosis of the main PA to the RV is accomplished via valved conduit or anastomosis of native (non-valved) PA-to-RV with patch augmentation. The Nikaidoh results in excellent outcomes with regard to the aortic valve and LV outflow tract, but reinterventions will be required for pulmonary regurgitation, as discussed with the Rastelli.

Clinical Pearl

A small number of children with d-TGA and significant LVOTO are not suitable for an ASO repair and instead require surgical repair with a Rastelli, Nikaidoh, or réparation à l'étage ventriculaire (REV) procedure.

What are the long-term issues, if any, in patients with repaired d-TGA?

Children with TGA-LVOTO who require repair with a Rastelli, REV, or Nikaidoh procedure will have some degree of residual disease, as previously discussed. However, the remainder of this discussion will concern children post-ASO.

Although uncommon, early mortality after the ASO is caused in large part by acute coronary events. Beyond 3 months post-ASO, coronary complications are relatively rare, despite angiographic or radiographic evidence of some degree of coronary stenosis or "insufficiency" in 3%–11% of patients. The rate of clinically symptomatic coronary pathology, however, is low, and there is no agreed upon consensus for standardized coronary surveillance as of 2018.

Despite refinements in surgical techniques, progressive right ventricular outflow tract obstruction (RVOTO) remains a relatively common long-term morbidity. The obstruction can be subvalvular, valvular, or supravalvular in nature or exist as multilevel obstruction. The precise cause of RVOTO in most patients is not clear. Classically, the ASO is accomplished utilizing the Lecompte maneuver, which involves moving the main and branch pulmonary arteries anterior to the aorta while the aorta is transected. This results in the pulmonary trunk and arteries laying overtop the aorta in a nonspiraled fashion, and while physiologically corrected, the lack of spiraling of the great vessels results in a different configuration from an embryologically normal heart. The Lecompte maneuver is done to prevent posterior compression of the PAs from the neoaortic root. However, it is postulated that larger aortic roots may actually increase stretching of the PAs, or indeed that the lack of spiraling changes flow dynamics, of which pulmonary artery stenosis becomes a long-term consequence.

Clinical Pearl

The most common cause of late reintervention post-ASO is to address RVOTO, often at the level of the branch pulmonary arteries.

Less common long-term morbidities include LVOTO, neoaortic root dilation, neoaortic valve regurgitation, compression of the tracheobronchial tree, and primary pulmonary hypertension. Arrhythmias and bundle branch blocks are uncommon after ASO, as this surgery usually avoids significant manipulation of the nodal and conducting cardiac tissue. However, closure of large VSDs or performance of any of the other non-ASO techniques (Senning, Mustard, REV, Nikaidoh, Rastelli) portend a higher risk of long-term arrhythmias.

What type of follow-up do these patients require after repair, and at what interval?

In addition to standard postoperative surgical follow-up, patients should have outpatient cardiology care at an interval recommended by the cardiologist. There are no current guidelines or recommendations for routine testing or follow-up in this patient population. The frequency of surveillance testing will generally be dependent on the presence of residual cardiac disease and could include annual electrocardiogram (ECG) and echocardiogram, with more dedicated imaging, such as cardiac magnetic resonance imaging, computed tomography angiography, or cardiac catheterization, based on the presence of symptoms or historical issues concerning for coronary, valvular, or overall cardiac function. On the other end of the spectrum, children with no evidence of residual cardiac disease may have infrequent cardiology visits.

The question of the maximal allowable time since last imaging or last cardiology visit prior to anesthesia for an elective procedure is difficult to define. In short, the child's family should be compliant with follow-up as recommended by his or her cardiologist. Additionally, if the child has new or progressive symptoms that are concerning for cardiac disease, consideration must be given to a cardiology visit or consultation prior to anesthesia, particularly for elective procedures.

Anesthetic Implications

What specific cardiac information should the preoperative assessment include?

In addition to the routine preoperative history and physical examination, the most recent echocardiogram should be reviewed to assess any residual right or left ventricular outflow tract obstruction, wall motion abnormalities, and biventricular function. An ECG can be reviewed for arrhythmias or the rare occurrence of ischemia, and records from the most recent cardiology visit should be reviewed when available. An assessment of current functional status can help gauge the degree of cardiopulmonary reserve and guide whether repeat imaging or further optimization of the child is necessary prior to elective surgery.

What are the signs, symptoms, and diagnostic criteria of pulmonary stenosis?

The diagnosis of pulmonary stenosis (PS) is based on echocardiographic Doppler measurements across the stenotic pulmonary valve or other level of outflow tract. Clinically, the child may be noted to have decreased exercise tolerance, shortness of breath and fatigue, chest pain, or poor growth. Findings on ECG may demonstrate RV hypertrophy with right axis deviation, a dominant R wave in V1, and deep S waves in V5 and V6.

Pulmonary stenosis is further characterized as mild, moderate, or severe, based on peak gradients of <40 mm Hg, 40–60 mm Hg, or >60 mm Hg, respectively. While these criteria generally apply to stenosis of the valve itself, the region of narrowing can occur anywhere along the RVOT, including superiorly to the branch pulmonary arteries. There is, however, a lack of agreement regarding optimal techniques to quantify and standardize data in these non-valvular regions. As such, clinical decision making for a child with possible multilevel RVOTO requires ongoing surveillance for changes and the development of symptoms over time to appropriately assess the need for intervention.

A peak gradient of 50 mm Hg or the presence of clinical symptoms is often used as a threshold for treatment of isolated PS. However, the treatment threshold is certainly multifactorial in a child with the development of postoperative PS that may exist at multiple levels and may require a more extensive surgical revision. Thus, the presence or severity of clinical symptoms, progression of RV hypertrophy, and rate of progression of PS will all be factors in assessing the need or timing for reintervention.

Clinical Pearl

Pulmonary stenosis is characterized as mild, moderate, or severe, based on peak gradients of <40 mm Hg, 40–60 mm Hg, or >60 mm Hg, respectively. The presence or severity of clinical symptoms, progression of RV hypertrophy, and rate of progression of PS are all factors in assessing the need or timing for reintervention.

How should patients and parents be counselled regarding their anesthetic risk?

Reporting from multiple centers and databases has implicated congenital and acquired cardiac disease as primary risk factors for anesthetic morbidity and mortality in children. However, congenital heart disease (CHD) clearly represents a wide range of disease types and surgical repairs. Subgroup analysis demonstrates that those patients with single ventricle physiology, obstructive left heart lesions, pulmonary hypertension, or cardiomyopathy appear to be most vulnerable. Although no long-term data are specifically reported for anesthetic risk in children or adults post-ASO, it is intuitive that children and adults with repaired CHD who are fit and have no residual defects are at low risk, with increasing risk correlating with the presence and severity of residual or comorbid disease. Ultimately, the child's American Society of Anesthesiologists physical status remains a strong predictor for the risk of anesthetic complications, emphasizing the importance of each patient's preoperative assessment.

What are the general anesthetic considerations for patients with PS?

Outflow tract obstructions cause an increase in ventricular afterload. The impact to the underlying ventricle, in this case the RV, depends on the severity and the rate of progression of stenosis. Slowly progressive PS results in gradual RV hypertrophy to compensate for the increased afterload, and the RV is typically well adapted to sustain physiologic demands, including exercise, despite the increased afterload. The child discussed in this chapter appears to fall into this category, with moderate to severe PS but preserved RV function and the ability to continue athletics, albeit with increased fatigue. With continued significant stenosis, progressive RV hypertrophy is eventually accompanied by impaired relaxation, a tenuous oxygen supply–demand relationship, and eventual risk of RV ischemia and failure. On the other hand, if a child has acute onset of severe PS, the risk of acute RV failure exists given that the RV has not had time to develop compensatory mechanisms to adapt to the severely increased afterload.

Anesthetic risk in the setting of PS, therefore, depends on the severity of PS and the underlying RV function, and many would consider RV function to directly correlate with risk of morbidity and mortality under anesthesia. Important goals during all phases of the anesthetic include normovolemia to maintain adequate preload, maintenance of normal sinus rhythm to optimize the atrial contribution to RV filling, and avoidance of tachycardia for optimization of both RV filling time and RV ejection across the stenosis. Special caution should be exercised during induction and emergence, as these times are more commonly fraught with hemodynamic instability.

of normovolemia for adequate preload, maintenance of normal sinus rhythm to optimize the atrial contribution to RV filling, and avoidance of tachycardia for optimization of both RV filling time and RV ejection across the stenosis.

Should additional monitors or invasive access be placed?

The use of a 5-lead ECG increases myocardial ischemia detection, is noninvasive, and as such is easily warranted for any patient at risk for ischemia under anesthesia. The need for and use of invasive monitors is dictated by both the surgical procedure and the presence of patient comorbidities. This child underwent a straightforward ASO repair and presents with PS, preserved RV function, and the ability to participate in sports. Given the short, noninvasive nature of the EGD and colonoscopy, invasive monitoring would not be warranted.

Are there any specific considerations for induction of anesthesia?

A patient with d-TGA post-ASO has normal anatomic circulation. Increased detection of myocardial ischemia can be obtained with a 5-lead ECG, but other specific considerations regarding the induction of anesthesia will depend on the presence of any residual cardiac disease, including outflow tract obstruction(s).

In this patient, the severity of his PS is the concerning cardiac manifestation, and anesthetic goals should be tailored as discussed earlier. Preload, afterload, and contractility are the key ingredients to maintain RV performance. Preload is managed with intravenous (IV) hydration. Further increases in RV afterload should be prevented, which means maintaining a low PVR via the normal mechanisms under anesthesia. Tachycardia may be reduced with administration of anxiolytic premedication if indicated and preoperative fluid hydration. Slow titration of anesthetic induction agents allows for close monitoring of hemodynamics and treatment if perfusion and oxygen delivery are compromised. The 10-year-old in this scenario will likely behave quite normally with a gentle inhalation or propofol-based induction. The child's history of vomiting must also be factored into the induction plan.

If the patient aspirated during induction, what are the specific risks in a child with PS?

In this case, the risk of aspiration is additive to the risk of PS. Aspiration of a large volume or particulate matter can cause obstruction of both the large and small airways, leading to atelectasis, hypoxemia, and hypercapnia. Each of these acutely increases PVR and risks abruptly increasing RV afterload and thus inducing RV strain or failure. Systemic hypoxemia further risks inadequate myocardial oxygen delivery, particularly in those with RV hypertrophy and elevated RV diastolic pressure (wall tension). While healthy children can be quite ill after a large-volume aspiration event, those with preexisting cardiopulmonary disease will likely fare worse.

Should positive pressure ventilation be avoided in this type of patient?

Positive pressure ventilation (PPV) decreases preload and increases RV afterload, which should be considered in those with existing RVOTO or RV dysfunction. On the other hand, hypoventilation with resultant hypercapnia and hypoxemia will increase PVR and also risk increasing the overall RV afterload. Thus, a reasonable approach is to allow spontaneous ventilation when appropriate for the procedure and when the patient is able to maintain adequate oxygenation or ventilation; if neither of these factors are met, it may be preferable to control ventilation. While the impact of PPV is a prudent question to consider in children with CHD, the impact is generally not a consideration for those with repaired defects, including repaired d-TGA, without residual cardiac abnormalities. In this case, the anesthesiologist must weigh the risks and benefits present, also considering the child's history of recurrent vomiting.

Is it appropriate to perform this case in a remote location?

Although the ASO for children with d-TGA provides anatomic correction with typically normal to near-normal physiologic function, there can be residual dysfunction as in this child. An understanding of the patient's current cardiac function, as well as the particular geographic constraints and proximity of the gastrointestinal (GI) suite to assistance, must be considered before agreeing to perform an anesthetic in a GI suite that may or may not be in a location remote from operative services. The appropriateness of care in a free-standing GI suite (not within a hospital) for patients with residual cardiac disease must be weighed with even greater caution.

Is outpatient surgery appropriate for this patient?

Overall, the appropriateness of outpatient surgery always depends on the presence of comorbidities, procedure type, need for postoperative pain management or physiologic support, and social issues at home. In this case, the 10-year-old boy has preserved RV function and is able to exercise, although with early fatigue. Nothing in this history is an absolute contraindication to outpatient care, especially considering the brevity and noninvasiveness of the procedure and lack of pain management requirements afterwards. A conservative but reasonable approach is to require a longer recovery period post-procedure, and if the anesthetic is uncomplicated and the child has "returned to baseline" without worrisome signs or symptoms, the child may be discharged home. Those with repaired d-TGA without residual cardiac comorbidities are certainly candidates for outpatient surgery, while those with signs of RV failure may require admission or prolonged observation post-procedure.

> **Clinical Pearl**
>
> *A conservative but reasonable approach is to require a longer recovery period post-procedure, and if the anesthetic is uncomplicated and the child has "returned to baseline" without worrisome signs or symptoms, the child may be discharged home.*

Suggested Reading

Angeli E., Raisky O., Bonnet D., et al. Late reoperations after neonatal arterial switch operation for transposition of the great arteries. *Eur J Cardiothorac Surg* 2008; **34**: 32–6.

Cohen M. S., Eidem B. W., Cetta F., et al. Multimodality imaging guidelines of patients with transposition of the great arteries from the American Society of Echocardiography developed in collaboration with the Society for Cardiovascular Magnetic Resonance and Society of Cardiovascular Computed Tomography. *J Am Soc Echocardiogr* 2016; **29**: 571–621.

Gottlieb E. A. and Andropoulos D. B. Anesthesia for the patient with congenital heart disease presenting for noncardiac surgery. *Curr Opin Anesth* 2013; **26**: 318–26.

Latham G. L., Joffe D. C., Eisses M. J., et al. Anesthetic considerations and management of transposition of the great arteries. *Semin Cardiothorac Vasc Anesth* 2015; **19**: 233–43.

Morgan C. T., Mertens L., Grotenhuis H., et al. Understanding the mechanism for branch pulmonary artery stenosis after the arterial switch operation for transposition of the great arteries. *Eur Heart J Cardiovasc Imaging* 2017; **18**: 180–5.

Warnes C. A., Williams R. G., Bashore T. M., et al. ACC/AHA 2008 Guidelines for the management of adults with congenital heart disease: a report of the American College of Cardiology/American Heart Association Task Force on practice guidelines (Writing Committee to develop guidelines on the management of adults with congenital heart disease). *Circulation* 2008; **118**: 714–833.

22

D-Transposition of the Great Arteries (Atrial Switch)

Denise C. Joffe and Michael J. Eisses

Case Scenario

A 35-year-old woman with dextro-transposition of the great arteries presented to the Adult Congenital Heart Disease clinic with a history of worsening exercise tolerance and shortness of breath. As a newborn she had a surgical balloon atrial septostomy performed, followed by a Mustard atrial switch procedure in infancy. A cardiac computed tomography scan now shows a possible small baffle leak, and thus she was scheduled for diagnostic cardiac catheterization with possible baffle leak closure.

Recent transthoracic echocardiogram shows:

- *Atrial switch repair of dextro-transposition of the great arteries*
- *Mildly depressed systemic right ventricular function*
- *No evidence of baffle stenosis or leaks*

Key Objectives

- Understand the anatomy of dextro-transposition of the great arteries and an atrial switch procedure.
- Describe the long-term sequelae of atrial switch anatomy in a patient with dextro-transposition.
- Describe the complications of an intraatrial baffle procedure.
- Describe the anesthetic considerations in patients with intraatrial baffle procedures who are undergoing noncardiac surgery and catheterization procedures.
- Describe the transesophageal echocardiogram in a patient with a Mustard procedure.

Pathophysiology

What is the anatomy of d-transposition of the great arteries?

In "simple" dextro-transposition of the great arteries (d-TGA) the great vessels originate from the wrong ventricle. The aortic valve is anterior and rightward of the pulmonic valve resulting in a discordant connection between the ventricles and the great arteries. Systemic blood return flows from the vena cavae to the right atrium (RA), right ventricle (RV), and aorta. Pulmonary venous blood flows from the left atrium (LA) to the left ventricle (LV) and exits the pulmonary artery (PA), returning again to the pulmonary veins. *Blood flows in a parallel fashion, with deoxygenated blood recirculating to the body and oxygenated blood recirculating to the lungs.* (See Chapter 21.) The resultant physiology is not compatible with life unless there is mixing between circulations. The most common source of mixing in simple d-TGA is an atrial septal defect (ASD), patent foramen ovale (PFO), or patent ductus arteriosus (PDA). In simple d-TGA there are no other associated cardiac defects.

What is the difference between an atrial switch and arterial switch procedure?

Although both procedures correct the abnormal physiology created by parallel circulations, they do so in significantly different ways. An *atrial switch* procedure reroutes atrial blood via a baffle to the correct great vessel, albeit via the wrong ventricle. (See Figure 22.1.) In contrast, in an *arterial switch* operation (ASO) the great vessels are transected and moved to the appropriate ventricle, and the coronary arteries are reimplanted into the neoaortic root, thereby correcting the anatomy. (Figure 21.4.) Importantly, in contrast to the atrial switch procedure, the LV becomes the systemic ventricle after an ASO.

Clinical Pearl

*An **atrial switch** procedure reroutes atrial blood via a baffle to the correct great vessel, albeit via the wrong ventricle. In contrast, in an **arterial switch** procedure the great vessels are transected and moved to the appropriate ventricle, and the coronary arteries are reimplanted into the neoaortic root, thereby correcting the anatomy. (See Figure 21.4.)*

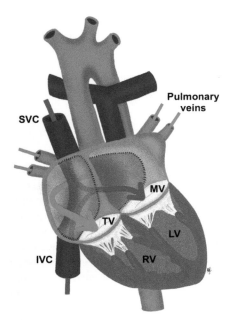

Figure 22.1 A Mustard repair for d-TGA. The SVC and IVC are baffled to form the SVP that directs blood to the MV and LV (blue arrow). Blood from the pulmonary veins enters posterior and to the right of the baffle, draining to the TV and RV (red arrow). IVC, inferior vena cava; LV, left ventricle; MV, mitral valve; RV, right ventricle; SVC, superior vena cava; TV, tricuspid valve. Courtesy of Michael Eisses, MD.

What is the history of management for patients with d-TGA?

Prior to the development of either the atrial switch or ASO, survival of neonates with d-TGA was improved by increasing intracardiac mixing of blood with a surgical atrial septostomy (Blalock–Hanlon–Thomas septostomy). Soon after, the introduction of the percutaneous balloon septostomy by Dr. Rashkind eliminated the need for surgery. However, a simple atrial septostomy did not eliminate shunts or correct the physiology, and patients succumbed early because of severe hypoxemia, congestive heart failure or pulmonary hypertension (PH). Survival beyond infancy came with the introduction of surgical repairs that corrected the discordant anatomy and eliminated the shunts. Although it was recognized from the outset that the optimal procedure to correct d-TGA was an ASO, the ability to transfer the coronary arteries required more sophisticated surgical techniques and equipment than was available at the time. In the late 1960s, Drs. Senning and Mustard developed ingenious but different ways of rerouting atrial blood to the opposite ventricle (see Figure 22.1), and atrial switch procedures became the procedure of choice for the next 15–20 years until the ASO became standard treatment for simple d-TGA. The atrial switch is no longer performed for

children with d-TGA, but as of 2008, there were an estimated 9000 adult congenital heart disease (ACHD) patients in the United States who had undergone atrial switch procedures performed for the correction of d-TGA.

Do any cardiac lesions still require an atrial switch procedure as part of the repair?

As previously described, an atrial switch is no longer performed in patients with d-TGA. An atrial switch or a hemi-atrial switch (also called a hemi-Mustard or hemi-Senning; the inferior vena cava (IVC) alone is baffled to the mitral valve while the superior vena cava (SVC) is utilized in a bidirectional Glenn shunt) may be necessary in a small subset of patients with complex congenital heart disease (CHD). For example, patients with levo-TGA (l-TGA) or heterotaxy syndrome may require an atrial switch or hemi-switch as part of their repair. (See Chapter 23.) Therefore, although the number of patients requiring an atrial switch procedure has decreased significantly in the past 30 years, these procedures are still occasionally performed.

> **Clinical Pearl**
>
> *Atrial switch procedures were historically performed in patients with d-TGA, and these patients are now between 35 and 60 years old. Atrial switch procedures are still occasionally performed in patients with complex anatomy such as levo-TGA and heterotaxy syndrome.*

What is the difference between a Mustard and a Senning procedure?

The Senning procedure uses complicated incisions and suturing of pericardium in situ to create the baffle, whereas the Mustard procedure uses the patient's excised pericardium to create the baffles and is an easier procedure to master. Although hard to conceptualize, the shape of the single piece of pericardium used in creating a Mustard baffle is rectangular. In both procedures, the baffles are fashioned so that the SVC and IVC limbs join together in what appears to be a "Y" connection, creating a systemic venous pathway that then directs blood to the left-sided mitral valve (MV), into the LV, and then to the PA. Oxygenated pulmonary venous blood remains on the posterior side of the baffle until it reaches the RA and the tricuspid valve (TV) and is then ejected from the RV into the aorta. Close inspection of Figures 22.1 and 22.2 demonstrates why these are referred to as atrial switch procedures. Blood returns to the correct circulation albeit via the wrong ventricle. The LV is also referred to as the subpulmonary ventricle and the RV as the subaortic ventricle. (See Figure 22.3.)

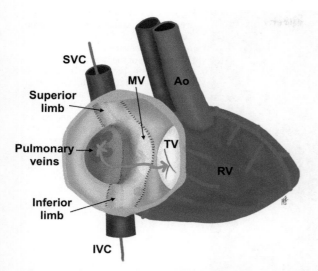

Figure 22.2 A Mustard procedure for d-TGA. A rectangular shaped baffle is used to create the SVP and PVP. The original interatrial septum is excised, and the baffle sutured as depicted creating the pathways. The PVP (red arrow) opens posteriorly and leads to the TV and RV. The SVP (blue arrow) is composed of the superior and inferior limbs that merge and are directed to the MV and LV. Ao, aorta; IVC, inferior vena cava; PA, pulmonary artery; RV, right ventricle; TV, tricuspid valve. Courtesy of Michael Eisses, MD.

It is impossible to distinguish the type of atrial switch using imaging techniques, but it is important to know whether the patient had a Mustard or Senning procedure because certain complications are more common depending on the procedure.

What are the long-term sequelae for patients with atrial switch anatomy after correction of d-TGA?

Common complications center around the constructed intraatrial baffles, including atrial arrhythmias, sinus node dysfunction, and baffle leaks and stenoses. Other long-term sequelae include systemic ventricular (RV) dysfunction and systemic atrioventricular valve regurgitation (for these patients, TR). (See Figure 22.4.)

Atrial arrhythmias (e.g., atrial flutter, supraventricular reentrant tachycardias) and sinus node dysfunction (e.g., junctional rhythm and atrioventricular block) are a common problem, occurring in up to 30% of patients by the age of 20 years. The etiology is likely multifactorial and includes extensive baffle suture lines across the atria with subsequent fibrosis, although injury to the sinus node artery itself during surgery is possible. Abnormal looping of the ventricles also contributes to heart block. Between 20% and 50% of patients are pacemaker-dependent by age 50 years,

with many requiring implantable cardioverter defibrillators (ICDs). Lead placement is backwards in these patients and can result in confusion, as leads are seen on the left side of the heart. The atrial lead is placed in the left atrial appendage and ventricular leads in the LV (subpulmonary atrium and ventricle), unlike the typical lead placement in the RA appendage and RV of a normal heart.

Symptoms of **baffle obstruction** depend on which venous pathway is affected. Systemic venous baffle obstruction is more common after the Mustard procedure whereas pulmonary venous baffle obstruction is more common after the Senning procedure. Obstruction of the systemic venous baffle occurs in up to 30% of patients. The superior limb is more susceptible because it is smaller than the inferior limb and also often has pacing leads. Patients usually have few signs and symptoms because obstruction generally develops over time, and the SVC can decompress via the azygous system to the inferior limb. Patients with obstruction of the inferior limb may present with ascites and liver dysfunction. Obstruction of the pulmonary venous baffle usually occurs at the distal end of the baffle as the pulmonary venous blood is directed into the TV. (See Figure 22.4.) Patients usually present with symptoms similar to those of mitral stenosis, including progressive shortness of breath (SOB), pulmonary edema, and PH. Although it might be difficult to identify the baffle obstruction with transthoracic echocardiography (TTE), indirect evidence of PH such as LV (subpulmonary) hypertrophy and elevated velocity of the MR jet should heighten the suspicion for obstruction and prompt further imaging investigation.

Baffle leaks are less common than baffle obstruction, but leaks occur in about 15% of patients. They result in a predominantly left-to-right shunt akin to an ASD from the higher pressure pulmonary venous pathway to the lower pressure systemic venous pathway, and cause symptoms of pulmonary overcirculation such as SOB and exercise intolerance. Most small defects are well tolerated and do not require closure as the hemodynamic burden is not significant. Some, however, may require closure in order to avoid systemic emboli when pacemaker or ICD leads are necessary. In the presence of systemic venous baffle stenosis and a proximal leak, patients can develop symptomatic right-to-left-shunting.

Clinical Pearl

Common complications center around the constructed intraatrial baffles, including atrial arrhythmias, sinus node dysfunction, and baffle leaks and stenoses. Other long-term sequelae include systemic ventricular (RV) dysfunction and systemic atrioventricular valve regurgitation (TR).

147

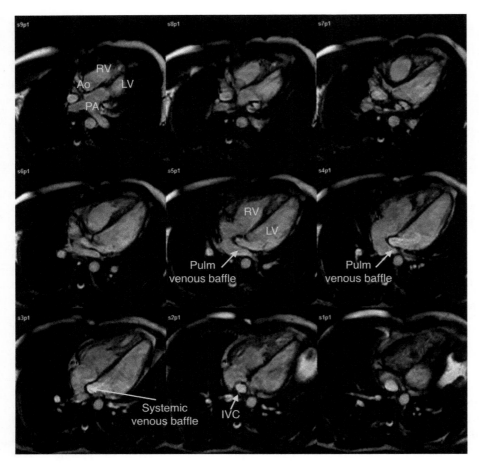

Figure 22.3 d-Transposition of the great arteries status post atrial baffle (Senning). Panel of four-chamber magnetic resonance imaging showing transposition of the great arteries status post atrial baffle procedure. The pulmonary veins are baffled to the right ventricle and the vena cavae are both baffled to the left ventricle. The resulting circulation is a systemic right ventricle connected to the aorta and a subpulmonary left ventricle connected to the pulmonary artery. Courtesy of Michael Taylor, MD.

Clinical Pearl

Between 20% and 50% of patients are pacemaker-dependent by age 50 years, with many requiring implantable cardioverter defibrillators. Lead placement is backwards in these patients and can result in confusion, since leads are seen on the left side of the heart. The atrial lead is placed in the left atrial appendage and ventricular leads in the LV (subpulmonary atrium and ventricle), unlike the typical lead placement in the RA appendage and RV of a normal heart.

How are baffle complications treated?

Whenever possible, transcatheter procedures such as balloon dilation, with or without stent placement, are used to treat baffle stenosis. In many cases of superior limb stenosis (i.e., SVC), the procedure is complicated by the presence of pacing leads entering the SVC. To place a stent, the pacing wires either have to be removed with laser therapy and then replaced, or the leads can be left in place and "jailed" by the stent. There are rare scenarios in which "jailing" leads may be indicated such as when the patient is being listed for heart transplant or if removing the leads poses prohibitive risk. Baffle leaks are treated with device closure. Surgical revisions are rarely necessary and have been plagued by a high operative mortality.

Although baffle-related complications may be difficult to identify by TTE, other noninvasive imaging techniques such as cardiovascular magnetic resonance imaging (CMRI) or cardiac computed tomography (CT) may offer improved visualization. In cases when the diagnosis remains unclear, such as the patient presented in the scenario, TEE performed during cardiac catheterization may confirm the diagnosis of a baffle complication and allow simultaneous treatment with a structural intervention.

How well does the RV function as the systemic ventricle?

Systemic RV function is largely preserved until the fourth decade of life, after which it begins to deteriorate. Causes of RV failure are multifactorial, including differences in

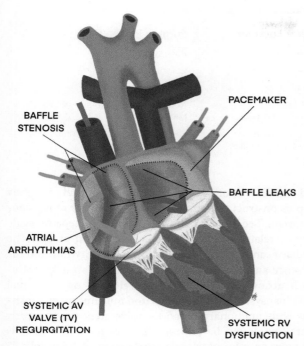

Figure 22.4 Common complications of a Mustard repair for d-TGA. Courtesy of Michael Eisses, MD.

geometric shape, coronary perfusion, and myocardial fiber orientation compared to the morphologic LV, with the end result that the RV is disadvantaged as a systemic ventricle. Also, the presence of TR significantly exacerbates systemic RV dysfunction, creating a cycle of worsening regurgitation and RV dysfunction.

> **Clinical Pearl**
>
> *Despite the fact that the RV is not well suited to perform as the systemic ventricle, RV function is mostly preserved until the fourth decade of life. Tricuspid regurgitation is poorly tolerated in patients with a systemic RV.*

How is RV function assessed?

With TTE, RV function is usually described in qualitative terms, ranging from normal to severely depressed function. However, the use of quantitative methods such as tricuspid annular plane systolic excursion (TAPSE), fractional area change, ejection fraction, and tissue Doppler may provide more objective assessment of RV function. The caveat is that echocardiography results are confounded by the frequent presence of significant TR, which can falsely infer good ventricular function as the aforementioned RV measures are preload and afterload dependent. These techniques are

also plagued by the difficulty of evaluating function because of the geometry of the RV (whether it be a normal RV or systemic RV). Three-dimensional strain echocardiography shows promise but has not been validated. Cardiac magnetic resonance imaging and/or cardiac CT are commonly used to provide a more reliable quantitative assessment of ventricular function using volume analysis and can provide an evaluation of anatomy. However, a significant number of patients are not eligible for CMRI due to the presence of a pacemaker.

> **Clinical Pearl**
>
> *Transthoracic echocardiography can overestimate right ventricular function in the presence of TR.*

What is the survival and functional status of patients after atrial switch procedures?

Historically, survival has been 80%–90% at 20 years and 68% at 40 years in patients with a Mustard procedure. Survival rates are marginally better in those with a Senning procedure. Most adults are in New York Heart Association Class I or II and are able to work and function quite normally. About half of deaths are sudden, suggesting an arrhythmogenic mechanism, with rapid atrial flutter or ventricular arrhythmias thought to be the likely mechanisms.

What is the recommended follow-up for patients who have undergone an atrial switch procedure?

According to the 2018 American Heart Association/ American College of Cardiology guidelines for the management of adults with CHD, follow-up is recommended annually, with TTE to be performed every 2–3 years. Echocardiography is also the primary diagnostic imaging modality in the event of new symptoms. Cardiac magnetic resonance imaging, cardiac CT, and cardiopulmonary exercise testing are also recommended every few years. Cardiac catheterization is performed on an as-needed basis. The incidence of complications, especially sinus node dysfunction with accompanying TR and systemic ventricular dysfunction, increases with age, mandating closer follow-up in older patients.

Despite these recommendations, in reality follow-up is often lacking due to a large number of factors, including poor transfer and coordination of care with appropriate ACHD specialists, lack of availability and expertise of ACHD in the community, insurance and financial issues, and poor patient compliance. A surprising proportion of

ACHD patients do not possess an adequate understanding of their cardiac disease or details of their repair and thus may struggle with self-advocacy and understanding the need for routine surveillance and care.

Unless the patient is in extremis, it is generally recommended that the ACHD patient with anything more than repaired simple CHD (ASD, VSD, or PDA) be followed by an ACHD cardiologist and cared for by ACHD specialists, including anesthesiologists, intensivists, and interventional radiologists.

In addition to the patient's CHD, it is equally important in the ACHD population to consider evaluation for acquired heart disease or other systemic diseases.

Clinical Pearl

Adult congenital heart disease patients frequently lack appropriate follow up surveillance and care. They should also be evaluated for acquired heart disease or other systemic diseases when indicated.

What key findings can be suggestive of potential complications?

Exercise tolerance is probably the best indicator of overall function in patients after an atrial switch procedure. Many symptoms develop gradually with decreasing cardiac function, so it is crucial to follow up with pointed questions, especially since poor conditioning can lead to similar symptoms. An overall decrease in exercise tolerance may be related to any aspect of abnormal anatomy from ventricular dysfunction to baffle complications. Specifically, paroxysmal dyspnea and orthopnea may point to pulmonary venous baffle obstruction or PH, and palpitations suggest atrial or ventricular arrhythmias. Syncope is very concerning, as it can be a symptom of malignant atrial or ventricular arrhythmias. Patients with ICDs should be asked if it has discharged; the device should be interrogated, and the history reviewed.

Clinical Pearl

Exercise tolerance is the best indicator of overall cardiac function. Poor exercise tolerance may be related to any of several important complications of an atrial switch and should be evaluated before anything but emergent surgery.

On physical examination, a low heart rate suggests sinus node dysfunction, and facial plethora may be related to obstruction of the SVC systemic venous baffle. Cyanosis is unusual and may suggest a combination of baffle stenosis

Table 22.1 Surgical Procedures and Scars Associated with d-TGA

Scar Location	Surgical Procedure
Midline	Atrial switch procedure
Left thoracotomy	Coarctation repair
Right thoracotomy	Surgical septostomy
Pacer in left subclavian pocket	Normal venous anatomy – normal pacer placement
Pacer in right subclavian pocket	Presence of left SVC or thrombosed right subclavian vein

and a baffle leak or PH. The location of surgical scars may help reconstruct the surgical history if the patient is a poor historian. (See Table 22.1.). The presence of hepatomegaly may be related to inferior baffle obstruction or PH. The cardiac examination should focus on rate, rhythm, and the presence and timing of murmurs, which can help distinguish atrioventricular valve regurgitation or a residual VSD (pansystolic) from the ejection murmur more consistent with pulmonary or aortic valve stenosis. However, heart sounds can be misleading, since the aortic valve is the more anterior of the two great vessels. A loud, split S2 may be normal and not a result of PH.

An electrocardiogram (ECG) should be performed or available. Right ventricular hypertrophy and right axis deviation are expected findings in patients with a systemic RV. Rate and rhythm can help determine sinus node function. If a pacemaker is present, paced beats should be noted, and formal pacemaker evaluation may be indicated if concerns arise from the history and physical examination. A chest radiograph will demonstrate sternal wires. In pacemaker-dependent patients, leads enter the left (subpulmonary) ventricle. Variable degrees of cardiomegaly and RV hypertrophy are usually present and consistent with a systemic RV.

Clinical Pearl

Red flags on physical examination may include lack of sinus rhythm, cyanosis, facial plethora, a pansystolic murmur (likely due to TR), and hepatomegaly.

Anesthetic Implications

What are the anesthetic considerations in patients who have undergone an atrial switch procedure?

The majority of ACHD patients are cared for in centers without specific expertise in CHD, so it is important for the anesthesiologist to have an understanding of the patient's disease and the previously described potential complications. A picture is worth a thousand words. Whenever possible, a copy of the patient's catheterization report or even a hand-sketched picture of the patient's heart often allows the anesthesiologist and other providers unfamiliar with the anatomy and repair to mentally reconstruct the direction of blood flow.

Clinical Pearls

Early consultation with an ACHD cardiologist is optimal for a patient with anything more than simple CHD; remote consultation may be necessary if no local provider is available. The most recent catheterization report with a picture of the patient's heart or a hand-drawn sketch of the anatomy and repair is extremely helpful to understand the direction of blood flow. Attaching it to the patient's bed or chart is very useful for all providers.

When transfer to a specialized center is not possible, the timing of the preoperative assessment should be planned to allow sufficient time before the procedure to obtain records from the patient's cardiologist. If records are not available, then a focused history and physical examination with an emphasis on exercise capacity can help classify the patient's condition. Even if the focused examination suggests good exercise capacity it is ideal to request a TTE in order to confirm the diagnosis and rule out any unexpected findings, since patients may not provide reliable histories. This sequence is suggested if no prior cardiology visits or TTE are available for reference. High-risk patients include those with limited exercise capacity, dyspnea (especially at rest), palpitations, presence of an ICD, RV dysfunction, TR, and evidence of PH. Elective surgery should be deferred pending a cardiology consultation in all high-risk patients.

If the patient is deemed stable, low-risk, and undergoing a low-risk procedure, then anesthesia should proceed in a standard fashion similar to that for any patient, with these caveats:

- Systemic RV function may not be as good as described in studies, especially in the presence of TR.
- The presence of TR is not as well tolerated in patients with a systemic RV.
- Pacemaker and ICD function may require reprogramming (similar to any patient with a pacemaker or ICD), and there should be a low threshold for placing defibrillator pads, even in the absence of a history of tachyarrhythmias, especially if the location of the surgical site will limit access to the chest.

A low threshold for utilization of monitors such as TEE should be considered as long as the echocardiographer understands the anatomy. If volume status and ventricular function are the primary objectives of monitoring, then it is possible to "ignore" the intraatrial anatomy and just focus on ventricular function and volume status using standard views, such as a four-chamber view or transgastric mid-papillary view, with the caveat that the RV is the systemic ventricle. The RV will appear more hypertrophied and dilated and the LV will appear compressed compared to normal anatomy. However, the technique for "eyeballing" function should be similar to that in a normal patient. Ideally, if the provider is able, the additional assessment of TR will permit a more accurate grading of "true" RV function as described previously.

Clinical Pearl

Transesophageal echocardiography can be used to monitor ventricular function and volume status even by those with only basic TEE training by ignoring intraatrial anatomy and with the caveat that the RV is the systemic ventricle.

What are the anesthetic considerations in high-risk patients presenting for noncardiac surgery?

A high-risk patient having a low-risk procedure should be managed like other high-risk cardiac patients with similar pathology. For example, an atrial switch patient with poor RV function and TR is analogous to a patient with severely decreased LV function and MR. A patient with an atrial switch and either PH or atrial arrhythmias requires management similar to that for patients with normal anatomy and similar pathology. The need for invasive monitoring will depend on both the procedure and the particular hemodynamic risks for that patient. There are no specific considerations for arterial access, and arterial lines should be placed for indications similar to those in other patients. There are special considerations for central venous access, as discussed in the next question. In general, there should be a low threshold for postoperative admission to intensive care, even after a low-risk procedure, especially in non-ACHD hospitals, given the lack of familiarity of most providers with the disease.

When a high-risk patient requires a high-risk procedure, the optimal scenario is to have it performed in a specialized center with cardiologists, cardiac anesthesiologists, and intensivists familiar with ACHD. All the considerations previously mentioned apply; in addition, the ability to perform and interpret intraoperative TEE should be available.

Options for advanced resuscitation with mechanical circulatory support (MCS) devices must be discussed in the context of the patient's anatomy. The choice of MCS device must consider the presence of intraatrial baffles and a systemic RV, which is morphologically distinct from an LV and may affect technical aspects of device placement. The preoperative visit should include determination of candidacy for MCS and whether the patient is a transplant candidate, as well as discussion of an advanced care directive.

What considerations exist when placing central venous lines in patients with an atrial switch?

If central venous access utilizing neck vessels is being considered due to patient or surgical factors, one must take into account the likely higher than normal risk of complications that could occur with line placement in a patient with a baffle. The use of fluoroscopy may facilitate placement, and the line should be placed by a proceduralist familiar with atrial baffle anatomy and knowledge of the expected course of the wire and catheter. The following factors should be considered prior to line placement:

1. *Knowledge of the primary lesion*: For example, if the atrial switch was performed for d-TGA, both superior (internal jugular or subclavian vein) and inferior (femoral) venous pressure measurements should be identical, since they reflect systemic venous pressures, that is, central venous pressure (CVP), whereas, if a hemi-Mustard is performed for l-TGA, an upper body CVL measures Glenn pressure, that is pulmonary artery pressure, and a femoral venous line measures CVP, which are not the same. (See Figure 22.5A and B.)

2. *Knowledge of the presence of baffle stenosis or leaks*: Known baffle stenosis can make line placement difficult and distort measurements. Baffle obstruction can be manifest by higher than expected pressure readings and a lack of phasic appearance if the line is superior to the obstruction. If there is resistance to advancement of the wire or catheter while placing a central venous line in the neck, there should be a low threshold to abandon placement, especially because obstruction of the superior limb of the atrial baffle is not uncommon, as discussed previously. Line placement through the femoral vein is also an option and avoids entering the heart and baffles.

Placing a central line in the neck in a patient with a baffle leak can result in inadvertent catheter misplacement or migration into the pulmonary venous baffle, which can theoretically extend the tear. In addition, pressure measurements will reflect pulmonary venous pressure, not systemic venous pressure. Also given that a leak usually results in a left-to-right shunt, intracardiac saturations (RA, PA) will be unreliable.

3. *The purpose of CVL placement*: If the line is being placed solely for volume resuscitation or medication infusion, then access via the femoral veins or a rapid infusion catheter (RIC) placed in a large upper extremity vein may be ideal, since it avoids the need to enter the heart. If the line is being placed for CVP measurement and/or medication infusions, femoral access may also be ideal, since it often allows accurate CVP measurement while avoiding the risk of entering the atrial baffles. When a PA catheter (PAC) is necessary to measure PA pressures or for cardiac output monitoring, the accuracy of some measurements (mixed venous or PA saturation and cardiac output) depends on the absence of baffle leaks or significant regurgitation of the subpulmonary atrioventricular valve (MR in the case of d-TGA and TR in the setting of l-TGA). Pulmonary artery catheter placement can be challenging, since it can be difficult to enter the PA from the LV, arguing for placement by an experienced provider using fluoroscopy. Pulmonary artery catheters should be used only when absolutely indicated for patient management.

What are the anesthetic considerations for cardiac catheterization procedures in a patient with an atrial switch?

In this population, a cardiac catheterization is typically performed to diagnose and treat a baffle problem, to diagnose PH and confirm its etiology, or as part of a pretransplant cardiac evaluation. Cardiac catheterizations may also be done as part of an electrophysiology procedure to treat arrythmias or to place or repair transvenous pacing or ICD systems.

Anesthetic management of ACHD patients in the catheterization laboratory depends on patient-related factors such as the diagnosis and severity of disease, the history of surgical procedures, and additional comorbidities. Many ACHD patients have significant anxiety and poor coping skills during medical procedures and prefer general anesthesia because that is what they received during their prior pediatric procedures. In addition, the need for TEE to guide device placement may mandate the use of general endotracheal anesthesia. When intracardiac echocardiography is used, the procedure can be performed with sedation alone, although even then a general anesthetic with a supraglottic device or endotracheal tube is frequently required for patient safety because of the duration or complexity of the case.

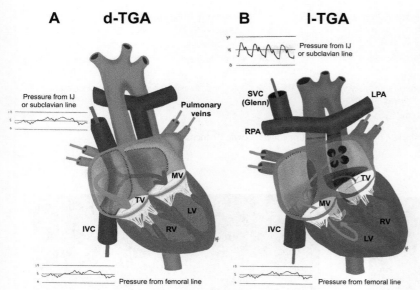

Figure 22.5 Central venous pressures. Depending on the original anatomy and the presence of a complete Mustard or hemi-Mustard, venous pressures from a central line in the neck versus a central femoral line may be different. In (A), both SVC and IVC pathways should reflect central venous pressure, whereas in (B), the IVC reflects central venous pressure and the SVC reflects PAP. IVC, inferior vena cava; LPA, left pulmonary artery; LV, left ventricle; MV, mitral valve; PAP, pulmonary artery pressure; RAP, right atrial pressure; RPA, right pulmonary artery; RV, right ventricle; SVC, superior vena cava; TV, tricuspid valve. Courtesy of Michael Eisses, MD.

Regarding vascular access, a peripheral intravenous catheter is all that is required for induction unless the patient's clinical status is precarious and necessitates a preinduction arterial line. The cardiologist usually places femoral arterial and venous lines for the majority of procedures, and the venous line can be accessed by large-bore extension tubing if needed. Placing separate invasive lines may be warranted if the patient requires pre- or postprocedural arterial blood pressure monitoring or ongoing central venous access. Replacing a relatively large femoral venous sheath used for the catheterization with a smaller CVL for use in the postoperative period may be complicated by unacceptable bleeding around the smaller line, necessitating placement at an alternate site. A more permanent CVL in the upper body can be performed with fluoroscopy at the conclusion of the procedure.

The procedure begins with a diagnostic catheterization of the systemic venous chambers, including the superior and inferior baffles and pathways, as well as the LV and PA. Saturation measurements in these locations are used to determine systemic and pulmonary cardiac outputs and assess for the presence of shunts. The patient should be maintained on room air in order to use the Fick equation for cardiac output and shunt calculations. Room air also allows baseline measurements of cardiac pressures. A left heart catheterization is performed in a retrograde fashion when indicated. When there is a concern for a baffle leak or obstruction, the complete TEE is performed concurrently with the catheterization in order to evaluate the baffle, help localize pathology, and guide the procedure when indicated.

The postoperative disposition of the patient varies with the severity of the patient's disease, and the procedure performed. In general, if the procedure is limited to a diagnostic catheterization, most patients are discharged home. If a therapeutic procedure with device placement is performed, the patient is usually admitted for observation and repeat TTE prior to discharge.

How can the baffle be evaluated using TEE?

A physician sonographer with advanced training in echocardiography should perform the examination and help guide the interventionalist. A general description of the echocardiographic evaluation is provided in the text that follows, since it helps non-CHD echocardiography trained providers understand the anatomy. When imaging a patient with an atrial switch using TEE, the optimal views include the mid-esophageal four-chamber view and an orthogonal (perpendicular) plane. Landmarks are used to identify the pathway being evaluated. (See Table 22.2.)

The four-chamber view provides qualitative assessment of biventricular and atrioventricular valve function and looks similar to that of a normal patient except the LV often appears flattened by a dilated and hypertrophied systemic RV. (See Figures 22.6 and 22.7.) The tricuspid and mitral valves are in their normal position and should be evaluated for regurgitation. In this view, the baffle and pathways are usually well seen. The more posterior pathway is the pulmonary venous baffle. The entire pathway can be seen by identifying the pulmonary veins using 2D and Doppler techniques and then following this pathway

Table 22.2 Landmarks Used to Identify the Systemic and Pulmonary Venous Pathways in Patients with d-TGA and Atrial Switch Procedures

Landmarks Used to Identify Pathway			
Systemic venous pathway	Find IVC and SVC and follow over to left	Pacer and defibrillator leads travel in pathway	Pathway in closest proximity and opening to the MV
Pulmonary venous pathway	Use color flow Doppler to find pulmonary vein (LUPV is easiest) and then follow pathway to the right.	The most posterior pathway	Pathway in closest proximity and opening to the TV

IVC, inferior vena cava; LUPV, left upper pulmonary vein; MV, mitral valve; SVC, superior vena cava; TV, tricuspid valve.

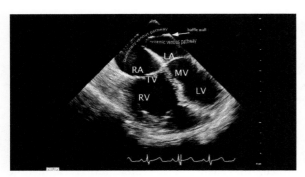

Figure 22.6 TEE ME four-chamber view. The ventricles appear in their usual position but note that the RV is larger than the LV, although the LV is slightly more dilated than expected because this patient has a significant baffle leak causing a left-to-right shunt similar to an ASD (causing LV dilation instead of RV dilation). In addition, there is right ventricular hypertrophy (the RV wall thickness is >5 mm). A baffle is seen in the atrium (labelled baffle wall). The pulmonary venous pathway is most posterior and is seen to empty into the TV. The systemic venous pathway is that portion of the LA in continuity with the MV. ASD, atrial septal defect; LA, left atrium; LV, left ventricle; ME, mid-esophageal; RV, right ventricle; TV, tricuspid valve.

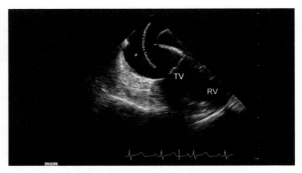

Figure 22.7 The image above is rotated to visualize the RV. The pulmonary venous pathway is seen to empty into the TV and RV. The asterisk marks a common location of obstruction in this pathway. RV, right ventricle; TV, tricuspid valve.

rightward toward the TV. In the four-chamber view, the systemic venous baffle is seen on the right side of the screen, anterior to the pulmonary venous baffle. It empties into the MV and LV. To follow the course of the systemic venous baffle, the probe is inserted into the stomach from the four-chamber view and turned to the right. The liver and the IVC are imaged enabling identification of the inferior portion of the superior venous pathway (SVP), and as the probe is withdrawn it is followed over to the left. (See Figure 22.8.)

When imaging in a plane orthogonal to the four-chamber view, the probe is rotated from right to left (counterclockwise). (See Figure 22.9.). Images depend on the cutting plane relative to the baffle. Starting with the probe rotated all the way to the right, the IVC drains to the inferior limb of the SVP. With further leftward rotation the superior (from SVC) and inferior (from IVC) limbs of the SVP are seen on either side of the pulmonary venous pathway (PVP), which courses

from posterior to anterior. This view is analogous to the mid-esophageal (ME) bicaval view with the SVC on the right of the screen and the IVC on the left. With further leftward rotation, the RV and aorta are visualized, and both limbs of the SVP are seen to merge in the center. A portion of the PVP is seen posterior to the merger, and another is seen close to the TV. Then, as the probe is rotated counterclockwise, the SVP is seen to merge completely. The RV and aorta disappear as the LV and PA are visualized. During rotation, the most posterior pathway and the one closest to the TV is always the PVP. The SVP is always closest to the mitral valve. In addition, as the probe is rotated, both ventricles, outflow tracts, and semilunar valves are seen in the long axis. As in a normal patient, the RV and tricuspid valve are first seen. The aorta originates from the RV. With further counterclockwise rotation the LV, MV, and PA are visualized.

Aliasing during color-flow Doppler examination is highly suggestive of baffle obstruction. Baffle leaks are occasionally large enough to be visible on 2D imaging, but caution is warranted to not confuse echo dropout with a defect. Echo dropout is created when the echo beam and structure of interest are almost parallel, resulting

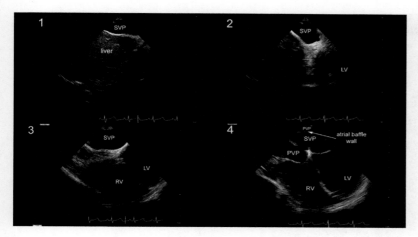

Figure 22.8 Sequence of TEE images during withdrawal from TG to ME levels and a sweep to the left at 0°. (1) TG position at the level of the liver. The IVC is visualized and identifies the SVP. (2–3) The pathway is kept in the center of the image as the probe is slowly withdrawn to the ME level and rotated to the left. (4) With the probe all the way to the left, the SVP opens to the MV. It is anterior to the PVP and is separated from it by the atrial baffle wall. IVC, inferior vena caval; ME, mid-esophageal; PVP, pulmonary venous pathway; SVP, superior venous pathway; TG, transgastric.

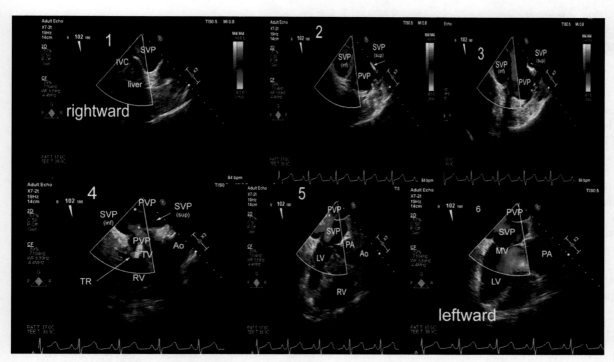

Figure 22.9 TEE color flow Doppler 102° rotation (orthogonal) sweep from the right to the left (counterclockwise). The right of the screen is superior, the left inferior, the bottom anterior, and the top posterior. (1) The IVC is located and allows identification of the inferior portions of the SVP. (2–3) The probe is withdrawn to the ME level and turned leftward. Both limbs of the SVP are seen on either side of the PVP. (4) The first ventricle visualized during the rotation is the RV. The RV, TV, and Ao are seen. Both limbs of the SVP are seen to merge. The PVP is seen posterior and closest to the TV valve. Mild to moderate TR is seen. Two baffle leaks are seen in this image (asterisks). (5) With further leftward rotation both ventricles are seen. The pathway closest to the MV is the SVP. The more posterior baffle leak is now seen between the PVP and SVP (asterisk). Note, the shunt here is left-to-right, which is the predominant overall direction of the shunt in this patient. (6) With the probe rotated all the way to the left, the LV and PA are seen, and no further shunt is visible. Ao, aorta, Inf, inferior; IVC, inferior vena cava; ME, mid-esophageal; PA, pulmonary artery; PVP, pulmonary venous pathway; RV, right ventricle; Sup, superior; SVP, superior venous pathway; TR, tricuspid regurgitation; TV, tricuspid valve.

in minimal return of echo signals and a void in the picture. A defect on 2D imaging, especially when it is an area parallel to beam, should always be verified in another view and with color-flow Doppler. (See Figure 22.10.)

When inconclusive, agitated saline can be used to verify a communication. Other supportive findings include dilation of the systemic venous atrium and ventricle (in this case the LA and LV).

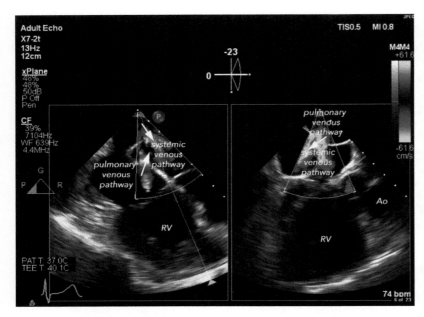

Figure 22.10 A TEE color flow Doppler ME four-chamber view and an orthogonal cut at the level of the posterior leak. This is easily performed using a TEE probe capable of biplane (X-plane) imaging. Both leaks are seen in the left-sided image, and the direction of flow is left-to-right (arrows). Although the dimensions are not measured in these images, they are quite large and measure at least 1 cm in this plane (based on the dots on the side of the image which are 1 cm apart). The right-sided image cuts through the more leftward and posterior defect only (see blue triangle at the bottom of the image and the location of the cutting plane). Ao, aorta; CFD, color flow Doppler; ME, mid-esophageal; RV, right ventricle.

Transcatheter procedures are used to treat baffle stenosis and leaks and have a high success rate. (See Figure 22.11.) TEE and fluoroscopy are used to guide the proceduralist and assess the results.

The majority of ACHD patients with atrial switch procedures initially had d-TGA, although atrial switch procedures are still occasionally performed for other complex lesions. It is necessary to understand the anatomy of the repair as well as the original lesion in order to appreciate all the anesthetic implications. Most patients remain a high-risk subgroup to anesthetize and given the complexity of the repair are best cared for in specialized centers.

Suggested Reading

Cohen M. S., Eidem B. W., Cetta F., et al. Multimodality imaging guidelines of patients with transposition of the great arteries: a report from the American Society of Echocardiography developed in collaboration with the Society for Cardiovascular Magnetic Resonance and the Society of Cardiovascular Computed Tomography. *J Am Soc Echocardiogr* 2016; **29**: 571–621.

Cuypers J. A., Eindhoven J. A., Slager M. A., et al. The natural and unnatural history of the Mustard procedure: long-term outcome up to 40 years. *Eur Heart J* 2014; **35**: 1666–74.

De Pasquale G. High prevalence of baffle leaks in adults after atrial switch operations for transposition of the great arteries. *Eur Heart J Cardiovasc Imaging* 2017; **18**: 531–5.

Dobson R., Dantan M., Nicola W., et al. The natural and unnatural history of the systemic right ventricle in

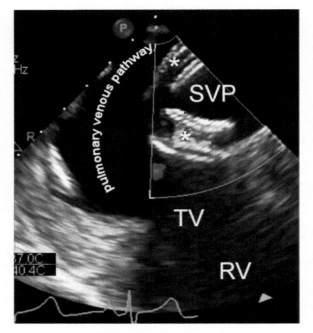

Figure 22.11 An ME four-chamber color flow Doppler view with the probe turned toward the right. This is a zoomed imaged similar to Figure 22.6. Two septal occlusion devices are visible (marked with an asterisks).

adult survivors. *J Thorac Cardiovasc Surg* 2013; **145**: 1493–50.

Haeffele C. and Lui G. K. Dextro-transposition of the great arteries: long-term sequelae of atrial and arterial switch. *Cardiol Clin* 2015; **33**: 543–58.

Joffe D. C., Krishnan S. K., Eisses M., et al. The use of transesophageal echocardiography in the management of baffles leaks in a patient with transposition of the great arteries. *AA Case Rep* 2018; 1–3.

Maxwell B. G., Wong J. K., Kin C., et al. Perioperative outcomes of major noncardiac surgery in adults with congenital heart disease. *Anesthesiology* 2013; **119**: 762–9.

Stout K. K., Daniels C. J., and Aboulhosn J. A. 2018 AHA/ACC guideline for the management of adults with congenital heart disease: a report of the American College of Cardiology/American Heart Association task force on clinical practice guidelines. *Circulation* 2018; **139**: e698–800.

Warnes C. A. Transposition of the great arteries. *Circulation* 2006; **114**: 2699–709.

Chapter 23

L-Transposition of the Great Arteries ("Corrected" Transposition)

Katie J. Roddy and Anna Kaiser

Case Scenario

A 12-year-old female presents with acute appendicitis, vomiting for more than 18 hours with minimal oral intake during this time. She has a history of levo-transposition of the great arteries diagnosed in utero and developed complete heart block requiring permanent pacemaker insertion at age 7 years. Her last outpatient cardiology appointment was 8 months ago. Her mother reports that since then she has been doing well and participating in normal activities. Cardiology was consulted, as outpatient records could not be obtained. Electrocardiogram shows a heart rate of 110 beats/minute with ventricular pacing spikes. Pacemaker interrogation revealed the following settings: DDD, intrinsic atrial rate 110 beats/minute, 0% atrial pacing, 100% ventricular pacing, and 3 years of pacemaker longevity remaining. Her current vital signs are heart rate 110 beats/minute, respiratory rate 20 breaths/minute, SpO_2 98% on room air, and blood pressure 95/55 mm Hg. Her abdomen is tender, but not distended. Her hemoglobin is 14 and hematocrit 42. Abdominal ultrasound is indicative of acute appendicitis. All other laboratory work is within normal limits.

Echocardiography reveals:

- *Mild right (systemic) ventricular dysfunction with ejection fraction 50%*
- *Moderate systemic atrioventricular valve regurgitation*
- *Dilation of the tricuspid valve annulus*

Key Objectives

- Describe the anatomy of levo (l-looped) transposition of the great arteries.
- Understand associated cardiac abnormalities and their clinical presentation.
- Identify long-term sequelae associated with uncorrected l-transposition.
- Describe the options for surgical repair to "correct" l-transposition.

- Discuss the preoperative assessment of patients with pacemakers.
- Describe intraoperative management and surgical considerations for this patient.
- Discuss whether a laparoscopic surgical approach is appropriate.
- Describe appropriate discharge criteria and disposition planning.

Pathophysiology

What are the anatomic characteristics of l-transposition of the great arteries?

Levo-transposition of the great arteries (l-TGA) is a rare anomaly, comprising less than 1% of all forms of congenital heart disease (CHD), and is characterized by both atrioventricular (AV) and ventriculoarterial (VA) discordance. In this anomaly, the right atrium (RA) connects via the mitral valve (MV) to the morphological left ventricle (LV), which supplies the pulmonary artery (PA). The left atrium (LA) connects via the tricuspid valve (TV) to the morphological right ventricle (RV), which supplies the aorta. (See Figure 23.1.) Because the TV and RV are connected to the aorta in l-TGA, they are also commonly referred as the systemic AV valve and systemic ventricle, respectively.

How does embryologic development affect the anatomy of l-TGA?

One of the crucial embryologic processes for correct anatomic alignment of the four chambers of the heart occurs during the third week of gestation. During this period the straight primitive heart tube "loops" to the right (dextro or d-loop), resulting in the normal morphologic position of the RV. However, looping to the left (levo or l-loop) leads to abnormal positioning of the ventricles and to abnormal

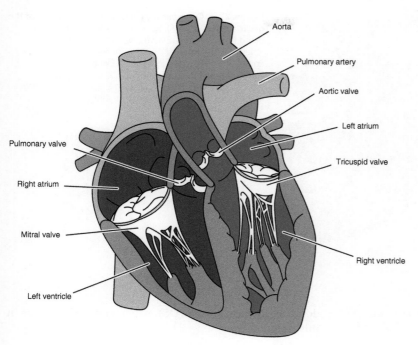

Aorta

Pulmonary artery

Aortic valve

Left atrium

Tricuspid valve

Pulmonary valve

Right atrium

Mitral valve

Right ventricle

Left ventricle

connections among the atrial, ventricular, and arterial segments of the heart.

What is the flow of deoxygenated and oxygenated blood in the heart of the l-TGA patient? Why is the term "congenitally corrected TGA" used in describing this lesion?

Deoxygenated systemic venous blood returns to the correctly positioned RA via the superior (SVC) and inferior vena cava (IVC). From the RA it flows to the discordant LV via the MV and into the lungs through the PA. Oxygenated blood from the lungs returns to the correctly positioned LA via the pulmonary veins. From the LA it flows to the discordant RV via the TV and returns to the systemic circulation through the aorta.

Based on the preceding description of blood flow, one can appreciate that the term "congenitally corrected TGA" is appropriate; despite ventriculoarterial discordance, oxygenated and deoxygenated blood flows in the correct physiologic direction resulting in normal oxygenation and perfusion. ʟ-transposition of the great arteries is also commonly referred to as "double discordance" or "ventricular inversion." (See Figure 23.2.)

What are the anatomic variations of l-TGA and the nomenclature for describing positions of the heart, atria, ventricles, and great arteries?

The most common anatomic arrangement of l-TGA is situs solitus with l-looping of the ventricles and with the aorta abnormally positioned anterior and leftward of the PA (S, L, L). Situs solitus refers to normal positioning of the thoracic and abdominal organs. Anatomically this means the heart is located in the left chest with a leftward pointing apex, with the morphologic RA located on the right and the morphologic LA located on the left. In a patient with normal cardiac anatomy, including situs solitus, d-looped ventricles, and normal great artery connections, the aorta is located rightward and posterior to the PA (S, D, D).

In a less common variation of l-TGA with situs solitus, the aorta is located anterior and rightward (S, L, D). An even less common variant of l-TGA includes dextrocardia, wherein the heart is positioned and oriented in the right chest, and situs inversus, where there is inversion of the abdominal viscera, including the liver, spleen, and stomach. It is an anatomic mirror image of l-TGA. Although the anatomy is different, the pathophysiology is the same, and thus it is also classified as l-TGA. Its designation is "I" (i.e., I, D, D) which describes situs inversus with d-looping

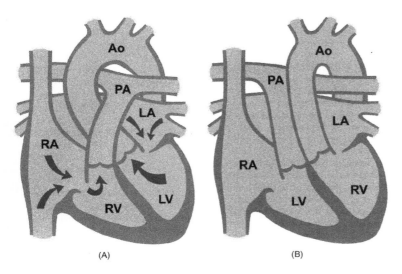

Figure 23.2 Congenitally corrected transposition of the great arteries (ccTGA). (A) Normal anatomy. (B) ccTGA – blood flow in corrected transposition. Ao, aorta; LA, left atrium; LV, left ventricle; PA, pulmonary artery; RA, right atrium; RV, right ventricle. From McEwan A. and Manolis M. Anesthesia for transposition of the great arteries. In Andropoulos D. B., Stayer S., Mossad E. B., et al., eds. *Anesthesia for Congenital Heart Surgery*, 3rd ed. John Wiley & Sons, 2015: 542–66. With permission.

of the ventricles, and the aorta positioned anterior and rightward of the PA.

> **Clinical Pearl**
>
> *Situs solitus refers to normal positioning of the thoracic and abdominal organs. Anatomically this means the heart is located in the left chest with a leftward pointing apex, with the morphologic RA located on the right and the morphologic LA located on the left. In a patient with normal cardiac anatomy, including situs solitus, d-looped ventricles, and normal great artery connections, the aorta is located rightward and posterior to the PA (S, D, D).*

How does coronary artery anatomy differ in l-TGA?

Coronary artery anatomy in patients with l-TGA is variable. The coronary arteries in l-TGA are inverted. Thus, the morphologic left coronary artery (LCA) arises from the patient's right-sided sinus and the morphologic right coronary artery (RCA) from the left sided sinus. The LCA (vessel originating from right-sided sinus) has a circumflex (left circumflex or LCX) and anterior descending (LAD) branch, while the RCA (vessel originating from the left-sided sinus) has an epicardial distribution. Although the above described coronary distributions are most common, many other variations have been described, including both RCA and LCA having a common single sinus origin, while other descriptions note hypoplasia of the left anterior descending branch. Ultimately, careful preoperative delineation of the coronary anatomy is important before the

double switch operation (DS), which is described later in this chapter.

> **Clinical Pearl**
>
> *The coronary arteries in l-TGA are inverted. Thus, the morphologic LCA arises from the patient's right-sided sinus and the morphologic RCA from the left-sided sinus.*

What is the typical clinical presentation of a patient with *isolated* l-TGA?

L-transposition occurs as an isolated defect in fewer than 10% of affected patients. Prenatal diagnosis is challenging and therefore often missed. Patients without other structural cardiac defects are asymptomatic at birth and during early childhood and usually present later in life, with some studies reporting lack of symptoms for up to 70–80 years. Older children and adults may present with signs and symptoms related to either cardiac conduction defects (bradycardia, fatigue, poor exercise tolerance) or systemic right heart failure (dyspnea, fatigue, fluid retention, decreased exercise tolerance).

Because the morphologic RV is not well suited to perform the workload of the systemic ventricle, progressive tricuspid regurgitation (TR) ensues. A controversial topic is whether poor RV function leads to TR or whether dysfunction is a result of long-standing TR. Either way, RV failure is a frequent sequel to systemic AV valve regurgitation, and surgical repair of the TV should be considered early, prior to onset of irreversible ventricular dysfunction. Tricuspid valve regurgitation increases volume overload and worsens ventricular failure. Additionally, the morphologic RV is perfused by a single coronary artery. Because the RV has higher systemic workload, it is hypothesized that its limited coronary arterial blood supply in relation to its demand places it at higher ischemic risk.

In l-TGA, the cardiac conduction system is often abnormal and unstable. The AV node and His–Purkinje conduction system (His bundle) have an unusual position and course, and many patients have dual AV nodes. The second anomalous AV node and bundle are usually located anteriorly, and the elongated bundle is vulnerable to fibrosis with advancing age. Thus, these patients are prone to developing complete heart block (CHB) and reentrant tachyarrhythmias (i.e., Wolff–Parkinson–White syndrome). The risk of developing CHB increases linearly with age; the progressive incidence is 2% per year.

Clinical Pearl

L-TGA occurs as an isolated defect in fewer than 10% of affected patients. They are asymptomatic at birth and during early childhood, and typically present later with either arrhythmias or systemic RV failure. Because their cardiac conduction system is often abnormal and unstable, they are prone to developing CHB and reentrant tachyarrhythmias.

What associated anatomic cardiac abnormalities exist for patients with l-TGA and how do these impact the physiology?

More than 90% of patients with l-TGA have additional cardiac anomalies. The most frequent are ventricular septal defects (VSD), pulmonary outflow tract obstruction, and abnormalities of the systemic (tricuspid) AV valve. The clinical presentation and course in this cohort of patients with l-TGA depends on the presence and nature of the associated defects.

- *Ventricular septal defects* occur in up to 80% of patients with l-TGA. Most commonly the VSD is a large, perimembranous outflow (subpulmonary) defect, although the defect can be located in any region of the ventricular septum. If the defect is small, or restrictive, a systolic murmur may be present, becoming evident once the pulmonary vascular resistance (PVR) sufficiently falls after birth. This results in left-to-right shunting, specifically shunting of blood from the morphologic RV (left-sided) to the morphologic LV (right-sided). Patients with a large or unrestrictive VSD usually present in infancy or childhood with congestive heart failure (CHF).

- *Pulmonary outflow tract obstruction* (used synonymously with LV outflow tract obstruction or LVOTO) occurs in approximately 30%–60% of patients with l-TGA and often accompanies a large VSD. The obstruction is commonly subpulmonary (subvalvular) and less frequently secondary to valvular pulmonary stenosis or atresia. Subpulmonary stenosis may be due to a fibromuscular membrane, fibrous tissue tags, or aneurysmal tissue of the interventricular septum. Neonates will often present with cyanosis if pulmonary outflow tract obstruction and concomitant VSD are present, as there is limited pulmonary blood flow (PBF) with significant pulmonary-to-systemic ventricular level shunting.

- *Tricuspid (systemic AV) valve abnormalities* have been reported in up to 90% of patients at autopsy, but not all clinically manifest during a patient's lifetime. Regurgitation is common and generally progressive. There is a wide range of variability in severity of the abnormality, with severe "Ebstein" anomaly being the worst, accounting for up to 55% of TV abnormalities. In these patients the systemic AV valve is inferiorly displaced, located closer to the cardiac apex. Additionally, these delicate valves are inherently prone to developing regurgitation, which is an additional burden for the systemic morphologic RV. If left uncorrected, systemic valve abnormalities lead to development of ventricular dysfunction and heart failure.

Clinical Pearl

The most commonly associated anatomic cardiac abnormalities in l-TGA are VSDs, pulmonary outflow tract obstruction, and TV abnormalities.

What are the surgical options to "correct" l-TGA?

There are several surgical options. Some focus on repairing the associated anatomic lesion (i.e., VSD, TV abnormality, pulmonary outflow tract obstruction) and others focus on definitive surgical intervention, with anatomic correction of the ventricular relationships. The presence of associated lesions remains the major determinant regarding the timing and surgical repair of l-TGA.

1. *Double switch*: The definitive option for anatomic repair offered to patients with l-TGA devoid of significant pulmonary outflow tract obstruction is the double switch operation (DS), which involves both atrial and arterial switch components. (See Figure 23.3.) An intraatrial baffle (Mustard or Senning

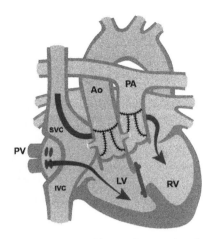

Figure 23.3 Double switch operation. Senning operation with the arterial switch procedure. Ao, aorta; IVC, inferior vena cava; LV, left ventricle; PA, pulmonary artery; PV, pulmonary veins; RV, right ventricle; SVC, superior vena cava. From McEwan A. and Manolis M. Anesthesia for transposition of the great arteries. In Andropoulos D. B., Stayer S., Mossad E. B., et al., eds. *Anesthesia for Congenital Heart Surgery*, 3rd ed. John Wiley & Sons, 2015: 542–66. With permission.

procedure) is created, which diverts deoxygenated systemic venous return into the morphologic RV and oxygenated pulmonary venous return into the morphologic LV. The arterial switch operation (ASO) involves the transection of both the PA and aorta, and translocation of the vessels to the opposite root, resulting in anastomosis of the PA to the morphologic RV, and aortic anastomosis to the morphologic LV. The DS operation establishes both AV and VA concordance. In other words, systemic deoxygenated blood returning to the RA is baffled across the atrial septum to the TV and into the morphologic RV, which is now connected to the PA, and into the pulmonary circulation. Additionally, oxygenated pulmonary venous blood returning to the LA is baffled across the atrial septum to the MV, into the morphologic LV, and then into the newly transposed aorta to the systemic circulation. The ASO also requires coronary artery transfer as part of the great artery transfer. (See Chapters 21 and 22.)

Clinical Pearl

The double switch operation offers anatomic repair of l-TGA, comprising both atrial and arterial switch components. Normal AV and VA concordance is established, which results in systemic deoxygenated blood returning to the RA to be rerouted to the RV and pulmonary circulation and pulmonary venous oxygenated blood returning to the LA to be rerouted to the LV and systemic circulation.

2. ***Senning–Rastelli procedure***: For l-TGA patients with a large VSD and pulmonary outflow tract obstruction, the Senning–Rastelli procedure is typically performed; it has two components. An intraatrial baffle (Senning tunnel) is created, diverting deoxygenated systemic venous return from the RA into the morphologic RV and oxygenated pulmonary venous return from the LA into the morphologic LV. Additionally, the Rastelli procedure is performed. This involves closure of the VSD with an intraventricular baffling technique so that blood from the right-sided morphologic LV courses across the ventricular septum into the aorta. Because the Rastelli baffle obliterates a possible pulmonary outflow tract, the main PA is transected from the morphologic LV, and an extracardiac conduit is placed between the morphologic RV and PA to restore PBF.

Clinical Pearl

The double switch operation is performed in patients without significant pulmonary outflow tract obstruction. The Senning–Rastelli operation is performed in patients with a large VSD and pulmonary outflow tract obstruction.

3. ***Physiologic repair***, also called "conventional" or "classical" repair, addresses only coexisting defects and does not lead to anatomic correction of l-TGA. The surgical techniques are dictated by the type and severity of associated lesions. Patients with a VSD may undergo only a VSD closure, while those with pulmonary outflow tract obstruction may undergo LV to PA conduit placement. Those with TR may undergo TV repair or replacement, which is ideally performed prior to onset of RV failure (defined as RV ejection fraction <40%).

4. ***Single ventricle palliation*** may be considered in the presence of complex straddling of AV valves across the ventricular septum or ventricular hypoplasia.

What long-term sequelae are associated with uncorrected l-TGA?

The long-term sequelae of patients with uncorrected l-TGA include RV dysfunction, systemic atrioventricular valve regurgitation, CHF, arrhythmias, and CHB. The natural history of l-TGA is largely determined by the presence of associated anatomic cardiac abnormalities and the progressive dysfunction of the morphologic RV as the systemic pump. Several studies have shown that a substantial number of unoperated patients with l-TGA have compromised function and a reduction in quality of life. Patients devoid of associated significant lesions may live normal lives into early adulthood, with many reports of women having successful pregnancies. However, by age 45 years, 67% of patients with l-TGA develop heart failure if they have associated cardiac lesions as opposed to a 25% incidence of heart failure in patients without significant lesions.

> **Clinical Pearl**
>
> *By age 45 years, 67% of patients with l-TGA develop heart failure if they have associated cardiac lesions, as opposed to a 25% incidence of heart failure in patients without significant lesions.*

What are indications for PA banding?

1. Infants with a ***large, unrestrictive VSD*** are at risk for developing heart failure secondary to excess PBF, which worsens as PVR falls during the first few weeks of life. These infants may require PA banding if unresponsive to medical management. The PA band, a surgically placed circumferential restriction of the PA, reduces PBF by mechanically increasing PVR, thereby improving heart failure symptoms.
2. Pulmonary artery banding is also used to ***"train" the underdeveloped morphologic LV*** in preparation for definitive surgical repair. Placing a PA band increases the PVR, placing a higher afterload on the LV. This exposure to near-systemic pressures results in gradually increasing LV posterior wall thickness or hypertrophy, thus preparing it for future anatomic repair or the DS operation. Pulmonary artery banding is usually done within the first few months to years of life, with timing of the subsequent DS operation variable. Studies report the median time from PA banding to the DS operation ranges from 2 to 14.5 months.
3. Pulmonary artery banding may also be indicated for patients with ***severe or progressive regurgitation of the systemic AV valve (TV)***, as it has been shown to stabilize systemic AV valve regurgitation and thus improve the systemic ventricular function.

What are the long-term outcomes for physiologic versus anatomic repair?

Early mortality for physiologic repair is low; however, long-term outcomes are poor due to progressive RV dysfunction and heart failure, with 84%, 75%, and 61% survival reported at 1, 5, and 15 years, respectively. Risk factors associated with poor outcome include TV replacement, preoperative RV dysfunction, postoperative CHB, subvalvular pulmonary stenosis, and Ebstein-like malformation of the TV.

In contrast, early mortality following anatomic repair remains high, up to 10%. However, long-term outcomes seem to be comparable or superior to those observed in physiologic repair patients. Since the DS and the Senning–Rastelli procedures were only introduced in the 1990s, long-term data are limited but growing. In the series of patients followed longest, the 20-year survival rates for patients following DS and Senning–Rastelli were similar (83% vs. 76%, respectively). The sequelae following anatomic correction are primarily due to conduction abnormalities (CHB and tachyarrhythmias), left ventricular dysfunction, and neoaortic valve regurgitation. In addition, some patients may experience baffle-associated complications, such as obstructions or leaks. Narrowing of the baffles created during the atrial switch procedure (i.e., Senning or Mustard) may present as chylothorax, SVC syndrome, or pulmonary venous congestion, depending on the site of the obstruction. Baffle leaks cause atrial level shunting, which may present as a simple cyanosis or in more severe cases as a cerebrovascular accident.

Up to 25% of patients following anatomic repair will require surgical reintervention. In the Senning–Rastelli group, RV–PA conduit replacements or interventional conduit procedures will be required; in the DS group, aortic valve replacements and intraatrial baffle interventions are more prevalent.

How can functional status be assessed in the pediatric patient with heart failure?

Heart failure (HF) in children is a progressive clinical and pathophysiologic syndrome with characteristic signs and symptoms that include edema, fatigue, respiratory distress, and growth failure. It is also accompanied by circulatory, neurohormonal, and molecular derangements. Heart failure is a risk factor for major adverse cardiac events after surgery. Even with minor procedures such as an appendectomy, patients with chronic stable HF have been shown to have increased morbidity and mortality. As the well-established New York Heart Association Heart Failure Classification is not applicable to most of the pediatric population, the Modified Ross Heart Failure Classification has been used in children. (See Table 23.1.)

It may be difficult to assess functional class in older children, especially teenagers who are excellent at masking their symptoms and limitations. Often questions like "What do you like to do for fun?", "What is your favorite activity in physical education?", or "Do you walk your dog?" provide more insight into functional capacity.

Heart failure in patients with unrepaired l-TGA is likely multifactorial but primarily attributed to the morphologic RV being structurally ill-equipped to perform the workload

163

Table 23.1 Modified Ross Classification for Pediatric Heart Failure

Class I	Asymptomatic
Class II	Mild tachypnea or diaphoresis with feeding in infants Dyspnea on exertion in older children
Class III	Marked tachypnea or diaphoresis with feeding in infants Prolonged feeding times with growth failure Marked dyspnea on exertion in older children
Class IV	Tachypnea, retractions, grunting, or diaphoresis at rest

Adapted from Ross R. D. *Pediatr Cardiol* 1992; 13: 72–5 and Ross R. D. *Pediatr Cardiol* 2012; **33**: 1295–300. With permission.

of the systemic ventricle. This can often be accentuated by volume overload from TR secondary to an abnormal TV. Additionally, the RV is supplied by a single coronary, whereas the LV has dual supply (LAD and LCX). This mismatch places the RV at higher ischemic risk, as it is functioning as the systemic ventricle. Finally, the TV support system has small, numerous papillary muscles originating from the septum as well as the free wall, making it poorly designed to handle RV dilation, leading to worsening TR.

Clinical Pearl

Heart failure in patients with unrepaired l-TGA is likely multifactorial but is primarily attributed to the morphologic RV being structurally ill equipped to perform the workload of the systemic ventricle. This can often be accentuated by volume overload from TR secondary to an abnormal TV.

Pacemaker/Implanted Device Management

What are the potential risks of surgery in a patient who is pacemaker-dependent or has an implantable cardioverter-defibrillator?

The most significant threat to the pacemaker (PM) and the patient is from electromagnetic interference (EMI), which may disrupt the operation of the device implanted in the patient if it is located in the area of the electromagnetic field. Electromagnetic interference is capable of precipitating pacing inhibition by oversensing. Electromagnetic waves are erroneously interpreted as the patient's intrinsic heart activity. This may lead to bradycardia or even asystole. In patients with an implantable cardioverter-defibrillator (ICD), EMI may be misinterpreted as tachyarrhythmias, resulting in either antitachycardia pacing or inappropriate shock therapy. Additionally, EMI may

stimulate the sensor for rate-responsive pacing, precipitating inappropriate tachycardia. It can activate "power on reset" of the device, reversing it to the factory program parameters such as VVI pacing at the lower rate. Finally, it can induce damage at the lead–tissue interface, worsening pacing thresholds or even causing direct damage to the device. Essential elements of preoperative evaluation of cardiovascular implantable electronic devices (CIEDs) are given in Table 23.2.

How can it be determined if a patient is PM dependent? What special precautions should be taken?

Determination of PM dependence can be difficult, especially if the interrogation report or reprogramming device is not available. It is prudent to obtain a 12-lead ECG or rhythm strip before surgery. If there are PM spikes in front of all or nearly all P waves and/or QRS complexes, assume dependency. Patients with a history of syncope or AV node ablation should be considered reliant on their PM. It is essential to have a backup pacing plan for these high-risk patients. At minimum, transcutaneous pacing and defibrillation pads should be placed in an anterior–posterior position, away from the generator, prior to draping. Standard American Society of Anesthesiologists (ASA) monitors and invasive monitoring (i.e., arterial line) aid in recognizing pacing inhibition. Plethysmography confirms a perfusing rhythm, while 5-lead ECG with appropriately adjusted gain allows for detection of pacing spikes.

Clinical Pearl

It is prudent to obtain a 12-lead ECG or rhythm strip before surgery. If there are PM spikes in front of all or almost all P waves and/or QRS complexes, assume dependency.

What are sources of EMI? How is the electrosurgical risk of cardiovascular implantable electronic devices interference minimized?

The most common source of EMI in the operating room is electrocautery. Other sources capable of interfering with CIEDs include external defibrillation, radiofrequency ablation, electroconvulsive therapy, and scanning systems for detecting retained surgical instruments, among others.

The ASA and the Heart Rhythm Association published a joint consensus statement on the perioperative management of patients with CIEDs, recommending programming the PM in asynchronous mode only if significant inhibition

Table 23.2 Essential Elements of Preoperative Evaluation of Cardiovascular Implantable Electronic Devices

Device type	Pacemaker (PM), implantable cardioverter defibrillator (ICD), chronic resynchronization therapy (CRT)
Date of last interrogation	<12 months for PM <6 months for ICD <3 months for CRT
Manufacturer and model	Chest radiograph may aid in identification if information not readily available
Device indication	PM: Sick sinus syndrome, atrioventricular block, syncope ICD: Primary or secondary prevention CRT: Heart failure
Device safety parameters	**Battery longevity** >3 months preferable **Capture threshold** <3 mV (the least amount of electrical stimulus required to consistently depolarize the myocardium) **Lead impedance** between 300 and 1200 Ohms **Sensitivity** >1.5 mV for P wave and > 4 mV for R wave detection (ability of the device to detect the patient's intrinsic rhythm; the greater the amplitude of the sensed complex, the higher likelihood of patient's own activity being sensed)
Leads	If implanted >3 months they are less susceptible to displacement
Programming essentials	**PM**: Mode, lower, and upper tracking rates **ICD**: Lowest heart rate for shock delivery, lowest heart rate for anti-tachycardia pacing **Rate adaptation**: Type of sensor (*mechanical* sensor detecting acceleration or *physiologic* sensor tracking minute ventilation)
Underlying rhythm/PM dependency	Determine underlying rhythm and information regarding ability to sustain adequate cardiac output
Magnet response	Will differ with type of device, manufacturer, and battery life Low battery life will cause pacing at lower rates What is magnet pacing rate? Does the device allow for magnet application function to be disabled to "no response"?

is observed, even in PM dependent patients. Certain steps can be taken to minimize EMI, such as keeping the presumed electric current path at least 6 inches away from the generator and/or the leads by properly positioning the electrocautery return pad. If not feasible, then bipolar cautery or short bursts of unipolar cautery at a lower power setting should be used (<5 seconds long with at least 2-second pauses between the bursts). In all cases, a magnet needs to be immediately available if preoperative reprogramming was not chosen or available.

Is magnet use always safe and feasible?

A magnet applied to the PM will prevent generator inhibition and avert inappropriate tracking or rate response by initiating asynchronous pacing.

Each pacemaker manufacturer has a slightly different magnet response, as follows:

- A *Medtronic* pacemaker will pace DOO or VOO at 85 bpm. However, if it is at the end of life or at elective replacement indicator, pacing drops to 65 bpm.
- A *St. Jude* device will pace at 100 bpm or 85 bpm depending on how much battery life is left. A response to the magnet should be confirmed preoperatively, because the response could be disabled in pacemakers manufactured by St. Jude Medical, Boston Scientific, or Biotronic.

- In the case of *ICDs*, a magnet will suspend tachyarrhythmia detection and therapy but will not affect the pacing. Therefore, EMI may cause oversensing and undesired inhibition of the ICD's PM function leading to inconsistent pacing. This may be catastrophic in patients with an ICD who are also PM dependent.

Generally, asynchronous pacing is well tolerated. However, in some patients magnet use may lead to deleterious hemodynamic effects. Pediatric patients, particularly those in HF, depend on AV synchrony and higher HR to maintain their cardiac output. Those with biventricular pacing for chronic resynchronization therapy should always be considered pacer dependent and not capable of tolerating asynchrony. For these high-risk patients preoperative reprogramming of their PM or ICD is preferred over using a magnet.

Clinical Pearl

A magnet applied to a pacemaker will prevent generator inhibition by initiating asynchronous pacing, but each pacemaker manufacturer has a slightly different magnet response. Magnet response should be confirmed preoperatively or the pacemaker should be reprogrammed.

Anesthetic Implications

What are the challenges of using a magnet during surgical procedures?

An essential element of safe and efficient management of patients with CIEDs is open communication between the surgical team, anesthesiologist, and CIED team (i.e., cardiologist, cardiac electrophysiologist). Surgical input should include procedure details such as site, positioning, possible sources of EMI, risk of fluid and electrolyte shifts, and need for blood transfusion. The magnet should be placed over the generator to elicit the desired response. If the surgical site is near the generator pocket and not readily accessible, a sterile magnet should be available on the surgical field, where it can be quickly placed if needed.

In pediatric patients with complex CHD, an epicardial pacing system is typically preferred to a transvenous system. Historically, the PM generator pocket has been formed in the abdominal wall within the rectus abdominus muscle sheath, often at the level of umbilicus. Other locations include subxiphoid and retrocostal approaches. Therefore, it is crucial to know the exact location of the generator pocket. Obtaining chest and abdominal radiographs is often indicated to confirm the PM location.

Which surgical approach, open or laparoscopic, is safer and more beneficial for this patient?

Benefits of laparoscopic surgery versus an open surgical procedure in children without CHD have been well established. Laparoscopic approaches have been associated with decreased morbidity and transfusion rates, as well as shorter length of stay. A recent retrospective cohort study from 2013–2014 National Surgical Quality Improvement Project-Pediatrics (NSQIP-P) data compared morbidity and mortality outcomes in children with minor, major, and severe CHD undergoing laparoscopic versus open procedures. Within the minor CHD group, laparoscopic procedures were associated with lower 30-day mortality, in-hospital mortality, and 30-day morbidity in comparison to open procedures. These benefits declined as the severity of CHD increased. Overall, analyzed outcomes were comparable between laparoscopic and open techniques. The risks of mortality and 30-day morbidity are significantly higher for patients with severe CHD (OR 12.31, 95% CI) and major CHD (OR 3.46, 95% CI). Patients with minor CHD have similar mortality as patients without CHD. However, the risks of increased morbidity (including reintubation, infection, and readmission) remained significantly higher even in the patients with minor CHD. Given that the patient in the aforementioned scenario has only mildly decreased RV function with good functional status, utilizing a laparoscopic approach is a reasonable surgical option for management of acute appendicitis. (See Table 23.3.)

What are the possible pitfalls of a laparoscopic approach?

Laparoscopy requires peritoneal insufflation of carbon dioxide (CO_2) resulting in increased intraabdominal pressure and $PaCO_2$. Pneumoperitoneum elevates the diaphragm, which worsens lung compliance, functional residual capacity, and atelectasis. Neonates and infants are particularly vulnerable to changes in respiratory mechanics. Hemodynamic changes such as diminished preload, rise in systemic vascular resistance (SVR), and a rise in PVR should be anticipated and treated accordingly. Patients with severe TR or significantly depressed RV function may not tolerate laparoscopy. Persistent hypoxia or hypotension may prompt conversion to an open procedure.

What are the perioperative considerations in anesthetizing a PM-dependent patient with unrepaired l-TGA presenting for emergent laparoscopic surgery?

A focused history and physical provides crucial information on a patient's functional status and severity of CHD, which

Table 23.3 NSQIP-P Definition and Classification of CHD Severity

Classifications	Definitions and Criteria
Minor CHD	• Cardiac condition with or without medication and maintenance, unrepaired (asymptomatic) • Repaired CHD with normal cardiovascular function and no medication
Major CHD	• Repaired or palliated CHD with residual hemodynamic abnormality with or without medications
Severe CHD	• Uncorrected cyanotic heart disease • Documented pulmonary hypertension • Ventricular dysfunction • Listed for heart transplant

CHD, congenital heart disease; NSQIP, National Surgical Quality Improvement Program.
Adapted from Faraoni D., et al. *J Am Coll Cardiol* 2016; **67**: 793–801. With permission.

aids in determining anesthetic, surgical, and disposition goals. Open communication between the surgeon, cardiologist, and anesthesiologist is essential in creating a safe and feasible plan.

To decide on magnet use versus reprogramming, assess the EMI risk with the surgeon and consult the cardiologist if the last PM interrogation was >12 months ago. If it is determined that the patient will tolerate either brief pacing inhibition, or asynchronous pacing, a sterile magnet should be available on the surgical field. The PM pocket location should be known to the surgical team and included in the prepped field. Reprogramming the PM prior to the procedure is not indicated in this patient scenario.

Another point of discussion with the surgeon should address laparoscopy. Despite being a safe and better option for this particular patient, laparoscopy may not be tolerated in every patient with major CHD. Criteria for conversion to open procedure need to be established a priori.

Clinical Pearl

To decide on magnet use versus reprogramming, assess the EMI risk with the surgeon and consult the cardiologist if the last PM interrogation was >12 months ago. If it is determined that the patient will tolerate either brief pacing inhibition, or asynchronous pacing, a sterile magnet should be available on the surgical field.

What methods are appropriate for induction and maintenance of anesthesia?

The anesthetic plan should address the issue of suboptimal preload due to prolonged fasting time and ongoing vomiting. Intravenous (IV) access should be established before induction to allow for sufficient rehydration, administration of IV premedication, and rapid sequence induction (RSI). Although our patient is in stable HF, the potential for hemodynamic instability should be expected and addressed. Ketamine or etomidate are both acceptable induction options in those with significant systemic AV valve regurgitation and compromised heart function. Inotropes (i.e., epinephrine, ephedrine, norepinephrine, and/or dopamine) should be readily available. Avoidance of both increases in SVR and decreases in heart rate is advisable, as these conditions worsen systemic AV valve regurgitation and lower cardiac output. Thus, inotropes with primarily α-adrenergic effects (i.e., phenylephrine and vasopressin) are discouraged as they will exacerbate systemic AV valve regurgitation, causing cardiac output to worsen. A backup pacing plan should be in place if the asynchronous rhythm becomes intolerable; place transcutaneous pacing pads away from the generator (anteroposterior position) prior to draping. For

this case standard ASA monitors, specifically plethysmography waveform (pulse oximetry), are sufficient for hemodynamic monitoring and detection of a nonperfusing rhythm. Arterial line placement is useful in assessing pacing effectiveness and pulsatility but is not required.

Is prophylaxis for prevention of bacterial endocarditis indicated for this patient?

According to the 2017 American Heart Association/American College of Cardiology Focused Update on antimicrobial prophylaxis for the prevention of bacterial endocarditis, antibiotic prophylaxis is recommended only in high-risk cardiac conditions, if ongoing gastrointestinal infection is present. The child in our scenario is in the low-risk category and therefore does not need prophylaxis. However, antibiotics should be administered if a surgical indication exists, for example, bowel perforation. (See Table 23.4.)

Should the patient's PM be reprogrammed or interrogated postoperatively?

Although reprogramming prior to the procedure is not necessary, postoperative interrogation may be needed if the patient experiences significant pacemaker-related intraoperative events (i.e., significant EMI, hemodynamic instability, cardiac arrest, need for defibrillation or transcutaneous pacing). If elected, postoperative interrogation must be completed prior to patient's discharge from telemetry. Follow-up with the patient's cardiologist within one month of discharge to complete PM interrogation is also recommended.

Clinical Pearl

Any pacemaker or ICD that has been reprogrammed preoperatively should be interrogated and reprogrammed to its preoperative or most optimal settings PRIOR to the patient's discharge from telemetry.

When is it safe to discharge a patient with uncorrected l-TGA following appendectomy?

Following surgery in this scenario, the unrepaired l-TGA patient with pacemaker should remain hospitalized overnight for observation. Close monitoring on telemetry would be warranted if any unusual perioperative events occurred or if the pacemaker was reprogrammed or affected in any way. For a scheduled or nonemergent procedure, same day discharge could be considered after an uneventful routine procedure assuming the patient is

Table 23.4 Indications for Antimicrobial Prophylaxis for the Prevention of Bacterial Endocarditis

Highest Risk Patients	Highest Risk Procedures
Prosthetic heart valves, including mechanical, bioprosthetic, and homograft valves (transcatheter-implanted as well as surgically implanted valves are included)	Dental procedures that involve manipulation of either gingival tissue or the periapical region of teeth or perforation of the oral mucosa; this includes routine dental cleaning
Prosthetic material used for cardiac valve repair, such as annuloplasty rings and chords	Procedures of the respiratory tract that involve incision or biopsy of the respiratory mucosa
A prior history of infective endocarditis	Gastrointestinal (GI) or genitourinary (GU) procedures in patients with ongoing GI or GU tract infection
Unrepaired cyanotic congenital heart disease	Procedures on infected skin, skin structure, or musculoskeletal tissue
Repaired congenital heart disease with residual shunts or valvular regurgitation at the site or adjacent to the site of the prosthetic patch or prosthetic device	Surgery to place prosthetic heart valves or prosthetic intravascular or intracardiac materials
Repaired congenital heart defects with catheter-based intervention involving an occlusion device or stent during the first 6 months after the procedure	
Valve regurgitation due to a structurally abnormal valve in a transplanted heart	

afebrile, tolerating a regular diet, and either free of pain or with pain well controlled on nonnarcotic agents.

Suggested Reading

Atallah J., Rutledge J. M., and Dyck J. D. Congenitally corrected transposition of the great arteries (atrioventricular and ventriculoarterial discordance). In Allen H., Driscoll D. J., Shaddy R. E., et al., eds. *Moss and Adams' Heart Disease in Infants, Children and Adolescents*, 8th ed. Philadelphia: Lippincott Williams & Wilkins; 2013, 1147–60.

Beauchesne L. M., Warnes C. A., Connolly H. M., et al. Outcome of the unoperated adult who presents with congenitally corrected transposition of the great arteries. *J Amer Coll Cardiol* 2002; **40**: 285–90.

Chu D. I., Tan J. M., Mattei P., et al. Mortality and morbidity after laparoscopic surgery in children with and without congenital heart disease. *J Pediatr* 2017; **185**: 88–93.

Crossley G. H., Poole J. E., Rozner M. A., et al. The Heart Rhythm Society (HRS)/American Society of Anesthesiologists (ASA) expert consensus statement on the perioperative management of patients with implantable defibrillators, pacemakers and arrhythmia monitors: facilities and patient management: this document was developed as a joint project with the American Society of Anesthesiologists (ASA), and in collaboration with the American Heart Association (AHA), and the Society of Thoracic Surgeons (STS). *Heart Rhythm* 2011; **8**: 1114–54.

Graham T. P., Bernard Y. D., Mellen B. G., et al. Long-term outcome in congenitally corrected transposition of the great arteries: a multi-institutional study. *J Am Coll Cardiol* 2000; **36**: 255–61.

Hornung T. S. and Calder L. Congenitally corrected transposition of the great arteries. *Heart* 2010; **96**: 1154–61.

McEwan A. and Manolis M. Anesthesia for transposition of the great arteries. In Andropoulos D. B., Stayer S., Mossad E. B. et al., eds. *Anesthesia for Congenital Heart Disease*, 3rd ed. Hoboken, NJ: John Wiley & Sons; 2015; 542–66.

Nishimura R. A., Otto C. M., Bonow R. O., et al. 2017 AHA/ACC focused update of the 2014 AHA/ACC guideline for the management of patients with valvular heart disease: a report of the American College of Cardiology/American Heart Association Task Force on Clinical Practice Guidelines. *J Am Coll Cardiol* 2017; **70**: 252–89.

Ross R. D. The Ross classification for heart failure in children after 25 years: a review and an age-stratified revision. *Pediatr Cardiol* 2012; **33**: 1295–300.

Warnes C. A. Transposition of the great arteries. *Circulation* 2006; **114**: 2699–709.

Total Anomalous Pulmonary Venous Return and Heterotaxy Syndrome

Anna E. Jankowska

Case Scenario

A 4-month-old female presents with feeding intolerance leading to abdominal distension. She was prenatally diagnosed with heterotaxy syndrome, atrioventricular septal defect, mild left ventricular hypoplasia, severe pulmonary stenosis, and total anomalous pulmonary venous return. Within 48 hours of birth, she demonstrated severe pulmonary venous obstruction and underwent emergent sutureless repair of obstructed pulmonary veins, as well as creation of a modified Blalock–Taussig shunt. At 2 months of age she required cardiac catheterization and balloon dilation of the pulmonary veins due to restenosis. Her current medications include acetylsalicylic acid. Postnatal abdominal imaging confirmed the presence of malrotation; thus a gastrostomy tube was placed and expectant management of malrotation was elected. Her current presenting symptoms are concerning for midgut volvulus necessitating an emergent intraabdominal exploration and a Ladd procedure.

Key Objectives

- Understand the clinical relevance and classification of total anomalous pulmonary venous return.
- Understand the salient features of heterotaxy syndrome.
- Understand that patients with total anomalous pulmonary venous return and heterotaxy can have either single-ventricle or two-ventricle physiology.
- Understand the pathophysiology of pulmonary venous obstruction in the setting of total anomalous pulmonary venous return.
- Describe the preoperative assessment and intraoperative management of a patient with recurrent pulmonary vein stenosis.

Pathophysiology

What is total anomalous pulmonary venous return?

Total anomalous pulmonary venous return (TAPVR) is a rare disorder that occurs in 2% of patients presenting with congenital heart anomalies. It is characterized by the lack of direct connection of the pulmonary veins to the left atrium (LA); instead, the pulmonary veins connect either directly to the right atrium (RA) or indirectly via a vein connected to the RA. This results in oxygenated blood ultimately draining into the RA and mixing with deoxygenated blood, necessitating a right-to-left (R-to-L) atrial shunt to survive.

Total anomalous pulmonary venous return is an isolated defect in approximately two-thirds of cases but can be associated with complex cardiac defects and frequently with heterotaxy syndrome in the remainder of patients. Patients with coexisting heterotaxy syndrome often have significant additional cardiac anomalies and may require single-ventricle palliation, as discussed in the text that follows. Despite improvements in prenatal diagnostics, isolated TAPVR continues to have one of the lowest rates for prenatal diagnosis compared to other CHD lesions (2%–10%). Conversely, TAPVR associated with complex heart disease has a high rate of prenatal diagnosis, up to 100% in those with heterotaxy and TAPVR.

The age at presentation depends on the presence or absence of associated cardiac anomalies. Most patients with isolated TAPVR present as neonates or infants with pulmonary overcirculation and evidence of heart failure due to the large left to right (L-to-R) shunt. However, when severe pulmonary venous obstruction (PVO) exists with limited atrial communication, patients present with hypoxemia, acidosis, and impending circulatory collapse shortly after birth. Total anomalous pulmonary venous return with severe PVO is one of the few congenital cardiac defects requiring emergent surgical intervention in the neonate with congenital heart disease. Because newborns with TAPVR associated with heterotaxy are routinely diagnosed prenatally, they should be born at or immediately transported to a hospital with a pediatric congenital heart program.

How is TAPVR classified?

There are four major anatomic subtypes of TAPVR and they can be associated with PVO of varying severity. (See Figure 24.1.) Classifications include supracardiac, infracardiac, cardiac, and mixed pulmonary venous return.

The *supracardiac* variant constitutes about 50% of cases of isolated TAPVR and 30% of those associated with heterotaxy [1]. All pulmonary veins enter the common confluence (a single vessel draining multiple pulmonary veins), which then empties into either the innominate vein or directly into the superior vena cava (SVC). Pulmonary venous obstruction in these patients usually results from compression of the ascending vein between the bronchi and the pulmonary artery or aorta, or from stenosis at the orifice of the vertical vein.

The *cardiac* type describes the common confluence draining into the coronary sinus or directly into the RA. Pulmonary venous obstruction is rare in these patients and usually occurs at the point of connection of the confluence with the coronary sinus.

The *infracardiac* variant accounts for about 25%–30% of patients, regardless of the presence or absence of heterotaxy. The confluence drains below the diaphragm to enter either the portal vein or the inferior vena cava (IVC) directly; PVO in this variant is very common. There may be stenosis at the point of intersection of the descending vein with the systemic venous system or some degree of flow limitation may exist in the portal venous system.

Mixed TAPVR describes pulmonary venous connections to more than one anomalous location, as discussed earlier.

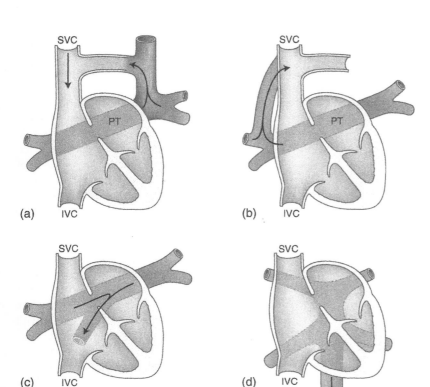

Figure 24.1 Total anomalous pulmonary venous connection (TAPVC) classified based on the site of pulmonary venous drainage (arrows). IVC, inferior vena cava; PT, pulmonary trunk; SVC, superior vena cava. (a) In type I/supracardiac connection, the four pulmonary veins drain via a common vein into the right SVC, left SVC, or their tributaries. (b) In type II/cardiac connection, the pulmonary veins connect directly to the right heart. (c) In type III/infracardiac connection, the common pulmonary vein travels down anterior to the esophagus through the diaphragm to connect to the portal venous system. (d) In type IV/mixed connections, the right and left pulmonary veins drain to different sites, such as left pulmonary veins into the left vertical vein to the left innominate, right pulmonary veins directly into the right atrium or coronary sinus. From G. Ottaviani and L. M. Buja. Congenital heart disease: pathology, natural history, and interventions. In Buja L. M. and Butany J., eds. *Cardiovascular Pathology*, 4th ed. Elsevier, 2015; 611–47. With permission.

Are there other defects associated with TAPVR?

Other than an atrial communication, two-thirds of patients with TAPVR have no other associated cardiac defects. Of the remaining one-third of patients, most have associated heterotaxy syndrome, and the majority of these will have single-ventricle (SV) physiology [1].

How is TAPVR surgically corrected?

The goal of surgical intervention is to establish the natural communication that should occur between the pulmonary veins and the LA. An anastomosis is created between either the pulmonary venous confluence or the posterior pericardium and the posterior wall of the LA. The procedure is performed on cardiopulmonary bypass, often with deep hypothermic circulatory arrest. A sutureless surgical technique was developed in an attempt to decrease the incidence of the recurrent PVO at the anastomotic sites. It involves creation of a pericardial well encasing the pulmonary venous confluence; the pericardial walls of this well are then anastomosed to the back of the LA [2].

Surgical considerations in children with heterotaxy syndrome are largely the same. Due to the presence of the atrioventricular septal defect (AVSD), the child in this scenario has a common atrium that therefore already allows mixing of oxygenated and deoxygenated venous return. Because of this, the L-to-R shunt from the TAPVR is irrelevant in the short term. However, due to the likelihood of partial or increasing obstruction to pulmonary venous blood flow in patients with supra- or infracardiac type TAPVR, patients with these anatomic variants are repaired soon after birth, while patients with intracardiac TAPVR may require surgical intervention only if a subsequent complete two-ventricle cardiac repair is pursued for their other cardiac anomalies.

What are possible postoperative sequelae of TAPVR repair?

Recurrent pulmonary venous stenosis occurs in up to 25% of patients with TAPVR, and the rate is thought to be significantly higher in patients with associated heterotaxy. Restenosis can occur at the anastomotic site or as a result of intimal hyperplasia involving the individual pulmonary veins. While the sutureless technique has decreased the rate of anastomotic site stenosis, intimal hyperplasia is a progressive disorder with limited treatment options and a poor prognosis. High long-term mortality is associated with PVO requiring reintervention, especially in patients with associated heterotaxy.

Sinus node dysfunction and other dysrhythmias occur frequently in this patient population. Ongoing follow-up with arrhythmia surveillance is recommended.

What is heterotaxy syndrome and how does it affect perioperative outcomes?

Heterotaxy, also known as *atrial isomerism*, is an embryologic disruption of right and left laterality of the thoracic and abdominal organs. It results in loss of the normal spatial relationship between the intraabdominal and intrathoracic organs. Constellations of cardiac manifestations are frequently seen in patients with heterotaxy syndrome, and they represent approximately 3% of patients with CHD. Cardiac manifestations are typically severe, leading to considerable morbidity and mortality. Children with heterotaxy and TAPVR have even higher rates of early and late morbidity and mortality. Patients with SV anatomy and TAPVR tend to have the least favorable outcomes because long-term SV outcomes are reliant on a compliant pulmonary vasculature and normal pulmonary vascular resistance (PVR). The presence of PVO elevates both morbidity and mortality rates.

Which organs are involved in heterotaxy syndrome?

In addition to congenital heart defects of varying types and severity, various intraabdominal organs may be involved including the stomach, intestines, liver, and spleen. Intestines may be malrotated, meaning that they do not loop correctly in the abdomen during fetal development. This can predispose the patient to intestinal volvulus. All babies with heterotaxy should be evaluated to rule out intestinal malrotation. Some children with heterotaxy syndrome can have biliary atresia. Patients may also have asplenia, where the spleen may be missing entirely, or polysplenia, where the spleen is divided into several smaller spleens with variable levels of function. Irregularities of the skeleton, central nervous system, and the urinary tract may also be present, albeit less commonly. (See Figure 24.2.)

How is heterotaxy classified?

Heterotaxy is classified into two types, right and left, based on atrial appendage morphology. Classification is important because right and left isomerisms are associated with markedly different anatomic findings of the affected organs, and these anatomic differences can be clinically significant.

Right atrial isomerism, sometimes referred to as *asplenia syndrome*, is associated with bilateral morphologically right atrial appendages. Other associated cardiac anomalies may include a constellation of some or all of the following: AVSD, TAPVR, transposition of the great arteries (discordant ventriculoarterial connections), side-by-side rather than spiraling of great arteries, bilateral SVCs, supraventricular tachycardia, bilateral trilobed lungs, central nervous system anomalies, and asplenia.

Left atrial isomerism is associated with bilateral morphologically left atrial appendages, as well as some or all of the following: AVSD, partial anomalous pulmonary venous return, interruption of the IVC, absence of the coronary sinus, mirror-image spiraling of great arteries, atrioventricular block (including complete heart block, necessitating insertion of a permanent pacemaker), bilaterally bilobed lungs, and asplenia or polysplenia.

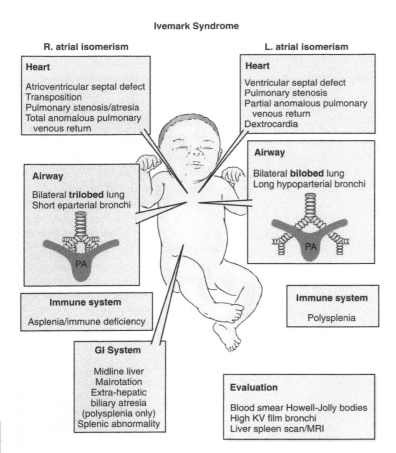

Figure 24.2 Associated defects of heterotaxy/Ivemark syndrome. From B. J. Landis and M. T. Lisi. Syndromes, genetics, and heritable heart disease. In Ungerleider R. M., Meliones J. N., McMillan K. N., et al., eds. *Critical Heart Disease in Infants and Children*, 3rd ed. Elsevier, 2019; 892–904. With permission.

Are there special infection-related precautions in heterotaxy patients?

Patients with the diagnosis of heterotaxy and uncertain splenic function should be started on antibiotic prophylaxis as soon as possible. Amoxicillin should be dosed at 20 mg/kg/day and can be divided into one or two doses per day. At 2 years of age, those with solitary spleen or polysplenia should undergo evaluation of splenic function. Antibiotic prophylaxis can be discontinued if the function is normal. For those in whom antibiotic prophylaxis is continued beyond the age of 2, it can be safely discontinued at the age of 5 years.

> **Clinical Pearl**
>
> *Patients with heterotaxy and uncertain splenic functional status should receive ongoing antibiotic prophylaxis until at least the age of 2 years.*

Anesthetic Implications

What is malrotation and how is it diagnosed and managed?

Malrotation is a congenital abnormal rotation of the midgut, frequently associated with heterotaxy syndrome. Malrotation increases the risk of midgut volvulus due to twisting of the abnormally fixed small bowel around a narrow-based mesentery and superior mesenteric artery. Presentation can vary from minor gastrointestinal distress and/or feeding difficulties to abdominal distention and bilious vomiting. Infants with CHD, particularly heterotaxy syndrome, have an incidence of malrotation as high as 40% to 90%. The diagnostic test of choice is an upper gastrointestinal bowel study with small bowel follow-through. Patients diagnosed with malrotation not associated with heterotaxy syndrome should be evaluated for intestinal atresia, trisomy 21, imperforate anus, Meckel's diverticulum, and cardiac anomalies.

The recommended surgical procedure is a Ladd procedure, performed via either an open or laparoscopic approach. The open procedure involves a right upper quadrant transverse incision or midline laparotomy. Intestinal contents are eviscerated and detorsed counterclockwise if volvulus is present. Grossly necrotic bowel is resected, and consideration is given to second look laparotomy if bowel viability is questionable. Ladd cecal bands (fibrous peritoneal bands that can cause intestinal obstruction) are released, the small intestine mesentery is broadened, and an incidental appendectomy is performed. The small bowel is placed on the right and the colon on the left, and the abdomen is then closed. With a laparoscopic approach three or four port sites (umbilical, right abdomen, left abdomen, +/− epigastric for liver retractor) are placed. All steps of the Ladd procedure except evisceration are performed. In the setting of acute volvulus, use of the laparoscopic approach is somewhat controversial.

Traditionally, a diagnosis of malrotation was followed by the Ladd procedure irrespective of symptoms. Currently performance of a prophylactic Ladd procedure in an asymptomatic patient is controversial, especially in children with multiple high-risk comorbidities. Many centers proceed with prophylactic Ladd procedure in children with heterotaxy with malrotation; however, this decision and the optimal timing remain controversial in this patient population. Single-ventricle physiology, regardless of the stage of palliation, places the patient at risk for increased perioperative morbidity. On the other hand, significant risk is clearly incurred in an infant with SV physiology who develops acute volvulus. In summary, perioperative risks due to the patient's current cardiopulmonary physiology and status must be weighed against the risk of acute or chronic abdominal pathology.

When a Ladd procedure is to be electively performed in a patient with SV physiology, an argument may be made for waiting until after Stage II palliation (superior cavopulmonary anastomosis, or bidirectional Glenn) has taken place, as surgical and anesthetic risk are lower at this stage than for patients with shunt-dependent physiology. However, this strategy does not address the risk of acute volvulus occurring in the first several months of life prior to the Stage II palliation procedure. (See Chapter 27.)

What anesthetic risks should be discussed with the perioperative care team and the child's family?

The care team and family should understand that there is considerable risk for a child with shunt-dependent or SV physiology undergoing a lengthy abdominal surgery that can be associated with significant fluid shifts. A child with SV physiology with a systemic artery-to-pulmonary artery shunt (such as a modified Blalock–Taussig [mBT] shunt) providing pulmonary blood flow (PBF) is at risk for imbalances in both pulmonary and systemic perfusion. As the SV works at near maximal capacity to provide both pulmonary and systemic output in the setting of the inherent inefficiencies of a mixing lesion, the infant is at risk for tenuous perfusion of the coronary arteries and thus myocardial ischemia, which in turn can result in decreased heart function acutely and in the long term. Surgical interventions also induce derangements in coagulation, making patients more prone to clotting. A systemic-to-pulmonary shunt is prone to thrombosis, and that risk is exacerbated by the surgical procedure and the inflammation caused by the intestinal malformations. The clinical risk associated with the Ladd procedure and systemic-to-pulmonary shunt occlusion in a patient with SV physiology and heterotaxy has been reported to be as high as 20% [3]. However, the anesthetic risk must be weighed against the risk presented by the abdominal pathology. In the setting of impending volvulus and resultant bowel ischemia, surgery must proceed, whereas proposed elective surgery necessitates a careful discussion of the optimal surgical time to mitigate perioperative risks. The patient in this stem is presenting with possible volvulus and must proceed to surgery.

How should this patient be evaluated preoperatively?

A focused history, including review of pertinent medical records, is necessary to appreciate the child's precise anatomy, physiology, disease course, interventions, and most recent test results. Records of all previous surgical interventions and details of prior anesthetics should be sought.

On physical examination, the current hemoglobin–oxygen saturation should be compared to recent historical numbers prior to the current illness. Decreases in hemoglobin–oxygen saturations from the expected baseline can be indicative of mBT shunt narrowing, respiratory insufficiency, and/or low cardiac output. The lungs should be auscultated, and work of breathing observed. Hypotension can signal the presence of significant abdominal pathology and sepsis.

Given the complexity of the cardiac anomalies associated with heterotaxy syndrome in this child, a recent echocardiogram should be available; if not, one should be obtained. Echocardiography should evaluate palliative shunts and ventricular function, valvular pathology, and evidence of intracardiac shunting. Echocardiography can also screen for the presence of PVO, which would be evidenced by turbulent flow at the anastomotic site as well as abnormal, high velocity, nonphasic flow on Doppler. In this scenario, it is also important to rule out progressive mBT shunt stenosis, worsening atrioventricular valve function, or reduced function of the predominant ventricle (in this case, the RV).

A cardiac catheterization is not usually required preoperatively, and certainly not prior to urgent or emergent surgery. However, if surgery is elective and there is evidence of PVO, then consideration must be given to cardiac catheterization with pulmonary vein angioplasty with or without

stent placement. While neither of these interventions have been found to have a high long-term success rate, they may delay the need for cardiac reoperation and, if recently performed with success, may decrease the degree of PVO at the time of the anesthetic for the Ladd procedure.

Given the high incidence of conduction anomalies associated with heterotaxy syndrome, an electrocardiogram (ECG) should be done. If the patient has congenital heart block and an epicardial pacemaker system, the pacemaker must be interrogated preoperatively, and intraoperative considerations for children with pacemakers must be considered. (See Chapters 23 and 49.)

The need for laboratory studies is guided by the child's history and physical exam and the surgery itself. An infant with complex heart disease should have at a minimum a complete blood count, electrolyte profile, and type and cross for packed red blood cells prior to abdominal surgery. A coagulation panel and liver function tests should also be considered.

What monitoring is appropriate for this patient?

In addition to standard American Society of Anesthesiologists recommended monitors, one should consider 5-lead ECG to enhance surveillance for arrhythmias, as well as ischemia during potential periods of hypoxemia and fluid shifts. The ECG can be adjusted to show pacer spikes in patients with pacemakers. Invasive arterial blood pressure monitoring can be of value both in open and laparoscopic procedures, but the decision to place an arterial line should depend on patient status. Adequate peripheral venous access is mandatory regardless of the surgical approach, but the need for central venous access depends on the overall status of the patient and the preference of the care team. The presence of a peripherally inserted central catheter can be invaluable should administration of inotropic medications become necessary. The monitoring of cerebral and systemic near-infrared spectroscopy can be beneficial for following trends in systemic oxygen delivery during anesthesia and surgery.

What methods are appropriate for induction and maintenance of anesthesia in this child?

In the setting of acute abdominal pathology from the child's malrotation, an intravenous (IV) induction should be performed. Depending on the degree of gastrointestinal symptomatology consideration should be given to a rapid or modified rapid sequence intubation. The child's current ventricular function and baseline hemoglobin–oxygen saturations will aid in determining the induction strategy.

The use of ketamine along with a narcotic (e.g., fentanyl) and an appropriate neuromuscular blocking agent would be appropriate.

This patient, palliated with an mBT shunt, currently has parallel circulations, and thus maintaining balance between the pulmonary and systemic circulations is essential. All anesthetic interventions should take into account their potential effects on both pulmonary and systemic vascular resistances in order to maintain this balance. Decreases in SVR will result in "steal" from the mBT shunt and reduce pulmonary blood flow, which may already be limited to some lung segments due to the presence of existing PVO. Inspired oxygen concentration (FiO_2) should be utilized as needed to maintain the infant's "normal" preoperative baseline saturation, and therefore the appropriate FiO_2 will likely vary during the course of the surgery with surgical manipulation, particularly if a laparoscopic approach is utilized.

> **Clinical Pearl**
>
> *In a patient who is palliated with an mBT shunt, anesthetic interventions should take into account potential effects on both pulmonary and systemic vascular resistances in order to maintain this balance. Inspired oxygen concentration (FiO_2) should be utilized as needed to maintain the infant's "normal" preoperative baseline saturation.*

How should this patient be ventilated?

Endotracheal intubation and the use of positive pressure ventilation (PPV) are necessary to perform the Ladd procedure. Maintenance of normal PVR is essential in order to maintain appropriate PBF.

- **If PVR is significantly decreased** via hyperoxygenation or hyperventilation, the child with PVO is at risk for pulmonary edema due to increased PBF in the setting of downstream obstruction. This is true for patients with either single- or two-ventricle physiology.
- **If PVR is increased**, this will compound the inherent resistance secondary to the PVO.
  - In a patient with biventricular anatomy this will result in right heart strain.
  - In a patient with an mBT shunt, significantly elevated PVR will reduce shunt flow and thus PBF, leading to hypoxemia.
- **Ventilatory goals** include the use of moderate tidal volumes (6–8 mL/kg) and short inspiratory times, favoring low mean airway pressures and PVR.

- Positive end expiratory pressure (PEEP) should be used in moderation; at optimal levels it helps to maintain functional residual capacity but at high levels can decrease PBF.
- Inspired oxygen concentrations should be titrated to maintain the patient's "normal" baseline oxygen saturations.

What other intraoperative concerns exist in patients with repaired TAPVR and PVO?

- **Fluid management**: In the setting of PVO, judicious IV fluid management is necessary. With obstruction in the pulmonary veins, an increase in intravascular hydrostatic pressure can lead to pulmonary edema. However, insensible fluid losses can be significant during the open Ladd procedure due to the sizable abdominal incision and evisceration of intestines and their exposure to ambient air. Replacement of those insensible losses must be performed diligently and may need to conservatively deviate from the recommended standard estimations and formulas. If a blood transfusion is required during the procedure, one should consider concurrent administration of a diuretic after consideration of the patient's overall volume status. Any change in pulmonary compliance as noted by trends in ventilator settings is important in assessing the development of pulmonary edema that could require additional PEEP to slow the alveolar exudative process.
- **Ventricular function**: Attention to ventricular function is paramount. As mentioned earlier, the predominant ventricle is already working at high capacity to maintain both pulmonary and systemic outputs (parallel circulations) with each stroke volume. Perturbations that acutely increase afterload, directly reduce contractility or heart rate, or reduce coronary blood flow risk the development of inadequate cardiac output to meet the demands of critical organs, including the heart. Inotropic support should be instituted if the ventricle is struggling to meet demands, while potentially causative mechanisms such as volume status, adequate hematocrit, and optimal oxygenation and ventilation are addressed.
- **Surgical approach**: Laparoscopic techniques often introduce additional challenges. Insufflation of CO_2 with resultant systemic absorption can increase ventilation requirements and negatively impact efforts to prevent hypercarbia and acidosis.

175

Increased intraabdominal pressures will require increased ventilatory pressures, which can have negative effects on venous return and ventricular function. Clear communication with the surgical team is essential should insufflation prove detrimental to the patient's ventilatory status and hemodynamics.

- *Electrolytes*: Patients with PVO are frequently treated with diuretics preoperatively as part of their medical therapy. This chronic use of loop or thiazide diuretics can lead to hypokalemia and hypochloremic metabolic alkalosis. One must be aware of the electrolyte shifts that can occur from intraoperative controlled ventilation in patients with acid–base derangements. For example, hyperventilation can further exacerbate hypokalemia and lead to an increased risk of dysrhythmias.

- *Airway*: Venous congestion in the airways can predispose patients to increased risk of endotracheal bleeding with suctioning. Suctioning should be performed gently and judiciously. If bleeding occurs, saline lavage should be performed, and the PEEP should be increased. One should then watchfully wait, as over time these maneuvers will frequently decrease and eventually stop the bleeding.

Clinical Pearl

In the setting of PVO, intraoperative goals include maintaining normal PVR to facilitate PBF and reduce right ventricular strain, and judicious fluid management to minimize the risk of pulmonary edema.

What is the most appropriate venue for postoperative management of this patient?

Patients with recurrent PVO are at high risk for postoperative complications, including mortality. This is especially true for patients with variants of SV anatomy in the setting of TAPVR and heterotaxy syndrome. Furthermore, major abdominal surgery in any infant requires inpatient management in a monitored bed due to the need to carefully manage nutrition, fluid shifts, and pain. A patient such as the one in this scenario requires care by a provider who understands their anatomy, physiology, and perioperative risk factors; therefore admission to the critical care setting postoperatively is most appropriate for this patient. Institutional preferences may vary between postoperative care in a cardiac intensive care unit setting versus a pediatric intensive care unit. The likely need for postoperative ventilation also warrants a planned intensive care bed.

When should the patient be extubated?

Timing of extubation depends on patient's clinical status as it relates to the underlying pathology and the intraoperative course. In the setting of PVO and SV physiology with an mBT shunt, excessive intraoperative fluid administration and/or the need for an intraoperative transfusion can lead to the development of pulmonary edema. The risk of pulmonary edema continues into the postoperative period, as third spacing of intravascular fluids continues, necessitating further fluid resuscitation. Patients successfully extubated in the operating room may be at risk for postoperative respiratory failure. Overall, it may be wise to keep any child intubated who has undergone a long surgery with major fluid shifts when concern exists for potential ongoing cardiopulmonary compromise. On the other hand, an older infant with two-ventricle physiology, or a patient with SV physiology who has been palliated with a superior cavopulmonary anastomosis (Glenn shunt) may be extubated if surgery was minimally invasive, fast and well tolerated from a cardiopulmonary standpoint.

How can postoperative pain management be optimized in this patient?

Regional or neuraxial techniques and nonopioid analgesics are encouraged. Both can facilitate early extubation and decrease the risk of hypoventilation and hypercarbia related to opioid administration.

Ileus is a frequent complication of the Ladd procedure regardless of surgical approach, and the use of opioid sparing techniques helps to limit opioid induced constipation and gut motility issues.

References

1. J. D. St. Louis, B. A. Harvey, J. S. Menk, et al. Repair of "simple" total anomalous pulmonary venous connection: a review from the Pediatric Cardiac Care Consortium. *Ann Thorac Surg* 2012; **94**: 133–7.

2. Y. Oshima, M. Yoshida, A. Maruo, et al. Modified primary sutureless repair of total anomalous pulmonary venous connection in heterotaxy. *Ann Thorac Surg* 2009; **888**: 1348–50.

3. S. Sen, J. Duchon, B. Lampl, et al. Heterotaxy syndrome infants are at risk for early shunt failure after Ladd procedure. *Ann Thorac Surg* 2015; **99**: 918–25.

Suggested Reading

Khan M. S., Bryant R., Kim S. H., et al. Contemporary outcomes of surgical repair of total anomalous pulmonary venous connection in patients with heterotaxy syndrome. *Ann Thorac Surg* 2015; **99**: 2134–9.

Loomba R. S., Morales D. L. S., and Redington A. Heterotaxy. In Ungerleider R. M., Meliones J. N., Nelson McMillan K. et al., eds. *Critical Heart Disease in Infants and Children*, 3rd ed. Philadelphia: Mosby Elsevier, 2019; 796–803.

Ryerson L. M., Pharis S., Pockett C., et al. Heterotaxy syndrome and intestinal abnormalities. *Pediatrics* 2018; **142**: e20174267.

St. Louis J., Molitor-Kirsch E., Shah S., et al. Total anomalous pulmonary venous return. In Ungerleider R. M., Meliones J. N., Nelson McMillan K., et al., eds. *Critical Heart Disease in Infants and Children*, 3rd ed. Philadelphia: Mosby Elsevier; 2019; 587–96.

25

Chapter

Truncus Arteriosus

Kelly Everhart and Faith J. Ross

Case Scenario

A 3-year-old female with a history of truncus arteriosus and DiGeorge syndrome presents for elective repair of a cleft palate. She was diagnosed prenatally with truncus arteriosus and underwent uncomplicated repair with placement of a right ventricle-to-pulmonary artery conduit at 5 days of age. She has been followed since that time and over the past year has developed a slowly increasing gradient across her conduit. A report from her cardiologist in her hometown 3 months ago described her conduit stenosis as moderate to severe. Her truncal valve was also mild to moderately regurgitant at that time. She has mild developmental delay and has recently begun to have some diminished exercise tolerance compared to her preschool classmates. On exam she has normal work of breathing with SpO$_2$ of 96% on room air. Heart rate and blood pressure are within normal limits.

Key Objectives

- Understand the anatomy and physiology of truncus arteriosus before and after surgical repair.
- Describe potential sequelae of truncus arteriosus repair.
- Describe the preoperative assessment of children with repaired congenital heart disease.
- Identify the anesthetic implications of DiGeorge syndrome.
- Describe the implications of cardiac disease in a patient undergoing cleft palate repair.

Pathophysiology

What is truncus arteriosus?

Truncus arteriosus (TA) is a rare form of cyanotic congenital heart disease (CHD) in which the embryologic separation of the arterial trunk remains incomplete. The primary anatomic lesion is a common arterial trunk that supplies the pulmonary, coronary, and systemic circulations. (See Figure 25.1.) A single semilunar "truncal valve," often with an abnormal number of cusps, takes the place of the aortic and pulmonic valves. (See Figure 25.2.) Nearly all cases of TA are associated with a ventricular septal defect (VSD); therefore, mixing of deoxygenated and oxygenated blood occurs both in the ventricular chambers and in the common arterial trunk [1, 2]. Truncus arteriosus accounts for up to 3% of congenital cardiac defects and is estimated to occur in 60 to 140 patients per million live births [3]. It is frequently prenatally diagnosed with routine fetal echocardiography [4, 5].

Clinical Pearl

The primary anatomic lesion is a common arterial trunk that supplies the pulmonary, coronary, and systemic circulations. A single semilunar "truncal valve," often with an abnormal number of cusps, takes the place of the aortic and pulmonic valves.

How are the anatomic variations classified?

Two classification systems are currently used to categorize anatomic variations of the pulmonary arteries (PAs) in TA.

Collett and Edwards (C & E) originally described four different variations, three of which are still in use.

- *Type 1*: The main PA originates from the common arterial trunk prior to bifurcation into the branch PAs.
- *Type 2*: The right and left PAs arise separately from the posterior aspect of the main arterial trunk.
- *Type 3*: The right and left PAs branch from the right- and left-lateral aspects of the main arterial trunk, respectively.

The *modified Van Praagh classification* [6] utilizes slightly different criteria.

- *Type 1* (analogous to C & E type 1): The main PA arises from the arterial trunk.
- *Type 2* (analogous to C & E types 2 and 3): The branch PAs arise separately from the arterial trunk.
- *Type 3*: Only one branch PA arises from the arterial trunk, and the other PA is supplied by the ductus arteriosus or collateral vessels.

178

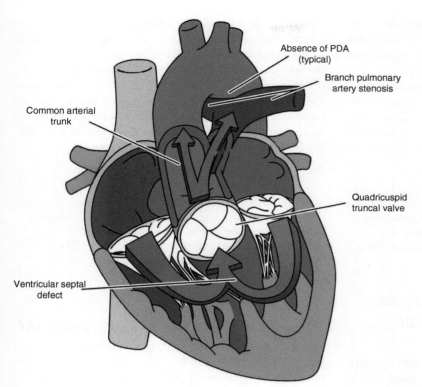

Figure 25.1 Truncus arteriosus. Drawing by Ryan Moore, MD, and Matt Nelson.

Absence of PDA (typical)

Branch pulmonary artery stenosis

Common arterial trunk

Quadricuspid truncal valve

Ventricular septal defect

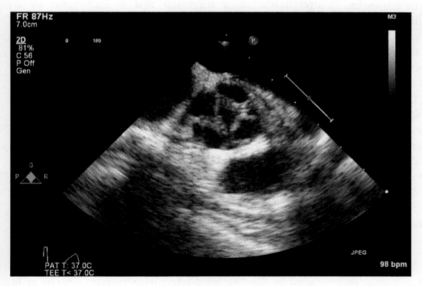

Figure 25.2 Quadrileaflet truncal valve, mid-esophageal short-axis image. Courtesy of Faith Ross, MD.

- A further subclassification denotes the presence (A) or absence (B) of a VSD.

In all cases of TA, a detailed understanding of the anatomy is important for surgical planning, but the physiologic principles remain largely the same.

What other congenital conditions are associated with TA?

Although TA can occur in isolation, it is commonly associated with comorbid cardiac and extracardiac congenital conditions. Patent foramen ovale (PFO) and other atrial

179

septal defects (ASDs) are the most common coexistent cardiac malformations, followed by anatomic variations in the coronary arteries and the aortic arch (right-sided or interrupted) [7].

The most common extracardiac congenital malformations associated with TA are those within the heterogeneous spectrum of 22q11 deletion syndrome (22q11DS), found in 30%–40% of cases [3, 8]. While the incidence of TA has significant correlation with trisomy 21, TA remains rare in this population.

Clinical Pearl

The most common extracardiac congenital malformations associated with TA are those within the heterogeneous spectrum of 22q11DS; they are found in 30%–40% of cases.

What is the distribution of pulmonary and systemic blood flow in a neonate with unrepaired TA?

In the neonate with unrepaired TA, the relative distribution of pulmonary (Q_p) and systemic (Q_s) blood flow is dynamically related to pulmonary vascular resistance (PVR) and systemic vascular resistance (SVR). This relationship is expressed as the ratio Q_p:Q_s. In the immediate peripartum period, PVR remains relatively high; thus, the distribution of blood flowing through the arterial trunk favors the systemic circulation (low Q_p:Q_s). With the physiologic decrease in PVR over the first hours, days, and weeks of life, the ratio of cardiac output entering the pulmonary circulation increases (increasing Q_p:Q_s).

Importantly, critical disruptions in the balance between Q_p and Q_s can precipitate rapid clinical deterioration, as in the setting of anesthetic induction or significant sympathetic stimulation. A dramatic rise in PVR or fall in SVR (very low Q_p:Q_s) will worsen hypoxemia, even to the point of critical systemic ischemia in the setting of right-to-left shunt. Alternatively, a substantial decrease in PVR (very high Q_p:Q_s) or rise in SVR is associated with pulmonary overcirculation and low systemic cardiac output that may be insufficient to meet systemic metabolic demands. The myocardium is at particular risk in this state, as low mixed venous oxygen saturation combined with low coronary perfusion pressure can severely impair the supply of oxygen to the myocardium.

What is the expected oxygen saturation in a neonate with TA? Why is this important?

Peripheral oxygen saturation in neonates with TA depends on the dynamic relationship between Q_p and Q_s. Oxygen saturations are often in the mid-80s shortly after birth, at which time PVR and SVR are relatively balanced. Saturations increase as PVR declines and may even reach the mid-to-high 90s if pulmonary overcirculation is severe. It is important to note that in this scenario, a saturation in the high 90s is not a reassuring sign, as it indicates severe pulmonary overcirculation and is thus concerning for accelerated decompensation toward congestive heart failure (CHF) and pulmonary vascular disease.

Clinical Pearl

Near-normal arterial saturation in a patient with unrepaired TA can be an indication of severe pulmonary overcirculation and is thus concerning for risk of inadequate systemic cardiac output and cardiac arrest, with intermediate to long-term risks of accelerated decompensation toward CHF and pulmonary vascular disease.

What is the natural history of unrepaired TA?

Patients with TA become symptomatic early in infancy because PVR falls over the first days to weeks of life, resulting in pulmonary overcirculation (high Q_p:Q_s). Ultimately, most patients with unrepaired TA succumb to high-output heart failure in the setting of pulmonary overcirculation, a condition that is accelerated by an incompetent truncal valve, which further loads the volume of the left ventricle and increases ventricular end-diastolic pressures. (See Figure 25.3.) The small number of patients who survive infancy develop severe pulmonary vascular disease, ultimately culminating in pulmonary hypertension. Pulmonary hypertension further contributes to critical changes in Q_p:Q_s that underlie the near-universal childhood mortality associated with unrepaired TA.

How are coronary blood flow and myocardial perfusion compromised in unrepaired TA?

Truncus arteriosus may be associated with abnormalities in the coronary arteries, such as single coronary artery, abnormally positioned coronary origins, coronary ostial stenosis, or intramural coronary arteries. In all variations of coronary anatomy, myocardial perfusion may be further compromised by diastolic steal into the pulmonary arteries or by low truncal root diastolic pressures in the setting of truncal valve insufficiency. Increased ventricular end-diastolic pressure in the setting of valve insufficiency and CHF further impairs myocardial perfusion. Finally, the risk is compounded by the baseline hypoxemia in the setting of a mixing lesion, and hypoxemia may be transiently worsened in the setting of an acute rise in right-to-left shunt.

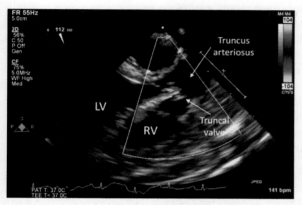

Figure 25.3 Truncal valve insufficiency and large ventricular septal defect, mid-esophageal long-axis image. Courtesy of Faith Ross, MD.

Clinical Pearl

In all variations of coronary anatomy, myocardial perfusion may be further compromised by diastolic runoff into the pulmonary arteries or by low truncal root diastolic pressures in the setting of truncal valve insufficiency.

At what age is TA typically repaired? Why is early repair important?

Ideally, TA is repaired within the first weeks of life. Patients with severe pulmonary overcirculation refractory to medical management or who require ongoing mechanical ventilation require repair in the first few days of life. Significant pulmonary overcirculation results in decreased systemic flow and low cardiac output (high Q_p:Q_s), myocardial ischemia, heart failure, and accelerated pulmonary vascular hypertensive disease, all of which can be improved with early surgical repair. Repair after 3 months of age carries increased risk for perioperative mortality.

What does the surgical repair of TA achieve?

Definitive repair of TA achieves three anatomic endpoints to restore separate pulmonary and systemic circuits:

- Removal of the pulmonary arteries from the arterial trunk such that the latter, now called the aorta, provides only systemic outflow
- Closure of the VSD
- Creation of a right ventricle to pulmonary artery (RV–PA) conduit

Truncal valve and aortic arch repair may occur during the same surgery if defects in either are likely to compromise

successful recovery from the initial repair, or these may be delayed until an older age if a "wait and watch" approach is appropriate. Truncal valve replacement is occasionally performed at the time of initial repair if truncal valve dysfunction is severe; however, due to the complications associated with frequent valve replacements in a growing child, a significant degree of truncal valve dysfunction is typically accepted before resorting to valve replacement.

What postoperative complications and long-term sequelae follow surgical repair of TA?

Fortunately, >90% of patients survive initial surgical repair of TA. Perioperative mortality increases with older age at intervention, additional cardiac defects, need for postoperative tracheostomy, and comorbid 22q11DS. An estimated 40%–60% of patients who survive to discharge may require subsequent surgical repair of the truncal valve, endovascular or surgical reintervention to decrease right ventricular outflow tract obstruction in the setting of RV–PA conduit stenosis, or surgical repair of residual defects of the aortic arch within the first decade of life [9]. Those with coronary artery anomalies have an increased risk of coronary insufficiency.

Clinical Pearl

Over 90% of children with TA survive their initial repair. Perioperative mortality increases with older age at intervention, additional cardiac defects, need for postoperative tracheostomy, and comorbid 22q11DS.

Anesthetic Implications

Apart from TA, what other anomalies are associated with 22q11DS?

There is substantial phenotypic heterogeneity in patients with 22q11DS, some of which are recognized constellations of multiorgan anomalies including DiGeorge, Catch-22, conotruncal facial, and velocardiofacial syndromes. 22q11 deletion syndrome is associated with immunodeficiency; hypocalcemia in the setting of parathyroid dysfunction; craniofacial abnormalities including cleft lip/palate; and cardiac defects including tetralogy of Fallot, interrupted aortic arch, VSD, and TA. Other anomalies of the genitourinary, renal, cognitive, endocrine, neurologic, and ophthalmologic organs are not uncommon in these patients.

How are these anomalies relevant to anesthetic management?

Even in the absence of CHD, features of 22q11DS can pose challenges to anesthesiologists. Neurodevelopmental delay may complicate the induction of anesthesia and necessitate careful preoperative anxiolysis. Dysmorphic facies, including micrognathia, retrognathia, palatal abnormalities, and laryngotracheomalacia, can impede airway management. Notably, Pierre Robin sequence is present in 10%–20% of patients with 22q11DS. In preparation for the cleft palate repair in this scenario, a thorough airway exam and review of previous anesthetic records are crucial to developing an appropriate plan for airway management in the setting of facial dysmorphology. Deficits in cell-mediated immunity necessitate irradiated blood products when transfusion is indicated. Limb hypoplasia and other malformations may make peripheral venous and arterial access challenging to obtain. Hypoparathyroidism may result in critical hypocalcemia requiring active replacement, especially in the setting of transfusion of citrated blood products [10].

Clinical Pearl

Patients with impaired cell-mediated immunity related to DiGeorge syndrome continue to require irradiated blood products throughout life, and blood products should be ordered well in advance to ensure adequate preparation time.

What clinical, laboratory, and imaging findings are critical to the preoperative evaluation of a patient with repaired TA prior to elective noncardiac surgery?

Assuming the child has fully recovered from the original cardiac surgical repair, the anesthesiologist should solicit a careful history of the patient's recent health, focusing on new or worsening symptoms of heart failure; valve insufficiency; or pulmonary vascular disease, including declines in exercise tolerance, diaphoresis, failure to thrive, syncopal episodes, unexpected weight gain or loss, or unusual shortness of breath. A physical exam complements the patient's history; increased work of breathing, new cyanosis, peripheral edema, a congested or tender liver, or changes in cardiac murmur are all concerning for complications of TA and its repair that may require intervention prior to elective noncardiac surgery.

The specific anatomy of the surgical repair and any reinterventions or complications in the interim must be appreciated. Recent imaging, such as transthoracic echocardiography, cardiac magnetic resonance imaging (CMRI), computed tomography, or cardiac catheterization will aid in the understanding of each individual's cardiac anatomy and physiology. A recent ECG may reveal inherent or acquired conduction abnormalities. Laboratory investigations should focus primarily on the appropriate type and screen of blood products if transfusion is likely, as these patients have often been exposed to blood products early in life and may have acquired sensitivity to uncommon red cell antigens.

Clinical Pearl

Patients with repaired TA should undergo routine cardiology follow-up throughout their lives. Patients should have a recent cardiology evaluation prior to any elective surgery. Evaluation should focus on identifying new or worsening signs or symptoms of heart failure, RV-PA conduit stenosis, valve incompetence, or pulmonary vascular disease.

When is preoperative consultation with cardiology indicated?

Consultation with the child's cardiologist may be warranted prior to an elective surgical procedure in several settings. Cardiology consultation is appropriate to determine the need for updated or clarified diagnostic imaging, including transthoracic echocardiography, CMRI, or heart catheterization, especially if relevant results are inaccessible or if there are new or worsening signs or symptoms of heart failure, valve incompetence, or pulmonary vascular disease. In all cases of concern, elective surgery should be delayed until complete cardiology evaluation and optimization.

The patient described in this scenario has some features that are concerning for increased anesthetic risk. Her RV–PA conduit gradient has progressed to the point where conduit intervention may be indicated prior to elective surgery, particularly as she is showing signs of decreased exercise tolerance. Moderate to even severe pulmonary stenosis can be reasonably well tolerated in children when the stenosis has developed gradually enough for the RV to compensate. However, it would be wise to determine that this is the case for this child. It is important to note the progression of the RV-PA conduit gradient over time and assess whether the RV function has remained normal on echocardiographic and/or CMRI examinations. Although her truncal valve has some insufficiency, this is often well tolerated under anesthesia. Overall, the child's cardiologist should at the very least be aware of the upcoming elective surgery and deem the timing acceptable.

Does this patient require infective endocarditis prophylaxis?

Yes. Current guidelines recommend endocarditis prophylaxis for patients with repaired CHD with bioprosthetic or homograft valves or with residual shunting or valvular incompetency at or near the site of bioprosthetic or homograft (e.g., conduit). Furthermore, although cleft palate repair is not a dental procedure per se, there is manipulation of the gingival mucosa that creates a risk for hematogenous seeding of oral bacteria. For these reasons, this patient should receive targeted antibiotic prophylaxis. Institutional guidelines often specify which antibiotic regimen is indicated for each patient, determined by the age, weight, and ability to take oral medications, but they often involve amoxicillin, cephalexin, clindamycin, or vancomycin. Note that when cefazolin is given for dual endocarditis and surgical prophylaxis, the recommended dose may be higher than for standard surgical prophylaxis [11].

Clinical Pearl

When cefazolin is given for dual endocarditis and surgical prophylaxis, the recommended dose may be higher than for standard surgical prophylaxis.

What are important features of a safe anesthetic plan for this patient?

In a well-compensated patient with repaired TA presenting for cleft palate repair, standard recommended American Society of Anesthesiologists monitors and routine peripheral venous access are sufficient. The details of the anesthetic plan should be tailored to the physiology of the individual patient, with special attention to optimizing PVR and SVR in patients with significant truncal valve insufficiency or RV–PA conduit stenosis. Effective preoperative anxiolysis can safely be employed to avoid unnecessary emotional upset, at the discretion of the anesthesia provider.

Induction of anesthesia and tracheal intubation should be swift and smooth, as hypercarbia, hypoxemia, and painful stimulation all increase PVR and can precipitate right heart failure in the setting of significant conduit stenosis, particularly if the PVR is reactive. Furthermore, increases in heart rate secondary to sympathetic stimulation impair filling of the hypertrophic and noncompliant RV. As craniofacial abnormalities can make rapid intubation a challenge at times, the anesthetic plan should include a skilled airway operator with all needed tools and personnel immediately available to them.

In this patient, who has both RV–PA conduit stenosis and truncal valve insufficiency, hemodynamic management must consider both of these conditions. Truncal valve insufficiency can be minimized by targeting low SVR and high-normal heart rate. However, as noted earlier, lower heart rates may be required to allow adequate right ventricular filling. These competing hemodynamic goals can make management of these patients challenging. These dueling priorities leave the anesthesiologist with the overarching goal of maintaining the child's baseline hemodynamics as much as possible, while of course providing supplemental oxygen. Cardiac output can be maintained close to baseline via a balanced anesthetic as well as the use of catecholaminergic drugs when necessary. The smooth induction of anesthesia may include the use of opioid medications, but these should be administered judiciously for the remainder of the procedure, as postoperative airway obstruction is a frequent complication of palate repair. Maintenance of euvolemia for these patients is also important especially when considering a hypertrophied and noncompliant RV.

Although postsurgical coronary artery pathology typically manifests in the first several months after repair, the possibility of coronary hypoperfusion in the setting of significant truncal valve insufficiency should be considered. Providers should pay close attention to diastolic blood pressure as this is the driving force for coronary perfusion.

What are the implications of RV–PA conduit stenosis and how does this finding affect the intraoperative anesthetic plan?

A frequent sequela of TA repair is stenosis of the RV–PA conduit. Right ventricular outflow tract obstruction (RVOTO) predisposes the patient to increased risk of RV failure. However, the low-pressure RV can withstand gradually increasing RVOTO for a long period of time in children, typically years, until there are clinical symptoms and/or signs of irreversible RV damage. Acute changes are more poorly tolerated. Acute rises in PVR, as can occur under anesthesia, contribute to an acutely increased RVOTO. However, clinically relevant increases in PVR are usually only mildly consequential when downstream from moderate to severe RV–PA conduit stenosis as in our patient.

Conversely, children with pulmonary hypertensive vascular disease or pulmonary hypertension are at risk for pulmonary hypertensive crises under anesthesia with subsequent acute RV failure, morbidity, and mortality.

As such, in addition to the features of the anesthetic plan described for all patients with repaired TA, anesthesia providers may choose to have the following immediately available:

- Agents to support right ventricular function (e.g., milrinone, epinephrine)
- Agents to provide pressor support without increasing PVR (e.g., vasopressin)
- Agents to decrease PVR (e.g., high FiO_2, inhaled nitric oxide) should there be concern for acute right heart failure in the setting of critically increased pulmonary artery pressures

Maintenance of euvolemia is also essential.

Clinical Pearl

A frequent long-term complication of TA repair is stenosis of the RV–PA conduit, which predisposes the patient to increased risk of RV failure. Right ventricular function may deteriorate under anesthesia due to increased afterload (PVR), tachycardia, or poor myocardial perfusion.

What is the appropriate level of immediate postoperative care for this child?

All children will be admitted to the hospital after palatal surgery. For a child with repaired TA and good functional capacity who underwent uncomplicated, routine cleft palate repair, the surgical floor is an appropriate disposition. However, if there is concern for right ventricular dysfunction, pulmonary vascular disease, or myocardial ischemia, the patient would likely benefit from close monitoring in an intensive care unit, as airway obstruction following oropharyngeal surgery may be so severe as to cause hypoxemia and hypercarbia, thus precipitating right heart failure in high-risk patients.

What are the options for analgesia after cleft palate repair? Why is effective analgesia important in the setting of RV–PA conduit stenosis?

Effective postoperative analgesia remains a vital component of perioperative care for all children, and especially in the setting of residual cardiopulmonary disease such as RV–PA conduit stenosis, for the reasons described earlier. Patient controlled opioid analgesia is an excellent option for patients who are old enough to effectively use this pain control strategy. Scheduled analgesia adjuvants, such as acetaminophen, are an effective opioid-sparing approach

to pain control, as is true for all postoperative patients. An acute pain specialist may provide tailored service and safe, timely adaptations of the pain control plan for some patients who experience particular discomfort. At centers with trained providers, regional anesthesia is an excellent option for some patients undergoing cleft palate repair [12].

Clinical Pearl

Analgesia following cleft palate repair in the setting of repaired TA should optimize regional and multimodal options, as hypercarbia related to airway obstruction and hypoventilation may exacerbate RVOTO and risk RV decompensation and failure.

References

1. R. W. Collett and J. E. Edwards. Persistent truncus arteriosus: a classification according to anatomic types. *Surg Clin North Am* 1949; **29**: 1245–70.

2. R. Van Praagh and S. Van Praagh. The anatomy of common aorticopulmonary trunk (truncus arteriosus communis) and its embryologic implications: a study of 57 necropsy cases. *Am J Cardiol* 1965; **16**: 406–25.

3. J. I. Hoffman, S. Kaplan, and R. R. Liberthson. Prevalence of congenital heart disease. *Am Heart J* 2004; **147**: 425–39.

4. J. S. Carvalho, E. Mavrides, E. A. Shinebourne, et al. Improving the effectiveness of routine prenatal screening for major congenital heart defects. *Heart* 2002; **88**: 387–91.

5. F. Gotsch, R. Romero, J. Espinoza, et al. Prenatal diagnosis of truncus arteriosus using multiplanar display in 4D ultrasonography. *J Matern Neonatal Med* 2010; **23**: 297–307.

6. M. L. Jacobs. Congenital Heart Surgery Nomenclature and Database Project: truncus arteriosus. *Ann Thorac Surg* 2000; **69**: 50–55.

7. R. Parikh, M. Eisses, G. L. Latham, et al. Perioperative and anesthetic considerations in truncus arteriosus. *Semin Cardiothorac Vasc Anesth* 2018; **22**: 285–93.

8. K. Momma. Cardiovascular anomalies associated with chromosome 22q11.2 deletion syndrome. *Am J Cardiol* 2010; **105**: 1617–24.

9. J. R. Buckley, V. Amula, P. Sassalos, et al. Multicenter analysis of early childhood outcomes after repair of truncus arteriosus. *Ann Thorac Surg* 2019; **107**: 553–9.

10. H. Yotsui-Tsuchimochi, K. Higa, M. Matsunaga, et al. Anesthetic management of a child with chromosome 22q11 deletion syndrome. *Pediatr Anesth* 2006; **16**: 454–7.

11. W. Wilson, K. A. Taubert, M. Gewitz, et al. Prevention of infective endocarditis. *Circulation* 2007; **116**: 1736–54.

12. J. Chiono, O. Raux, S. Bringuier, et al. Bilateral suprazygomatic maxillary nerve block for cleft palate repair in children. *Anesthesiology* 2014; **120**: 132–69.

Suggested Reading

Buckley J. R., Amula V., Sassalos P., et al. Multicenter analysis of early childhood outcomes after repair of truncus arteriosus. *Ann Thorac Surg* 2019; **107**: 553–59.

O'Byrne M. L., Mercer-Rosa L., Zhao H., et al. Morbidity in children and adolescents after surgical correction of truncus arteriosus communis. *Am Heart J* 2013; **166**: 512–18.

Parikh R., Eisses M., Latham G. J., et al. Perioperative and anesthetic considerations in truncus arteriosus. *Semin Cardiothorac Vasc Anesth* 2018; **22**: 285–93.

Yotsui-Tsuchimochi H., Higa K., Matsunaga M., et al. Anesthetic management of a child with chromosome 22q11 deletion syndrome. *Pediatr Anesth* 2006; **16**: 454–7.

Chapter

26

Stage I Palliation, Hypoplastic Left Heart Syndrome

Bishr Haydar

Case Scenario

A 6-week-old infant weighing 4 kg is scheduled for laparoscopic Nissen fundoplication with gastrostomy tube placement. She was born at term with hypoplastic left heart syndrome, for which she underwent a Stage I palliation (Norwood procedure) with a Sano modification at age 5 days. Her initial postoperative course was uncomplicated, but she has had persistent difficulty feeding and has failed to gain weight. She was discharged from the hospital on furosemide and aspirin.

Transthoracic echocardiogram at the time of discharge 3 weeks earlier showed the following:

- *Mild-to-moderate tricuspid regurgitation*
- *Mildly diminished right ventricular systolic function*
- *A patent Sano (right ventricular to pulmonary artery) shunt with a 40 mm Hg peak gradient*

Despite placement of a nasogastric tube for feeding, she has gained little weight and has persistent reflux. She appears alert, although small and thin, with a heart rate of 150 beats/minute, respiratory rate of 40 breaths/minute, and SpO$_2$ 86% on room air. Her cardiologist would like surgery to take place as soon as possible.

Key Objectives

- Describe the anatomy and physiology of hypoplastic left heart syndrome.
- Describe available options for the initial palliation of hypoplastic left heart syndrome.
- Describe the anatomy and physiology of a patient who has undergone surgical Stage I palliation.
- Describe an appropriate plan for perioperative anesthetic management of this infant.
- Identify markers of inadequate pulmonary or systemic blood flow in infants after Stage I palliation.
- Describe the physiology of laparoscopy as it pertains to this population.
- Discuss perioperative complications related to this population.

Pathophysiology

What is hypoplastic left heart syndrome?

The term "hypoplastic left heart syndrome" (HLHS) is used to describe a spectrum of congenital cardiac abnormalities involving underdevelopment of left-sided heart structures. Findings may include mitral valve stenosis or atresia, aortic stenosis or atresia, hypoplasia or absence of the left ventricle (LV), and hypoplasia of the ascending aorta and aortic arch. Hypoplastic left heart syndrome occurs relatively commonly (approximately 1 in 4000 births).

The combination of these defects results in single-ventricle physiology, wherein a single ventricle, in this case the right ventricle (RV), is required to support both pulmonary and systemic circulations. Single-ventricle physiology requires complete intracardiac mixing of pulmonary venous and systemic venous blood that is then supplied to parallel pulmonary and systemic circuits.

Clinical Pearl

Hypoplastic left heart syndrome is a spectrum of congenital cardiac abnormalities involving underdevelopment of left-sided heart structures and resulting in physiology wherein a single ventricle, in this case the RV, is required to support both pulmonary and systemic circulations.

What is the circulatory pattern in patients with HLHS after birth and what does "ductal-dependent" mean?

In patients with HLHS, due to the inadequacy of the left-sided heart structures, blood flow through the native LV outflow tract is limited and therefore flow to the systemic circulation after birth is dependent on flow provided via the patent ductus arteriosus (PDA). In patients with aortic atresia, the child is completely dependent on the PDA for blood flow to the coronary and cerebral circulations and significant hypotension may be poorly tolerated. It is therefore necessary for patients with HLHS to be placed on continuous prostaglandin E_1 (PGE_1) infusions after birth to assure continued patency of the ductus arteriosus and flow to the systemic circulation. Hypoplastic left heart syndrome is therefore known as a "ductal-dependent" cardiac lesion. (See Figure 26.1.)

> **Clinical Pearl**
>
> *In patients with HLHS, due to the inadequacy of the left-sided heart structures, flow to the systemic circulation after birth is dependent on flow provided via the PDA.*

What is a "series" circulation as opposed to a "parallel" circulation?

In a normal two-ventricle heart the systemic and pulmonary circulations exist in series, with each circulation supported by its own ventricle. In HLHS patients, prior to and immediately after Stage I palliation, blood flow to both systemic and pulmonary circulations is supplied in parallel by the single ventricle. The single ventricle therefore has to perform increased work in order to maintain flow to both the systemic and the pulmonary circulations.

Once patients undergo Stage II palliation (hemi-Fontan or bidirectional Glenn, see Chapter 27) followed by the Fontan procedure (see Chapters 28–30) their systemic and pulmonary circulations then exist in series, meaning that blood pumped by the single ventricle will pass through both circulations before returning to the heart.

> **Clinical Pearl**
>
> *In HLHS patients, prior to and immediately after Stage I palliation, blood flow to both systemic and pulmonary circulations is supplied in parallel by the single ventricle.*

When do patients undergo Stage I palliation?

The use of PGE_1 is associated with a variety of dose-dependent side effects which can commonly include hypotension and apnea, and thus the lowest effective dose is utilized to minimize these side effects. Additionally, the natural decrease in pulmonary vascular resistance (PVR) after birth compared to systemic vascular resistance (SVR) means that pulmonary overcirculation will occur as blood preferentially flows to the circulation with lower resistance. In an infant with parallel circulations this increase in pulmonary blood flow (PBF) will come at the expense of systemic blood flow and oxygen delivery. For these reasons, unless other issues delay surgery it is preferable to proceed with the Stage I palliative surgery within the first week of life when possible.

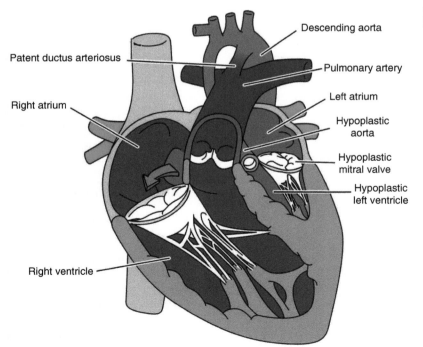

Figure 26.1 Hypoplastic left heart syndrome.
Drawing by Ryan Moore, MD, and Matt Nelson.

Descending aorta

Patent ductus arteriosus

Pulmonary artery

Right atrium

Left atrium

Hypoplastic aorta

Hypoplastic mitral valve

Hypoplastic left ventricle

Right ventricle

What is a "Stage I" palliation and what are the surgical goals?

A Stage I palliation for HLHS is often referred to as the "Norwood procedure," after surgeon William I. Norwood, who first successfully performed the procedure in Boston in 1983 [1]. Although a Stage I palliation for HLHS is a complicated procedure, it may be more easily understood if broken down into the individual goals the surgery must achieve.

1. ***Creation of an unobstructed source of systemic blood flow (aortic reconstruction)***: In HLHS patients the aorta is diminutive or hypoplastic, and prior to Stage I palliation distal flow to the aorta is provided via the PDA. Initial surgical palliation will utilize the patient's native pulmonary outlet, and utilizing autologous tissue supplemented with patch material for augmentation will adjoin it to the patient's hypoplastic aortic outlet, creating a single ventricular outlet, or "neo-aorta." Going forward this will serve as the systemic outflow tract. To utilize the pulmonary root for aortic reconstruction the main pulmonary artery will be transected and oversewn, so it is then necessary to create a source of PBF.

2. ***Creation of a PBF source***: As the main pulmonary artery is transected and oversewn in order to utilize the pulmonary outlet for reconstruction of the hypoplastic aorta, a new source of PBF must be established, with the goal of providing adequate but not excessive PBF. This systemic-to-pulmonary shunt may take one of several forms.

   a. *Modified Blalock-Taussig (mBT) shunt*. A GORE-TEX® tube graft (generally 3.5 mm) is interposed between the right subclavian or innominate artery and the pulmonary artery (PA) to provide PBF. As PA diastolic pressures are lower than aortic diastolic pressure, this shunt is associated with increased flow during diastole, leading to lower aortic diastolic pressure. This may result in diastolic hypotension and coronary ischemia. (See Figure 26.2.)

   b. *Sano shunt*. An alternate approach preferred by some centers involves creation of a graft between the single RV and the PA, known as a Sano shunt. The RV–PA shunt maintains higher diastolic pressure with presumably better coronary blood flow and is associated with better early surgical outcomes in certain types of HLHS [2] (See Figure 26.3.)

   c. *Central shunt*. Aortic-to-pulmonary shunts are less commonly utilized.

3. ***Ensure complete atrial mixing***: Going forward the patient's heart will function as a single atrium and a single ventricle. Therefore, an atrial septectomy is necessary to allow complete mixing of oxygenated pulmonary venous return and deoxygenated systemic

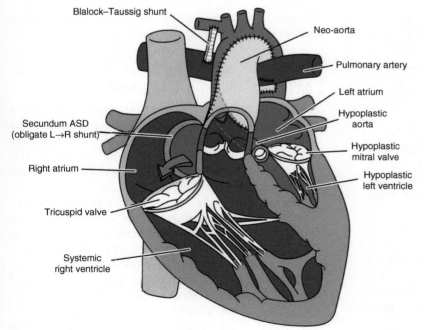

Blalock–Taussig shunt
Neo-aorta
Pulmonary artery
Left atrium
Hypoplastic aorta
Secundum ASD (obligate L→R shunt)
Hypoplastic mitral valve
Right atrium
Hypoplastic left ventricle
Tricuspid valve
Systemic right ventricle

Figure 26.2 HLHS Stage I palliation with modified Blalock-Taussig shunt. Drawing by Ryan Moore, MD, and Matt Nelson.

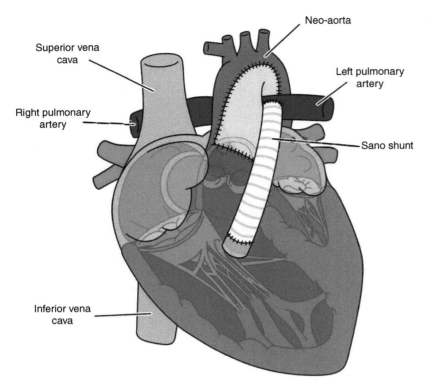

Superior vena cava

Right pulmonary artery

Inferior vena cava

Neo-aorta

Left pulmonary artery

Sano shunt

Figure 26.3 HLHS Stage I palliation with Sano shunt. Drawing by Ryan Moore, MD, and Matt Nelson.

venous return. Because of this mixing, the patient's expected oxygen saturations will be 75–85% after Stage I palliation.

Clinical Pearl

Due to mixing of pulmonary and systemic venous return in the common atrium, the patient's expected oxygen saturations will be 75%–85% after Stage I palliation.

What is the new pattern of blood flow in a patient after a Stage I procedure?

- Systemic and pulmonary venous return mix in the common atrium.
- Blood flows through the atrioventricular valve (tricuspid valve in the case of HLHS).
- The single systemic ventricle pumps blood into the newly constructed "neo-aorta."
- Systemic blood flow is provided via the neoaorta.
- A surgically created shunt (either an mBT or Sano) provides PBF.

Therefore, blood ejected from the single ventricle can enter *either* the pulmonary or systemic circulation. The ratio of

pulmonary to systemic blood flow (Q_p:Q_s) therefore varies depending on resistance in each circulation (PVR and SVR). As PVR is generally lower than SVR, the risk for excessive PBF is high. Mechanical restriction to pulmonary blood flow is achieved by using an appropriately sized shunt.

What is the "hybrid approach" to Stage I palliation? When is it utilized?

The hybrid approach refers to the combined use of surgical and interventional cardiology techniques to achieve the desired goals and is performed in the cardiac catheterization laboratory or in a specially designed "hybrid" operating room. It is performed via sternotomy but without the use of cardiopulmonary bypass (CPB).

The hybrid procedure is preferred for patients who may be at higher than normal risk for a traditional Stage I procedure and might be expected to have a poor outcome. This often includes patients weighing <2 kg, including those who are premature and small for gestational age. It is also utilized in patients whose families wish to avoid blood transfusion, such as Jehovah's Witnesses. Hybrid procedures may also be used to limit PBF in other forms of congenital heart disease. This approach allows the patient to grow until their size is more appropriate for surgical repair or until cardiac transplantation, depending on their disease.

What are the goals of a hybrid procedure?

Goals of a hybrid procedure are similar to the Stage I Norwood procedure. (See Figures 26.2 and 26.3.)

- **Systemic blood flow provision**: Rather than continuing to rely on PGE_1 to maintain ductal patency, the surgeon and interventional cardiologist **place a stent directly into the PDA** via a sheath in the PA. The stented PDA will allow continued provision of systemic blood flow via the distal aorta. Surgical reconstruction of the aorta will take place at the time of the Stage II palliative procedure.

- **Pulmonary blood flow** is supplied via the pulmonary arteries, and in order to prevent pulmonary overcirculation, **restrictive bands are placed on the left and right pulmonary arteries.** The degree of restriction is titrated based on oxygen saturation and direct pressure measurements measured via the pulmonary artery sheath and transesophageal echocardiography.

What surgical stages are generally involved in complete palliation of an HLHS patient?

The ultimate goal of single-ventricle palliation is utilization of the single ventricle to provide systemic blood flow. Pulmonary blood flow is supplied by passive blood flow of systemic venous return directly to the lungs.

Stage I palliation involves the creation of a single atrium by performing an atrial septectomy, reconstructing the aorta as the outflow tract of the single ventricle and creating a surgical shunt for PBF. Because this circulatory arrangement involves complete mixing of systemic and pulmonary venous return the patient remains cyanotic after Stage I pallation.

As the fixed size of either an mBT or a Sano shunt means that the infant will become increasingly cyanotic with growth, **Stage II palliation** is usually performed between 3 and 6 months of age, allowing PVR to continue to decrease prior to this surgery. In Stage II palliation the initial mBT or Sano shunt is taken down, and a new source of PBF is created either by anastomosis of the superior vena cava (SVC) directly to the PA via a bidirectional Glenn procedure (BDG) or through creation of an atrial baffle with a hemi-Fontan procedure. After the Stage II surgery deoxygenated blood from the inferior vena cava (IVC) still mixes with oxygenated blood from the pulmonary veins in the atrium, so the patient continues to be cyanotic. (See Chapter 27.)

The Fontan procedure – the final stage – creates a connection between the IVC and the PA, either through an extracardiac tube graft or by creating a lateral tunnel via revision of the atrial baffle [3]. The systemic and pulmonary circulations are now separated and oxygen saturations are usually in the 90s. (See Chapters 28–30.)

What is the Q_p:Q_s ratio and what is its significance?

Pulmonary blood flow is denoted by Q_p, and systemic blood flow by Q_s. The Q_p:Q_s ratio represents the ratio of pulmonary blood flow to systemic blood flow. In a normal biventricular heart this ratio is 1.

How do changes in the balance of Q_p and Q_s affect the patient?

In a single-ventricle (parallel) circulation, blood ejected by the ventricle can flow through either the systemic (Q_s) or pulmonary arterial (Q_p) system.

- A marked decrease in PVR or a sudden increase in SVR will cause increased Q_p at the cost of Q_s, resulting in hypotension and signs of poor perfusion.

- A marked decrease in SVR will cause increased Q_s at the cost of Q_p and result in increased cyanosis.

Diminished cardiac output, whether from myocardial dysfunction, ischemia, or atrioventricular (AV) valve regurgitation, can result in reduced flows to both circulations, causing both hypotension and desaturation.

What is the optimal Q_p:Q_s in a patient with Stage I physiology and what oxygen saturation does this typically reflect?

An oxygen saturation of 75%–85% as measured by pulse oximetry appears to be optimal for most patients with Stage I physiology, as higher saturations may indicate pulmonary overcirculation, placing increased demands on the single ventricle as it provides flow to both circulations. These saturations typically reflect a Q_p:Q_s ratio of 0.7–1.0 [4].

What factors allow optimization of Stage I palliation physiology?

Optimization of the patient's physiology focuses on maximizing cardiac output and oxygen delivery. Atrioventricular valve regurgitation and dysrhythmias are poorly tolerated as they reduce cardiac output. Marked changes in either pulmonary or systemic vascular resistance may cause an imbalance of Q_p:Q_s. As increased oxygen carrying capacity is desirable, a higher hematocrit is utilized to maintain adequate oxygen delivery. Cyanotic patients typically require a hematocrit of 40% or greater.

Anesthetic Implications

What is the significance of this patient's failure to thrive?

Feeding and digestion require relatively high metabolic demand in infants as compared to their resting state and so both failure to thrive and gastroesophageal reflux are frequently seen in this patient population. They can be manifestations of the inability to mount an appropriate cardiac or pulmonary response to increased metabolic demand. Vocal cord dysfunction can occur as a result of recurrent laryngeal nerve injury during aortic arch reconstruction or as a result of prolonged intubation and may also result in feeding intolerance. Approximately 15%–30% of patients with HLHS have other genetic abnormalities, and reflux and failure to thrive may also be symptoms of other congenital abnormalities or syndromes.

What preoperative assessment should be performed for this patient?

A thorough preoperative chart review, interview, and physical exam are essential. Initial assessment should include review of a recent echocardiogram, focusing on ventricular function, AV valve regurgitation and shunt patency. Anesthetic records and hospital discharge summaries should be reviewed for complications associated with Stage I surgery and hospitalization. Perioperative and postoperative complications can also include nervous system injury, shunt malfunction, arterial or central venous occlusion, and renal dysfunction. The most recent cardiology notes and laboratory studies, especially hematocrit, should be reviewed as well. Blood type and antibody screening should be up to date, as patients have usually been previously transfused and may require transfusion to maintain a hematocrit in the preferred range above 40%.

Preoperative evaluation should include assessment for adequacy of cardiac output. Infants experience peak metabolic demand while feeding and digesting which can produce transient symptoms of inadequate cardiac output. These can include tachypnea, interruption of feeding, sweating, and worsened cyanosis. This may result in poor weight gain; severely inadequate cardiac output may result in lethargy. Home oxygen saturation values should be reviewed. In this patient, a baseline oxygen saturation of 86% may reflect pulmonary overcirculation, especially in this child with poor feeding. Aspirin is often continued in the perioperative period while diuretics are typically held during fasting.

> **Clinical Pearl**
>
> *Specific echocardiographic findings indicate patients at increased risk for adverse outcomes. These include impaired ventricular function, significant valvular regurgitation and coronary artery pathology. Patients with mBT shunts are at greater risk for diastolic hypotension and myocardial ischemia than those with Sano shunts.*

How should parents be counselled about anesthetic risk?

Infants with Stage I physiology are at markedly increased risk for perioperative complications compared to healthy infants and older patients. They have reduced respiratory reserve owing to their baseline desaturation, as well as limited cardiac reserve. Hypotension necessitating intraoperative inotropic support is, unfortunately, not uncommon. The presence of a common atrium may allow any intravenous (IV) air bubble to enter the arterial tree and result in stroke. Because of the risk of perioperative hemodynamic and respiratory instability, most Stage I patients are routinely taken to an intensive care unit (ICU) for postoperative management. At some centers they are routinely transferred to the ICU while still intubated, allowing the intensivists to carefully monitor for adequate perfusion, ventilation, and full awakening prior to extubation.

An increase in afterload or decrease in cardiac output may result in sluggish shunt flow, which can result in shunt thrombosis. This may require emergent initiation of extracorporeal membrane oxygenation (ECMO) for survival. Intensive care units allow for more rapid initiation of ECMO compared to the recovery room or hospital ward.

Parents should therefore be counseled on the potential need for inotropic support and blood transfusion, and the likelihood of postoperative intubation following the procedure. The risk of stroke, cardiac arrest, and shunt thrombosis requiring ECMO cannulation are significantly higher compared to children without heart disease, though they are still uncommon.

What vascular access and monitoring is advisable for this procedure?

For this procedure, a peripheral IV line in the upper extremity is preferred, in case of IVC obstruction due to insufflation or injury during dissection. However, it is best to avoid internal jugular or subclavian central venous access, as this may cause venous stenosis that could subsequently negatively impact successful Stage II palliation. If upper extremity central access is needed, a peripherally inserted central catheter along with large-bore peripheral IV access would be preferable and may prove beneficial if use of vasopressor and/or inotropic therapy is likely.

It is generally advisable to have two peripheral IV lines at a minimum to administer fluids, blood if necessary, and vasoactive drugs if needed. The gradient between $PaCO_2$ and $ETCO_2$ increases during laparoscopic procedures, and this increase is magnified in patients with cyanotic heart disease. Measuring instantaneous blood pressure with an arterial catheter is advantageous and placement of an arterial line is generally prudent. However, this must be balanced against the difficulty of placing arterial access in an infant who has recently had an arterial line and will require future arterial lines; patient status and the expected length of surgery can aid the practitioner in making this decision. Other factors to consider when determining the need for invasive monitors include potential blood loss, patient-specific bleeding and/or transfusion risk factors, postoperative monitoring needs, long-term venous access, and postoperative disposition.

What method of induction is preferable and what are the hemodynamic goals during induction?

Although induction can be achieved via inhalational or intravenous routes, an IV induction would be safest for this patient. For any patient with poor cardiopulmonary reserve, IV induction provides optimal hemodynamic control, the option for correction of fluid deficits prior to induction and immediate access for resuscitation. It also makes rapid sequence induction possible, if deemed

necessary. Preferred induction medications may include ketamine, fentanyl, and etomidate along with neuromuscular blocking agents.

Cardiac output is best maintained through ensuring adequate preload and judicious dosing of anesthetic agents. Decreases in PVR must be avoided and supplemental oxygen should be used sparingly, immediately before laryngoscopy or when a patient becomes hypoxemic. Oxygen saturations should be maintained at or near the baseline preoperative value.

The initiation of positive pressure ventilation (PPV) and/or administration of high-dose sevoflurane can lead to anesthetic overdose. Volatile anesthetic agents can cause myocardial depression and should be used judiciously. Even with the use of neuromuscular blockade and reduced dosing of inhaled anesthetics hemodynamic instability is not uncommon.

What are the anesthetic considerations for a patient whose PBF is provided via a systemic-to-pulmonary shunt?

Inhalational induction may be prolonged in patients with cyanotic heart disease and an IV induction of anesthesia would be recommended for this patient. These patients can be extremely sensitive to reductions in PVR that result in excess Q_p, which in turn compromises Q_s. Efforts should be made to maintain oxygen saturations at the preoperative baseline level. After endotracheal intubation this often means utilizing an inspired oxygen concentration (FiO_2) at or near 0.21. Once insufflation has commenced it is generally necessary to adjust ventilator settings to compensate for the increase in $ETCO_2$ and it may also be necessary to increase FiO_2 at that time if oxygen saturations have decreased appreciably from baseline.

Patients with Stage I single-ventricle physiology have increased ventricular volume work and afterload relative to normal biventricular hearts. Alterations in preload due to prolonged preoperative fasting and/or the effects of decreased cardiac contractility due to anesthetic agents may therefore be more deleterious. Hypotension is very common and may require the judicious replacement of fluids, administration of blood products, or in some cases inotropic therapy. Paradoxical emboli are a major concern, as anything that enters systemic venous return can be immediately transmitted to the systemic arterial circulation due to the complete mixing of the circulations.

Patients are frequently taking antiplatelet or anticoagulant medications to prevent shunt thrombosis or treat previous vascular occlusions due to cardiac catheterization or prolonged central venous or arterial catheter use. If present, long-standing polycythemia can result in a reduction in plasma clotting factor compensation which may further increase bleeding risk.

Cyanotic patients and those with surgical grafts are also at increased risk for infective endocarditis and should receive appropriate antibiotic prophylaxis.

Lastly, any precipitous fall in SpO_2 that fails to respond to the appropriate manipulations of increased FiO_2, volume administration and vasoactive medications necessitates an emergent echocardiogram. Shunt thrombosis, particularly in a patient with an mBT shunt, is a catastrophic occurrence and can require the emergent initiation of ECMO.

Clinical Pearl

Any precipitous fall in SpO_2 that fails to respond to the appropriate manipulations of increased FiO_2, volume administration and vasoactive medications necessitates an emergent echocardiogram to rule out shunt thrombosis.

How can anesthetics and PPV alter the balance of systemic and pulmonary blood flow?

In patients with normal pulmonary compliance, PVR can be readily reduced with mechanical ventilation. Accidental hyperventilation and hyperoxia are, unfortunately, common. Volatile anesthetics reduce blood pressure in a dose-dependent fashion through reductions in contractility, stroke volume, cardiac output, and SVR. This may result in a reduction in both Q_s and Q_p. Dexmedetomidine may reduce the need for anesthetics implicated in possible anesthetic neurotoxicity to the developing brain, but it should be noted that rapid boluses may result in a greater increase in SVR relative to PVR as well as bradycardia.

What are signs of inadequate Q_s? What are the likely causes and best initial treatments?

Inadequate Q_s can be identified by hypotension, mottled appearance, hepatomegaly, lactic acidosis, and low mixed venous oxygen content. This can result from either low

PVR resulting in excess Q_p at the cost of Q_s, diminished total cardiac output, or both. Pulmonary blood flow may be reduced with ventilatory maneuvers such as decreasing FiO_2 and permissive hypercarbia to increase PVR. Cardiac output can be augmented by use of volume expansion and inotropic agents. Intraoperatively the most likely causes of inadequate systemic flow are diminished cardiac output due to anesthetic agents and excess reduction in PVR from excess ventilation or hyperoxia.

Clinical Pearl

Inadequate Q_s can be identified by hypotension, mottled appearance, hepatomegaly, lactic acidosis, and low mixed venous oxygen content. This can result from low PVR causing excess Q_p at the cost of Q_s, or through diminished total cardiac output, or both.

What are signs of inadequate Q_p? What are the likely causes and best initial treatments?

Inadequate Q_p is often marked by cyanosis and desaturation, as well as a possible increase in the gradient between $ETCO_2$ and $PaCO_2$. This may be related to globally reduced cardiac output, increased PVR, or reduced SVR. Treatments can include PVR reduction, increasing cardiac output and treatment of reduced SVR.

Pulmonary vascular resistance can be reduced with lung recruitment, increased FiO_2, and treatment of pain and/or acidosis. Treatment of low SVR often begins with vasopressors such as epinephrine or phenylephrine that increase SVR more than PVR. However, vasopressors must be used cautiously, as they may reduce end-organ perfusion, resulting in lactic acidosis and further impairing myocardial performance. Cardiac output can be increased through volume expansion and inotropic therapies.

What are other causes of desaturation besides decreased Q_p?

In addition to decreased Q_p, other contributing causes to desaturation can include pulmonary derecruitment and atelectasis, congestive heart failure with pulmonary edema, and inadequate oxygen delivery leading to low mixed venous oxygen saturation. Increasing oxygen delivery either via transfusion and/or increasing cardiac output can raise mixed venous oxygen saturation, resulting in increased arterial oxygen saturation. Anatomic obstruction to Q_p must also be considered. Shunt stenosis due to kinking or thrombosis is, unfortunately, common. Another less likely cause is obstruction to pulmonary venous return, which can be caused directly by pulmonary venous stenosis or downstream by a restrictive atrial septum resulting in high left atrial pressure.

What are signs of simultaneously inadequate systemic and pulmonary blood flow and what treatments are indicated?

Patients may manifest any combination of the symptoms mentioned earlier. Treatment will require increased flow which may involve volume expansion including transfusion, along with inotropes and possibly inodilators such as milrinone to maximize perfusion. Veno-arterial extracorporeal membrane oxygenation (VA-ECMO) may be required if the above fail to improve oxygen saturation and perfusion.

What are the likely causes and initial treatment for hypoxemia and *hyper*tension?

Intraoperatively the onset of hypoxemia without hypotension or signs of reduced cardiac output is often the result of atelectasis. When hypoxemia is associated with hypertension, elevation in PVR causing a reduction in Q_p relative to Q_s is likely. Elevated PVR may result in sluggish shunt flow and should therefore be addressed. Reduction in PVR through utilization of anesthetic or analgesic agents and treatment of acidosis and hyperthermia may be helpful. Oxygen supplementation should be used judiciously in order to avoid hyperoxia and excessive Q_p. Hypoxemia may also reflect low mixed venous oxygen saturation. In this situation volume expansion, transfusion and inotropic therapy may also be required. Should hypoxemia and hypertension persist despite therapy, consideration should be given to the occurrence of a potential pulmonary hypertensive crisis, in which case inhaled nitric oxide would prove useful.

What physiologic changes occur with laparoscopy?

In healthy children, insufflation pressures of 6 mm Hg are not associated with hemodynamic changes by transesophageal echocardiography. However, insufflation pressures of 10 mm Hg reduced aortic blood flow and increased SVR without changes in blood pressure. Insufflation with pressures of 12 mm Hg reduced systemic ventricular systolic function and cardiac index. Insufflation also decreases lung compliance in children [5, 6].

During insufflation carbon dioxide (CO_2) uptake into the circulation occurs at a greater rate in children as compared to adults. Minute ventilation typically needs to be increased 20%–30% to offset some of this uptake. However, some of the CO_2 is buffered and released postoperatively, resulting in a sustained need for increased minute ventilation to prevent hypercapnia postoperatively [7]. Cyanotic patients normally have a greater difference between $PaCO_2$ and $ETCO_2$ than acyanotic patients due to reduced PBF and increased alveolar dead space. Insufflation worsens both of these factors. This results in an approximate doubling of the $PaCO_2$-$ETCO_2$ difference during laparoscopy [8].

Would it be safer to perform this procedure with an open laparotomy?

In patients with CHD, multiple retrospective studies have shown fewer complications and lower mortality in patients undergoing laparoscopic procedures [9]. A study using national surgery quality data revealed lower morbidity and a trend toward lower mortality in patients with minor CHD undergoing laparoscopic procedures, but no difference in those with severe or major CHD. Laparoscopic procedures were associated with shorter length of stay and less transfusion. Patients with CHD have a higher rate of reintubation, infection, readmission, and mortality, with a roughly fourfold higher rate as compared to healthy patients. Laparoscopy in all patients with CHD appears to have a mortality of 20%–30% [10–13].

Regarding patients with single-ventricle physiology in particular, an older case series with open fundoplication described instances of hemodynamic instability, some requiring VA-ECMO cannulation and/or resulting in postoperative death [14]. A subsequent case series evaluating laparoscopic procedures found no such major complications. The need for empiric blood transfusion to increase hematocrit to >45% and occurrence of infection were quite common. In another subsequent case series, hemodynamic instability was very common, with one patient requiring VA-ECMO cannulation for shunt thrombosis [15]. For Nissen fundoplication in particular, surgical dissection near the diaphragm results in increased mediastinal and pleural pressures, worsening lung compliance and potentially further increasing intraoperative $PaCO_2$ [11].

> **Clinical Pearl**
>
> *Laparoscopic procedures in patients with Stage I physiology may be technically challenging. Abdominal insufflation and positioning changes should be applied in a graded fashion to ensure patient tolerance.*

If the patient developed refractory hypoxemia, what additional cause should be considered?

Shunt thrombosis is a life-threatening emergency that results in marked reduction or cessation of PBF. The ensuing hypoxemia and hypercarbia cause rapid deterioration of cardiac performance, shock, and cardiac arrest. Initial hypoxemia is associated with marked reduction and then loss of $ETCO_2$. Auscultation of the heart may reveal the loss of the characteristic shunt murmur. Bradycardia and ST segment changes are often the first manifestations of inadequate myocardial oxygen delivery.

Immediate treatments include:

- Administration of heparin, typically 100 units/kg IV
- Stat call for echocardiography to assess shunt flow
- Epinephrine boluses to attempt to dislodge thrombus
- Emergent consultations to cardiology and cardiac surgery for shunt recannulation in the catheterization lab or revision in the operating room
- Initiation of VA-ECMO cannulation

In patients with an open chest or a recent sternotomy that can be safely and rapidly reopened, direct massage of the shunt may dislodge the thrombus. Patients who develop cardiac arrest related to complete shunt obstruction may have no PBF and cannot be resuscitated without restoration of shunt flow or an alternative means of oxygenation, namely VA-ECMO.

> **Clinical Pearl**
>
> *Decreases in cardiac output can precipitate shunt thrombosis, which is life-threatening and may require initiation of VA-ECMO and emergent cardiac catheterization or surgery to restore blood flow. Anesthetics, positioning, and laparoscopic insufflation may each independently cause reductions in cardiac output.*

What are the intraoperative and postoperative analgesic options for this patient?

After confirming the absence of anticoagulation, neuraxial techniques including single shot and continuous caudal analgesia have been successfully used for in this patient population. Abdominal wall blocks may also be considered, and, at a minimum, local anesthetic should be infiltrated near incisions. Intravenous acetaminophen may also reduce postoperative opioid analgesic requirements. In young infants, the combination of non-steroidal anti-inflammatory drugs and acetaminophen may not reduce pain scores or opioid consumption compared to acetaminophen alone. The use of nonsteroidal antiinflammatory drugs is controversial, owing to their effects on platelet and renal function. Repeated dosing in young infants has also been associated with increased postoperative bleeding [16].

If postoperative ventilation is required, dexmedetomidine may provide both sedation and analgesia.

Adequate analgesia is essential as inadequate pain control can cause increased oxygen consumption and subsequently desaturation.

What is the appropriate postoperative disposition for this patient?

A discussion including the patient's primary cardiologist, surgeon, the intensivist who may receive the patient, and the anesthesiologist should occur preoperatively regarding postoperative disposition.

Some hospitals require ICU admission following general anesthesia for all Stage I patients, owing to their fragile physiology and significantly elevated mortality as compared to other phases of single-ventricle palliation. At a minimum, patients with risk factors for increased morbidity and mortality or evidence of poor cardiopulmonary reserve must be scheduled for ICU. Any patient with Stage I physiology undergoing elective or semielective procedures under general anesthesia should have an ICU bed readily available for postoperative care, as perhaps 25% of patients experience an escalation of care such as unplanned ICU admission [12]. Even with an uneventful perioperative course postoperative observation in an ICU setting would be recommended for this patient.

Should this patient be immediately extubated at the conclusion of surgery?

After fundoplication, patients exhibit impaired diaphragmatic function, which reduces pulmonary reserve. After laparoscopy or thoracoscopy, patients have transiently increased pulmonary demand to eliminate CO_2

that was absorbed and buffered during insufflation. Patients with tachypnea and other signs of inadequate cardiopulmonary reserve at baseline may benefit from mechanical ventilation until excess CO_2 is eliminated and adequate postoperative analgesia and hemodynamics have been proven. However, the negative aspects of mechanical ventilation are numerous. Positive pressure ventilation impairs venous return and requires sedation, which may result in hypotension. Admission to the ICU and postoperative mechanical ventilation is associated with increased cost and length of stay. As presented, this patient is a candidate for extubation at the end of surgery should the perioperative course prove uneventful although he should still be admitted to an ICU setting.

Can this patient have this surgery at a hospital that does not have ECMO capability?

A known complication for a patient with shunt-dependent single-ventricle physiology having a Nissen fundoplication is the need to resuscitate using ECMO in the event of shunt thrombosis. Therefore, it would be prudent to have the procedure performed in a center with ECMO capability, although the ability to put the patient on CPB during resuscitation might be an alternative.

References

1. W. I. Norwood, P. Lang, and D. D. Hansen. Physiologic repair of aortic atresia-hypoplastic left heart syndrome. *N Engl J Med* 1983; **308**: 23–6.

2. S. Sano, K. Ishino, M. Kawada, et al. Right ventricle-pulmonary artery shunt in first-stage palliation of hypoplastic left heart syndrome. *J Thorac Cardiovasc Surg* 2003; **126**: 504–9.

3. J. M. Pearl, D. P. Nelson, S. M. Schwartz, et al. First-stage palliation for hypoplastic left heart syndrome in the twenty-first century. *Ann Thorac Surg* 2002; **73**: 331–39.

4. S. C. Nicolson, J. M. Steven, L. K. Diaz, et al. Anesthesia for the patient with a single ventricle. In Andropoulos D. B., Stayer S., Mossad E. B. et al., eds. *Anesthesia for Congenital Heart Disease*, 3rd ed. Hoboken, NJ: John Wiley & Sons, 2015; 567–97.

5. S. G. Sakka, E. Huettemann, G. Petrat, et al. Transesophageal echocardiographic assessment of haemodynamic changes during laparoscopic herniorrhaphy in small children. *Br J Anaesth* 2000; **84**: 330–4.

6. P. Y. Gueugniaud, M. Abisseror, M. Moussa, et al. The hemodynamic effects of pneumoperitoneum during laparoscopic surgery in healthy infants: assessment by continuous esophageal aortic blood flow echo-Doppler. *Anesth Analg* 1998; **86**: 290–3.

7. J. H. Pennant. Anesthesia for laparoscopy in the pediatric patient. *Anesthesiol Clin North Am* 2001; **19**: 69–88.

8. M. L. Wulkan and S. A. Vasudevan. Is end-tidal CO_2 an accurate measure of arterial CO_2 during laparoscopic procedures in children and neonates with cyanotic congenital heart disease? *J Pediatr Surg* 2001; **36**: 1234–6.

9. J. Kim, Z. Sun, B. R. Englum, et al. Laparoscopy is safe in infants and neonates with congenital heart disease: a national study of 3684 patients. *J Laparoendosc Adv Surg Tech A* 2016; **26**: 836–9.

10. B. Slater, S. Rangel, C. Ramamoorthy, et al. Outcomes after laparoscopic surgery in neonates with hypoplastic left heart syndrome. *J Pediatr Surg* 2007; **42**: 1118–21.

11. B. C. H. Gulack and O. O. Adibe. Laparoscopic antireflux surgery in infants with single ventricle physiology: a review. *J Laparoendosc Adv Surg Tech A* 2013; **23**: 733–7.

12. D. I. Chu, J. M. Tan, P. Mattei, et al. Mortality and morbidity after laparoscopic surgery in children with and without congenital heart disease. *J Pediatr* 2017; **185**: 88–93.

13. L. A. Gillory, M. L. Megison, C. M. Harmon, et al. Laparoscopic surgery in children with congenital heart disease. *J Pediatr Surg* 2012; **47**: 1084–8.

14. C. L. Garey, C. A. Laituri, P. Aguayo, et al. Outcomes in children with hypoplastic left heart syndrome undergoing open fundoplication. *J Pediatr Surg* 2011; **46**: 859–62.

15. B. T. Craig, E. J. Rellinger, B. A. Metter, et al. Laparoscopic Nissen fundoplication in infants with hypoplastic left heart syndrome. *J Pediatr Surg* 2016; **51**: 76–80.

16. A. Gupta, C. Daggett, S. Drant, et al. Prospective randomized trial of ketorolac after congenital heart surgery. *J Cardiothorac Vasc Anesth* 2004; **18**: 454–7.

Suggested Reading

Chu D. I., Tan J. M., Mattei P., et al. Outcomes of laparoscopic and open surgery in children with and without congenital heart disease. *J Pediatr Surg* 2018; **53**: 1980–8.

Nicolson S. C., Steven J. M., Diaz L. K., et al. Anesthesia for the patient with a single ventricle. In Andropoulos D. B., Stayer S. A., Mossad E. B., et al., eds. *Anesthesia for Congenital Heart Disease*, 3rd ed. Hoboken, NJ: John Wiley & Sons, 2015; 356–72.

Quintessenza J., DeSena H. C., Justice L., et al. Hypoplastic left heart syndrome. In Ungerleider R. M., Meliones J. N., Nelson McMillan K. et al., eds. *Critical Heart Disease in Infants and Children*, 3rd ed. Philadelphia: Mosby Elsevier, 2019; 778–95.

Short J. A., Paris S. T., Booker P. D., et al. Arterial to end-tidal carbon dioxide tension difference in children with congenital heart disease. *Br J Anaesth* 2001; **86**: 349–53.

Watkins S., Morrow S. E., McNew B. S., et al. Perioperative management of infants undergoing fundoplication and gastrostomy after stage I palliation of hypoplastic left heart syndrome. *Pediatr Cardiol* 2012; **33**: 697–704.

Bidirectional Glenn

Amanpreet S. Kalsi

Case Scenario

A 9-month-old male infant weighing 8.4 kg presents for a complex hypospadias repair. His past medical history is significant for hypoplastic left heart syndrome. He has undergone two previous surgeries: a Stage I palliation (Norwood procedure) shortly after birth and three months earlier a bidirectional Glenn procedure or Stage II palliation. The history obtained from the parents reveals that he is doing well and developing appropriately and has no other significant medical problems. He is regularly seen as an outpatient by his pediatric cardiologist and his only current medication is acetylsalicylic acid. Current vital signs are: SpO$_2$ 79% on room air, heart rate 115 beats/minute, blood pressure 80/48 mm Hg, and temperature 36.8°C. The operative time is expected to be approximately 3 hours.

His last transthoracic echocardiogram revealed the following:

- *A mildly dilated right ventricle with normal function*
- *Trivial atrioventricular valve regurgitation*

Key Objectives

- Understand the anatomy and physiology of a Stage II palliation or bidirectional Glenn procedure.
- Describe the path of blood flow in these patients.
- Understand how the manipulation of pulmonary and systemic vascular resistances affect systemic oxygen delivery.
- Understand the potential effects of different anesthetic perioperative management plans.
- Discuss the importance of ventilatory strategies in patients with a bidirectional Glenn procedure.

Pathophysiology

What is hypoplastic left heart syndrome?

Hypoplastic left heart syndrome (HLHS) encompasses an array of cardiac anomalies in which the development of the left ventricle (LV) and/or the mitral valve, systemic outflow tract, and ascending aorta are hindered in utero. While some institutions treat this lesion with primary heart transplantation, it is most commonly treated via a three-stage palliative pathway. Stage I is often referred to as the Norwood procedure and includes aortic reconstruction along with creation of a systemic-to-pulmonary artery shunt to provide pulmonary blood flow (PBF). Stage II palliation involves the creation of either a bidirectional Glenn shunt or a hemi-Fontan, replacing the systemic-to-pulmonary artery shunt with a superior cavopulmonary anastomosis (SCPA) to provide PBF. The third or final palliative stage is known as the Fontan procedure, and it routes inferior vena cava (IVC) flow directly to the pulmonary vascular bed. (See Chapter 26.) After completion of the Fontan procedure all PBF is now passively supplied to the pulmonary vascular bed, allowing the single ventricle to provide systemic blood flow.

What is a bidirectional Glenn shunt?

The Glenn shunt is a form of SCPA named for William Glenn, the surgeon who first performed the procedure in 1958. It routes deoxygenated blood from the superior vena cava (SVC) to the right pulmonary artery. A modification of the Glenn shunt was developed in 1973 by Dr. Gaetano Azzolina to facilitate flow to both the left and right pulmonary arteries, leading to the term "bidirectional" Glenn (BDG) shunt. This procedure is now the second stage of the three-stage palliation for HLHS.

Why are single-ventricle palliative surgeries staged in this way?

Following Stage I Norwood palliation for HLHS the RV has a volume burden, as it supports both the pulmonary and systemic circulations in parallel. Over time, this can adversely affect ventricular function and manifest as RV dysfunction accompanied by tricuspid regurgitation (TR) due to malcoaptation of the valve leaflets secondary to distortion of the tricuspid annulus. During Stage I palliation the pulmonary vasculature is also exposed to excessive pressures due to blood flow from the shunt: either systemic arterial (modified Blalock–Taussig shunt) or ventricular (Sano shunt).

Low pulmonary vascular resistance (PVR) is required for passive PBF via either the BDG or hemi-Fontan to be successful, and therefore the Stage II procedure is usually performed around 3–6 months of age. At this point in the infant's development, the pulmonary vasculature has matured and PVR has fallen to sufficiently low levels to permit adequate passive PBF. Completion of this stage reduces the volume loading on the heart and wall stress on the RV, which over time allows for RV remodeling. Subsequently, improvement of RV function should occur along with reduction of TR from improved tricuspid valve leaflet coaptation. These factors are important for the long-term function of the single RV.

Stage III (Fontan completion) surgery is completed usually around the age of 18 months to 4 years, and baffles IVC flow into the pulmonary circulation such that all systemic venous return now directly enters the pulmonary bed.

Is a superior cavopulmonary anastomosis performed only for HLHS patients?

Congenital cardiac patients with functionally univentricular hearts that are not suitable for biventricular repair can also be palliated via the single-ventricle pathway. In these patients, one of the ventricles is hypoplastic. The dominant ventricle could be either the LV, the RV, or of indeterminate morphology. All of these groups may undergo single-ventricle pathway palliation.

Why is a Stage II palliation performed and how are the goals achieved?

Physiologic objectives of second stage palliation are twofold:

- Creation of a lower pressure source of PBF that will grow with the patient
- Reduction of the volume burden on the single ventricle

Following this surgery, the single ventricle only needs to support the systemic cardiac output as blood flow to the lungs is now passive.

The systemic-to-pulmonary artery shunt (high-pressure arterial) that was created during the Stage I palliation is ligated. The SVC is then anastomosed to the pulmonary artery (PA), establishing the new source of PBF. The resulting circulation establishes passive flow of deoxygenated blood from the upper body via the SVC to the pulmonary arteries as the source of PBF.

> **Clinical Pearl**
>
> *Anastomosis of the SVC to the PA establishes passive flow of deoxygenated blood from the upper body via the SVC to the pulmonary arteries as the source of PBF.*

How does the BDG procedure differ from the hemi-Fontan?

Although the physiologic goals are the same, with provision of SVC blood to the pulmonary vascular bed, the BDG and hemi-Fontan differ anatomically. (See Figure 27.1.)

- *Bidirectional Glenn procedure* (see Figure 27.2):

1. The SVC is divided from the RA at the superior cavoatrial junction and the atrial end is oversewn.
2. The RPA is incised, and the posterior wall of the SVC is anastomosed to the superior edge of the PA.

Following a BDG, the completion Fontan operation typically involves the creation of an *extracardiac conduit* wherein the IVC is anastomosed to the PA or distal SVC.

- *Hemi-Fontan procedure* (see Figure 27.3):

1. The natural SVC-to-RA confluence is preserved, and a side-to-side anastomosis is used to join the SVC and RPA.
2. Homograft tissue is used to augment the branch pulmonary arteries, creating a dam across the superior cavoatrial junction, and preventing blood flow between the SVC and RA.
3. The SVC-RA junction is also enlarged to match the size of the IVC.

The hemi-Fontan addresses any PA hypoplasia, and later simplifies the completion of a *lateral tunnel Fontan*. At the time of Fontan completion, the dam is excised, and a polytetrafluoroethylene patch is used to create a division in the atrium such that IVC flow is tunneled toward the pulmonary arteries and pulmonary venous return is directed across the atrioventricular valve.

What is the circulatory path for blood after Stage II palliation?

Deoxygenated blood from the lower body enters the common atrium via the IVC. Deoxygenated blood from the upper extremities, head, and neck passively drains via the SVC into the pulmonary artery. It then traverses the pulmonary vasculature and becomes oxygenated. This oxygenated blood drains via the pulmonary veins into the common atrium and mixes with the deoxygenated blood from the IVC. Blood then passes via the atrioventricular valve into the ventricle. The dominant ventricle (the RV in

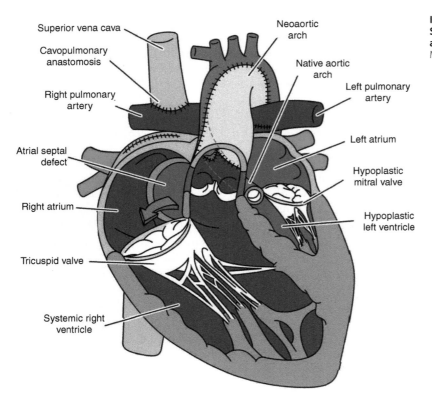

Superior vena cava

Cavopulmonary anastomosis

Right pulmonary artery

Atrial septal defect

Right atrium

Tricuspid valve

Systemic right ventricle

Neoaortic arch

Native aortic arch

Left pulmonary artery

Left atrium

Hypoplastic mitral valve

Hypoplastic left ventricle

Figure 27.1 Hypoplastic left heart syndrome, Stage II palliation, superior cavopulmonary anastomosis (bidirectional Glenn). Drawing by Ryan Moore, MD, and Matt Nelson.

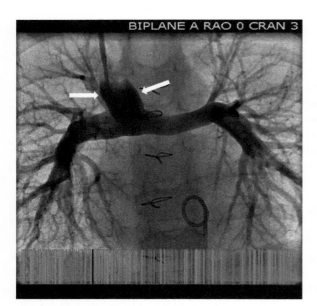

Figure 27.2 Bidirectional Glenn procedure. An angiogram is performed in AP projection in the SVC in a patient with a Glenn shunt. The direct anastomosis of the SVC to the pulmonary artery is noted (arrows). Courtesy of Russel Hirsch, MD.

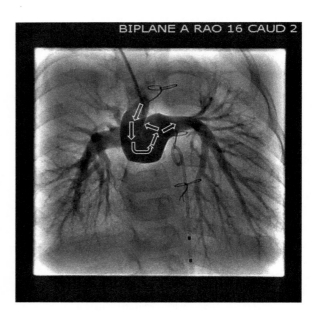

Figure 27.3 Hemi-Fontan. An angiogram is performed in AP projection in the SVC in a patient with a hemi-Fontan. The angiogram demonstrates the anterior course of the SVC with reversed curve anastomosis into the pulmonary arteries. The arrows demonstrate the direction of blood flow. Courtesy of Russel Hirsch, MD.

patients with HLHS) then ejects blood into the systemic circulation.

What are the expected oxygen saturations in patients with a bidirectional Glenn shunt?

The superior systemic venous circulation and the pulmonary circulation are in series; therefore only blood from the SVC travels to the lungs and is oxygenated. Due to the atrial septectomy that has been previously performed in these patients, oxygenated blood returning to the atrium via the pulmonary veins mixes with deoxygenated systemic venous return from the IVC. This mixing results in systemic oxygen saturations in the range of 75%–85%. Therefore, oxygen saturations after Stage II palliation do not differ significantly from saturations prior to Stage II palliation.

Over time, patients with SCPA connections may form veno-venous collaterals and pulmonary-venous connections, which can result in worsening cyanosis [1]. Prior to an anesthetic it is important to be aware of these as possible causes when greater than expected levels of hypoxemia are observed in BDG patients. In addition to the formation of collaterals, a persistent left SVC to coronary sinus connection may also be a cause of cyanosis. Cardiac catheterization and echocardiography data should be assessed in patients who have lower than expected systemic saturations to elucidate the cause.

Clinical Pearl

Oxygenated blood returning to the common atrium via the pulmonary veins mixes with deoxygenated systemic venous return from the IVC. This mixing results in systemic oxygen saturations ranging from 75% to 85%. Therefore, oxygen saturations after Stage II palliation do not differ significantly from saturations prior to Stage II palliation.

Anesthetic Implications

What specific areas should be evaluated in the preoperative assessment?

In addition to a thorough anesthetic preoperative assessment, attention should focus on establishing an understanding of the primary congenital cardiac lesion, the anatomy, and the level and direction of both intracardiac and extracardiac shunts. Furthermore, it is crucial to successful perioperative management to understand and appreciate the effects on systemic tissue oxygen delivery of manipulating both the pulmonary and systemic vascular resistances.

Previous anesthetic records, if available, should also be reviewed with particular attention to the airway management history. Previous intubations and the duration of time spent intubated after previous surgeries, particularly if prolonged, can increase the risk of subglottic stenosis.

How is functional status assessed?

Functional assessment involves evaluating appropriate development, weight gain, attainment of milestones, and reviewing for signs of heart failure. Heart failure can result when the heart is either pressure and/or volume overloaded. These signs differ with age. An infant in heart failure may present with poor feeding, failure to gain weight, and hepatomegaly. Signs that are common to all ages include tachypnea, tachycardia, diaphoresis, and cool extremities.

What should be done if the patient has a respiratory tract infection?

Pediatric patients with recent or active respiratory tract infections are at increased risk for perioperative respiratory complications [2]. In patients with a BDG, the presence of upper or lower respiratory tract infections can have additional hemodynamic ramifications, as infections can increase airway reactivity and reduce pulmonary compliance. Both are poorly tolerated and can lead to intraoperative complications that may arise from difficulty maintaining adequate PBF. Acute increases in PVR resulting from bronchospasm in a patient with an SCPA will present as increased cyanosis, coupled with hypotension from reduced preload. Elective surgery should not be undertaken in the presence of a significant upper or lower respiratory infection, and the case should be rescheduled for 4–6 weeks after resolution of symptoms, allowing airway reactivity to return to normal.

Clinical Pearl

In patients with a BDG, the presence of upper or lower respiratory tract infections can have additional hemodynamic ramifications as they can increase airway reactivity and reduce pulmonary compliance. Both are poorly tolerated and can lead to complications intraoperatively that may arise from difficulty maintaining adequate PBF.

What medications might the child be taking? Which medications should be withheld prior to surgery?

Polycythemia resulting from chronic cyanosis increases whole blood viscosity, reducing blood flow in small arterioles and capillaries. This places these patients at an increased risk of thrombus formation. As a result, patients with a BDG shunt are often taking antiplatelet agents or anticoagulants.

Antiarrhythmic agents, diuretics, and antihypertensives are also frequently used in patients with congenital heart disease (CHD). In particular, angiotensin converting enzyme inhibitors (ACEi) are frequently prescribed for patients with single-ventricle physiology. Evidence for preoperatively withholding these in children is lacking and as a result most guidelines regarding the perioperative administration of ACEi in pediatric patients have been adapted from adult practice. As such, most ACEi are withheld on the morning of surgery.

When considering which medications to continue or withhold, it is advisable to review each case on an individual basis. Advice from the child's pediatric cardiologist should be sought should questions arise.

What preoperative investigations are required?

All available preexisting cardiac data for the patient should be reviewed, including a recent echocardiogram and any cardiac catheterization data. Specific areas of interest on the echocardiogram include assessment of ventricular systolic function (ejection fraction) and atrioventricular valve competence. The patient should also be in compliance with requested cardiology follow-up visits.

An electrocardiogram (ECG) should be evaluated to assess for normal sinus rhythm and conduction abnormalities. Arrhythmias are generally poorly tolerated in patients with CHD, particularly those with single-ventricle physiology. Furthermore, single-ventricle patients with ventricular ectopy have an approximately 30% higher incidence of intraoperative arrythmias resulting in mortality and adverse outcomes [3]. Therefore, the patient with an abnormal ECG should be considered at an increased risk of developing intraoperative arrhythmias.

Available laboratory data should be reviewed. If not recently performed, it is reasonable to obtain a basic metabolic profile and a complete blood count prior to surgery. Although significant blood loss would not be anticipated in this surgery, it is booked for 3 hours.

What is the expected hematocrit and why might it be higher than normally expected?

Polycythemia as a result of ongoing cyanosis is expected, and therefore a hematocrit in the range of 40%–45% is often seen. The transfusion threshold for patients with single-ventricle physiology should be lower than that in a noncyanotic patient; in order to preserve oxygen carrying capacity and tissue oxygen delivery the desired hematocrit

is greater than 40%. Maintaining a higher hematocrit also increases the arterial oxygen saturation in a child with this physiology by improving the mixed venous saturation.

Clinical Pearl

The target hematocrit for patients with Stage II physiology is 40%–45%.

Are there specific preoperative fasting considerations?

While no specific changes should be made to the institutional and nationally accepted preoperative fasting times in a patient with a BDG, normal preload is important for maintenance of stable hemodynamics. Therefore, fasting for clear fluids should be minimized, and if prolonged fasting times are unavoidable, the preoperative institution of intravenous (IV) fluids should be considered. Dehydration should be avoided, as cyanotic patients become polycythemic as an adaptive response, which can cause hyperviscosity and increased risk for thrombus formation.

Should anxiolytic premedication be utilized?

At 9 months of age, infants are not generally likely to experience separation anxiety from the parents or caregivers and often respond well to simple maneuvers such as being held and hearing soothing voices. Therefore, routine premedication in this age group may not be necessary. However, cases should be assessed on an individual basis. If premedication is deemed necessary, patients with BDG shunts can be safely premedicated with an oral or intranasally administered benzodiazepine.

The use of premedication can be helpful in the extremely anxious child as it can aid in decreasing oxygen consumption. In addition, it may reduce the dose of induction agent required, which in turn limits the decrease in systemic vascular resistance (SVR) associated with some anesthetic induction agents.

Is endocarditis prophylaxis required?

In 2017, a focused update of the 2014 guidelines released by the American College of Cardiology and American Heart Association Task Force stated that in the absence of active infection there is no evidence to suggest any benefit from the routine use of antimicrobial agents for infective endocarditis (IE) prophylaxis in gastrointestinal or genitourinary procedures. However, it is their consensus opinion that the use of antimicrobial prophylaxis in patient populations who are either at increased risk of developing IE or at a higher risk of adverse outcomes from contracting IE is not unreasonable. Patients with CHD, either unrepaired or repaired, who have shunts or valvular regurgitation at or adjacent to a prosthetic patch or device would be considered appropriate for IE prophylaxis when undergoing certain dental procedures [4].

What intraoperative monitors should be used? Are invasive pressure monitors required?

Stable BDG patients with normal ventricular function do not require invasive monitors for hypospadias repairs, and the use of standard recommended American Society of Anesthesiologists monitors is appropriate.

During other major surgical procedures, should the use of invasive monitoring be required, placement of arterial access in the upper extremity on the ipsilateral side as a previous modified Blalock–Taussig shunt should be avoided. Residual stenosis may exist at the site of the previous shunt that can cause an erroneously low blood pressure reading. Should central venous access be required it should be remembered that placement of an internal jugular line will yield PA and not atrial pressures. Institutional preferences exist, and some centers may prefer to avoid utilizing the internal jugular and subclavian vessels to mitigate the risk of causing thrombosis or stenosis and reducing SVC drainage into the pulmonary arteries.

Clinical Pearl

Should central venous access be required in a patient with an SCPA it should be remembered that placement of an internal jugular line will yield PA and not atrial pressures.

What are the intraoperative management goals for a child with a BDG?

General goals for the intraoperative management of HLHS patients post Stage II palliation are:

- *Maintain adequate preload.* Should hypotension be encountered intraoperatively, this should be treated initially with IV fluids. Insensible fluid losses, fluid deficit from preoperative fasting, and ongoing blood loss should be accounted for and replaced.
- *Maintain low PVR* to maximize passive PBF. In addition, a high-normal pCO_2 results in cerebral vasodilatation and therefore augments cerebral blood flow, in turn increasing venous return to the pulmonary vasculature via the SVC. When using mild

hypoventilation, it is important to avoid significant acidosis, which increases PVR.

- *Avoid acute increases in PVR and SVR* from sympathetic surges resulting from noxious stimuli.
- *Preserve cardiac contractility* and maintain a normal or low SVR. Using a balanced anesthetic technique is preferable when aiming to achieve stable hemodynamics.
- *Maintain coronary perfusion pressure* and preserve myocardial O_2 supply/demand balance.
- *Avoidance of air embolus* (paradoxical air embolus). All IV administration lines and connectors should be deaired, and medication administration sites should be free of air.
- *Maintain normal sinus rhythm* and avoid arrhythmias.

Clinical Pearl

A high normal pCO_2 results in cerebral vasodilatation and therefore augments cerebral blood flow, in turn increasing venous return to the pulmonary vasculature via the SVC. When using mild hypoventilation, it is important to avoid significant acidosis, which increases PVR.

Does the SCPA affect cerebral perfusion pressure in single-ventricle patients?

In single-ventricle patients, cerebral autoregulation remains intact. However, the modification to the venous return pathway from brain to the heart via the SVC to PA anastomosis has implications for cerebral perfusion pressure (CPP). Cerebral perfusion pressure has typically been described as mean arterial pressure minus intracranial pressure (ICP); jugular venous pressure or CVP can be used in place of ICP if their numerical values are higher. In the SCPA circulation, the following equation more accurately depicts CPP (if PAP is higher than ICP):

$$CPP = MAP - mPAP,$$

where CPP = cerebral perfusion pressure; MAP = mean arterial pressure; and mPAP = mean pulmonary arterial pressure. It can be seen from this equation that factors that decrease MAP or increase ICP and PAP will decrease CPP. Infants with SCPA usually have low PVR and therefore low PA pressures. In infants with a BDG or hemi-Fontan who have low pulmonary pressures, CBF can be increased by maintaining slight hypercarbia, which dilates cerebral blood vessels and promotes greater blood flow in the SVC, thus increasing oxygenated venous return to the heart. However, in all Stage II single-ventricle palliation patients, to maintain adequate CPP and adequate systemic oxygenation, PAP should be kept low and MAP maintained near normal.

Occasionally a patient is unable to progress past the BDG circulation to Stage III (Fontan) palliation due to elevated PA pressures. In these patients, the presence of elevated PA pressures and low MAP places them at significant risk of cerebral ischemia intraoperatively from inadequate cerebral perfusion. In this scenario, it is crucial to avoid decreases in SVR and PVR should be kept as low as possible. Older patients with SCPA should be assumed to have elevated PA pressure and should be cared for in specialist centers.

Clinical Pearl

Factors that decrease MAP or increase ICP and PA pressures will decrease cerebral perfusion pressures in the patient with a BDG. To maintain adequate cerebral perfusion pressure and adequate systemic oxygenation, PA pressures should be kept low and MAP maintained near normal.

Which pharmacologic agents are suitable for induction of anesthesia?

Either inhalational induction or IV induction of anesthesia is suitable. The exact choice of inhalational or IV induction agent matters less than the expertise by which it is administered.

Inhalational induction with sevoflurane and an air/oxygen mixture is appropriate. The use of nitrous oxide is not contraindicated, but many anesthesiologists avoid its use in congenital cardiac patients with shunts. First, it can cause gas bubble expansion, which can potentiate the harmful effects of inadvertent intravenous gas embolus. Second, it can cause constriction of pulmonary vascular smooth muscle, and so may increase PVR.

Propofol decreases SVR and MAP. In children with CHD, this can worsen right-to-left shunting and reduce systemic oxygen saturations. Furthermore, the reduction in MAP can decrease coronary perfusion pressure, which, if significant enough, can impair myocardial function and precipitate arrhythmias. However, with awareness of the potential detrimental effects and the use of smaller doses, it can be used safely in this patient group in patients with normal ventricular function.

Other induction agents such as etomidate and ketamine, barbiturates, and volatile agents such as isoflurane and desflurane can be used safely in this patient population with awareness of their mechanisms of action, influence on PVR and SVR, and adverse effects.

How can PVR be manipulated?

In patients with single-ventricle physiology who have undergone a BDG, the sole source of PBF is passive drainage from the SVC. As a result, an understanding of how to manipulate PVR is of the utmost importance intraoperatively as increases in PVR or intrathoracic pressure will negatively impact PBF.

Pulmonary vascular resistance is influenced by pCO_2, pO_2, pH, temperature, mean airway pressure, atelectasis, and sympathetic stimulus. Factors increasing PVR include acidosis, high pCO_2, high mean airway pressure, hypothermia, basal atelectasis, increased sympathetic stimulus, and a low pO_2. To maintain a low PVR use a higher inspired O_2 concentration, avoid significant hypoventilation and acidosis, maintain low mean airway pressures and normothermia, and avoid sympathetic surges.

Clinical Pearl

Optimal pulmonary blood flow in patients with a BDG occurs when the PVR is low. Factors negatively impacting PVR include acidosis, high pCO_2, high mean airway pressure, hypothermia, basal atelectasis, increased sympathetic stimulus, and a low pO_2.

How should ventilation be managed?

The key to successful management of ventilation in HLHS patients with a BDG shunt is understanding that in this patient population, PBF occurs passively. With this in mind, it becomes clear that factors that influence PVR and intrathoracic pressure gradients have a major role in influencing PBF.

Spontaneous ventilation is beneficial as the negative intrathoracic pressure generated by inspiration augments venous return via the SVC to the PA, improving PBF. However, the use of a spontaneous breathing technique may be limited by the duration and type of operative procedure and patient positioning. The eventual loss of alveolar recruitment and basal atelectasis over long cases needs to be considered when formulating an appropriate ventilation strategy.

The use of positive pressure ventilation (PPV) is possible in individuals with a BDG. Although using this technique will eliminate the augmentation of PBF associated with spontaneous inspiration, it allows for greater control over the end-tidal carbon dioxide ($ETCO_2$) concentration and enables the anesthesiologist to optimize positive end-expiratory pressure (PEEP) and maintain alveolar recruitment. Ideally, low peak inspiratory pressures should be maintained by ventilating on the optimal (steep) part of the compliance curve. Maintaining low peak inspiratory pressures and using a slightly prolonged expiratory phase will help to facilitate PBF, which occurs during expiration with PPV [5].

In the patient with a BDG, maintaining slight hypercarbia (ETCO$_2$ concentration of 45–55 mm Hg) results in vasodilation of cerebral blood vessels and increases cerebral blood flow [6], which in turn increases the volume of deoxygenated blood returning to the PAs via the SVC. It appears that the additional PBF that results from mild hypercarbia induced cerebral vasodilation outweighs the negative effects of the mild acidosis on increasing the PVR.

In summary, when PPV is employed, the following principles should be used:

- Maintain low PVR.
- Maintain low intrathoracic pressure.
- Maintain a target ETCO$_2$ of 40–45 mm Hg.
- Use a slightly prolonged expiratory time to allow extra time for PBF to occur.
- Optimize tidal volumes and PEEP to achieve optimal compliance of gas exchanging units.
- Maintain adequate minute ventilation.

Clinical Pearl

Although spontaneous ventilation can be beneficial, the use of a spontaneous breathing technique may be limited by the duration and type of operative procedure and patient positioning. The eventual loss of alveolar recruitment and basal atelectasis over long cases needs to be considered when formulating an appropriate ventilation strategy.

Can a laryngeal mask airway be used?

General anesthesia with spontaneous ventilation via a laryngeal mask airway (LMA) can be effectively used in HLHS patients with BDG shunts. It provides the advantage of maintaining the negative intrathoracic pressure associated with inspiration which in turn helps augment PBF in patients with a BDG shunt. However, this needs to be balanced against the duration of surgery and the inevitable derecruitment and atelectasis that can occur over prolonged cases with spontaneous ventilation and LMA usage. In addition, many anesthesiologists prefer not to use supraglottic airway devices in infants.

What happens if laryngospasm or bronchospasm occurs?

In BDG patients the source of preload for the heart is derived from two sources: deoxygenated blood from the IVC and blood from the SVC which has become oxygenated after passing through the pulmonary vasculature. Laryngospasm or bronchospasm will cause an acute and abrupt increase in PVR with a resultant decrease in PBF. In the patient with a BDG, both hypotension and marked oxygen desaturation will be evident, resulting from the reduction in oxygenated preload. However, in the BDG circulation, the heart will still receive some preload in the form of deoxygenated blood from the IVC. Thus, both laryngospasm and bronchospasm should be aggressively managed in order to restore the passive flow of oxygenated blood from the pulmonary vasculature.

What are the analgesic options for this patient?

Intravenous analgesics are suitable, preferably a multimodal strategy, which will help reduce the total opiate dose. Postoperative respiratory depression in children with BDG shunts should be avoided, as it will lead to hypoxia from alveolar hypoventilation and hypercarbia. This in turn will raise the PVR and further impede PBF.

Local anesthetics are also a very useful adjunct. Caudal or penile blocks are both appropriate for hypospadias repairs and provide excellent intraoperative and postoperative analgesia. Prior to considering any regional or neuraxial analgesic technique, the anticoagulant medication history should be reviewed to ensure there are no contraindications to performing the procedure. Local and national guidelines regarding safety of regional anesthesia in patients on anticoagulants and antiplatelet agents should be followed.

Are there any specific considerations for emergence from anesthesia?

While tracheal extubation is generally performed with the patient awake, if an LMA was utilized it may often be safely removed with the child still in a deep plane of anesthesia. As with the initial choice of airway utilized for the procedure, decision making regarding the timing of airway removal at the end of the procedure should be individualized and based on the child's airway characteristics as noted during induction, the duration of surgery, and the intraoperative course. Should the decision be made to remove either an endotracheal tube or an LMA with the patient "deep," most practitioners then elect to remain in the operating room until the patient has emerged from anesthesia. If doubt exists regarding any of these factors, the airway should be removed with the patient awake in the operating room environment.

What are the discharge criteria for patients with Stage II palliation?

Standard local guidelines should be used when determining if pediatric patients meet discharge criteria following surgical intervention. Additional considerations for BDG patients that could result in an adverse outcome include residual sedation and poor tolerance of hypovolemia from emesis and/or poor oral intake. If the infant has returned to baseline, has good analgesia, and is tolerating feeds appropriately, they may be appropriate for discharge. However, the length of the surgical procedure is an important factor to consider, and with a complex repair of 3 or more hours duration it would be reasonable to admit for overnight observation following the procedure. Of note, a careful handoff of care should be completed with recovery staff and expected vitals and ranges for blood pressure, heart rate, and oxygen saturations (75%–85%) should be discussed.

References

1. R. M. Freedom, D. Nykanen, and L. N. Benson. The physiology of the bidirectional cavopulmonary connection. *Ann Thorac Surg* 1998; **66**: 664–7.

2. B. S. Von Ungern-Sternberg, K. Boda, N. A. Chambers, et al. Risk assessment for respiratory complications in paediatric anaesthesia: a prospective cohort study. *Lancet* 2010; **376**: 773–83.

3. M. C. White and J. M. Peyton. Anaesthetic management of children with congenital heart disease for non-cardiac surgery. *Cont Educ Anesth Crit Care Pain* 2012; **12**: 17–22.

4. R. A. Nishimura, C. M. Otto, R. O. Bonow, et al. AHA/ACC focused update of the 2014 AHA/ACC guideline for the management of patients with valvular heart disease: a report of the American College of Cardiology/American Heart Association Task Force on Clinical Practice Guidelines. *Circulation* 2017; **135**: e1159–95.

5. A. Al-Eyadhy. Mechanical ventilation strategy following Glenn and Fontan surgeries: on going challenge! *J Saudi Heart Assoc* 2009; **21**: 153–7.

6. S. M. Bradley, J. M. Simsic, and D. M. Mulvihill. Hypoventilation improves oxygenation after bidirectional superior cavopulmonary connection. *J Thorac Cardiovasc Surg* 2003; **126**: 1033–9.

Suggested Reading

Feinstein J. A., Benson D. W., Dubin A. M., et al. Hypoplastic left heart syndrome: current considerations and expectations. *J Am Coll Cardiol* 2012; **59**: S1–42.

Freedom R. M., Nykanen D., and Benson L. N. The physiology of the bidirectional cavopulmonary connection. *Ann Thorac Surg* 1998; **66**: 664–7.

Gupta B., Gupta A., Agarwal M., et al. Glenn shunt: anaesthetic concerns for a non-cardiac surgery. *North J ISA* 2017; **2**: 36–42.

White M. C. and Peyton J. M. Anaesthetic management of children with congenital heart disease for non-cardiac surgery. *Cont Educ Anesth Crit Care Pain* 2012; **12**: 17–22.

Chapter
28
Lateral Tunnel Fenestrated Fontan

Wenyu Bai

Case Scenario

A 14-year-old girl, weighing 53 kg, with severe thoracic scoliosis (Cobb angle 54°) is scheduled to undergo a posterior spinal fusion from level T4 to L1. She was born with tricuspid atresia, and initially underwent placement of a modified Blalock–Taussig shunt, followed by a bidirectional Glenn procedure and ultimately completion of her palliation with a lateral tunnel, fenestrated Fontan procedure. During a recent cardiac catheterization her Fontan pressure was 14 mm Hg and two stents were placed in her left pulmonary artery. Current medications include iron supplements 65 mg once a day, enalapril 5 mg once a day, and acetylsalicylic acid 81 mg once a day, with the latter discontinued 5 days prior to surgery. Recent laboratory evaluation revealed a hemoglobin of 12.5 g/dL, a hematocrit of 35%, and a platelet count of 165 K/μL. Coagulation studies (prothrombin time, international normalized ratio, and partial thromboplastin time) were within normal ranges. Two 250-mL aliquots of autologous blood were collected on two occasions prior to her spine surgery.

Transthoracic echocardiography 4 weeks prior to surgery showed the following:

• *Normal left ventricular function*
• *A patent Fontan fenestration with minimal right-to-left shunting*
• *An unobstructed Fontan pathway*

Key Objectives

• Understand Fontan physiology and the major determinants of Fontan circulation.
• Describe the anesthetic management of patients with Fontan physiology for noncardiac surgery.
• Discuss blood-saving strategies during posterior spinal fusion in patients with Fontan physiology.
• Describe perioperative complications in patients with Fontan physiology for spinal fusion.

Pathophysiology
What is tricuspid atresia?

Tricuspid atresia is a cyanotic congenital heart defect in which the tricuspid valve (TV) is underdeveloped, resulting in complete obstruction of blood flow from the right atrium (RA) into either ventricle, (See Figure 28.1.)

Characteristics of TA include the following:

• A lack of communication between the RA and the morphologic right ventricle (RV)
• An interatrial communication
• An enlarged left-sided atrioventricular (AV) valve
• Absence of the RV inlet with varying deficiency of the trabecular RV

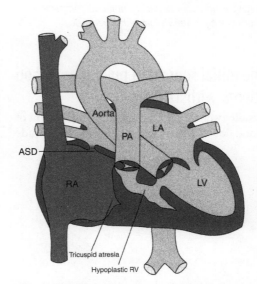

Figure 28.1 Tricuspid atresia. Diagram illustrating tricuspid atresia, atrial septal defect, and hypoplastic right ventricle. ASD, atrial septal defect; LA, left atrium; LV, left ventricle; PA, pulmonary artery; RA, right atrium; RV, right ventricle. In V. G. Nasr and J. A. DiNardo, *The Pediatric Cardiac Anesthesia Handbook*, 1st ed. John Wiley & Sons, 2017; 195–8. With permission.

The RV is often underdeveloped, ranging from near total absence to varying degrees of hypoplasia. Other abnormalities including pulmonary stenosis (PS) may be present as well. A bulboventricular foramen or ventricular septal defect (VSD) is present in nearly all cases. Depending on the size of the VSD and the degree of PS (if present), antegrade pulmonary blood flow may occur via the VSD from the left ventricle (LV) to the RV to the pulmonary artery.

After birth an unrestrictive interatrial communication, in the form of either a patent foramen ovale (PFO) or an atrial septal defect (ASD), is crucial to provide mixing between systemic and pulmonary venous blood, as systemic venous return cannot proceed from the RA to the RV. If not present, an urgent atrial septostomy must be performed to open the atrial septum and allow blood flow from the RA to LA; this is generally performed in the cardiac catheterization laboratory.

Tricuspid atresia has three major variants based on the associated relationship of the great vessels. Type I is characterized by normally related great arteries; pulmonary obstruction is most common in type I TA. Type II is characterized by dextro (d)-transposition of the great vessels and these patients generally have unobstructed pulmonary blood flow. Type III TA is characterized by levo (l)-transposition of the great arteries.

Clinical Pearl

Tricuspid atresia is a cyanotic congenital heart defect in which the tricuspid valve is underdeveloped, resulting in complete obstruction from the right atrium into either ventricle.

What are the initial sources of pulmonary blood flow in patients with TA?

The pathophysiology of TA is determined by the amount of pulmonary blood flow (PBF). Initial sources of PBF include flow via the patent ductus arteriosus (PDA) and antegrade flow provided via the VSD to the RV and pulmonary arteries. Depending on the size of the VSD and the degree of PS (if any) initial PBF may be decreased, balanced, or increased. Patients with decreased PBF will require placement of a systemic-to-pulmonary artery shunt as their initial surgical procedure. (See Figure 28.2.)

Clinical Pearl

The pathophysiology of TA is determined by the amount of PBF. Initial sources of PBF include flow via the PDA and antegrade flow provided via the VSD to the RV and pulmonary arteries.

What was the path of blood flow in this patient with TA at birth?

Systemic venous return from the vena cavae entered the RA and traveled via a PFO or ASD to the LA, where it mixed with pulmonary venous blood. From there it flowed via the mitral valve into the left ventricle (LV). It then traveled either via a small VSD to the RV or was ejected via the aorta. The majority of PBF was initially provided via the PDA. Ductal patency was maintained with a prostaglandin (PGE_1) infusion in the neonatal period until a modified Blalock–Taussig (mBT) shunt was placed surgically to provide PBF.

What cardiac surgical procedures do patients with TA undergo?

In tricuspid atresia the RV is often hypoplastic, leaving the LV as the systemic ventricle. Since the left ventricular outflow tract is normal in TA, a traditional Norwood procedure including aortic reconstruction is not necessary as it would be for a patient with hypoplastic left heart syndrome. A stable source of PBF is required, and thus the

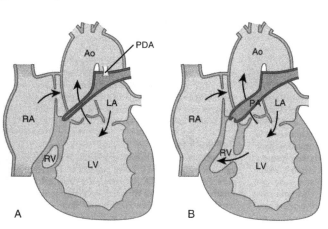
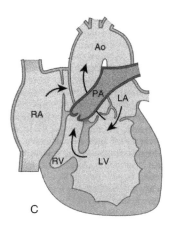

Figure 28.2 Anatomy and blood flow in tricuspid atresia Type I. Type 1A: Pulmonary atresia with pulmonary blood flow via patent ductus arteriosus or major aortopulmonary collateral arteries (MAPCAs). Type 1B: Small ventricular septal defect and pulmonary stenosis. Type 1C: Large ventricular septal defect and no pulmonary stenosis. From DiNardo J. A., Shukla A. C., and McGowan, F. X., Jr. Anesthesia for congenital heart surgery. In Davis P. J. and Cladis F. P., eds. *Smith's Anesthesia for Infants and Children*, 9th ed. Elsevier; 2017: 635–98. With permission.

first surgery for these patients is generally a systemic-to-pulmonary artery or mBT shunt.

Initial palliation with an mBT shunt allows the infant to grow while pulmonary vascular resistance (PVR) falls in the months following birth. Ultimately the pulmonary and systemic circulations are separated using two-staged operations for single-ventricle palliation. The first, performed at 3–6 months of age, is a hemi-Fontan or a bidirectional Glenn (BDG) procedure, which connects the superior vena cava (SVC) to the pulmonary artery, taking the place of the mBT shunt. Venous return from the SVC will now flow directly to the pulmonary circulation while venous return from the inferior vena cava (IVC) continues to mix with oxygenated pulmonary venous return in the atrium. At age 2–4 years this is followed by the Fontan procedure, which completes the separation of the pulmonary and systemic circulations by baffling IVC blood directly into the pulmonary vascular bed. (See Chapters 27, 29, and 30 for details of single-ventricle staged palliative procedures.)

What is the Fontan operation?

The Fontan operation completes the separation of the pulmonary and systemic circulations in a patient with single-ventricle physiology. Usually performed at 2–4 years of age, the Fontan procedure connects IVC blood directly to the pulmonary arteries or to the previously created superior cavopulmonary anastomosis (SCPA), allowing all systemic venous blood to flow directly to the lungs. The single ventricle (for patients with TA, the LV) then pumps oxygenated blood systemically. In addition to providing better systemic oxygenation (usual $SpO_2 > 90\%$), the Fontan procedure also reduces volume loading of the systemic ventricle and reduces the risk of paradoxical embolism.

There have been several modifications to the original Fontan procedure and currently the connection between the vena cavae is established either via placement of an extracardiac conduit (**extracardiac Fontan**) or an intraatrial baffle (**lateral tunnel Fontan**; see Figure 28.3). A communication or fenestration may be created between the Fontan conduit or baffle and the common atrium. This serves as a "pop-off" during times of high PVR, allowing right-to-left shunting to occur, augmenting ventricular filling and maintaining cardiac output, albeit at the cost of desaturation.

Clinical Pearl

A communication or fenestration may be made between the Fontan conduit or baffle and the common atrium. This serves as a "pop-off" during times of high PVR, allowing right-to-left shunting to occur, augmenting ventricular filling and maintaining cardiac output, albeit at the cost of desaturation.

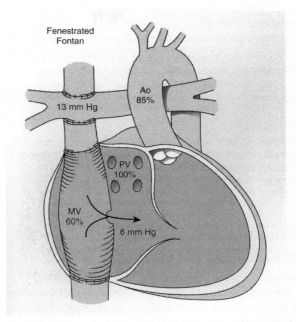

Figure 28.3 Lateral tunnel Fontan with patent fenestration. Ao, Aortic saturation; MV, mixed venous saturation; PV, pulmonary vein saturation. From B. D. Kussman, A. J. Powell, and F. X. McGowan Jr. Congenital cardiac anesthesia nonbypass procedures. In Davis P. J. and Cladis F. P., eds. *Smith's Anesthesia for Infants and Children*, 9th ed. Elsevier; 2017: 699–743. With permission.

What are the major determinants of the Fontan circulation?

The **transpulmonary gradient** (TPG) may be defined as the pressure difference between the systemic venous system and the common atrial pressure. After Fontan completion, the TPG across the Fontan pathway is the driving force to maintain blood flow through the pulmonary vasculature to maintain adequate oxygenation and cardiac output.

Important determinants of the function of the Fontan circulation include the following:

- Systemic ventricular function
- Atrioventricular valve competency
- Cardiac rhythm
- Systemic venous pressure and volume status
- Pulmonary vascular pressure and resistance

Alterations in any of these factors, alone or in combination, may compromise systemic cardiac output. One of the key features of a Fontan circulation is the higher central venous pressure (CVP), usually 10–14 mm Hg, required to maintain the pulmonary circulation and cardiac output.

Survival has significantly improved in patients with a Fontan circulation over the past two decades; a recently published study demonstrated a 26-year survival rate of

89% in patients with a lateral tunnel Fontan [1]. This success has created a growing population of children and adults with single-ventricle physiology who may require additional surgical procedures to address other comorbid conditions, including spine surgeries.

> **Clinical Pearl**
>
> *The transpulmonary gradient is defined as the pressure difference between the central venous system (PA pressure) and the common atrial pressure. Patients with Fontan circulation have higher CVPs (10–14 mm Hg) which are required to maintain pulmonary circulation and cardiac output.*

What is scoliosis and what are the different types and incidence of scoliosis in children?

Scoliosis is defined as a lateral curvature of the spine >10° on an anterior–posterior standing radiograph. The location of the scoliotic curve varies and can be thoracic, lumbar, or thoracolumbar. Scoliosis is classified as idiopathic, congenital, or neuromuscular, based on the etiologies.

Idiopathic scoliosis is the most common subtype. However, multiple studies have reported the incidence of scoliosis in patients with CHD and a history of cardiothoracic surgery to be higher, and a prevalence of 9.8% has been reported in patients with Fontan circulation [2, 3]. Congenital scoliosis arises as a result of congenital malformations of the spine. Neuromuscular scoliosis occurs due to neurologic or muscular disorders. These patients, who often have impaired respiratory and cardiac function, are more clinically complex than patients with idiopathic scoliosis due to their neurologic disease.

How is the severity of scoliosis measured and what are the surgical treatment options?

The Cobb angle, a measurement of the degree of side-to-side spinal curvature, is used to define the severity of the scoliosis and determine the appropriate treatment. Spinal fusion is recommended for patients with a Cobb angle above 45–50 degrees at mature skeletal growth to decrease the curve progression and ongoing impairment of pulmonary function.

Early onset of congenital scoliosis, and some types of neuromuscular scoliosis, can cause significant adverse effects on lung development, predisposing these patients to impaired gas exchange and pulmonary hypertension. In these patients the use of growing rods or vertical expandable prosthetic titanium ribs provides the option to correct spine and chest wall abnormalities while allowing the spine to continue to grow.

Anesthetic Implications

How should this patient be assessed preoperatively?

Preoperatively, the anesthesiologist should focus on past medical history, changes in recent health status, exercise capacity, pulmonary function, and current medications. Any history of changes in recent health or exercise capacity in Fontan patients warrant additional investigation.

A recent visit with pediatric cardiology is essential, and electrocardiogram, echocardiogram, cardiac catheterization, and/or cardiac magnetic resonance imaging findings should be reviewed. Important considerations include the evaluation and review of cardiac anatomy, single-ventricle function, Fontan pathway, transpulmonary gradient, the status of the fenestration (open vs. closed), and baseline oxygen saturation. For patients with severe scoliosis, pulmonary function testing is often helpful to guide intraoperative and postoperative ventilatory management. A preoperative consultation with a pediatric electrophysiologist is recommended for patients who have a history of arrhythmias or a pacemaker.

The physical examination should encompass the airway, heart and lungs, overall perfusion, and evaluation for potential difficulties with vascular access. The physical examination of a well-functioning Fontan patient should be notable for a baseline $SpO_2 > 90$. It is also important to document preoperative neurologic function due to the risk of perioperative neurologic complications.

Laboratory tests should include a complete blood count (including platelet count), basic metabolic panel, liver panel, and coagulation profile. Normal results are anticipated in well compensated Fontan patients who are not on anticoagulant medications.

> **Clinical Pearl**
>
> *Important considerations include the evaluation and review of cardiac anatomy, single-ventricle function, Fontan pathway, transpulmonary gradient, fenestration status, and baseline oxygen saturation. Normal laboratory results are anticipated in well compensated Fontan patients who are not on anticoagulant medications.*

Is multidisciplinary preoperative collaboration important for this patient?

Due to the complex perioperative management considerations involved in patients with Fontan physiology who are undergoing a major surgery such as a PSF, close collaboration among pediatric orthopedists, cardiologists, neurophysiologists, anesthesiologists, and postoperative intensivists is essential. Pediatric cardiologists can clarify specific issues regarding the anatomy and physiology of the Fontan patient, as well as consult and assist postoperatively in medical management. Pediatric orthopedic surgeons should be involved in discussions about potential intraoperative blood loss, which can be higher than normally anticipated due to the higher CVPs and coagulation issues that exist in Fontan patients. The need to optimize blood pressure to minimize surgical blood loss must be balanced with maintaining adequate cardiac output, and this should also be discussed with the surgeons. The surgeons may opt to minimize operative time and choose a moderate curve correction.

Neurophysiology specialists should be involved in preoperative discussions regarding the effects of anesthetic medications on neuromonitoring, as well as plans to treat potential decreases or loss of neuromonitoring signals, including the necessity for an intraoperative wake-up test. It is important to rehearse the potential intraoperative wake-up test with the patient during the preoperative visit to psychologically prepare the patient and family.

What medications are generally taken by patients with Fontan physiology and how should they be managed perioperatively?

Acetylsalicylic acid (ASA), warfarin and angiotensin converting enzyme inhibitors (ACEi) are the most commonly administered medications in patients with well-compensated Fontan physiology.

Most patients receive ASA or warfarin for chronic thrombotic prophylaxis. Cardiologists recommend stopping ASA or warfarin 5–7 days before the surgery to facilitate a normally functioning coagulation system. For individuals who are advised to continue ASA preoperatively, the surgeon and anesthesiologist should be made aware of this due to the potential effects on platelet function. Appropriate blood products should be prepared preoperatively.

Angiotensin converting enzyme inhibitors are used to reduce afterload and minimize strain on the single ventricle. However, with general anesthesia they may result in severe hypotension refractory to treatment with adrenergic agonists. It is recommended that the patient not take ACEi on the morning of surgery. Refractory intraoperative hypotension may be treated with intravenous vasopressin.

What premedication options exist for this patient?

A benzodiazepine may be administered either orally or intravenously for anxiolysis and should be well tolerated in a patient with Fontan physiology, but should probably be utilized judiciously and as a single agent. Heavy sedation or combinations of multiple sedative medications may cause hypoventilation and hypercarbia with subsequent increases in PVR, which is undesirable in patients with a Fontan circulation. In a teenager, the administration of oral midazolam prior to placement of a peripheral intravenous (IV) line may be helpful if the patient is excessively anxious.

Acetaminophen (10–15 mg/kg, maximal dose of 1 g) may be administered orally in the preoperative area. Gabapentin, an anticonvulsant medication used to treat partial seizures and neuropathic and perioperative pain, may also be used as an adjunct for perioperative pain control in a dosage of 10 mg/kg administered orally.

What considerations exist for anesthetic induction?

Although either inhalational or IV techniques can be safely used for anesthetic induction in a well-compensated Fontan patient, ideally IV medications with minimal cardiac depressive effects (etomidate, ketamine, midazolam, and/or opioids) should be used for patients with Fontan physiology. Although propofol may be used, in larger doses it may cause myocardial depression, afterload reduction and venous dilation which may not be well tolerated by these patients. If propofol is used, it is imperative to titrate to effect with careful monitoring during induction. When IV access is not obtained preoperatively, careful titration of sevoflurane is commonly used for anesthetic induction. A fentanyl bolus given IV before intubation can blunt the increase in PVR associated with laryngoscopy and endotracheal tube placement. Either a short-acting neuromuscular blocking agent or rocuronium, an agent that can be reversed by sugammadex prior to initiating neuromonitoring, should be administered to facilitate intubation. The anesthesiologist should carefully plan the induction, choosing the approach most likely to maintain hemodynamic stability in this patient with unique physiology and limited cardiac reserve.

Clinical Pearl

Either intravenous or inhalational agents can be safely used for induction in a well-compensated Fontan patient. Induction agents and techniques should not cause increases in PVR or depression of the systemic ventricle, and preload should be optimized prior to anesthetic induction.

How should intraoperative fluids be managed?

Adequate preload is essential to maintain normal cardiac output and compensate for possible peripheral vasodilatation during induction. A patient with Fontan physiology should avoid excessive preoperative fasting and should be encouraged to drink clear liquids up to 2 hours before surgery. Fluids should be administered as soon as IV access is established, if possible before induction of anesthesia. A crystalloid bolus of 5–10 mL/kg before or during induction may be given to maintain hemodynamic stability. Intraoperative fluid management should be guided by patient's hemodynamics, fasting time, blood and third space fluid loss, urine output, and laboratory measurements. It is crucial to have adequate IV access with at least two large-bore peripheral IV lines, as rapid fluid or blood administration is often necessary during this surgery. It is important to remember that the maintenance of adequate CVP is critical for providing PBF, and that hypovolemia is poorly tolerated. Meticulous attention to removal of bubbles from IV lines is absolutely necessary as Fontan patients may have an open atrial fenestration or other arterial-venous connections that put them at risk for systemic embolism of air.

Clinical Pearl

Meticulous removal of bubbles from IV lines when administering medications is absolutely necessary as Fontan patients may have an open atrial fenestration or other arterial-venous connections that put them at risk for systemic embolism of any air.

What are the effects of spontaneous versus mechanical ventilation in a patient with a Fontan circulation?

During most uncomplicated surgeries spontaneous ventilation is preferentially used whenever possible in Fontan patients. Negative intrathoracic pressure during inspiration enhances venous return and hemodynamic performance. Mechanical positive pressure ventilation (PPV) can lead to less favorable hemodynamics due to increased intrathoracic pressure leading to decreased central venous return. However, during a spinal fusion, when the patient is prone for several hours, spontaneous ventilation is not possible. Hypoventilation with associated hypercarbia, hypoxia, and atelectasis, all of which can lead to increased PVR, should be avoided in patients with Fontan physiology. Mechanical ventilation with maintenance of low mean airway pressures and normocarbia should be the goal.

Tidal volumes of 6–8 mL/kg along with physiologic use of positive end-expiratory pressure (PEEP) is generally appropriate.

Clinical Pearl

Mechanical ventilation with maintenance of low mean airway pressures and normocarbia should be the goal. Tidal volumes of 6–8 mL/kg along with physiologic use of PEEP is generally appropriate.

What routine monitoring is utilized for patients undergoing PSF?

Constant vigilance to hemodynamics, respiratory mechanics, and the surgical field to rapidly identify and treat derangements during spinal surgery is essential, particularly in a single-ventricle patient. Potential difficulties include significant blood loss with hemodynamic derangements, fluid shifts, and neurologic injury. In addition to standard American Society of Anesthesiologists recommended monitors, an arterial line, urinary catheter, and neuromonitoring should be used. Neuromonitoring may include somatosensory-evoked potential (SSEP), transcranial motor-evoked potentials (TcMEPs), and electromyography (EMG). Somatosensory-evoked potentials monitor the somatosensory pathway and TcMEPs monitor the corticospinal tract or motor activity. A decrease in amplitude of 50% and increase in latency of >10% in SSEPs are considered significant changes that may require anesthetic or surgical intervention. Many anesthetic medications, including both IV and inhalational agents, prolong latency or reduce amplitude at varying doses. Electromyography is used to evaluate spinal nerve root injury and is frequently used during pedicle screw placement. Both EMG and TcMEPs are inaccurate with the use of neuromuscular blocking agents, so these should be avoided except during induction. Preferences for anesthetic management should be discussed with the neuromonitoring team in advance, particularly as institutional preferences may vary slightly. In general, a balanced anesthetic or total intravenous anesthetic technique is preferred.

Is there a need for additional monitoring?

Intraoperative CVP monitoring, transesophageal echocardiography (TEE) and near-infrared spectroscopy may be utilized as well for optimal hemodynamic monitoring, depending on the status of the patient.

While a CVP line may not always be utilized for a PSF in a healthy two-ventricle patient with idiopathic scoliosis, it is advisable to place a CVP line in patients with Fontan physiology undergoing PSF. The ability to follow CVP trends is not only useful for guiding volume and blood replacement therapy but can also be helpful for administration of vasoactive drugs if necessary. Central venous pressure increases when a patient is prone due to IVC compression, decreased cardiac compliance, and an increase in intrathoracic pressure, with one study showing an average increase in CVP when prone of 9 mm Hg [4]. The CVP in a patient with Fontan physiology may need to be in the high teens or low 20s to provide adequate cardiac output in the prone position. It is critical to monitor CVP trends, especially once the patient has been turned prone.

Although CVP monitoring can provide valuable information, it is not without risks. It should be noted that the CVP in a Fontan patient actually reflects mean pulmonary artery pressure, since the SVC and IVC are directly connected to the pulmonary arteries. Placement of a central venous catheter can result in pulmonary artery injury, paradoxical air emboli, Fontan pathway thrombus, and central line associated blood stream infection. The length of central venous line in the internal jugular vein must be carefully assessed. To reduce complication risks the CVP catheter should be removed postoperatively as soon as hemodynamics are stabilized. Alternatively, TEE is an excellent tool for intraoperative monitoring of ventricular function, ventricular preload, the Fontan pathway, any cardiac shunting (baffle leak or fenestration), and venous air embolism, but its use often depends on the availability of a pediatric cardiologist to perform and interpret the TEE. Near-infrared spectroscopy may be a useful tool to monitor cardiac output, cerebral perfusion, and tissue oxygenation in Fontan patients, especially when CVP is elevated due to prone positioning during posterior spinal fusion [5].

It is important to know whether the patient had a previous mBT shunt, and if so, where it was located (right or left side; right-sided mBT shunt being most common). A noninvasive blood pressure cuff or an arterial catheter placed on or in the ipsilateral side where the previous mBT shunt existed may measure falsely low systemic blood pressure due to vessel stenosis near the shunt take-down. If there is no alternative but to use the arm on the ipsilateral side of the previous mBT shunt, the blood pressure in that arm should first be verified to be the same as in other extremities.

Clinical Pearl

Central venous pressure in a patient with Fontan circulation may need to be in the high teens or low 20s to provide adequate cardiac output in the prone position. It is critical to monitor the CVP trends, especially when the patient is turned prone. It should be noted that the CVP in a Fontan patient reflects mean pulmonary artery pressure as the SVC and IVC are directly connected to the pulmonary arteries.

What are the general anesthetic principles for managing a patient with Fontan physiology for noncardiac surgery?

Guiding principles include maximizing preload, minimizing myocardial depression caused by medications and/or inhalational agents, maintaining sinus rhythm, and avoiding increases in PVR which can be caused by hypoxia, hypercarbia, acidosis, high peak inspiratory pressures with mechanical ventilation, and poorly controlled pain or surgical stimulation.

How should temperature be managed intraoperatively for this patient?

It is challenging to keep a PSF patient normothermic during surgery, but intraoperative hypothermia can lead to increases in PVR and decreases in cardiac output which are particularly detrimental to a Fontan patient. Lower temperatures shift the oxyhemoglobin dissociation curve to the left, reducing oxygen availability to the tissues. Therefore, active warming should begin during induction of anesthesia. There is potential for the patient to lose significant heat, particularly during prone positioning and in the time before surgical incision. An underbody convection warmer may be used under the patient in the preoperative area and turned on during induction. Core temperature should be monitored during the surgery using a nasal, esophageal, or bladder temperature probe.

What issues are associated with surgery in the prone position in a Fontan patient?

Prone positioning during anesthesia can elicit a variety of respiratory and cardiovascular responses. There may be a decrease in cardiac index and ventricular compliance, varying degrees of increased pressure in the IVC, and increased peak airway pressures (dependent on the type of operating frame used) when patients are in the prone position [6]. While these changes may be tolerated in otherwise healthy patients they often present challenges in patients with Fontan physiology.

Extensive padding is necessary to prevent a wide spectrum of compression and stretch injuries as well as to keep the abdomen free from impeding ventilation. In Fontan patients, it is of particular importance to ensure free diaphragmatic movement as increases in intraabdominal pressure may impair ventilation and cause IVC compression. In turn this can result in a decrease in systemic venous return to the Fontan circuit and a reduction in preload to the systemic ventricle. Impaired ventilation can lead to increases in PVR and further elevations in systemic venous

213

pressure, and then, as a consequence, increases in epidural venous pressure and intraoperative bleeding. Careful positioning is essential to minimize these risks. A Jackson table with abdominal free 4-point pads has the least effect on cardiac performance and if available should be considered for patients with Fontan physiology.

Clinical Pearl

Care should be taken during positioning to ensure that lung excursion is unimpeded and padding of pressure points is optimal. Increases in intraabdominal pressure may impair ventilation, cause IVC compression, and decrease preload and cardiac output. Increased intraabdominal pressure may also further elevate systemic venous pressure, which may in turn increase epidural venous pressure and intraoperative bleeding.

What is the differential diagnosis and treatment for intraoperative hypoxemia in this patient?

The differential diagnosis for acute oxygen desaturation in a Fontan patient includes the common airway-related causes such as accidental extubation during prone positioning, endobronchial intubation, bronchospasm, endotracheal obstruction, and atelectasis. Additionally, in a Fontan patient, an acute elevation of PVR causing right-to-left shunting across a fenestration or baffle leak should be considered. Intraoperative TEE is a valuable tool to assist in this clinical diagnosis and guide treatment. Techniques to decrease PVR and improve oxygenation include optimizing mechanical ventilation (increasing FiO_2, correcting hypercarbia, and avoiding excessive positive pressure), correcting hypothermia and acidosis, and administering phosphodiesterase inhibitors such as milrinone and/or utilizing inhaled nitric oxide.

What techniques can be used to minimize intraoperative blood loss and use of allogeneic transfusion in this patient?

Intraoperative bleeding during PSF is primarily venous, with the average blood loss in the range of 800–1200 mL for children and adolescents with idiopathic scoliosis. Children with Fontan physiology may have significantly higher intraoperative blood loss, which may be in excess of an entire blood volume [7, 8].

Techniques to minimize intraoperative blood loss and allogeneic transfusion in patients having a PSF include preoperative or intraoperative autologous blood donation, appropriate prone positioning, an appropriate operating table, intraoperative blood salvage, controlled hypotension,

and use of intravenous antifibrinolytic agents (ε-aminocaproic acid or tranexamic acid). Due to the higher baseline CVP required to maintain the Fontan circulation and diminished cardiac functional reserve, controlled hypotension is not recommended in single-ventricle patients. Goals include keeping hematocrit ≥30% and mean arterial pressure ≥60–65 mm Hg.

Clinical Pearl

Keep hematocrit ≥30% and mean arterial pressure ≥60–65 mm Hg. Controlled hypotension is not recommended in single-ventricle patients.

The surgeon reports profuse oozing in the surgical field. The patient's current blood pressure is 79/40 mm Hg (mean 48), with a CVP trending from 20 to 16 mm Hg. What are the differential diagnoses and potential therapies?

This clinical presentation strongly suggests intravascular volume depletion which is a common scenario in a Fontan patient having a PSF. Sequential arterial blood gases (ABGs) with hematocrit should be obtained to provide information to help confirm the diagnosis and guide appropriate therapy and fluid management. Posterior spinal fusion in Fontan patients is associated with major intraoperative blood loss with means of 64–84 mL/kg or higher [7]. Appropriate volume replacement given expeditiously to maintain adequate preload and cardiac output is absolutely fundamental. Balanced salt solutions, followed by 5% albumin, are suitable to replace blood loss initially. The transfusion threshold is lower in patients with Fontan physiology and it is recommended to keep the hematocrit ≥30 [5, 7]. In addition to transfusing autologous blood and blood from intraoperative cell savage, allogeneic whole blood or packed red blood cells are commonly used to replace intraoperative volume depletion caused by surgical bleeding. Other blood products such as fresh frozen plasma, platelets, and cryoprecipitate are also frequently needed, guided by intraoperative coagulation testing, including rotational thromboelastometry or thromboelastography. Massive intraoperative bleeding may require use of a rapid transfusion system and/or activation of the massive transfusion protocol.

Diminished ventricular function may also be a cause of hypotension, especially if anesthetics with cardiac depressant effects are used. Ventricular function and cardiac filling can be evaluated by CVP trends and TEE. The dynamic visualization of cardiac function and venous return by TEE is more helpful than CVP monitoring [9]. If cardiac function is compromised, the use of inotropic medications should be considered. Drugs such as the phosphodiesterase inhibitor milrinone can be used to improve both systolic and diastolic function without increasing PVR. Catecholamine inotropic agents, which improve systolic function, may worsen diastolic function by impairing ventricular relaxation. However, epinephrine in low doses (0.02–0.04 mcg/kg/minute) can be considered for refractory hypotension.

Cardiac arrhythmias are not uncommon in patients with a Fontan circulation. The onset of atrial tachycardia may produce hemodynamic compromise and necessitate antiarrhythmic therapy immediately, including direct current cardioversion. Should this occur the electrophysiology team should be contacted immediately. Defibrillator pads should be placed on the patient before incision.

Clinical Pearl

Massive intraoperative bleeding may require the use of a rapid transfusion system and activation of the massive transfusion protocol. If cardiac function is compromised, the phosphodiesterase inhibitor milrinone should be considered. Epinephrine in low doses (0.02–0.04 mcg/kg/minute) should be considered for refractory hypotension, assuming hypotension is not secondary to hypovolemia.

How should a sudden change in SSEPs be managed in this patient?

It is important to have a plan should sudden changes in neuromonitoring occur to prevent new-onset neurological deficits. When neuromonitoring signals are changed or lost, anesthetic techniques which could compromise oxygen delivery should be adjusted or corrected immediately. This may include transfusing blood to increase the hematocrit and raising the mean arterial blood pressure to optimize tissue perfusion and increase oxygen delivery to the spinal cord. An ABG should be measured in order to correct metabolic acidosis and adjust the partial pressure of carbon dioxide to help improve oxygen supply to the spinal cord. Also, medications administered just prior to the signal changes should be considered as a potential cause for the signal changes.

At a time of potential neurologic compromise it is critical for the entire patient care team to communicate and collaborate to lessen the risk of neurologic damage. Neuromonitoring specialists should recheck the signals, electrodes, and connections to determine the pattern and timing of signal changes. The surgeon should review the surgical steps that occurred prior the signal changes and consider adjusting the distraction, removing rods and screws, and using intraoperative imaging to evaluate and prevent the possibility of spinal cord compression or ischemia.

Although neuromonitoring can be helpful to prevent permanent spinal cord damage, an intraoperative wake-up test may be needed to make a formal diagnosis and conclusively rule out permanent neurologic damage. Ideally a wake-up test should have been carefully planned, discussed, and rehearsed with the patient before the surgery. Still, it can be associated with severe complications. A Fontan patient with a pacemaker was reported to have suffered ventricular tachycardia during a wake-up test that necessitated intraoperative CPR for resuscitation [10]. Continuous dexmedetomidine, a highly selective α_2-adrenergic receptor agonist, along with an amnestic such as midazolam, may provide adequate sedation for the patient during the wake-up test.

What perioperative analgesic plans could be suggested for this patient?

Inadequate pain control may cause anxiety, hypertension, and increases in SVR and PVR and should be avoided. However, pain relief with heavy sedative effects should also be avoided due to potential risks of hypoventilation, hypoxia, and hypercarbia.

Multimodal pain control combining opioids and a variety of nonopioid medications is optimal in patients with Fontan physiology. Opioids can be given orally, intravenously and via the epidural space. Medications such as acetaminophen, nonsteroidal antiinflammatory drugs (NSAIDs), gabapentin, ketamine, and methadone may be administered as adjuncts for pain control perioperatively.

Epidural analgesia with local anesthetics and opioid infusion has been used successfully in Fontan patients but the use of ongoing anticoagulant therapies in many Fontan patients may preclude or limit the use of epidural or other regional analgesia techniques. If utilized, local anesthetic dosing, with lidocaine or bupivacaine, should be titrated and monitored carefully to minimize sympatholytic effects and to facilitate postoperative neurologic examinations. Augmenting preload with IV fluids before epidural dosing is prudent. Patient-controlled analgesia is another option.

Intrathecal morphine (6 mcg/kg, maximal 600 mcg for patients receiving gabapentin and 8 mcg/kg, maximal 800 mcg for patients without gabapentin) administered by the anesthesiologist after induction, before incision, may also be utilized. The patient could also receive oral gabapentin preoperatively, IV acetaminophen intraoperatively and in the first 24 hours postoperatively, followed by oral opioids and NSAIDs during the next 2–3 days.

What is an appropriate plan for extubation in this patient?

Extubation in the operating room at the end of the surgery is optimal for a patient with Fontan physiology, assuming an uneventful intraoperative course. The shift from mechanical to spontaneous ventilation should improve hemodynamics and decrease the risks of ventilator-associated sedation. An awake patient can facilitate accurate postoperative neurologic exams as well. When a Fontan patient has other severe comorbidities such as severe restrictive lung disease or unstable hemodynamics, delayed extubation may be necessary, and appropriate pain management and sedation strategies should be utilized. Hypertension associated with inadequate pain control may add extra strain to the systemic ventricle and should be avoided. Intravenous midazolam and opioids are commonly used medications for postoperative pain control and sedation. Additionally, dexmedetomidine has been shown be an excellent sedative in the intensive care unit.

What are the possible postoperative complications in patients with Fontan physiology undergoing PSF?

Postoperative complications can be severe in these patients and can include continuous bleeding with hypotension requiring vasoactive medications, prolonged intubation, acute renal dysfunction, pleural effusions, Horner syndrome, superior mesenteric artery syndrome, and delayed neurologic damage [7, 8, 10]. Postoperative bleeding may be significant and death has been reported due to hypovolemic shock and dysrhythmias which started during surgery and continued in the immediate postoperative period [8]. This emphasizes the need for continuous close monitoring with early intervention or resuscitation of Fontan patients in the immediate postoperative period either in a pediatric intensive care unit or a cardiac intensive care unit.

As Fontan patients are at risk for thromboembolic events, cardiologists often recommend continuation of anticoagulation therapies, particularly ASA or low-molecular-weight heparin throughout the perioperative period. Pneumatic compression boots for deep vein thrombosis prophylaxis are also important, especially in the immediate postoperative period for patients with limited ambulation.

References

1. C. Schilling, K. Dalsiel, R. Nunn, et al. The Fontan epidemic: population projections from Australia and New Zealand Fontan registry. *Int J Cardiol* 2016; **219**: 14–19.

2. J. A. Herrera Soto, K. L. Vander Hare, P. Barry-Lane, et al. Retrospective study on the development of spinal deformities following sternotomy for congenital heart disease. *Spine* 2007; **32**: 1998–2004.

3. M. Kadhim, C. Pizarro, L. Holmes, et al. Prevalence of scoliosis in patients with Fontan circulation. *Arch Dis Child* 2013; **98**: 170–5.

4. D. E. Soliman, A. D. Maslow, P. M. Bokesch, et al. Transesophageal echocardiography during scoliosis repair: comparison with CVP monitoring. *Can J Anaesth* 1998; **45**: 925–32.

5. C. Walker, D. Martin, J. Klamar, et al. Perioperative management of a patient with Fontan physiology for posterior spinal fusion. *J Med Cases* 2014; **5**: 392–6.

6. Z. E. Brown, M. Görges, E. Cooke, et al. Changes in cardiac index and blood pressure on positioning children prone for scoliosis surgery. *Anaesthesia* 2013; **68**: 742–6.

7. M. B. Rafique, E. A. Stuth, J. C. Tassone. Increased blood loss during posterior spinal fusion for idiopathic scoliosis in an adolescent with Fontan physiology. *Pediatr Anesth* 2006; **16**: 206–12.

8. C. P. C. Macarrón, E. S. Ruiz, J. B. Flores, et al. Spinal surgery in the univentricular heart – is it viable? *Cardiol Young* 2014; **24**: 73–8.

9. D. Vischoff, L. P. Fortier, E. Villeneuve, et al. Anaesthetic management of an adolescent for scoliosis surgery with a Fontan circulation. *Paediatr Anaesth* 2001; **11**: 607–10.

10. C. I. Leichtle, M. Kumpf, M. Gass, et al. Surgical correction of scoliosis in children with congenital heart failure (Fontan circulation): case report and literature review. *Eur Spine J* 2008; **17**: 312–17.

Suggested Reading

Edgcombe H., Carter K., and Yarrow S. Anaesthesia in the prone position. *Br J Anaesth* 2008; **100**: 165–83.

Kadhim M., Pizarro C., Holmes L., et al. Prevalence of scoliosis in patients with Fontan circulation. *Arch Dis Child* 2013; **98**: 170–5.

Macarrón C. P. C., Ruiz E. S., Flores J. B., et al. Spinal surgery in the univentricular heart – is it viable? *Cardiol Young* 2014; **24**: 73–8.

Walker C., Martin D., Klamar J., et al. Perioperative management of a patient with Fontan physiology for posterior spinal fusion. *J Med Cases* 2014; **5**: 392–6.

Extracardiac Fontan

Chinwe Unegbu and Nina Deutsch

Case Scenario

A 15-year-old teenager presents for excision of a lipoma on her back. She was born with complex single-ventricle anatomy consisting of dextro-transposition of the great arteries, pulmonary atresia, and a hypoplastic left ventricle. As a neonate, she underwent placement of a modified Blalock–Taussig shunt. Subsequently, she had a bidirectional Glenn procedure at 6 months of age, followed by an extracardiac Fontan procedure at 2 years of age. She has been doing well at home and her cardiologist has been seeing her every 6 months. She reports some difficulty keeping up with her peers in gym class but no significant change over the past several years. Her current medications are aspirin and enalapril. Vital signs are heart rate 84 beats/minute, respiratory rate 18 breaths/minute, and SpO$_2$ 95% on room air. Hemoglobin is 15 g/dL and all other laboratory values are within normal limits.

Echocardiography reveals:

- *Mildly depressed right ventricular function*
- *Mild tricuspid regurgitation*

Key Objectives

- Describe this patient's complex single-ventricle anatomy.
- Review the palliative surgeries that culminate in Fontan physiology.
- Describe the preoperative assessment of a patient with Fontan physiology.
- Review the intraoperative monitoring and management goals for a patient with Fontan physiology.
- Discuss postoperative disposition in patients with Fontan physiology having noncardiac surgery.

Pathophysiology

How can this patient's cardiac anatomy at birth be described?

The patient's cardiac anatomy and underlying physiology must be considered based on the two primary cardiac

lesions: dextro (d)-transposition of the great arteries (d-TGA) and the hypoplastic left ventricle (LV).

- In d-TGA, a normal relationship exists between the heart's atrial and ventricular connections (*atrioventricular concordance*) but the ventricles and great arteries are incorrectly connected (*ventriculoarterial discordance*). (See Chapter 21.) Blood from the superior and inferior vena cavae (IVC) enters the right atrium (RA), passes through the tricuspid valve into the right ventricle (RV), and then into a right-sided and anterior aorta. On the other side of the heart, the left atrium (LA) connects to the LV via the mitral valve. From there, blood passes into the left-sided, posterior pulmonary artery.

  ○ With d-TGA blood flow in the pulmonary and systemic circulations exists in parallel (deoxygenated blood incorrectly flows to the systemic circulation and oxygenated blood returns to the pulmonary circulation, which is incompatible with life) rather than in series as normally occurs.

  ○ For the infant to survive after birth, a connection between the two circulations, such as a patent foramen ovale, atrial septal defect (ASD) or ventricular septal defect, must be present to allow for mixing and delivery of oxygenated blood to the rest of the body.

  ○ If an inadequate atrial connection is present, an urgent balloon atrial septostomy must be performed to create an ASD. This is typically performed either in the intensive care unit (ICU) with ultrasound guidance or in the cardiac catheterization lab with fluoroscopy. The femoral vein is accessed and a balloon-tipped catheter is passed into the RA, across the foramen ovale, and into the LA. With the balloon inflated, the catheter is then forcefully withdrawn back into the RA, thereby increasing the size of the atrial septal connection and allowing for improved mixing of atrial blood.

- This patient was also born with pulmonary atresia and a hypoplastic LV, which means that the main pulmonary artery and the LV were underdeveloped. Pulmonary atresia anatomy varies and can range from a fused trileaflet valve to a long segment of atresia, with all variations causing complete pulmonary outflow tract obstruction requiring an alternate source of pulmonary blood flow (PBF), which in this case was the patent ductus arteriosus (PDA). The PDA supplied blood to the pulmonary arteries from the aorta. Generally a prostaglandin (PGE₁) infusion is required to maintain patency of the PDA until a surgical source of blood flow (such as a modified Blalock–Taussig [mBT] shunt) can be created. Hypoplasia of the LV means that the LV cannot support cardiac output (CO) and the patient therefore will require single-ventricle palliation. Because of the transposition, the aorta originated from the RV, the only functional ventricle for this infant.

What was the first step in cardiac surgical palliation for this patient?

During the neonatal period, this patient required an mBT shunt, an artificial tube graft sewn between the subclavian or innominate artery and the pulmonary artery in order to supply blood flow to the pulmonary arteries. The patient's PDA was then ligated. This procedure may or may not require cardiopulmonary bypass (CPB) depending on individual patient factors. Because the aorta was of normal size, this patient did not require a Norwood procedure (which would have included aortic reconstruction) for her first surgery; she required only an mBT shunt to provide PBF.

Clinical Pearl

Because her aorta was of normal size, this patient did not require a Norwood procedure which includes aortic reconstruction for her first surgery; she required only an mBT shunt to provide pulmonary blood flow.

What are the benefits of an mBT shunt and how does it affect pulmonary blood flow?

Anatomically, the mBT shunt is similar to the PDA in that it provides blood flow to the pulmonary arteries. Unlike a PDA, it provides a stable source of PBF that is not dependent on a prostaglandin infusion. The mBT shunt size is usually 3.5–4.0 mm, depending on patient size and the size of the shunt relative to the size of the aorta and pulmonary arteries. The length of the mBT shunt and the location of the arterial anastomosis (subclavian vs. innominate) also determines the amount of PBF provided. As pulmonary vascular resistance (PVR)

is lower than systemic vascular resistance (SVR), this promotes PBF through the mBT shunt while limiting pulmonary overcirculation. Ultimately, the goal is to have a balanced $Q_p:Q_s$ (clinically indicated by an oxygen saturation of 75%–85%) and to have flow to both pulmonary arteries allowing for symmetrical growth. (See Chapter 1 for $Q_p:Q_s$ discussion.)

The patient's arterial oxygen saturation is determined by the oxygen saturation of systemic venous blood returning to the RA (mixed venous saturation), the oxygen saturation of pulmonary venous blood entering the RA across the ASD, and the amount of flow returning to the heart from both of these circulations. If an adequate ASD is not present, it will be necessary to perform either a balloon atrial septostomy or an atrial septectomy to ensure adequate mixing of oxygenated and deoxygenated blood. Unlike a balloon atrial septostomy, an atrial septectomy requires the use of CPB.

Clinical Pearl

Factors determining the patient's arterial oxygen saturation include the saturation of systemic venous blood returning to the right atrium (mixed venous oxygenation), the saturation of pulmonary venous blood entering the right atrium across the ASD, and the amount of flow returning to the heart from both of these circulations.

What monitoring concerns exist in patients who have had mBT shunts?

After the mBT shunt is taken down there can subsequently be distortion, stenosis, or aneurysmal dilation at the site of the proximal shunt insertion on the subclavian artery which could limit blood flow through the vessel. More rarely, the subclavian artery is sacrificed when the mBT shunt is taken down. Thrombosis of the artery is also possible. In each case, blood pressure measurements may not be accurate in the ipsilateral arm. Usually it is best to avoid the affected arm, but if it is necessary to use the ipsilateral arm for blood pressure measurements, comparison with measurements on other extremities is advised.

Clinical Pearl

In a patient with a history of an mBT shunt, blood pressure measurements may not be accurate on the affected side due to distortion, stenosis, or thrombosis of the subclavian vessel. This applies to both noninvasive and direct arterial blood pressure measurements.

What is a bidirectional Glenn procedure and what criteria must be met before proceeding with it?

The bidirectional Glenn is also known as a *superior cavopulmonary anastomosis* (SCPA) wherein the superior vena cava (SVC) is anastomosed to the pulmonary artery (PA); this is usually the second stage of single-ventricle palliation. (See Chapter 27.) This procedure is performed using CPB. To allow time for PVR to decrease from the higher levels seen in neonates, a BDG is usually not performed before 3 months of age. Low PVR is essential for the success of the BDG, as PBF will now be passively supplied via the SVC–PA anastomosis.

Once on CPB, the mBT shunt is taken down. The SVC is disconnected from the RA and reanastomosed to the right pulmonary artery so that all venous flow from the upper body, including cerebral and upper extremity drainage, bypasses the heart and passively drains directly into the pulmonary circulation. Because the pulmonary arteries are in continuity, both lungs are supplied with blood as it flows from the SVC into the right and left pulmonary artery, hence the term "bidirectional."

What are the expected oxygen saturations and hematocrit for patients following a BDG?

When the BDG is performed the previous mBT shunt is replaced with a new shunt: the SVC-to-PA anastomosis. Because deoxygenated blood from the IVC returns to the common atrium and mixes with oxygenated pulmonary venous return, the patient's oxygen saturations do not change significantly after the BDG and remain 75%–85%. This persistent cyanosis triggers a compensatory increase in red blood cell production and oxygen carrying capacity leading to expected hematocrits of 40%–45%.

What is the Fontan procedure?

The Fontan procedure, also known as a *total cavopulmonary anastomosis*, is the final palliative stage for patients with single-ventricle physiology. In this procedure IVC blood flow is baffled to the pulmonary arteries and therefore, given the previous BDG, all systemic venous blood return now bypasses the RA and flows directly into the pulmonary circulation.

In this era the Fontan procedure is most commonly performed using an extracardiac conduit that consists of a tubular GORE-TEX® graft directing IVC flow to the pulmonary arteries; thus all systemic venous return is now passively directed to the pulmonary circulation. Pulmonary blood flow then returns from the lungs to the

heart via the pulmonary veins, passes through the common atrium into the single RV, and (owing to the d-TGA) is pumped out of the aorta. The pulmonary and systemic circulations are now separated and a series circulation exists. Pulmonary blood flow depends on the pressure gradient between the central venous pressure (CVP) and the pressure in the common atrium, which is called the transpulmonary pressure or *transpulmonary gradient (TPG)*. This pressure difference allows blood flow to move through the lungs without the assistance of the pumping action of the heart. (See further details of single-ventricle palliative procedures in Chapters 26, 28, and 30.)

> **Clinical Pearl**
>
> *After a Fontan procedure PBF depends on the pressure gradient between the central venous pressure and the pressure in the atrium, which is called the transpulmonary gradient. This pressure difference allows blood flow to move through the lungs without the assistance of the pumping action of the heart.*

What surgical techniques can be used for the Fontan procedure?

Two main types of Fontan procedures are currently performed by surgeons, either the lateral tunnel or the extracardiac conduit, both of which result in similar physiology.

- The *lateral tunnel Fontan* is usually preceded by a hemi-Fontan procedure (HF) which is a modification of the BDG. The HF incorporates part of the RA into the connection between the SVC and the PA but is otherwise physiologically similar to a BDG. An advantage to the HF for the lateral tunnel Fontan sequence is that after the atrial anastomosis during the HF, creating the lateral tunnel baffle in the RA is often a more straightforward and shorter procedure than creating an extracardiac conduit. The lateral tunnel Fontan allows for direct placement of a fenestration allowing flow between the Fontan pathway and the common atrium. (See Chapter 28.)

- In an *extracardiac Fontan*, the RA is bypassed completely and all systemic venous flow (SVC and IVC) is directed to the pulmonary arteries. An advantage to the extracardiac Fontan is that since the atrium is not part of the connection and thus does not see significantly elevated central pressures, the incidence of atrial arrhythmias may be lower than observed with the lateral tunnel Fontan. Additionally, there is minimal suturing of atrial tissue in the

(a)

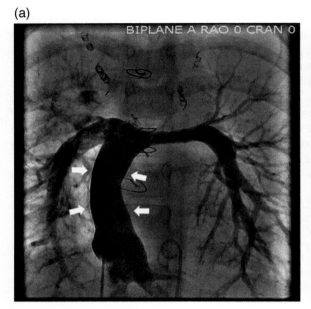

(b)

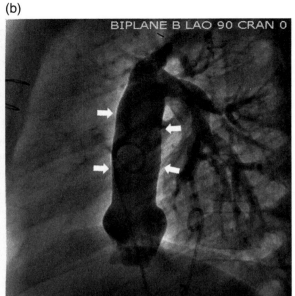

Figure 29.1 (A, B) Extracardiac Fontan. An angiogram is performed in the AP and lateral projection in the lower aspect of the extracardiac Fontan connection (white arrows). The Fontan connection is tube-like and smooth walled. Courtesy of Russel Hirsch, MD.

extracardiac conduit, which may further decrease the risk of arrhythmias. (See Figure 29.1A and B.)

Clinical Pearl

An advantage to the extracardiac Fontan procedure is that since the atrium is not part of the connection and thus does not see significantly elevated central pressures, the incidence of atrial arrhythmias may be lower than observed with the lateral tunnel Fontan.

What is a fenestration and what potential advantage does it offer?

In a patient with a newly created Fontan pathway, it is essential that PVR remain low. If the pulmonary impedance increases, this can result in a reduction of blood flow through the pulmonary vascular bed. A fenestration is a surgically created 4 mm hole in the lateral tunnel baffle, created to allow systemic venous blood to "pop-off" into the atrium when pulmonary impedance increases, resulting in a right-to-left shunt. This "pop-off" helps to maintain CO in the presence of higher resistance in the pulmonary bed, but it can also cause arterial desaturation due to the blood moving from the right (deoxygenated) side to the left (oxygenated). Once the pulmonary vascular bed has adapted to the new physiology, the fenestration can be closed in the cardiac catheterization lab, with the timing dependent on the patient's clinical condition.

While the fenestration is straightforward to place when creating a lateral tunnel Fontan, it is slightly less so in the extracardiac conduit and hence the intra/extra-cardiac conduit Fontan procedure was developed [1]. An extracardiac conduit is used so the atrium is not subjected to the higher pressures that can be seen with the lateral tunnel Fontan. However, in some patients, a small portion of the atrium is connected to the conduit and called a fenestration. Importantly, this fenestration is not placed near the sinus node, which decreases the risk of atrial arrhythmias.

Clinical Pearl

A fenestration in a lateral tunnel Fontan can behave as a "pop-off" by allowing right-to-left shunting from the IVC to the atrium. This helps to maintain CO in the presence of higher resistance in the pulmonary bed but can cause arterial desaturation due to the blood moving from the right (deoxygenated) side to the left (oxygenated).

What should the patient's expected oxygen saturations be if a fenestration is open? If it is closed?

With Fontan physiology and an open fenestration, arterial oxygen saturations can be expected to be in the range of 80%–90% depending on the degree of shunting occurring.

Without a fenestration (as in this patient) or once the fenestration is closed, saturations should be above 90%.

> **Clinical Pearl**
>
> *Patients with a fenestrated Fontan can have oxygen saturations in the range of 80%–90%. Once closed, oxygen saturations should be near normal, in the upper 90s.*

What are the considerations regarding PVR in a patient with Fontan physiology undergoing noncardiac surgery?

In a patient with a Fontan palliation, CO must traverse the pulmonary vascular bed without the advantage of a pumping ventricle, which makes maintenance of low PVR critical. Elevations in PVR can compromise both oxygen saturation and CO. Intraoperatively, it is important to avoid hypoxia, hypercarbia, hypothermia, acidosis, and inadequate anesthesia, in order to keep PVR low and maintain flow through the Fontan pathway. Priority should be given to correcting respiratory or metabolic acidosis, as pH is a potent effector of pulmonary vascular tone. In patients with a fenestrated Fontan, oxygen saturation is a simple method to evaluate the degree of right-to-left shunt, as more flow across the fenestration (which could indicate increased PVR) will lead to more systemic oxygen desaturation. Elevations in PVR are not well tolerated in patients with Fontan physiology and should be minimized.

> **Clinical Pearl**
>
> *Elevations in PVR can compromise both oxygen saturation and CO as CO must traverse the pulmonary vascular bed without the advantage of a pumping ventricle.*

What potential issues can develop in patients with long-standing Fontan physiology?

Long-term issues can develop in patients with Fontan physiology and the likelihood of complications increases with age. Potential issues include Fontan failure, end-organ failure, arrhythmias, and thrombosis. *Atrial arrhythmias* are common in Fontan physiology, and the incidence increases with age. This may be due to stretching of the atrium secondary to both high pressures and the proximity of the Fontan connection to the sinus node. Older Fontan patients may require ablation procedures or require a pacemaker or implantable cardioverter-defibrillator.

Significant risk exists for the development of *vascular thrombosis* secondary to potentially poor cardiac function, dilated atria, nonpulsatile PBF, arrhythmias, and coagulation abnormalities. Many patients are on antithrombotic medications, such as aspirin, which may also contribute to perioperative coagulation abnormalities.

About 70% of patients with Fontan circulation develop *myocardial dysfunction* and failure at the 10-year mark as the systemic ventricle becomes dilated, hypertrophic, and hypocontractile, with deterioration in both systolic and diastolic function. A patient with Fontan failure may have signs of chronic systemic venous congestion affecting multiple organ systems, including hepatomegaly, splenomegaly, ascites, and exercise intolerance. Fontan failure may present as *protein-losing enteropathy (PLE)*, in which patients lose proteins and coagulation factors through their intestinal tract resulting in severe diarrhea, electrolyte abnormalities, hypercoagulability, hypocalcemia, hypomagnesemia, and ascites. About 13% of patients have PLE at 10-year follow-up, and the prognosis is poor, with an approximately 60% five-year survival after diagnosis [2]. *Plastic bronchitis* is another manifestation of Fontan failure, in which mucofibrinous bronchial casts form in the airways and can cause potentially life-threatening airway obstruction. Additionally, end-organ damage to the liver, kidneys, or lungs can develop separately from overt heart failure. This end-organ damage is thought to be multifactorial and may be secondary to high central venous pressures, poor tissue oxygenation, and/or lack of pulsatility of PBF. (See Chapter 30.)

> **Clinical Pearl**
>
> *Older patients with Fontan physiology are at increased risk for long-term complications including decreased CO, hepatic dysfunction, atrial arrhythmias, and thrombosis. Preoperative evaluation should evaluate for these sequelae. This includes review of a recent echocardiogram and electrocardiogram, as well as laboratory testing including coagulation studies.*

Anesthetic Implications

What fasting instructions should be given to the patient and family?

The American Society of Anesthesiologists (ASA) guidelines for preoperative fasting should be followed in all patients, including those with Fontan physiology. These guidelines mandate that the fasting times for children be 6 hours for formula and solids, 4 hours for breast milk, and

2 hours for clear liquids. In patients with Fontan circulation, intravascular volume is a major determinant of central venous pressure and flow through the pulmonary vasculature, thus hypovolemia from prolonged fasting is poorly tolerated. Patients, with help from their families, should be strongly encouraged to continue clear liquids until 2 hours before the start of the anesthetic. This often necessitates that the procedure be scheduled as first case of the day to minimize schedule delays. If fasting is prolonged or case start time is unpredictable, consideration should be given to preoperative intravenous (IV) fluid administration.

Clinical Pearl

In patients with Fontan circulation, intravascular volume is a major determinant of central venous pressure and flow through the pulmonary vasculature; thus hypovolemia from prolonged fasting is poorly tolerated. Patients, with help from their families, should be strongly encouraged to continue clear liquids until 2 hours before the start of the anesthetic.

Should this patient's enalapril and aspirin be withheld preoperatively?

Many patients with Fontan palliation take angiotensin converting enzyme inhibitors (ACEi) for afterload reduction of the systemic ventricle. These medications have been associated with hemodynamic lability, refractory hypotension, and vasoplegia under anesthesia, especially in the adult population [3, 4]. The half-life of enalapril is <12 hours; it is generally advised to hold the morning dose on the day of surgery. The decision whether to discontinue this medication before a procedure should be carefully considered and discussion with the patient's cardiologist may be useful. If the procedure is emergent or the patient did not follow instructions to hold the morning dose, the case would usually not be delayed or cancelled. However, vasopressin (0.04 units/kg intravenously or 0.5 milliunits/kg/minute infusion) should be readily available to counteract refractory hypotension.

Patients with Fontan circulation are often on antiplatelet agents or anticoagulants due to their increased risk for thromboembolism. Depending on the anticipated procedure, antiplatelet therapy may be temporarily withheld perioperatively. Bridging therapy with a shorter acting anticoagulant may be needed for patients on warfarin until treatment can be continued, with the timing depending on the procedure. The precise timeline for discontinuation and reinitiation of therapy should include a thoughtful discussion and agreement between the surgeon, cardiologist, and anesthesiologist.

What preoperative testing is required for this patient?

Due to the multisystem organ effects of Fontan physiology, a comprehensive metabolic panel within a year of the scheduled procedure is advisable in Fontan patients. In addition, a complete blood count should also be reviewed, recognizing that high hemoglobin and hematocrit are consistent with chronic cyanosis. At a minimum a 12-lead electrocardiogram (ECG) should be performed to assess rhythm disturbances, and a recent echocardiogram should be available to assess pathways, and valvular and cardiac function within 12 months of the surgical date. Repeat studies would be warranted prior to surgery if the patient has developed new symptomatology or a change in exercise tolerance in the interim.

Clinical Pearl

Repeat studies would be warranted prior to surgery if the patient has developed new symptomatology or a change in exercise tolerance in the interim since the last study.

Should a cardiology visit be scheduled preoperatively?

Most Fontan patients are closely followed by their cardiologist. Depending on the patient's functional status and the nature and invasiveness of the planned surgery, no additional testing may be required preoperatively. However, if the patient has been lost to follow-up or has not visited their cardiologist recently a careful history and physical to determine functional status is crucial. If evidence of decreased exercise tolerance or other concerning cardiac signs or symptoms are found in a patient with minimal or limited cardiology follow-up, the surgery should be rescheduled until a patient has seen a cardiologist. Ideally all patients with Fontan physiology having an anesthetic should have been seen by a cardiologist within the past 12 months. In patients who have routine cardiology visits, the cardiologist should be informed of the planned procedure so they have the opportunity to convey any concerns not made immediately evident by imaging and laboratory studies.

Clinical Pearl

If evidence of decreased exercise tolerance or other concerning cardiac signs or symptoms are found in a patient with minimal or limited cardiology follow-up, the surgery should be rescheduled until a patient has seen a cardiologist. Ideally all patients with Fontan physiology undergoing an anesthetic should have been seen by a cardiologist within the past 12 months.

What aspects of the echocardiogram are most important to review?

The anesthesiologist should review the most recent echocardiogram or magnetic resonance imaging study, ideally dated within 6–12 months of the planned procedure. During review of the echocardiogram, one should note systemic ventricular systolic and diastolic performance, atrioventricular and aortic valve function, atrioventricular or aortic valve obstruction, ventricular outflow obstruction including coarctation, patency of the Fontan pathway, pulmonary artery patency, and atrial septal communication. Particular attention should be focused on the function of the single ventricle.

Can or should this patient have this procedure done at a freestanding outpatient center?

An elective procedure under anesthesia in a patient with Fontan physiology should ideally be performed at a hospital with appropriate personnel, equipment, and resources in the event of an adverse event. This would include clinicians who understand the physiology and implications of a Fontan circulation. In most circumstances, this would not be at a freestanding center.

Is prophylaxis for infective endocarditis indicated for this procedure?

Infective endocarditis (IE) prophylaxis may be required in a patient with Fontan circulation presenting for noncardiac surgery if they have a residual lesion. If this patient does not have such lesions, she would not require IE prophylaxis.

What monitoring should be recommended?

Standard monitoring as recommended by the ASA guidelines, including pulse oximetry, 5-lead ECG, noninvasive blood pressure, temperature, and end-tidal carbon dioxide (CO_2) monitoring are highly recommended for all cases in patients with Fontan circulation. This patient should only require standard monitors for this particular surgery.

Clinical Pearl

Standard ASA monitors with a 5-lead ECG should provide an adequate level of monitoring for patients undergoing low or moderate risk surgery. Patients with a poorly functioning Fontan circulation who are undergoing high-risk surgery should have an arterial line and central venous catheter placed for continuous blood pressure monitoring, assessment of volume status, and potential delivery of inotropic agents.

When might more invasive monitoring might be recommended?

When a Fontan patient has decreased ventricular function or is undergoing major surgery, particularly where significant volume shifts are expected, invasive arterial and CVP monitoring are strongly recommended. An arterial pressure line allows for continuous blood pressure monitoring and blood gas sampling. Monitoring the CVP trend can aid in assessment of volume status. It is important to remember that a central venous catheter with the tip in the SVC will not measure ventricular filling pressure, but instead will measure mean PA pressure since the SVC is connected to the PA in a patient with Fontan physiology. Obtaining a ventricular filling pressure during a noncardiac procedure in this patient will be impossible since there is no percutaneous method of accessing the atrium in a Fontan patient. Central venous pressure trends are followed as a reasonable alternative, recognizing that CVP in a Fontan patient is higher than a typical CVP in a patient with a normal heart.

Clinical Pearl

A central venous catheter with the tip in the SVC will not measure ventricular filling pressure but instead will measure mean pulmonary artery pressure, since the SVC is connected to the pulmonary artery in a patient with Fontan physiology.

What is the TPG and what is its relationship to the CVP in a Fontan patient?

In patients with a Fontan circulation, the TPG is the primary driving force promoting PBF and subsequent CO. The TPG is defined as the difference between CVP and pulmonary venous atrial pressure. In a well-compensated Fontan, CVP is usually 10–15 mm Hg and pulmonary venous atrial pressure is usually 5–10 mm Hg, giving an ideal TPG of about 5–8 mm Hg. In addition to CVP trend, transesophageal echocardiography can be used for intraoperative assessment of ventricular preload and function as well as to monitor for the presence of emboli.

Clinical Pearl

In a well-compensated Fontan, CVP is usually 10–15 mm Hg and pulmonary venous atrial pressure is usually 5–10 mm Hg, giving an ideal TPG of about 5–8 mm Hg.

What are the anesthetic goals for this surgery in this patient?

The main goals for anesthetic management in a patient with well-functioning Fontan physiology are the following:

- Maintain adequate preload: replace fasting volume appropriately and keep abreast of third space loss and blood loss.
- Avoid agents that significantly depress myocardial contractility.
- Maintain sinus rhythm.
- Avoid increases in PVR.

What are the options for induction of anesthesia in this patient?

Given the patient's age and physiology a peripheral IV line should be placed for induction of anesthesia. Induction agents with minimal effect on myocardial contractility, CO and PBF should be selected. Etomidate and ketamine are both good choices for induction as they preserve myocardial contractility and vascular tone with little to no effect on PVR. Propofol should be administered judiciously, as it may cause both profound decreases in venous return and myocardial depression. If a muscle relaxant is necessary, avoid those with histamine-releasing properties, as they can result in hypotension and tachycardia. Rocuronium, vecuronium, cisatracurium, and succinylcholine are all good selections because of their stable hemodynamic properties. One must also be cognizant during induction that airway obstruction and/or difficult ventilation or intubation can lead to acute elevations in partial pressure of CO_2 which can increase PVR and negatively impact CO.

What are the effects of spontaneous ventilation on Fontan physiology? What are the considerations for this patient for this procedure?

Since PBF is dependent on passive venous drainage from the SVC and IVC into the pulmonary circulation, any ventilation strategy impeding intrathoracic venous return will have a negative effect on PBF and subsequently CO. During spontaneous ventilation, negative intrathoracic pressure increases antegrade flow from the SVC, IVC, and hepatic venous circulation into the pulmonary arterial tree, allowing more blood to be available for gas exchange. The benefits of spontaneous ventilation must be compared to the risks of hypoventilation and hypercarbia under anesthesia with sedatives. For this surgery, the patient will need to be prone; therefore spontaneous ventilation either with or without a definitive airway device may be contraindicated. A discussion with the surgeon is warranted to determine the length of the procedure and if, in this case, the position can be altered from prone to lateral. A short procedure or a change in position from prone may make spontaneous ventilation a better option for this patient.

> **Clinical Pearl**
>
> *Since PBF is dependent on passive venous drainage from the SVC and IVC into the pulmonary circulation, any ventilation strategy impeding intrathoracic venous return will have a negative effect on PBF and subsequently CO.*

What are the effects of positive pressure ventilation on this patient physiology?

Positive pressure ventilation (PPV) via an endotracheal tube can increase intrathoracic pressure, diminish venous return, PBF, and CO in patients with Fontan physiology. High peak inspiratory pressures and high positive end-expiratory pressures (PEEP) can decrease venous return and inhibit PBF. If PPV is indicated because of patient or procedural factors, the ventilatory goals should be as follows: low tidal volumes (6–8 mL/kg), low respiratory rates, short inspiratory times, and low (physiologic) PEEP. This ventilation strategy will optimize Fontan flow and CO.

What considerations are important during the maintenance phase of anesthesia?

Preservation of CO is a key goal during the maintenance of anesthesia. This is accomplished by ensuring adequate preload for good ventricular filling, minimizing agents which decrease contractility, and avoiding increases in PVR which can compromise ventricular filling and CO. Hypoxia, hypercarbia, acidosis, hypothermia, inadequate analgesia or anesthesia, excessive mean airway pressure, and PEEP can all increase PVR and should be minimized or avoided. A balanced anesthetic is ideal for maintenance. A low concentration of inhalational agent in conjunction with opioids, benzodiazepines, and/or dexmedetomidine should provide hemodynamic stability.

Is regional anesthesia feasible or useful in patients with Fontan physiology?

The risk-benefit profile of regional anesthesia should be examined critically and executed with caution. Close attention should be paid to any existing coagulopathy as well as the use of antiplatelet agents or anticoagulants. Epidural anesthesia has been successfully employed in patients with Fontan circulation; however, a spinal anesthetic is not recommended due to the hypotension and bradycardia that may accompany the sympathectomy occurring with spinal local anesthetics. Adequate monitoring and appropriate fluid administration are recommended if a neuraxial procedure is performed [5].

What are the options for treatment if pulmonary artery pressures acutely increase intraoperatively?

Treatment for an acute increase in PA pressure in a patient with Fontan physiology under anesthesia includes administration of 100% oxygen, fluid, and pulmonary vasodilators such as inhaled nitric oxide and inhaled prostacyclin analogues.

Are patients with Fontan circulation candidates for laparoscopic surgery?

Patients with a Fontan circulation have successfully undergone laparoscopic abdominal surgery. Key goals include keeping intraabdominal pressure during insufflation at or <10 mm Hg, ensuring adequate ventilation, and maintaining intravascular volume during the procedure. Potential complications due to the induced pneumoperitoneum include hypercarbia, gas embolism, hypotension, pneumothorax, and mediastinal emphysema. Additionally, if there is a fenestration in the Fontan circuit, there is a risk of paradoxical CO_2 embolism. If unrecognized, these complications may be potentially catastrophic. With careful management, most patients with a well-functioning Fontan circulation can tolerate laparoscopic abdominal surgery, which allows them to benefit from the reduced postoperative pain and recovery time compared with open surgery.

What is the appropriate postoperative disposition in this patient after this surgery?

This patient, with a well-functioning Fontan and minimal comorbidities, should be able to have outpatient surgery. She can be discharged home after an uneventful anesthetic once she is tolerating fluids by mouth, pain issues are addressed, and when she meets post-anesthesia care unit discharge criteria. If any instability or adverse events occur

during the anesthetic, consideration must be given to admitting her for further observation, depending on the nature of the event.

What is the long-term prognosis for this patient?

With improvements in surgical techniques and overall management of patients following the Fontan procedure, long-term survival continues to improve as well. However, overall survival for patients with Fontan physiology is significantly lower than that of the general population due to the development of complications as described above. Recent reports indicate that approximately 74% of Fontan patients will survive without transplantation and the 30-year transplant-free survival rate is only 43% [2].

References

1. R. A. Jonas. The intra/extracardiac conduit fenestrated Fontan. *Semin Thorac Cardiovasc Surg Pediatr Card Surg Annual* 2011; **14**: 11–18.

2. A. Kay, T. Moe, B. Suter, et al. Long term consequences of the Fontan procedure and how to manage them. *Prog Cardiovasc Dis* 2018; **61**: 365–76.

3. C. C. Ajuba-Iwuji, S. Puttreddy, B. G. Maxwell, et al. Effect of preoperative angiotensin-converting enzyme inhibitor and angiotensin II receptor blocker use on hemodynamic variables in pediatric patients undergoing cardiopulmonary bypass. *World J Pediatr Congenit Heart Surg* 2014; **5**: 515–21.

4. C. Hollmann, N. L. Fernandes, and B. M. Biccard. A systematic review of outcomes associated with withholding or continuing angiotensin-converting enzyme inhibitors and angiotensin receptor blockers before noncardiac surgery. *Anesth Analg* 2018; **127**: 678–87.

5. M. Tiouririne, D. G. De Souza, K. T. Beers, et al. Anesthetic management of parturients with a Fontan circulation: a review of published case reports. *Semin Cardiothorac Vasc Anesth* 2015; **19**: 203–9.

Suggested Reading

Kiran U., Aggarwal S., Choudhary A., et al. The Blalock and Taussig shunt revisited. *Ann Card Anaesth* 2017; **20**: 323–30.

McClain C. D., McGowan F. X., and Kovatsis P. G. Laparoscopic surgery in a patient with Fontan physiology. *Anesth Analg* 2006; **103**: 856–8.

Nayak S. and Booker P. The Fontan circulation. *Cont Educ Anaesth Crit Care Pain* 2008; **8**: 26–30.

Failing Fontan

Maricarmen Roche Rodriguez and Viviane G. Nasr

Case Scenario

A 20-year-old female with a past medical history of anxiety and hypoplastic left heart syndrome palliated to a fenestrated lateral tunnel Fontan presents for wisdom teeth extraction. She underwent Fontan completion at age 3 years, with her initial postoperative course complicated by chylous effusions requiring chest tube placement and postoperative sinoatrial node dysfunction requiring placement of a dual chamber pacemaker. Two years ago, she was admitted with severe cyanosis and found to have restrictive flow across the intraatrial Fontan baffle at the level of the anastomosis with the inferior vena cava. She underwent stenting of the obstruction without recurrence and since then has maintained appropriate follow-up with her cardiologist.

She states that she has been doing well and denies syncopal episodes, chest pain, or palpitations. Pulse oximetry shows a room air saturation of 91%. On examination, she is alert but anxious. Electrocardiogram shows a paced rhythm at 70 beats/minute. Recent cardiac catheterization confirmed the echocardiographic findings and noted a small patent baffle fenestration. Fontan pressure was measured as 20 mm Hg and several systemic-pulmonary venous collateral vessels were coiled.

A recent echocardiogram shows:

- *A morphologic right ventricle*
- *Mild tricuspid valve regurgitation*
- *Mildly impaired systolic function, ejection fraction 40%*
- *An unobstructed stented lateral tunnel Fontan*

Key Objectives

- Understand the Fontan procedure and physiology.
- Recognize symptoms, signs, and outcomes of failing Fontan physiology.
- Discuss preoperative assessment of Fontan patients.
- Develop a perioperative management plan for a patient with a failing Fontan.
- Discuss the postoperative disposition of Fontan patients.

Pathophysiology

What is Fontan physiology?

Initially proposed by Francis Fontan and Eugene Baudet as a surgical palliation for tricuspid atresia, the Fontan procedure has since been adapted as a palliation for a variety of congenital heart diseases resulting in single-ventricle (SV) physiology. Improvements in surgical technique and medical management have led to increased survival, making it more likely that these patients will present for a variety of noncardiac procedures. In general, patients with congenital heart disease (CHD) have an increased risk of 30-day mortality when compared to healthy cohorts [1]. To provide a safe perioperative course, it is essential to understand Fontan physiology.

In a normal circulation each ventricle pumps against one resistance, either pulmonary or systemic. The Fontan procedure directly routes systemic venous return to the pulmonary arteries, creating a series circulation whereby cardiac output (CO) is dependent on three elements: pulmonary blood flow (PBF), the transpulmonary gradient (TPG), and the single ventricle. In other words, the single ventricle must provide the energy for blood to flow across three resistance beds: the systemic vascular bed, the cavopulmonary connection, and the pulmonary vascular bed. A reduction in PBF therefore results in both decreased CO and systemic deoxygenation. (See Chapters 26–29 for further details of single-ventricle palliation and Fontan physiology.)

Clinical Pearl

In a normal circulation each ventricle pumps against one resistance, either pulmonary or systemic. Cardiac output in a patient with Fontan physiology is dependent on maximizing blood flow across three resistances (systemic vascular, cavopulmonary connection, and pulmonary vascular) with one ventricle.

What makes a "good" Fontan candidate?

Requirements for an ideal Fontan circulation can be divided into cardiac and pulmonary components.

- *Cardiac requirements*
  - Sinus rhythm
  - Atrioventricular valve competency
  - Good ventricular function
  - Unobstructed systemic outflow from the single ventricle
- *Pulmonary requirements*
  - Nonrestrictive, unobstructed Fontan connection from the systemic veins to the pulmonary arteries
  - Adequately sized pulmonary arteries without anatomic distortion
  - Near-normal pulmonary vascular resistance (PVR)
  - Unobstructed pulmonary venous return

In other words, the pulmonary artery pressure (PAP) should be low (ideally <15 mm Hg). The transpulmonary gradient (the difference between mean PAP and LA pressure) should also be low, below 7 mm Hg. It may be elevated when there is increased pulmonary venous pressure, which will impair adequate flow across the Fontan circulation. Pulmonary vascular resistance should be <4 Wood units/m^2. These measurements are indicators of potential pulmonary vascular disease.

What are the different types of Fontan procedure?

Over time several different anatomic variations of the Fontan have been performed and are outlined below in chronological order. Although the atriopulmonary Fontan is no longer performed, older surviving patients may still display this anatomic connection.

1. *Atriopulmonary Fontan.* Performed after a "classic" Glenn procedure, this method has become obsolete as a surgical option. A "classic Glenn" procedure anastomoses the superior vena cava (SVC) to the distal end of the right pulmonary artery (RPA). An atriopulmonary connection is then established between the proximal end of the divided RPA and the anatomic right atrium (RA). The atrial septal defect is closed and IVC blood flow is now directed toward the left PA to perfuse the left lung. The main PA is ligated, allowing blood to bypass the nonfunctional ventricle. (See Figure 30.1A.)
2. *Total cavopulmonary anastomosis (TCPA).* This may be performed after EITHER a bidirectional Glenn (BDG) or hemi-Fontan (HF) Stage II procedure. The

BDG and HF are both procedures performed by surgically connecting the SVC and the pulmonary arteries, thus providing a source of PBF. *Although they differ anatomically, the physiologic result is the same.*

- The *BDG* is created by dividing the SVC at its junction with the RA, oversewing the atrial end, and creating an end-to-side anastomosis between the SVC and the RPA.
- The *HF*, in contrast, keeps the SVC and RA in continuity when the SVC is connected to the RPA. However, homograft tissue is sewn across the superior cavoatrial junction to prevent blood flow from the SVC to the RA.

The TCPA or "completion Fontan" is then generally performed 1–3 years after either the BDG or HF procedure. This completion adds IVC flow directly into the pulmonary bed as well, and commonly takes one of two forms as listed below. An opening, or a *fenestration*, is often created between the RA and the conduit or baffle. This allows right to left (R-to-L) shunting in the setting of any increases in PVR and hence a means of increasing CO, albeit at the cost of normal oxygen saturations, as oxygenated and deoxygenated blood are then allowed to mix.

- *Lateral tunnel Fontan.* (See Figure 30.1B.) The RA is septated and an intraatrial baffle is placed in order to direct blood from the IVC to the RPA.
- *Extracardiac Fontan.* (See Figure 30.1C.) The IVC is disconnected from the RA and anastomosed using a conduit to the RPA.

Clinical Pearl

An opening, or fenestration, is often created between the RA and the conduit or baffle during the Fontan procedure, allowing a R-to-L shunt to occur in the setting of any increases in pulmonary vascular resistance. This results in increased systemic blood flow, albeit at the cost of normal oxygen saturations, as oxygenated and deoxygenated blood are then allowed to mix.

What are the advantages of a TCPA versus atriopulmonary Fontan?

It was initially thought that the atriopulmonary Fontan improved PBF secondary to a pulsatile atrium. However, over time the thin-walled atrial portion becomes dilated from exposure to higher than normal systemic venous pressures, leading to impaired contractility and energy loss. The atrium also becomes a site for the development of atrial arrhythmia and thrombus formation due to stasis.

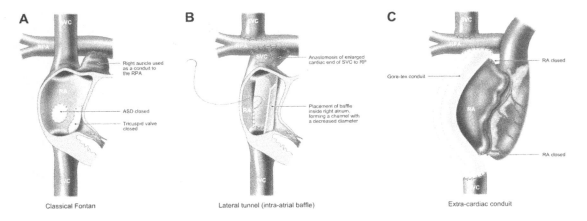

Figure 30.1 Fontan surgical techniques. (A) Classical atriopulmonary connection. (B) Lateral tunnel cavopulmonary connection. (C) Extracardiac cavopulmonary connection. From Y. d'Udekem et al. The Fontan procedure: contemporary techniques have improved long-term outcomes. *Circulation* 2007; **116**: I-157–64. With permission.

Patient's age (years)

	20	25	30	35	40	45	50	55	60
ASD	25	26	32	38	42	47	52	57	61
Valvar disease	29	31	36	40	45	49	54	59	63
VSD	28	30	36	40	44	49	53	59	63
Aortic coarctation	32	33	38	43	47	52	56	62	66
AVSD	33	34	39	44	48	52	57	62	66
Marfan syndrome	37	38	42	46	50	54	59	64	68
Tetralogy of Fallot	37	38	42	47	50	54	60	65	69
Ebstein anomaly	42	43	47	51	54	59	63	68	72
Systemic RV	46	48	51	55	59	63	67	72	76
Eisenmenager syndrome	57	58	62	65	69	73	77	81	84
Complex CHD	58	59	63	67	70	74	78	82	85
Fontan	64	65	68	72	75	78	82	86	91

Age difference:
- >40
- 30–40
- 20–30
- 10–20
- 5–10
- 2–5
- <2

Figure 30.2 The numbers represent the equivalent age having similar 5-year mortality rates. Colors reflect the difference between the relative age and the actual age of patients. ASD, atrial septal defect; AVSD, atrioventricular septal defect; CHD, congenital heart disease; RV, right ventricle; VSD, ventricular septal defect. From G. Diller et al. Survival prospects and circumstances of death in contemporary adult congenital heart disease patients under follow-up at a large tertiary centre. *Circulation* 2015; **132**: 2118–25. With permission.

Patients with TCPA have demonstrated improved outcomes and also have a decreased risk over time of atrial arrhythmias and thrombosis compared to patients with atriopulmonary Fontans. The lateral tunnel method includes the lateral wall of the RA, which allows for growth as the child grows. The extracardiac conduit decreases suture lines within the atrium and because it excludes atrial tissue, dilation is limited. This decreases arrhythmogenic foci. However, the graft used does not allow for growth potential, so this method is usually performed in patients large enough to accept a graft of adequate size for adult IVC flow.

Does the presence of CHD affect the onset of heart failure?

The progression of symptomatic heart failure in congenital heart patients, particularly patients with SV physiology, occurs decades before failure in patients with acquired heart disease. This is illustrated in Figure 30.2, where the equivalent age for adult patients with CHD is compared to that of patients without CHD [2]. For example, the 5-year mortality rate of a 35-year-old Fontan patient is equivalent to the 5-year mortality rate of a 72-year-old from the general population!

What is Fontan failure and what are the signs and symptoms?

Signs and symptoms of Fontan failure may include fatigue, dyspnea, growth failure, exercise intolerance, decreased activity level, syncopal/presyncopal episodes, palpitations, cyanosis, weight gain, edema, ascites, and cough with expectoration of mucoid cast-like material. These can be secondary to ventricular dysfunction, systemic atrioventricular valve insufficiency, atrial and/or ventricular arrhythmias, renal failure, hepatic insufficiency, protein losing enteropathy (PLE), and plastic bronchitis [3, 4].

Cardiac

- *Ventricular function.* Systemic ventricular dysfunction is a common problem encountered over time and may be due to a history of ventriculotomy during staged palliative procedures or chronic hypoxemia. *Patients with a morphologic systemic RV experience a greater decline in ventricular function compared to those patients with systemic left ventricles.* Low CO can present as a decline in exercise tolerance and resting or exercise desaturation. Decreasing exercise tolerance may also result from a decreased response to β-stimulation secondary to limited preload reserve [5]. These patients show an abnormal response to increased heart rate, including a diminished contractile response and impaired diastolic filling [6]. Additional causes of low CO may be related to low flow across the Fontan pathway from physical obstruction across the pulmonary arteries, compression of pulmonary venous return, elevations in PVR, or atrioventricular (AV) valve dysfunction. Atrioventricular valve dysfunction results in elevated atrial pressures that may cause atrial dysrhythmias and decreased CO. Aortic stenosis will lead to ventricular hypertrophy and reduced ventricular compliance, while aortic regurgitation creates volume overload and systemic ventricular failure.
- *Rhythm disturbances.* Fontan patients may suffer from a multitude of rhythm disturbances including sinus node dysfunction, junctional rhythm, AV block, and supraventricular or ventricular arrhythmias. Risk factors include atrial suture lines, myocardial fibrosis, atrial dilation, AV valve regurgitation, and ventricular failure. Atrioventricular conduction block may occur due to intrinsic conduction abnormalities or as a consequence of surgery. If pacemaker implantation is necessary, epicardial pacemakers are used most commonly due to limited venous access to the atrium and the risk of endocardial lead thrombosis. It is imperative to maintain sinus rhythm in Fontan patients, as nonsinus rhythm can cause an acute elevation in atrial pressures with each ventricular contraction and is associated with decreased CO and long-term hepatic fibrosis [6, 7].
- *Oxygen saturation.* Cyanosis may occur from persistent R-to-L shunting and pulmonary venous desaturation.
  - *R-to-L shunting* can occur secondary to excessive flow across a fenestration, a baffle leak, and/or veno-

venous or veno-arterial decompressing collateral vessels. The formation of decompressing vessels (such as veno-venous collaterals) is not unusual in a Fontan patient where systemic venous pressure becomes elevated. This compensatory process alleviates pressure in the venous return pathway, while maintaining systemic ventricular preload. Patients who become desaturated may form aortopulmonary collaterals, which are vessels that carry oxygenated blood from the aorta to the pulmonary vascular bed in patients with poor PBF. These not only decrease systemic CO and but also cause volume overload on the single ventricle. If volume overload is significant, the patient may present for hemodynamic cardiac catheterization and possible coiling of decompressing vessels.
  - *Pulmonary venous desaturation* may occur due to intrinsic lung disease, pulmonary arteriovenous malformations, pleural effusions, or plastic bronchitis. Plastic bronchitis presents as tachypnea, cough, wheezing, and expectoration of bronchial casts. Leakage of proteinaceous material into the airways lead to cast formation and potential obstruction of the airways. It is a poor prognostic sign and an indication for transplant.
  - *Pulmonary thromboembolic events* can contribute to hypoxemia.

Hepatorenal

Chronic elevated systemic venous pressure, low CO, and end-organ hypoperfusion lead to hepatic and renal dysfunction. Patients may have mild elevations in bilirubin and abnormally elevated liver enzymes.

- *Hypoalbuminemia* and increased risk of hepatocellular carcinoma may occur.
- *Protein losing enteropathy* is characterized by lymphatic dysfunction with persistent hypoalbuminemia in the absence of renal or liver disease, with manifestations of ascites, peripheral edema, pleural effusions, and fat malabsorption. The etiology is not well known; theories include low CO, mesenteric vascular flow anomalies and elevated pressures, or autoimmune/inflammatory reactions. Initial management includes adjustments to existing anticongestive therapy, parenteral albumin, sodium restriction and diet modification, immunoglobulin replacement, or steroid therapy. Patients with obstructive lesions within the Fontan circuit are evaluated and obstructions may need to be relieved via transcatheter approach or surgical management. The presence of PLE is a poor prognostic sign and may be an indication for transplant.

Hematologic

Hematologic disturbances may arise, including possible sequestration of platelets by the liver and spleen resulting in thrombocytopenia. *Thromboembolism* may occur due to atrial dilation, reduced CO, slow-moving venous flow, anatomic obstructions within the Fontan circuit, and arrhythmias. For this reason, patients are usually on anticoagulation medications [3, 4].

Table 30.1 summarizes the clinical manifestations of failing Fontan physiology along with possible etiologies.

What potential etiologies exist for the lower oxygen saturation in this patient?

Systemic oxygen saturation in a well-functioning Fontan patient should be between 90% and 95%. Potential causes of hypoxemia in the Fontan population include persistent R-to-L shunting and pulmonary venous desaturation.

What does an oxygen saturation of 100% indicate in a patient with a fenestrated Fontan?

A fenestration is often created between an extracardiac or lateral tunnel Fontan and the atrium to maintain ventricular preload while reducing elevated pressure in the Fontan circuit. This fenestration helps preserve systemic preload and CO when PVR is elevated and/or PBF is decreased. Decreased PBF may occur when there is an obstruction within the Fontan circulation or an increase in PVR. This occurs at the expense of systemic desaturation, as the systemic venous return will bypass the pulmonary circulation. An oxygen saturation of 100% raises the suspicion for obstruction or thrombus formation at the level of the fenestration.

> **Clinical Pearl**
>
> *The systemic oxygen saturation in a patient with Fontan physiology is usually between 90% and 95%. Desaturation is abnormal and could indicate a failing Fontan, while saturation of 100% in a fenestrated Fontan could indicate thrombosis or obstruction at the level of the fenestration.*

Anesthetic Implications

How can clinical status be assessed in a patient with Fontan physiology?

The preoperative evaluation of patients with Fontan physiology involves a thorough history and physical examination with attention to recent changes in health status, exercise capacity, hospital admissions, current medications, and additional comorbid conditions. Recent respiratory tract infections are of special concern, as they can lead to an increased incidence of bronchospasm or laryngospasm with increased airway resistance and PVR, resulting in lower PBF and CO. Physical evaluation should focus on the airway, heart, and lungs, as well as extremities. The assessment of the extremities allows for the evaluation of cyanosis, edema, and vascular access.

The patient with a well-functioning Fontan is warm, well perfused, and acyanotic. Auscultation of the heart should be without murmurs and oxygen saturation is typically between 90% and 95%. However, in a patient with a failing Fontan signs of systemic venous and hepatic congestion are often present. Vascular access may prove challenging due to previous surgeries and interventions. Preoperative hematologic studies including blood counts, electrolytes, and hepatic and renal function studies should be considered depending on the type of surgery. Table 30.2 describes possible laboratory findings in a patient with failing Fontan physiology [6, 8, 9].

Table 30.1 Laboratory Abnormalities in the Failing Fontan

Cardiac	Elevated brain natriuretic peptide (BNP)
Hepatic	Liver function tests Hyperbilirubinemia
Renal	Elevated creatinine
Hematologic	Anemia Polycythemia Lymphopenia Immunoglobulin deficiency Decreased or prolonged PT, PTT, INR
Electrolyte abnormalities	Hyponatremia Hyperglycemia
Protein-losing enteropathy	Hypoproteinemia Hypoalbuminemia Hypocalcemia + stool α_1-antitrypsin

INR, international normalized ratio; PT, prothrombin time; PTT, partial thromboplastin time.

> **Clinical Pearl**
>
> *The functional status and comorbidities in patients with Fontan physiology can vary widely, from patients who are well-compensated to those with a failing circulation.*

Table 30.2 Failing Fontan

Complications	Etiology
Growth failure	Suboptimal cardiac output
Exercise intolerance	Chronotropic incompetence, abnormal pulmonary compliance with exertion, atrial distention
Depression	Limitations in functional status
Arrhythmias	Sinus node dysfunction, predominant junctional rhythm, AV block, supraventricular tachycardia/atrial tachycardia, ventricular tachycardia
Diminished cardiac output	Obstruction: Atriopulmonary, pulmonary arterial, pulmonary venous obstruction, AV valve inflow or ventricular outflow AV valve dysfunction Ventricular dysfunction: due to atrial distortion or dilation, AV valve dysfunction, chronic arrhythmias, impaired myocardial perfusion, abnormal ventricular morphology, prolonged cyanosis, or volume overload Thrombosis: systemic venous, atrial, or pulmonary
Cyanosis	Intracardiac right-to-left shunt, veno-venous collaterals, pulmonary AVMs, progressive increase in PVR
Pleural effusions	Elevated Fontan pressures
Plastic bronchitis	Unknown
Protein losing enteropathy	Unknown
Hepato-renal insufficiency	Low cardiac output, sepsis
Ascites	Portal hypertension from obstruction, hepatic failure, cirrhosis
Metabolic derangements	Decreased albumin, thrombocytopenia, hyperbilirubinemia, coagulopathy

AV, atrioventricular; AVM, arteriovenous malformation; PVR, pulmonary vascular resistance.

The patient's medications include albuterol, aspirin, enalapril, fluoxetine, and spironolactone. What preoperative considerations are involved?

Preoperative assessment includes knowledge of the current medication regimen and any recent changes consistent with worsening clinical status. Patients are frequently taking diuretics, digoxin, antihypertensives, antiarrhythmics, and anticoagulants.

Most cardiac medications should be continued up to the time of anesthetic induction. No consensus exists for preoperative diuretics. They are typically continued for low-risk surgery but withheld for higher-risk surgeries due to the risk of potential dehydration. Of note, patients on diuretic therapy may have electrolyte abnormalities that should be evaluated with preoperative laboratory studies. Angiotensin converting enzyme inhibitors (ACEi) are commonly withheld prior to surgical procedures requiring general anesthesia due to intraoperative hypotension that can be difficult to manage. If a patient is taking an ACEi prior to surgery, the recommendation at our institution is to stop the ACEi 24 hours prior to the procedure. If the patient took their ACEi on the day of the procedure, the decision to proceed with surgery is determined by the type and urgency of the surgical

procedure: a procedure with the potential for large volume shifts and hemodynamic instability should be postponed if possible.

Aspirin is usually continued to prevent thrombosis, and patients on warfarin may need preoperative admission for monitoring and bridging to intravenous heparin. The patient's cardiologist and surgeon should be involved in discussions regarding the perioperative management of antithrombotic medications.

Clinical Pearl

The patient's cardiologist and surgeon should be involved in discussions regarding the perioperative management of antithrombotic medications.

What are the major preoperative anesthetic concerns for this patient?

Patients with failing Fontan physiology often have poor ventricular systolic function at baseline and are vasoconstricted in order to maximally augment their preload. These patients are also at risk for hemodynamically significant atrial arrhythmias. The patient in this scenario has RV dysfunction in addition to AV valve regurgitation. Her

Table 30.3 Diagnostic Modalities and Their Utility in the Evaluation of the Failing Fontan

Diagnostic Modality	Evaluation
Electrocardiogram	• Rhythm • Pacing dependence
Echocardiography	• Ventricular function • AV valve function • Fontan pathway patency • Fenestration status/gradient
Cardiac catheterization	• Fontan conduit pressure/resistance • Quantification of ventricular function • Ventricular end-diastolic pressure • Quantification of PVR • Presence/embolization of collateral vessels or arteriovenous malformations
Chest radiography	• Heart size • Pleural effusions • Pulmonary edema

AV, atrioventricular; PVR, pulmonary vascular resistance.

cardiac catheterization demonstrated elevated Fontan pressures, which could indicate an obstruction to flow or significant myocardial dysfunction. Finally, in addition to the risk of arrhythmia secondary to the Fontan pathway, she is pacemaker-dependent and will thus require pacemaker management in the perioperative period.

Baseline hematologic and biochemical studies are important in the preoperative evaluation. In addition, several imaging and diagnostic modalities are required. These are summarized in Table 30.3.

With a history of complete heart block and a pacemaker, what considerations are important?

The management of any permanent pacemaker (PPM) or implantable cardioverter-defibrillator (ICD) device requires knowing the indication for placement, pacing mode, pacing rate, battery life, underlying rhythm, and any cardioversion or defibrillation events. For that reason, it is necessary to consult the electrophysiology team and to interrogate these devices in the preoperative setting.

The potential effects of electromagnetic interference (EMI) on device function are of concern in pacemaker-dependent patients. Possible sources of EMI include electrocautery (especially monopolar electrocautery), evoked potential monitors, nerve stimulators, external defibrillation,

radiofrequency ablation, and extracorporeal shock wave lithotripsy. Electromagnetic interference may be misinterpreted as intrinsic cardiac signals, resulting in oversensing and inhibition of pacing in PPMs. In pacemaker-dependent patients, inappropriate inhibition of pacing due to EMI can cause bradycardia, sinus arrest, or ventricular standstill. In ICDs, EMI can cause noise, potentially resulting in inappropriate cardioversion/defibrillation. (See Chapters 23 and 49 for details of intraoperative pacemaker management.)

> **Clinical Pearl**
>
> *The management of any PPM or ICD requires the knowledge of the indication for placement, pacing mode, pacing rate, battery life, underlying rhythm, and any cardioversion or defibrillation events. In pacemaker-dependent patients, inappropriate inhibition of pacing due to EMI can cause bradycardia, sinus arrest, or ventricular standstill. In ICDs, EMI can cause noise, which causes inappropriate cardioversion/defibrillation.*

What anesthetic options exist for this patient?

General anesthesia, regional anesthesia, or sedation can be used in Fontan patients. In this case, the safest option is the use of local anesthesia and supplementation with intravenous anxiolytics such as midazolam. Spontaneous ventilation allows for optimal PBF without the need for positive pressure ventilation (PPV), and avoidance of general anesthesia prevents the potential risk of hemodynamic instability from systemic vasodilation. Intravenous fentanyl may be used to supplement sedation and as an adjunct for procedural discomfort. However, it is important to keep in mind that a diminished respiratory drive with subsequent increased carbon dioxide levels may lead to hemodynamically significant elevations in PVR.

Due to her extreme anxiety the patient desires general anesthesia. What is an appropriate plan?

Intravenous (IV) anesthetic agents may cause vasodilation, decreased preload, and myocardial depression. Due to her diminished ventricular function, a peripheral IV line should be placed prior to induction in this patient. For patients with severely diminished ventricular function it may be advisable to start inotropic support prior to induction. Although in patients with well-compensated physiology an inhalation induction may be performed safely if necessary, in a teenage or adult patient with decreased ventricular function an IV induction is preferable.

This patient requires endotracheal intubation to protect the airway while providing general anesthesia. While the surgical team generally prefers nasotracheal intubation over orotracheal intubation for ease of access to the oral cavity, the need for nasotracheal intubation should be discussed with the proceduralist as these patients are at high risk for bleeding secondary to elevated venous pressures, hepatic dysfunction and preoperative use of anticoagulants, and the use of an oral endotracheal tube is often acceptable in light of these risks.

During anesthetic maintenance, the use of high concentration of volatile agents should be avoided due to the increased risk of arrhythmias and myocardial depression. Using low concentrations of inhalational agent in combination with the intermittent use of opioid or a short-acting opioid infusion can provide a hemodynamically stable anesthetic. Neuromuscular blocking agents are a useful adjunct for intubation and may be used as long as there is adequate reversal since residual weakness can lead to hypoventilation and hypercarbia, which are poorly tolerated. Finally, perioperative pain control in Fontan patients should be adequate, as uncontrolled pain increases catecholamine release and thus increases PVR. Useful adjuncts in this case can include the use of local anesthetic by the surgical team and intravenous acetaminophen if deemed appropriate.

Potential anesthetic problems can include intraoperative hypotension, thromboembolic events, unstable arrhythmias, significant bleeding, and coagulopathy.

Clinical Pearl

While the surgical team generally prefers nasotracheal intubation over orotracheal intubation for ease of access to the oral cavity, the need for nasotracheal intubation should be discussed preoperatively as Fontan patients are at high risk for bleeding secondary to elevated venous pressures, hepatic dysfunction, and preoperative use of anticoagulants. The use of an oral endotracheal tube is often acceptable in light of these risks.

What type of monitoring should be utilized?

Standard monitors should be placed prior to the induction of general anesthesia, including 5-lead ECG, noninvasive blood pressure monitoring, and pulse oximetry. Blood pressure measurements should be assessed in all four extremities, as discrepancies may exist due to prior surgical procedures or previous arterial cut-down attempts. For example, the presence of a previous classic Blalock–Taussig shunt may cause altered blood pressure readings in the upper extremity when compared to the contralateral side.

The use of invasive monitors depends on patient-specific conditions including pre-existing ventricular dysfunction, as well as procedure-specific factors, and should not be necessary for this case. The use of invasive arterial blood pressure monitoring and central line placement for central venous pressure (CVP) monitoring may be useful in managing large fluid shifts during major surgery. Monitoring CVP trends can help in assessing intravascular volume status but it is important to remember that this number will be a reflection of main PA pressure and not ventricular preload. Central venous access may also be beneficial to provide inotropic support. The routine use of central lines for noncardiac procedures is rare, as the risks of infection, thrombosis, and impaired venous return within the Fontan circulation may outweigh any potential benefits. Transesophageal echocardiography can be used for the assessment of ventricular preload and function when appropriate.

Due to the history of pacemaker-dependent sinus node dysfunction and the risk for arrhythmias, intraoperative placement of transcutaneous defibrillator pads is advised. The placement of invasive arterial blood pressure monitoring prior to the start of the case is not necessary since the upper extremities are readily accessible should the patient become unstable. Finally, a neuromuscular twitch monitor should be used to assure adequate reversal of neuromuscular blockade prior to endotracheal extubation.

Clinical Pearl

The routine use of central lines for minor noncardiac procedures is rare, as the risks of infection, thrombosis, and impaired venous return within the Fontan circulation may outweigh any potential benefits.

Should endocarditis prophylaxis be administered?

The need for bacterial endocarditis prophylaxis in Fontan patients is based on the type of surgical procedure. Current American Heart Association guidelines state that prophylaxis should be administered during dental procedures involving manipulation of gingival tissue, manipulation of the periapical region of teeth, or perforation of the oral mucosa in patients with the following [10]:

- Prosthetic cardiac valves, including transcatheter-implanted prostheses and homografts
- Prosthetic material used for cardiac valve repair, such as annuloplasty rings and chords

- Previous endocarditis
- Congenital heart disease in the following categories:
  - Unrepaired cyanotic CHD, including palliative shunts and conduits
  - Completely repaired CHD with prosthetic material or device, whether placed by surgery or catheter intervention, during the first 6 months after the procedure
  - Repaired CHD with residual shunts or valvular regurgitation at the site or adjacent to the site of a prosthetic patch or prosthetic device
- Cardiac transplantation recipients with valvular regurgitation due to a structurally abnormal valve

In this case, the patient will require endocarditis prophylaxis because of her tricuspid regurgitation and the surgical palliation using prosthetic material within the lateral tunnel. Appropriate intramuscular (IM) or intravenous (IV) endocarditis prophylaxis consists of either ampicillin 2 g OR the choice of cefazolin or ceftriaxone 1 g. If the patient is allergic to penicillin, then clindamycin 600 mg should be used and can be administered either IM or IV.

What are the hemodynamic goals during anesthesia?

Intraoperative management goals include the following:
- *Maintain sinus rhythm.*
- *Maintain adequate preload* to enhance PBF and CO. Dehydration can prove to be hemodynamically significant and detrimental for Fontan patients. Fasting intervals should be minimized to ensure adequate preoperative hydration and when possible Fontan patients should be scheduled as the first case of the day. Clear liquid intake should be allowed until 2 hours prior to surgery. In older patients, preoperative placement of IV access and IV fluid administration should be considered, particularly if the case is scheduled later in the day.
- *Avoid or minimize increases in PVR,* as increased PVR can compromise ventricular filling and CO. Hypoxia, hypercarbia, acidosis, hypothermia, inadequate analgesia or anesthesia, vasoactive drug use, excessive mean airway pressure, or compression of the lung by pleural effusion can all result in increased PVR.
- *Support of ventricular function.* Intraoperative management involves maintenance of adequate perfusion pressures with the use of inotropic support if necessary.
- *Minimize afterload.*

Induction is uneventful, but as the case progresses the patient has persistent hypotension only transiently responsive to repeated fluid boluses. What is the differential diagnosis and what potential therapies should be considered?

The differential diagnosis for hypotension in this patient includes hypovolemia, vasodilation, cardiac depression, arrhythmia, and/or obstruction to flow across the Fontan circulation. This patient is susceptible to hypotension due to her preexisting depressed right ventricular function and elevated Fontan pressure. These factors are exacerbated by hypovolemia and any cause of decreased blood flow through the Fontan circulation. Fluid boluses may be required to counteract decreased preload. However, if the patient is no longer responding to fluid boluses it is appropriate to initiate inotropic support for persistent hypotension.

The initiation of PPV after intubation can also result in hypotension, as PPV can result in decreased PBF and CO due to decreased systemic venous return with increased intrathoracic pressure and an increase in PVR. Appropriate ventilatory parameters during PPV include moderately elevated tidal volumes, low respiratory rate, a long expiratory time, and minimal positive end-expiratory pressure to maintain low PVR and mean airway pressure. It would be beneficial to reassess ventilation strategies and consider starting inotropic support if necessary. A summary of common agents used for hemodynamic support and their effects on the Fontan circulation is presented in Table 30.4.

The patient in this scenario is also pacemaker-dependent and sudden loss of capture can lead to hypotension. Other potential arrhythmias include junctional rhythm and atrial arrhythmias such as flutter or fibrillation. Acute episodes of atrial tachycardia should be terminated early due to the risk of rapid deterioration. In the case of refractory hypotension, potential obstruction across the Fontan pathway due to thrombus formation should be considered. In this case, it is likely that the patient will also experience significant hypoxemia. If thrombus formation is suspected, then the patient should be urgently anticoagulated with heparin, taken for cardiac catheterization, and if necessary extracorporeal membrane oxygenation (ECMO) support may be considered.

Clinical Pearl

The first step in managing intraoperative hypotension should be intravenous fluid replacement. Should hypotension persist the initiation of inotropic therapies should be considered.

Table 30.4 Agents for the Hemodynamic Management of the Failing Fontan

Agent	Effects
Oxygen	Lowers PVR
Dobutamine α-antagonist, β-agonist	Inodilator Lowers PVR, SVR Easily titratable
Dopamine α- and β-agonist	Inotropy and vasoconstriction Increased SVR and PVR (greater than epinephrine) Tachycardia/arrhythmogenic
Epinephrine α- and β-agonist	Inotropy and vasoconstriction Increased SVR and PVR Tachycardia/arrhythmogenic
Milrinone Phosphodiesterase type 3 inhibitor	Lusitropy Lowers PVR and SVR Not easily titratable
Inhaled nitric oxide	Decreases PVR
Nitroglycerin/nitroprusside	Decrease SVR Decreases preload

PVR, pulmonary vascular resistance; SVR, systemic vascular resistance.

The ECG rhythm changes abruptly to atrial flutter with a rapid ventricular response. What management options exist?

The acute management of atrial tachyarrhythmias is dependent on the hemodynamic status of the patient. In a stable patient, management includes rate control and cardioversion and, if persistent, anticoagulation to prevent thromboembolism. Options for rate control include ß-blockers, calcium channel blockers, or amiodarone. In unstable patients, atrial tachyarrhythmias can be terminated by electrical cardioversion, overdrive pacing, or drug therapy. Pharmacologic cardioversion can be used acutely. Amiodarone is the medication used most often; however, ibutilide or sotalol may also be used. Intraoperative atrial tachyarrhythmia management, particularly if the patient becomes unstable, can be supported by guidance from the cardiac electrophysiologist. Once a patient has experienced an atrial arrhythmia, recurrences are common, thus rhythm control is generally recommended.

Atrial tachyarrhythmias occur in 40%–50% of patients with a Fontan pathway, and these patients have an increased risk of sudden death, stroke, and heart failure [7]. The occurrence of atrial arrhythmias following Fontan surgery is determined by the type of Fontan procedure, with a lower incidence of atrial arrhythmias following the lateral tunnel and extracardiac operations compared to the classic atriopulmonary Fontan [11]. Risk factors for the development of tachyarrhythmias include atriopulmonary connection, right atrial dilation, history of AV valve surgery and/or AV valve regurgitation, and a history of immediate postoperative arrhythmias.

Patients with CHD, and Fontan physiology in particular, have anatomic and physiologic factors that can make conventional cardiopulmonary resuscitation (CPR) ineffective. In general, CPR may provide 10%–30% of normal blood flow to the heart and 30%–40% of normal blood flow to the brain. These numbers are lower in those patients with already compromised pulmonary and systemic blood flows and cerebral perfusion. Critical components of high-quality CPR include minimal interruptions in chest compressions, compressions of adequate rate and depth, avoidance of leaning between compressions, and avoidance of excessive ventilation. Finally, the early use of extracorporeal life support in patients who have failed CPR has been useful when the etiology of arrest is thought to potentially be from reversible causes [12].

Clinical Pearl

Patients with Fontan physiology have anatomic and physiologic factors that can make conventional CPR ineffective. The early use of extracorporeal life support has been useful in patients in whom the etiology of arrest is thought to be from potentially reversible causes.

What considerations exist with emergent surgery as opposed to a scheduled procedure?

Understanding the proposed surgery and its implications is important to provide a safe perioperative course. If a Fontan patient has to undergo emergency surgery without time for total optimization, it is important to do a preoperative evaluation of the patient's current status and a dedicated assessment of ventricular function. These patients will require both IV hydration and resuscitation before induction of anesthesia and intraoperative monitoring of volume and acid–base status. Transfusions may be necessary depending on the type of surgery.

Postoperative pain control may present a challenge in Fontan patients undergoing major surgery. Although epidural anesthesia has been successfully used, coagulation status should be evaluated prior to its implementation. Subarachnoid block is not recommended because of associated sympathectomy, hypotension, and bradycardia, which are poorly tolerated in Fontan patients. Some centers have implemented erector spinae plane blocks for thoracic pain coverage in patients who are either coagulopathic or who have received intraoperative anticoagulation. These blocks are believed to be safer options, as they are performed in a superficial plane, with lower risk of neurologic sequelae from hematoma formation [13].

How should postoperative care be managed?

Postoperative management of the Fontan patient is similar to management throughout the intraoperative period. It is imperative to maintain adequate intravascular volume and ventilation, normal acid–base status and CO during the immediate recovery period. Finally, adequate analgesia is necessary to avoid increases in catecholamines potentially leading to increases in PVR. However, analgesics should be carefully titrated to avoid hypoventilation. Patients with a pacemaker should have the pacemaker reevaluated by a member of the electrophysiology team prior to discharge.

> **Clinical Pearl**
>
> *Hemodynamic goals for postoperative care include maintaining adequate CO and avoiding increases in PVR. Adequate postoperative analgesia can assist in achieving these goals.*

What is the most appropriate discharge disposition for this patient?

Due to her new onset atrial arrhythmia, this patient should be admitted to an intensive care unit for monitoring postoperatively. In general, the recovery location should be discussed with the patient's cardiologist and surgeon, and arrangements should be made prior to the day of surgery. The postoperative disposition will depend on the patient's overall preoperative status, the type of surgery performed, and the perioperative course. A Fontan patient with well-compensated physiology undergoing wisdom teeth extraction can be considered for same day discharge if the perioperative course remains uncomplicated. If there is concern that the patient will be unable to maintain an adequate volume status and CO due to nausea, vomiting, or the inability to take fluids orally, then the patient should be admitted to an inpatient unit for IV hydration. On the other hand, patients with failing Fontan circulation undergoing a low-risk procedure such as this should still be considered for inpatient recovery despite an uncomplicated perioperative course. Escalation of care should depend on the patient's ventricular function, comorbid conditions, and intraoperative course.

Should this procedure be performed at an outpatient facility or ambulatory care center?

Although wisdom teeth extractions can be safely performed at an outpatient facility, in the case of the patient with failing Fontan, surgery should take place at a facility with an appropriate support system including cardiologists, nurses, and ancillary staff comfortable managing patients with CHD, in particular those with Fontan physiology.

When would a failing Fontan be considered for heart transplant?

Patients referred for transplant due to failing Fontan circulation have two different modes of presentation. These patients are categorized into those with systolic ventricular dysfunction and those with relatively preserved systolic ventricular function but suffering from the complications of the failed Fontan circulation. The primary indication for heart transplantation is systolic ventricular dysfunction. However, despite preserved ventricular function patients who demonstrate sequelae of a failed Fontan prior to transplant are at high risk of mortality, with a greater than threefold risk of death within one year after transplant compared to those with ventricular dysfunction [14].

Conclusion

Patients with Fontan circulation are experiencing improved long-term outcomes and longer life expectancy, and hence present more often for noncardiac surgery. A comprehensive understanding of the Fontan circulation is required to provide safe care to both well-functioning and failing Fontan patients in the perioperative period.

References

1. V. G. Nasr, S.J. Staffa, D. Zurakowski, et al. Pediatric risk stratification is improved by integrating both patient comorbidities and intrinsic surgical risk. *Anesthesiology* 2019; **130**: 971–80.

2. G. P. Diller, A. Kempny, R. Alonso-Gonzalez, et al. Survival prospects and circumstances of death in contemporary adult congenital heart disease patients under follow-up at a large tertiary centre. *Circulation* 2015; **132**: 2118–25.

3. B. J. Deal and M. L. Jacobs. Management of the failing Fontan circulation. *Heart* 2012; **98**: 1098–104.

4. D. J. Goldberg, R. E. Shaddy, C. Ravishankar, et al. The failing Fontan: etiology, diagnosis and management. *Expert Rev Cardiovasc Ther* 2011; **9**: 785–93.

5. H. Senzaki, S. Masutani, H. Ishido, et al. Cardiac rest and reserve function in patients with Fontan circulation. *J Am Coll Cardiol* 2006; **47**: 2528–35.

6. S. S. Eagle and S. M. Daves. The adult with Fontan physiology: systematic approach to perioperative management for noncardiac surgery. *J Cardiothorac Vasc Anesth* 2011; **25**: 320–34.

7. A. Karbassi, K. Nair, L. Harris, et al. Atrial tachyarrhythmia in adult congenital heart disease. *World J Cardiol* 2017; **9**: 496–507.

8. A. D. Pitkin, M. C. Wesley, K.J. Guleserian, et al. Perioperative management of a patient with failed Fontan physiology. *Semin Cardiothorac Vasc Anesth* 2013; **17**: 61–5.

9. P. D. Bailey and D. R. Jobes. The Fontan patient. *Anesth Clin* 2009; **27**: 285–300.

10. W. Wilson, K. A. Taubert, M. Gewitz, et al. Prevention of infective endocarditis: guidelines from the American Heart Association: a guideline from the American Heart Association Rheumatic Fever, Endocarditis and Kawasaki Disease Committee, Council on Cardiovascular Disease in the Young, and the Council on Clinical Cardiology, Council on Cardiovascular Surgery and Anesthesia, and the Quality of Care and Outcomes Research Interdisciplinary Working Group. *J Am Dent Assoc* 2008; **139**: 3S–24S.

11. S. Ovroutski, I. Dahnert, V. Alexi-Meskishvili, et al. Preliminary analysis of arrhythmias after the Fontan operation with extracardiac conduit compared with intra-atrial lateral tunnel. *Thorac Cardiovasc Surg* 2001; **49**: 334–7.

12. B. S. Marino, S. Tabbutt, G. MacLaren, et al. Cardiopulmonary resuscitation in infants and children with cardiac disease: a scientific statement from the American Heart Association. *Circulation* 2018; **137**: e691–782.

13. C. Noss, K. J. Anderson, and A. J. Gregory. Erector spinae plane block for open-heart surgery: a potential tool for improved analgesia. *J Cardiothorac Vasc Anesth* 2019; **33**: 376–7.

14. E. R. Griffiths, A. K. Kaza, M. C. Wyler von Ballmoos, et al. Evaluating failing Fontans for heart transplantation: predictors of death. *Ann Thorac Surg* 2009; **88**: 558–64.

Suggested Reading

Jolley M., Colan S. D., Rhodes J., et al. Fontan physiology revisited. *Anesth Anal* 2015; **121**: 172–82.

Windsor J., Townsley M. M., Briston D., et al. Fontan palliation for single-ventricle physiology: perioperative management for noncardiac surgery and analysis of outcomes. *J Cardiothorac Vasc Anesth* 2017; **31**: 2296–303.

Chapter

31

Duchenne Muscular Dystrophy

Elizabeth R. Vogel and Annette Y. Schure

Case Scenario

A 20-year-old male with Duchenne muscular dystrophy presents to the cardiac catheterization laboratory for automatic implantable cardioverter defibrillator insertion. He was recently evaluated for palpitations and found to have intermittent runs of nonsustained ventricular tachycardia. He follows up annually with his cardiologist. He had spine surgery at age 12 years for scoliosis, is no longer ambulatory, and uses a wheelchair. He is also followed by a pulmonologist. Pulmonary function tests 2 weeks earlier were consistent with severe restrictive lung disease with forced expiratory volume 10% predicted, forced vital capacity 8% predicted, and pCO_2 100 mm Hg. He was started on bilevel positive airway pressure respiratory support at night, which he tolerates. His current vital signs are heart rate 110 beats/minute, respiratory rate 20 breaths/minute, blood pressure 102/64, and SpO_2 93% on room air.

His last echocardiogram, performed 11 months ago, demonstrated the following:

- *Moderate-to-severe left ventricular dysfunction (ejection fraction 30%)*
- *Posterolateral akinesis*

Key Objectives

- Discuss the cardiopulmonary morbidity associated with Duchenne muscular dystrophy.
- Describe the preoperative assessment of patients with Duchenne muscular dystrophy.
- Understand important considerations for the anesthetic management of these patients.
- Evaluate various strategies for intra- and postoperative cardiac and respiratory support of patients with Duchenne muscular dystrophy.

Pathophysiology

What is Duchenne muscular dystrophy and what is the underlying pathophysiology?

Duchenne muscular dystrophy (DMD) is a progressive neuromuscular disorder that is inherited in an X-linked recessive pattern, therefore predominantly affecting the male offspring of maternal carriers. However, nearly 30% of cases are due to random mutation rather than hereditary transmission. The incidence is approximately 1:5000 to 1:3500 live births. Duchenne muscular dystrophy is caused by a mutation on Xp21 that results in the absence of dystrophin, a structural protein critical to the dystroglycan complex found in skeletal and cardiac muscle cells. This complex stabilizes the muscle cell membrane during contraction. Without the dystroglycan complex, the cellular membrane is fragile, leading to cell damage and eventual necrosis over time. The subsequent scarring with fatty infiltration and fibrosis results in progressive muscular weakness and dysfunction.

What is the typical timeline for presentation and progression of symptoms in patients with DMD?

Duchenne muscular dystrophy is characterized by progressive muscle weakness and damage that impacts both skeletal and cardiac muscle tissue. Symptoms typically manifest as clumsiness, weakness, or failure to meet gross motor milestones by 3–5 years of age. Loss of ability to ambulate usually occurs around age 12 years. Cardiac muscle damage and fibrosis lead to clinically evident cardiomyopathy in the mid-to-late teen years, though evidence of cardiac damage can be seen much earlier on cardiac magnetic resonance imaging (MRI) and electrocardiogram (ECG) evaluations. Chest wall and diaphragmatic weakness eventually result in respiratory insufficiency and the need for respiratory support in the late teens to early 20s. In the past, respiratory insufficiency and infections were the leading cause of death for patients with DMD, but now, with early noninvasive respiratory support, heart failure and arrhythmias are often life limiting.

Clinical Pearl

In the past, respiratory insufficiency and infections were the leading cause of death for patients with DMD, but now, with early noninvasive respiratory support, heart failure and arrhythmias are often life limiting.

239

What are the cardiac implications of DMD?

The absence of dystrophin in cardiac muscle cells causes gradual damage and destruction of cardiac muscle fibers and increasing fibrosis. Patients develop a progressive form of cardiomyopathy with a steady decline in cardiac function and ejection fraction (EF). Diagnostic studies can reveal early myocardial changes in asymptomatic children. For instance, ECG abnormalities have been noted in >50% of children <5 years of age. Early fibrosis and decrease in cardiac strain capacity can be seen on cardiac MRI within a similar age group. Echocardiographic and clinical evidence of cardiomyopathy typically present in 50% of patients by age 15, though clinical symptoms are not always readily apparent in nonambulatory patients. More than 90% of patients will have clinically significant cardiomyopathy by age 18.

The dilated cardiomyopathy seen in patients with DMD is characterized by systolic and diastolic dysfunction. Diastolic dysfunction usually precedes systolic dysfunction and may be present even in young children. Over time, EF decreases and cardiac output (CO) falls. The ventricles are often dilated with elevated left atrial and ventricular end-diastolic pressures, potentially resulting in valvular dysfunction (mitral or tricuspid regurgitation). The myocardium may also become increasingly arrhythmogenic; this can manifest as simple ectopy, atrial or ventricular dysrhythmias, and heart block.

What is the current treatment for patients with DMD? Are there special considerations for the perioperative period?

The cardiomyopathy associated with DMD is often treated with a variety of medications. These can include cardioselective ß-blockers to prevent excessive sympathetic activation, angiotensin converting enzyme inhibitors (ACEi) or angiotensin receptor blockers (ARBs) for afterload reduction, diuretics to reduce volume overload, antiarrhythmics, and occasionally inotropic support.

- *Corticosteroids* are used to preserve muscle strength and prolong functional abilities such as walking. Depending on the dose, duration, and dosing regimen, they can be associated with numerous side effects, including iatrogenic adrenal insufficiency and fracture risk. For more invasive procedures, use of a perioperative stress dose of steroids should be considered.
- *ß-blocker*: ß-blocker therapy should be continued in the perioperative period to avoid reflex tachycardia, unless discontinued by the electrophysiologist in preparation for the procedure.

- *Afterload reduction*: ACEi or ARBs should be withheld for 24 hours prior to anesthesia or sedation to prevent hypotension.
- *Diuretics*: Chronic diuretic therapy can lead to significant electrolyte disturbances, especially hypokalemia, and should prompt preoperative electrolyte checks. Vasodilation during anesthesia or sedation often unmasks latent hypovolemia and can result in significant hypotension, requiring careful fluid resuscitation and temporary vasoconstrictor therapy.
- *Antiarrhythmics*: Generally, antiarrhythmics should be continued in the perioperative period, but occasionally electrophysiologists prefer to withhold longer acting medications to facilitate testing during the procedure. Close communication with the cardiologist is important.
- *Inotropic support*: Some patients are on long-term home inotropic support with milrinone, which can cause platelet dysfunction. If possible, central access dedicated to this medication should not be disconnected or used for anesthesia induction, as an inadvertent milrinone bolus can result in significant hypotension that is difficult to treat.
- *Destination therapy with left ventricular (LV) assist devices*: While DMD patients are not candidates for heart transplantation, under special circumstances ventricular assist devices may be implanted to improve the remaining quality of life.

What are the pulmonary implications of DMD?

Duchenne muscular dystrophy causes progressive destruction and weakness of the respiratory muscles, a decline in total lung capacity, and eventually the inability to maintain adequate tidal volumes. As the disease advances, patients typically require noninvasive respiratory support only at night initially, but later it may also be necessary during the day. The need for continuous respiratory support may prompt placement of a tracheostomy for ongoing mechanical ventilatory support. It is important to clarify the patient's respiratory status at the time of surgery and discuss their plans for future respiratory support.

Cough and airway clearance ability are frequently impaired. Some patients use cough assist devices to prevent atelectasis and mucous plugs. Weakness of the oropharyngeal muscles results in decreased ability to manage secretions and increased risk of aspiration. Patients with DMD frequently suffer from recurrent pneumonias and respiratory tract infections.

Anesthetic Implications

How should this patient's cardiac function be evaluated preoperatively? What abnormalities might be expected?

Preoperative evaluation of cardiac function should include a baseline ECG to screen for arrhythmias or conduction abnormalities and a recent echocardiogram or cardiac MRI to assess ventricular and valvular function.

Left ventricular hypertrophy is the most common finding in young DMD patients, with the ECG demonstrating Q-waves in lead III or V6. Older patients typically have deep Q waves in leads I, aVL, V5, and V6 with right ventricular (RV) hypertrophy and a shortened PR interval. A pseudo-infarction pattern consistent with a posterior or posterolateral infarct is common. Many patients develop persistent sinus tachycardia, defined as a heart rate >100 beats/minute after 12 years of age. This tachycardia is termed "disordered automaticity" and is presumably due to a sympathetic imbalance or impaired autonomic function. Atrial fibrillation, atrial flutter, and ventricular tachyarrhythmias are also common.

An echocardiogram should be performed to evaluate the degree of ventricular dysfunction and potential valvular involvement. Left ventricular posterior wall thinning, posterolateral akinesis, LV dilation and decreased shortening/ejection fraction are typical findings. However, many DMD patients are technically challenging to scan, as thoracic deformities result in poor acoustic windows and suboptimal image quality.

A cardiac MRI (CMR) is currently the preferred imaging modality for basic cardiac assessment in patients with DMD. It can provide more detailed information about ventricular function and myocardial strain patterns, and, with late gadolinium enhancement, allow for early detection of myocardial fibrosis, well before the onset of clinical manifestations. Furthermore, unlike echocardiography, CMR is not affected by acoustic windows or lung artifact. Unfortunately, previous spine surgery with extensive instrumentation often prevents adequate CMR imaging in many DMD patients.

Preoperative assessment should also include a discussion with the patient about any recent functional changes, cardiac symptoms, or alterations to their medication regimen. It is important to note, however, that even when significant cardiomyopathy is noted on imaging studies symptoms are often absent due to the patient's limited ambulation and physical activity.

> **Clinical Pearl**
>
> *Many patients develop persistent sinus tachycardia, defined as a heart rate >100 beats/minute after 12 years of age. This tachycardia is termed "disordered automaticity" and is presumably due to a sympathetic imbalance or impaired autonomic function. Atrial fibrillation, atrial flutter, and ventricular tachyarrhythmias are also common.*

How should this patient's pulmonary function be evaluated?

Preoperative assessment of pulmonary function should include a thorough discussion of the patient's current respiratory status, their baseline requirement for respiratory support and oxygen therapy, and their ability to lie flat.

Baseline oxygenation and gas exchange, lung volumes, and the patient's ability to cough and clear the airway have significant implications for perioperative management. Oxygenation can be assessed using pulse oximetry. Inadequate oxygen saturations on room air may be an early sign of respiratory insufficiency and an indication for initiation of ventilatory support. Oxyhemoglobin saturations lower than 95% on room air should prompt further evaluation. Awake carbon dioxide tension measured with capnography or blood gas sampling (arterial or venous) can determine the presence of hypoventilation with hypercarbia.

In addition, spirometric pulmonary function tests (PFTs) should document forced vital capacity (FVC), forced expiratory volume (FEV_1), maximal mid-expiratory flow rate, maximum inspiratory and expiratory pressures, and peak cough flow. According to the American College of Chest Physicians consensus statement on respiratory support in DMD, a decreased FVC may be associated with an increased risk of postoperative respiratory failure. Patients with an FVC < 50% predicted have an increased risk of respiratory complications while those with an FVC < 30% predicted are at high risk of complications. For high-risk DMD patients, preoperative training in noninvasive ventilation should be considered to facilitate extubation and the transition to noninvasive positive pressure ventilation (NPPV) following surgery. A measured peak cough flow <270 L/minute identifies patients with ineffective airway clearance who could benefit from cough assistance techniques and should also be preoperatively trained with a mechanical insufflation–exsufflation device.

Are there other implications for DMD patients?

Many patients with DMD also suffer from gastrointestinal symptoms and can present with poor nutritional status. Gastric paresis and intestinal dysmotility lead to frequent vomiting, inadequate oral intake, and constipation. Adequate nutrition is important for respiratory function (increased work of breathing) and for wound healing. In bilevel positive airway pressure dependent patients, it can often be achieved only with special enteral formulations administered through a gastrostomy tube.

Significant contractures and poor mobility can result in development of pressure ulcers and increased risk for fractures. Positioning can be very difficult and requires careful attention to adequate padding of all pressure points.

What other issues should be discussed with the patient/family?

The preoperative discussion should address goals of care and resuscitation preferences. The patient's wishes regarding prolonged dependence on mechanical ventilation should be documented and respected. If not already done, this is also the appropriate time to offer assistance with advanced directives, living wills, and the identification of a medical proxy. Ideally the discussion should include both the patient and their designated medical proxy to avoid any confusion or uncertainty. Finally, prior to any procedure, there should be a clear understanding and agreement between members of the patient's care team whether advanced resuscitative techniques and hemodynamic support options such as extracorporeal membrane oxygenation (ECMO) and/or LV assist device placement are medically possible and desired by the patient and family.

Do patients with DMD carry an increased risk for developing malignant hyperthermia?

There is no association between DMD and risk of malignant hyperthermia. Patients with DMD have the same risk of malignant hyperthermia as the general population. However, DMD is associated with a significant risk of rhabdomyolysis and hyperkalemia during exposure to volatile anesthetics and succinylcholine. Use of volatile anesthetics in this patient population remains controversial. While numerous case reports of rhabdomyolysis with even low-level volatile anesthetics have been published, many volatile anesthetics have been performed in patients with DMD without any evidence of rhabdomyolysis. The exact mechanism is unknown, but it is possible that volatile anesthetics can induce additional destabilization of the cellular membrane in patients with DMD. The risk of rhabdomyolysis seems to decrease with increasing age, most likely due to loss of muscle mass and increasing fibrosis.

Given the risk of rhabdomyolysis and hyperkalemia, volatile anesthetics are generally avoided in this population. Succinylcholine should never be administered to a patient with DMD because of the likelihood of a hyperkalemic cardiac arrest. Total intravenous anesthesia is the preferred technique. If intravenous (IV) access is unattainable, even with oral or intramuscular premedication and nitrous oxide (which is safe), a short exposure to a volatile anesthetic for induction and venous access may be acceptable after careful risk/benefit evaluation. Prolonged exposure, however, is not recommended.

What are some of the considerations for using monitored anesthesia care for this procedure?

Automatic implantable cardioverter–defibrillator (AICD) insertion is a minimally invasive procedure that typically requires transvenous access to the heart via the subclavian or cephalic vein as well as the creation of a subcutaneous pocket for the generator. This can often be performed under local anesthesia with IV sedation as needed. The duration of the procedure can vary significantly, depending on the time it takes to find acceptable myocardial sites for the intracardiac electrodes and the testing of the system. Occasionally, the presence of extensive myocardial fibrosis, an "irritable" myocardium, and poor cardiac function necessitate multiple attempts. Furthermore, rescue defibrillations can have a negative impact on the already borderline cardiac function.

Depending on the patient's baseline functional status and whether she or he is amenable, the administration of minimal sedation with midazolam, ketamine, or dexmedetomidine, and local anesthetic infiltration by the proceduralist may allow for device placement without significant negative impact on cardiopulmonary function. However, this patient is 20 years old and has experienced significant progression of his neuromuscular disease, currently requiring noninvasive respiratory support overnight. His baseline SpO_2 on room air is only 93%, a sign of borderline respiratory function. His preoperative PFT results clearly put him in a high-risk category for respiratory complications. Any level of sedation can further impair his respiratory status by decreasing his upper airway muscle tone and leading to airway obstruction. During a procedure in the supine position requiring sedation for device testing he will benefit from the use of NPPV. The potential need for more invasive ventilation strategies (i.e., intubation) in response to complications should be discussed during the preoperative evaluation and consent process.

From a cardiac perspective, patients with heart failure often require elevated levels of circulating catecholamines to maintain cardiac output. Even minimal sedation can decrease sympathetic activation and result in inadequate perfusion. The circulation time is often prolonged, and the onset of medication effects can be delayed. Sedatives should be given in small increments and carefully titrated to effect. Some patients may require low-dose inotropic support (e.g., epinephrine 0.02 mcg/kg/minute) to allow for adequate sedation. On the other hand, untreated anxiety and pain can cause increases in afterload and/or ectopy that would be poorly tolerated by a failing ventricle.

Clinical Pearl

Patients with cardiomyopathy can have a significantly prolonged circulation time and thus the onset of medication effects is often delayed. Sedatives should be given in small increments and carefully titrated to effect.

What kind of vascular access and monitoring is indicated?

Severe muscle atrophy and contractures can complicate peripheral vascular access. Anesthesia providers should allow for additional time and be prepared to use ultrasound guided techniques. The placement of additional vascular access for inotropic support should always be considered, especially in the catheterization laboratory, where access to the patient is extremely limited once the procedure has begun. Ultrasound guidance can also be useful to identify possible central venous or ECMO cannulation sites in the event of complications.

The need for invasive monitoring depends on the patient's respiratory and cardiac status. An arterial line provides accurate blood pressure readings during prolonged periods of ectopy or low cardiac output states and facilitates respiratory monitoring.

What are the considerations for induction and maintenance of a general anesthetic if this patient is unable to tolerate the procedure under sedation?

The need for general anesthesia in case of failed sedation and/or procedural complications should always be anticipated. Some patients, especially if untrained, are unable to tolerate the facemask for NPPV. Syringe pumps with the IV anesthetic(s) of choice, vasoactive infusions, and intubation equipment should be readily accessible. Given the limited access to the patient in the catheterization lab, it is best to make the decision to induce general anesthesia before the patient is fully draped and positioned, otherwise the procedure should be stopped and access to the patient optimized. Preoxygenation with 100% FiO_2 either via facemask or the noninvasive ventilation device is very important. The primary goal during anesthetic induction is maintenance of cardiac output by avoiding ventricular depression, hypotension, and tachycardia. Depending on the patient's cardiac status, it may be beneficial to start inotropic support prior to induction. Owing to their relatively minimal hemodynamic effects, ketamine and etomidate are commonly used induction agents. It is important to note that ketamine, while typically well tolerated, does have direct myocardial depressant effects that can manifest in patients with significant cardiomyopathy and chronic sympathetic activation. Propofol is an alternative but should be titrated slowly in small doses to effect to minimize its vasodilating and cardiodepressant properties. Anesthetic maintenance can be accomplished with a total IV anesthetic technique using a carefully titrated propofol infusion. Adjuvant dexmedetomidine or ketamine infusions can be helpful to decrease propofol requirements. If local anesthesia is not providing adequate analgesia, a short-acting opioid infusion such as remifentanil can be added.

What options exist for respiratory management of this patient intraoperatively under sedation or general anesthesia?

If the patient is not at increased risk for aspiration, tolerates the facemask, and has adequate ventilation and gas exchange with acceptable pressure support, a noninvasive ventilation device can be used. Patients who use NPPV at home should always be instructed to bring their system to the hospital to use in the perioperative period when allowed.

In case of airway obstruction due to poor upper airway muscle tone or inadequate mask seal, a laryngeal mask airway (LMA) could be an alternative. For prolonged and more invasive procedures, and/or patients who are at risk for aspiration or have restrictive lung disease, a secure airway with an endotracheal tube is the best option, as it also allows clearance of secretions and mucus.

Are there any concerns about intubation in patients with DMD?

Compared to the general population, patients with DMD are at increased risk for difficult laryngoscopy. Progressive fibrotic infiltration of oropharyngeal and cervical muscles can lead to tongue hypertrophy, restricted mouth opening, and limited neck movement. Difficult airway equipment such as a video laryngoscope or a flexible fiberoptic bronchoscope should be readily available.

What are the implications of utilizing neuromuscular blocking drugs in patients with DMD?

Depolarizing neuromuscular blocking drugs such as succinylcholine are absolutely contraindicated in patients with DMD due to the risk of hyperkalemic cardiac arrest secondary to profound rhabdomyolysis. Nondepolarizing neuromuscular blocking drugs may be used with caution if muscle relaxation is necessary. The onset, duration, and time to recovery is significantly prolonged in patients with DMD. Given the increased risk of respiratory insufficiency after anesthesia, maintenance and full recovery of the remaining muscle function are critical. Therefore, neuromuscular blockade is often avoided. Adequate intubating conditions can be achieved with propofol and remifentanil. Alternatively, for patients with severe cardiomyopathy who are unable to tolerate intubating doses of propofol, rocuronium can be used, but the onset of full relaxation will be delayed. Several case reports have described the successful use of sugammadex for reversal of rocuronium-induced neuromuscular blockade in patients with DMD.

What intraoperative hemodynamic changes should be anticipated?

Even minimal sedation can lead to hemodynamic instability in a patient with significant cardiomyopathy. Endogenous catecholamine secretion is typically elevated at baseline and can be affected by sedative medications or general anesthesia resulting in decreased cardiac output, vasodilation, and hypotension. Early inotropic support may be required; consider epinephrine (0.02–0.04 mcg/kg/minute), dopamine (5–10 mcg/kg/minute), or milrinone (0.25–0.5 mcg/kg/minute). However, depending on the extent of myocardial fibrosis and cardiomyopathy, the heart may have limited ability to increase contractility.

Although beneficial from a respiratory standpoint, positive pressure ventilation can decrease LV wall tension and preload to the RV. Depending on the patient's volume status and the degree of diastolic dysfunction, slow and careful fluid resuscitation may be necessary.

What complications may occur during pacemaker or AICD placement?

Possible complications during the procedure may be divided into access- and device-related problems:

- *Access-related complications* can include pneumo- or hemothorax, air embolism, and later, thrombosis. The risk of intraoperative pneumothorax varies from 0.6% to 5% (average 2%) depending on the procedural approach. The highest risk of pneumothorax occurs with a blind subclavian approach. Use of fluoroscopy during subclavian access somewhat decreases this risk. Vascular access via the cephalic vein, axillary vein, internal jugular vein, or femoral vein carries a lower risk. Given the impaired respiratory status of patients with DMD, pneumothorax is poorly tolerated and must be recognized and treated expeditiously.

- *Device-related complications* can be caused by the leads or the generator. Arrhythmias during lead placement are common but generally self-limited. Recurrent arrhythmias without adequate recovery periods (e.g., during the testing phase) can lead to significant hemodynamic compromise and may require treatment. In rare occasions, perforation of the atrial or ventricular wall by the pacing wires cause pericardial effusion and possible tamponade. The risk is increased during the placement of atrial (thin wall) or biventricular leads for cardiac resynchronization therapy.

What are the postoperative respiratory risks for patients with DMD? How can these be mitigated?

Patients with DMD are at high risk of postoperative respiratory failure. The lowest level of sedation necessary should be used during the procedure. Whenever possible, pain control should be achieved with local anesthesia and regional techniques to limit the use of opioids and the risk of respiratory depression. Noninvasive respiratory support can be extended into the postoperative period until the patient returns to his baseline level of respiratory function. If intubation or LMA placement was necessary, transition to NPPV should occur immediately after removal of the airway device for patients who use NPPV chronically. For all other patients, transition to NPPV after extubation or LMA removal should be strongly considered, particularly for those with FVC <50% predicted. Supplemental oxygen should be carefully titrated to the lowest level necessary to maintain adequate saturations; otherwise, hypoventilation, poor clearance of secretions, and atelectasis are easily masked.

Does this patient require an intensive care bed postoperatively?

The level of care during the postoperative recovery strongly depends on the degree of residual sedation, analgesic requirements, and need for respiratory or hemodynamic support. A back-up intensive care unit (ICU) bed should be available. If the patient was able to tolerate the procedure with minimal sedation and returns to his baseline status, extended recovery and inpatient overnight observation for late cardiac or respiratory complications is reasonable. Many hospitals will allow patients on stable chronic noninvasive respiratory support to return to the floor. Patients who required intubation or LMA placement and were extubated to NPPV support should be admitted to an ICU or stepdown unit where therapeutic respiratory modalities are more readily available. For some patients, the surgical procedure may unmask the need for a higher level of respiratory support with mechanical ventilation or prolonged NPPV.

How should postoperative pain be treated?

The use of opioids should be minimized whenever possible to reduce respiratory depression and cough suppression. A multimodal analgesic approach to pain control is optimal, using acetaminophen, nonsteroidal antiinflammatory agents, and local anesthesia. Pectus or intercostal nerve blocks can be useful regional anesthesia techniques to provide long-lasting analgesia after pacemaker placement.

Suggested Reading

Allen H. D., Thrush P. T., Hoffman T. M., et al. Cardiac management in neuromuscular diseases. *Phys Med Rehabil Clin N Am* 2012; **23**: 855–68.

Birnkrant D. J., Panitch H. B., Benditt J. O., et al. American College of Chest Physicians consensus statement on the respiratory and related management of patients with Duchenne muscular dystrophy undergoing anesthesia or sedation. *Chest* 2007; **132**: 1977–86.

Cripe L. H. and Tobias J. D. Cardiac considerations in the operative management of the patient with Duchenne or Becker muscular dystrophy. *Paediatr Anaesth* 2013; **23**: 777–84.

Hayes J., Veyckemans F., and Bissonnette B. Duchenne muscular dystrophy: an old anesthesia problem revisited. *Paediatr Anaesth* 2008; **18**: 100–6.

Ing R. J., Ames W. A., and Chambers N. A. Paediatric cardiomyopathy and anaesthesia. *Br J Anaesth* 2012; **108**: 4–12.

Kamdar F. and Garry D. J. Dystrophin-deficient cardiomyopathy. *J Am Coll Cardiol* 2016; **67**: 2533–46.

Kotsakou M., Kioumis I., Lazaridis G., et al. Pacemaker insertion. *Ann Transl Med* 2015; **3**: 42.

Dilated Cardiomyopathy

Stephen Alcos and Andreas W. Loepke

Key Objectives

- Describe the pathophysiology and presentation of dilated cardiomyopathy.
- Specify how it differs from other forms of cardiomyopathy.
- Identify preprocedural assessment for patients with dilated cardiomyopathy.
- Discuss anesthetic options and risks for the patient in this scenario.

Pathophysiology

How is dilated cardiomyopathy defined?

Cardiomyopathy is a disease of the myocardium associated with cardiac dysfunction that cannot be explained by abnormal loading conditions or congenital heart disease. Dilated cardiomyopathy (DCM) is a phenotypic class of cardiomyopathy that is defined by ventricular chamber dilation with dysfunction that is secondary to ineffective systolic shortening. One or both ventricles can be affected. It is frequently associated with increased myocardial mass but decreased wall thickness.

What causes DCM?

In children without known structural heart abnormalities DCM is the most common cause of congestive heart failure (CHF), with the highest incidence noted in infancy. While two-thirds of cases are idiopathic, it is imperative to search for underlying causes, especially in infants who are more likely to have metabolic disease that can be treatable. Identifiable causes of DCM include myocarditis, neuro-muscular disorders, familial and metabolic disorders, and toxin exposure. Viral infections are the most common cause of myocarditis. Anthracycline exposure is a risk factor for the development of cardiomyopathy in patients who have been treated with this chemotherapeutic agent for neoplastic disease.

How do other forms of cardiomyopathy differ from DCM?

Other cardiomyopathy phenotypes include the following:

- ***Hypertrophic cardiomyopathy*** is characterized by abnormal left and/or right ventricular hypertrophy that occurs in the absence of an obvious stimulus. Ventricular volumes are normal or diminished.

Hypertrophy is usually asymmetrical, with the interventricular septal wall being thicker than the free wall. Obstructions to left or right ventricular outflow tracts are common because of septal hypertrophy. Systolic ventricular function is normal, or even hyperdynamic, until later in the disease process. Familial predisposition and idiopathic origins are most prevalent. It is a leading cause of sudden death in young people.

- **Restrictive cardiomyopathy** is primarily idiopathic in nature and characterized by diastolic dysfunction with normal or reduced ventricular volume and normal ventricular wall thickness. Systolic function is normal in the early phases of the disease and progressively worsens. Atrial enlargement may be present along with elevated atrial and ventricular end-diastolic pressures.
- **Left ventricular noncompaction cardiomyopathy** is caused by the abnormal development of deep myocardial trabeculations, predominantly in the apex of the left ventricle (LV), but right ventricular (RV) involvement can also occur. It is frequently associated with a neuromuscular disorder.
- **Arrhythmogenic RV dysplasia** is characterized by fatty and fibrous infiltration of the myocardium that creates loci for spontaneous arrhythmia development. There is typically regional hypokinesis on echocardiogram. The RV free wall is most often involved, but recent evidence suggests the LV wall can also be affected.

How does DCM present clinically?

Children with DCM most often present with signs and symptoms of CHF, which can be variable and nonspecific. Therefore, diagnosis requires a high index of clinical suspicion. Presenting symptoms also vary with age of the patient. Infants commonly present with feeding intolerance and failure to thrive. Respiratory complaints include tachypnea, shortness of breath, and increased work of breathing. For older children, a low cardiac output state can manifest as poor exercise capacity and gastrointestinal complaints of abdominal pain, nausea, and/or vomiting. Additionally, patients with DCM caused by viral myocarditis may also present with a classic prodrome of fever and myalgias in addition to respiratory and gastrointestinal symptoms.

Clinical Pearl

Dilated cardiomyopathy often presents with signs of CHF, such as failure to thrive, gastrointestinal distress, diminished exercise tolerance, or pulmonary edema. Manifestations may differ depending on the age at presentation.

What does a focused physical exam reveal?

Patients with nonfulminant heart failure can actually present with normal findings on physical examination. Further confounding the matter, examination findings can overlap with other conditions such as gastroenteritis, asthma, or pneumonia. Common physical examination findings are listed in Table 32.1. Hypotension is generally a late and ominous finding, as it implies that the body's compensatory mechanisms have been exhausted. Weak peripheral pulses and cool distal extremities with poor capillary refill are also suggestive of decompensated heart failure.

Clinical Pearl

Hypotension is generally a late and ominous finding, as it implies that the body's compensatory mechanisms have been exhausted.

What is the prognosis of DCM in children?

The outcome of patients presenting with DCM is variable, with some children presenting with fulminant heart failure requiring mechanical circulatory support and transplantation while others recover normal function. Transplant-free survival rates for 5 years post-diagnosis range from 60% to 75% [1]. Factors associated with worse outcomes include older age at diagnosis (>6 years of age), lower shortening fraction, greater LV dilation, and elevated LV end-diastolic pressure (>20–25 mm Hg) [2]. Congestive heart failure at the time of presentation is associated with a higher risk of death or transplantation only in infants <1 year of age. Transplant waitlist mortality is 11%, except in patients who are mechanically ventilated or on mechanical circulatory support [3]. In patients in whom DCM represents part of a multisystem process the underlying disease can also impact patient outcome. Sudden death in children with DCM is quite uncommon.

Table 32.1 Dilated Cardiomyopathy Physical Exam Findings by System

Respiratory	Gastrointestinal	Cardiac
Tachypnea	Hepatomegaly	Tachycardia
Hypoxia	Poor weight gain	Hypotension
Crackles/rales/ wheezing		Murmur/gallop
Retractions		Cool extremities
Increased work of breathing		Delayed capillary refill
		Jugular venous distention

What are the hemodynamic features of DCM?

The primary pathophysiologic features of DCM are ventricular dilation with systolic and diastolic dysfunction, decreased ejection fraction, and decreased cardiac output (CO). The diastolic dysfunction affects both active relaxation and passive compliance, thereby reducing ventricular filling and elevating end-diastolic pressures. Atrial and LV filling pressures are usually elevated. Associated mitral valve regurgitation, tricuspid valve regurgitation, or both often exist. The dilated heart chambers also have the potential to be arrhythmogenic.

What diagnostic modalities are generally utilized?

An echocardiogram is typically diagnostic and essential to quantify systolic and diastolic function, LV end-diastolic dimension, and LV volume. Patients typically have global systolic hypokinesis but may have segmental wall motion abnormalities as well. Atrioventricular valve regurgitation from annular dilation and additional anatomic abnormalities (i.e., outflow obstruction, coarctation, coronary anomalies) can also be identified. In patients with a low cardiac ejection fraction, intracardiac thrombi may be detected.

Electrocardiogram findings are usually nonspecific. A chest radiograph typically demonstrates cardiomegaly and there may be evidence of pulmonary edema. A cardiac magnetic resonance imaging study may show myocardial fibrosis and inflammation in addition to the assessment of myocardial volumes, contractile function, and wall thickness. While brain natriuretic peptide levels are routinely measured in adults for risk stratification of patients in acute decompensated heart failure, their utility in the pediatric population remains unclear. There is some evidence that levels greater than 300 pg/mL are associated with worse outcomes, including death, hospitalization for heart failure, and transplantation [4].

When treating new-onset heart failure in children, it is also important to simultaneously look for underlying metabolic, congenital, or acquired causes. Thus, in this patient, viral titers were sent to rule out myocarditis, and the echocardiogram was also reviewed for structural anomalies such as abnormal coronary artery anatomy.

What pharmacologic therapies are used in DCM patients?

Therapeutic guidelines have largely been extrapolated from adult data as high-quality pediatric studies are lacking. Commonly used chronic heart failure medications used in symptomatic pediatric patients with ventricular dysfunction include angiotensin-converting enzyme inhibitors (ACEi), angiotensin receptor antagonists, and ß-blockers. Diuretics are used therapeutically for treatment of both acute and chronic volume overload and are a mainstay therapy for acute decompensated heart failure. Digoxin has also been used to treat myocardial dysfunction and volume overload in children.

Inotropic support is reserved for low CO states or ongoing hypotension. Milrinone (an inodilator), dobutamine, or low-dose epinephrine may be titrated to effect. However, it is important to keep in mind that a patient with end-stage cardiomyopathy may not show significant improvement with inotropic therapy.

What other treatment options exist?

Children with end-stage heart failure unresponsive to inotropic support may require mechanical circulatory support, either with extracorporeal membrane oxygenation (ECMO) or with a ventricular assist device (VAD). This support may be utilized as a bridge to either recovery (in cases of myocarditis) or heart transplantation. Survival at 10 years post transplantation is 72% [3].

Anesthetic Implications

What are the preoperative considerations?

A thorough history and physical exam along with a review of current medications aids in establishing the patient's current functional baseline. A review of the most recent echocardiogram, chest radiograph, and other available imaging facilitates preanesthetic risk assessment. The patient's cardiologist is also an excellent source of information regarding the patient's clinical status.

Patients on diuretic therapy should have their potassium level checked and normalized if necessary. Most anesthesia providers advocate withholding ACEi on the morning of the procedure to avoid intraoperative hypotension. Patients with an implantable device for biventricular pacing as part of their medical therapy should have their device interrogated to ensure functionality.

What should the parents be told about anesthetic risk?

The anesthetic management of patients with severe cardiomyopathies is associated with high morbidity and mortality. Patients with DCM may suffer from significant cardiopulmonary instability secondary to administration of anesthetic agents, intubation and mechanical ventilation, and noxious stimulation. Life-threatening ventricular arrhythmias may also occur during the perioperative period. For these reasons, parents must have a thorough understanding of the patient's high-risk condition when consent is obtained. Discussions of rescue strategies including mechanical circulatory support should take place prior to the procedure.

What are the intraoperative hemodynamic considerations?

The intraoperative hemodynamic goal for DCM patients is simply to maintain cardiac output while minimizing any increases in oxygen consumption.

This can be achieved by the following:

- Maintain preload.
- Avoid increases in heart rate above baseline (excessive tachycardia).
- Avoid elevations in systemic vascular resistance (SVR).
- Preserve myocardial contractility.
- Optimize coronary perfusion.

A significantly dysfunctional ventricle will not be able to maintain CO in the face of increased SVR, so inotropic support may be needed to optimize contractility.

How might the anesthetic be conducted for this child? How should the airway be managed?

There is no single best approach for induction or maintenance of anesthesia in this patient population. It is advisable to establish reliable intravenous (IV) access prior to induction. Although this patient currently has vascular access, as he is receiving milrinone, it is always advisable to have separate, dedicated IV access for administration of anesthetic and sedative medications. It is important to keep the hemodynamic goals in mind and to titrate anesthetic

agents accordingly. Circulation time can be substantially slowed given the low CO state in many of these patients, so sufficient time should be given for divided doses of medications to take effect. If the patient is receiving IV inotropic and/or vasodilator therapy, these should be continued, and care should be taken to neither interrupt nor inadvertently bolus these medications.

In a child presenting without IV access, oral premedication may be helpful to attenuate anxiety and facilitate separation from the parents. Premedication can also facilitate securing IV access in the operating room or procedure room prior to induction. Oral midazolam 0.25–0.5 mg/kg and, if needed, oral ketamine 4–6 mg/kg is usually adequate. Patients with existing IV access can be premedicated with IV midazolam in titrated doses (0.03–0.05 mg/kg) or IV ketamine in doses of 0.5–1.0 mg/kg if necessary for severe anxiety. Decisions regarding premedication in patients with severe ventricular dysfunction should be made on an individualized basis, and medications should be carefully titrated while the patient is being monitored.

For placement of a peripherally inserted central catheter (PICC), infiltration of the insertion site with local anesthesia can blunt hemodynamic responses to noxious stimulation without causing undue myocardial depression, vasodilation, or hypotension. For this particular case, carefully titrated doses of ketamine 0.5–1.0 mg/kg in combination with titrated doses of dexmedetomidine 0.5–1.0 mcg/kg are often sufficient and can be used for both induction and maintenance. With this technique, spontaneous ventilation can be maintained without necessitating the use of an invasive airway. Supplemental oxygen via nasal cannula is often required to maintain appropriate levels of oxygenation; it is also useful for monitoring of end-tidal CO_2.

For more invasive cases or if endotracheal intubation and mechanical ventilation are necessary, induction of anesthesia with etomidate (0.3 mg/kg) can avert hemodynamic instability. Ketamine (2–4 mg/kg) avoids hypotension, *except for patients with end-stage heart failure*, in whom it can lead to myocardial depression. In general, the anesthetic induction phase must be monitored carefully as patients can swiftly deteriorate due to anesthetic-induced vasodilation. The initiation of low-dose inotropic therapy may be warranted in fragile patients prior to anesthetic induction.

The use of inhaled agents for maintenance of anesthesia should be managed judiciously to avoid hemodynamic instability in light of failing cardiac function. Alternately, a combination of propofol and ketamine infusions can also be used. Caution must also be exercised when opioids are used in conjunction with benzodiazepines, as these medications act synergistically in producing side effects of increased venous capacitance and decreased SVR.

What are the specific risks for a child with DCM undergoing anesthesia?

Generally speaking, children are not as cooperative as adults and therefore require moderate-to-deep sedation or general anesthesia, even for diagnostic procedures. A deeper level of anesthesia inherently exposes the patient to a greater myocardial depressant effect, which is generally not well tolerated in a patient with severe ventricular dysfunction. Children with cardiomyopathy undergoing noncardiac surgery have a high complication rate, with hypotension requiring inotropic therapy occurring in 61% of patients [5]. The Pediatric Perioperative Cardiac Arrest (POCA) registry reports a mortality rate of 50% in children with cardiomyopathy who sustain a perioperative cardiac arrest [6]. Therefore, it is recommended that hemodynamic support, invasive monitoring, and postoperative cardiac intensive care monitoring should be available for patients with severe DCM undergoing anesthetic procedures. In some cases, intraoperative echocardiography may be helpful in determining real-time function and volume status. The availability of ECMO and the patient's suitability for ECMO or mechanical circulatory support options should also be discussed with both the family and the surgical team pre-procedure.

What are the considerations if hemodynamic instability occurs?

Episodes of hemodynamic compromise must be responded to swiftly in a patient with DCM. During a bradycardic event, atropine should be used cautiously because it may initiate tachycardia which can result in compromised subendocardial perfusion. Ephedrine, a direct and indirect-acting α- and β-agonist dosed at 0.03–0.07 mg/kg, is a reliable agent to increase heart rate without compromising diastolic coronary perfusion. In addition, the augmentation in diastolic blood pressure is beneficial when hypotension accompanies bradycardia.

Excessive tachycardia is detrimental for patients with DCM as it can cause subendocardial ischemia and hemodynamic compromise, but many patients may have tachycardia at baseline due to their heart failure. The cause of the tachycardia must be identified and addressed, and anesthesia depth is increased if indicated. β-blockers should be used very selectively intraoperatively considering the patient's severely depressed systolic function.

If hypotension due to reduced SVR occurs, volume infusion (5–10 mL/kg) to increase preload to preinduction levels or the use of incremental doses of phenylephrine (0.5–1.5 mcg/kg) will usually correct the problem. Phenylephrine reliably increases SVR, but caution must be exercised in DCM patients with severe systolic dysfunction since excessive use of phenylephrine will increase afterload and reduce stroke volume. If the patient fails to respond with a prompt increase in systemic blood pressure, an inotropic agent should be started to avoid a downward spiral of acute heart failure manifested by ventricular dilatation, increased wall stress, reduced stroke volume, and worsening hypotension. Dopamine 3–5 mcg/kg/minute or epinephrine 0.03–0.05 mcg/kg/minute would be reasonable choices in this situation.

What is the appropriate postoperative disposition for this patient?

This patient should return directly to the intensive care unit on completion of the procedure. For patients with less severe cardiac dysfunction, postoperative disposition should be predicated on their stability during the procedure and any ongoing concerns regarding airway or hemodynamic stability.

References

1. T. M. Lee, D.T. Hsu, P. Kantor, et al. Pediatric cardiomyopathies. *Circ Res* 2017; **121**: 855–73.

2. D. T. Hsu, C. E. Canter. Dilated cardiomyopathy and heart failure in children. *Heart Fail Clin* 2010; **6**: 415–32.

3. R. Kirk, D. Naftel, T. M. Hoffman, et al. Outcome of pediatric patients with dilated cardiomyopathy listed for transplant: a multi-institutional study. *J Heart Lung Transplant* 2009; **28**: 1322–8.

4. J. F. Price, A. K. Thomas, M. Grenier, et al. B-type natriuretic peptide predicts adverse cardiovascular events in pediatric outpatients with chronic left ventricular systolic dysfunction. *Circulation* 2006; **114**: 1063–9.

5. A. K. Kipps, C. Ramamoorthy, D. N. Rosenthal, et al. Children with cardiomyopathy: complications after noncardiac procedures with general anesthesia. *Paediatr Anaesth* 2007; **17**: 775–81.

6. C. Ramamoorthy, C. Haberkern, S. Bhananker, et al. Anesthesia-related cardiac arrest in children with heart disease: data from the Pediatric Perioperative Cardiac Arrest (POCA) registry. *Anesth Analg* 2010; **110**: 1376–82.

Suggested Reading

Ing R. J., Ames W. A., and Chambers N. A. Paediatric cardiomyopathy and anaesthesia. *Br J Anaesth* 2012; **108**: 4–12.

Williams G. D. and Hammer G. B. Cardiomyopathy in childhood. *Curr Opin Anesthesiol* 2011; **24**: 289–300.

33

Mixed Cardiomyopathy

Adam C. Adler

Case Scenario

A 3-year-old male weighing 11 kg presents for semielective inguinal hernia repair following recurrent bowel incarceration. The past medical history includes arthrogryposis and severe kyphoscoliosis in addition to complex heart disease. Home medications include metoprolol. The patient is asymptomatic but is wheelchair bound due to limb deformities. The parents are requesting information regarding the safety of anesthesia for their child and the anesthetic options.

Recent transthoracic echocardiogram revealed the following:

- *Severe mixed cardiomyopathy with hypertrophic and restrictive physiology*
- *Severe biventricular hypertrophic cardiomyopathy with near complete cavitary obliteration*
- *Left ventricular diastolic septal thickness consistent with a z-score of +19*
- *Right and left ventricular outflow tract obstruction (see Figure 33.1)*
- *Ejection fraction 74%*
- *Dynamic left ventricular outflow tract obstruction from systolic anterior motion of the mitral valve*
- *Prominent reversal of flow in the hepatic veins and inferior vena cava*

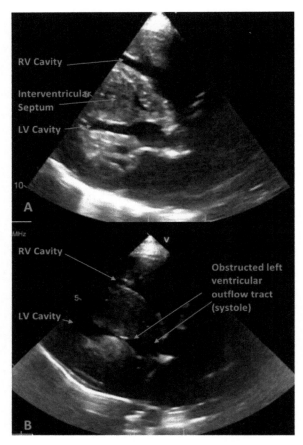

Figure 33.1 Preoperative transthoracic echocardiography in parasternal long axis view demonstrating (A) severe right and left ventricular cavity obliteration from thickened ventricular free wall and interventricular septum and (B) dynamic obstruction of the left ventricular outflow track. Courtesy of Adam C. Adler, MD.

Key Objectives

- Identify the subtypes of pediatric cardiomyopathies.
- Review the pathophysiology and clinical presentation for pediatric cardiomyopathies.
- Formulate a safe anesthetic plan for children with severe cardiomyopathy.

Pathophysiology

What are the subtypes of pediatric cardiomyopathy?

Pediatric cardiomyopathy subtypes include:

- Dilated cardiomyopathy (DCM)
- Hypertrophic cardiomyopathy (HCM)
- Restrictive cardiomyopathy (RCM)
- Noncompaction cardiomyopathy (NCM)
- Arrhythmogenic right ventricular dysplasia (ARVD)

While distinct classifications exist, in practice, the variants occur in combination. However, there is generally a predominant phenotype diagnosed by echocardiography that allows multicenter registries to track epidemiology, management, and outcomes related to pediatric cardiomyopathy. This chapter will focus on mixed hypertrophic and restrictive forms of cardiomyopathy. (See Chapter 32.)

> **Clinical Pearl**
>
> *While distinct types of cardiomyopathy exist, patients often present clinically with mixed types and physiology.*

What is the incidence of pediatric cardiomyopathy?

The overall incidence of pediatric cardiomyopathy is estimated to be around 1–1.5 cases per 100,000 patients. Dilated cardiomyopathy accounts for more than 50% of all cases. Hypertrophic cardiomyopathy is the second leading cause, with restrictive cardiomyopathy being the least common.

Hypertrophic Cardiomyopathy

What is hypertrophic cardiomyopathy?

Hypertrophic cardiomyopathy (HCM) is a disease of the myocardial sarcomere characterized by thickening of the myocardium. It occurs either sporadically or as part of a familial (genetic) disorder or metabolic syndrome. On echocardiography, HCM appears as increased muscle mass without ventricular dilation. Histologically, HCM appears as myocyte disarray and fibrosis, which is best thought of as an increase in poorly or nonfunctioning myocardium.

What are primary and secondary hypertrophic cardiomyopathy and how do they differ?

- *Primary HCM* (most common) reflects an autosomal dominant pattern of inheritance and is characterized by left ventricular hypertrophy (LVH) with rare RV involvement. Primary HCM results from a genetic mutation affecting different elements of the muscle sarcomere. More than 1000 genetic mutations have been identified for primary HCM. The primary form of HCM typically develops in childhood or adolescence.
- *Secondary HCM* is generally "secondary" to a variety of metabolic and mitochondrial disorders and syndromes and is generally not isolated to the cardiac muscle. Manifestation of secondary HCM occurs in infancy and commonly affects both right and left ventricles. Some disorders associated with secondary HCM include mitochondrial diseases such as Friedreich's ataxia and metabolic disorders such as Fabry and Pompe disease.

What are the anatomic manifestations of HCM and the resultant pathophysiology?

While the phenotypic expression of HCM varies, the pattern of LVH typically involves the basal and mid-interventricular septum. Generally, the ratio of septal wall to inferolateral wall thickness is >60%. Severe septal hypertrophy often displaces the mitral valve apparatus and obstructs the left ventricular outflow tract (LVOT) in the subaortic region. This septal hypertrophy results in dynamic obstruction to the LVOT during mid-systole when the septal wall moves toward the mitral apparatus. (See Figure 33.2.) In addition to LVOT obstruction, significant diastolic dysfunction occurs with

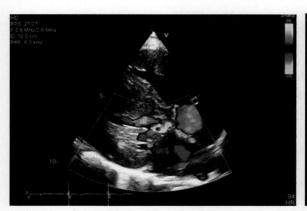
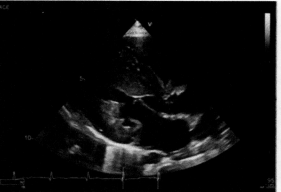

Figure 33.2 Transthoracic long axis view showing significant flow acceleration at the LV outflow tract (left) and dynamic LV outflow obstruction due to systolic anterior motion of the mitral valve (right). Courtesy of Adam C. Adler, MD.

HCM, even in patients with mild disease. Although the LV cavity size is normal, myocardial dysfunction results in impaired LV relaxation and distensibility. Additionally, patients with HCM are prone to developing coronary ischemia. In addition to the increased myocardial oxygen demand (from increased myocardial mass), intramural coronary vasculature is often affected by the myocardial wall stress. Lastly, elevated LV end-diastolic pressure results in subendocardial ischemia.

What is the typical clinical presentation for patients with HCM?

The range of symptoms seen in patients with primary HCM varies from asymptomatic to severe, including sudden death. Most often patients have dyspnea due to LV diastolic dysfunction. Additionally, many patients experience syncope, particularly with exertion. This occurs as a result of LVOT obstruction with impedance of coronary and systemic perfusion, in addition to the multifactorial effects on the distal coronaries as noted earlier.

What management options exist for patients with HCM?

Treatment strategies for HCM include medical therapy in addition to interventional and surgical approaches. For those with mild HCM, medical management with ß-blockers and/or calcium channel blockers is initiated and guided by patient symptoms or performance on stress testing. For patients with advanced disease as evidenced by symptomatology, poor ventricular function, or a history of arrhythmias, automated implantable cardioverter-defibrillators are placed to prevent sudden death. Patients with advanced disease may be suitable for surgical septal myectomy. Surgical candidacy is guided by symptomatology (arrhythmias, dyspnea, angina, syncope) and echocardiographic findings (LVOT gradient >50 mm Hg). Patients with end-stage heart failure are often evaluated for orthotopic heart transplantation.

Restrictive Cardiomyopathy

What is restrictive cardiomyopathy?

Isolated RCM is rare, encompassing approximately 5% of pediatric cardiomyopathies. More often, more common forms of cardiomyopathy (i.e., HCM) appear in conjunction with restrictive physiology as opposed to isolated RCM.

> **Clinical Pearl**
>
> *Restrictive cardiomyopathy is a disease process with isolated diastolic heart failure. It is distinct from other forms of cardiomyopathy that may also result in diastolic failure and restrictive physiology.*

What are the common presenting signs and symptoms in patients with RCM?

Most of the presenting symptomatology results from prolonged elevation of ventricular filling pressures. Elevated end-diastolic pressure results in pulmonary edema and pulmonary hypertension, peripheral edema, hepatomegaly, and weight gain. Not uncommonly, patients present after undergoing an unrevealing workup for reactive airway disease. Restrictive cardiomyopathy may also be diagnosed during evaluation for a variety of diseases (see later). Syncope is an ominous presenting sign and is associated with a higher risk of sudden death.

What is the etiology and pathophysiology of RCM?

Restrictive cardiomyopathy is characterized by abnormal diastolic compliance or filling with normal or decreased diastolic volume in the setting of normal systolic function. Increased myocardial stiffness results in impaired myocardial relaxation and ventricular noncompliance. The resulting noncompliance causes elevated diastolic pressure in both ventricles and atria. Over time, atrial dilation occurs and may lead to arrhythmias. (See Figure 33.3.) In late stages, systolic function may also fail. Echocardiography and/or cardiac magnetic resonance imaging (MRI) can be used to differentiate RCM from constrictive pericarditis that can occur in patients with RCM, specifically those with deposition-related disorders (see later).

Although the exact etiology is unknown, RCM can be secondary to medication or chest radiation, or associated with the following diseases:

Metabolic syndromes/disorders

- Carcinoid syndrome
- Fabry disease
- Gaucher disease
- Glycogen storage disease
- Hurler syndrome

Deposition-based disorders

- Amyloidosis
- Hemosiderosis

- Hemochromatosis
- Loeffler syndrome – hypereosinophilia

What are the management options and prognosis for patients with RCM?

Unfortunately, there are no medical management strategies that directly target diastolic dysfunction. Treatment is aimed at decreasing volume overload with diuretics, reducing systemic and pulmonary venous congestion. Antiarrhythmics are used, as abnormal rhythms frequently occur with

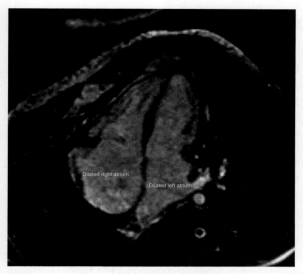

Figure 33.3 Restrictive cardiomyopathy. Four-chamber magnetic resonance imaging showing markedly dilated atria with normal ventricular sizes. The systolic function is usually normal, but diastolic relaxation is severely impaired resulting in restrictive filling of both ventricles. Courtesy of Michael Taylor, MD

progressive atrial enlargement. Many patients require anticoagulation due to the risk of thromboembolism, particularly in the atria.

Outcomes for patients with pediatric RCM remain poor, with a transplant-free survival rate of approximately 50% at 1 year post-diagnosis. Thus, patients are referred early for cardiac transplantation. Patients with mixed RCM/HCM have a better prognosis for transplant-free survival compared to those with isolated RCM.

Left Ventricular Noncompaction Cardiomyopathy

What is LV noncompaction cardiomyopathy?

Noncompaction cardiomyopathy (NCM) is the result of a failed process in ventricular development. Typically, the fetal LV trabeculations fill in during the course of development to form complete and circumferential ventricular cardiac smooth muscle, a process known as compaction. When compaction does not occur, the LV has deep trabeculations that are unsuited to the needs of a systemic ventricle. (See Figure 33.4.) These trabeculations result in poor subendocardial perfusion and ischemia.

The NCM subtype is associated with Barth syndrome and a variety of other genetic anomalies and syndromes (trisomy 13, 18, 21; Turner, Soto, and Marfan syndromes) along with neuromuscular dystrophies (Duchenne, Becker, multiminicore, and limb-girdle).

Noncompaction cardiomyopathy is associated with a progressive decline in systolic and/or diastolic function, multifactorial arrhythmias, and elevated risk of thromboembolism. In many cases, NCM occurs in association with other forms of cardiomyopathy, especially hypertrophic or dilated phenotypes.

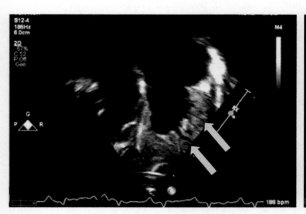
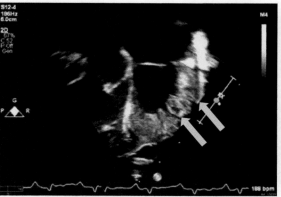

Figure 33.4 Transthoracic four-chamber view identifying deep trabeculations (yellow arrows) that are classic for LV noncompaction cardiomyopathy. Courtesy of Adam C. Adler, MD.

255

Anesthetic Implications

What are the preoperative anesthetic considerations for patients with cardiomyopathy?

In addition to the perioperative considerations related to any underlying illness, preoperative evaluation in this patient population should focus on signs and symptoms associated with cardiomyopathy.

- *Physical examination*: Specifically, the focus should be on determining the presence and severity of dyspnea, angina, exercise tolerance, weight gain, and syncopal episodes (including frequency).
- *Echocardiography*: A recent echocardiogram should be reviewed. Echocardiographic findings differ in patients with HCM versus RCM, but there can be overlap (e.g., HCM with restrictive physiology).
- *Systolic function*: Many patients with HCM have hyperdynamic ventricular function. While the ejection fraction (EF) may be normal or even supranormal, this should be considered in association with the other findings (a small obliterated cavity, as seen in Figure 33.5, may completely empty, providing a normal EF despite a minuscule stroke volume). Assessment of function should also be considered given the high risk of coronary ischemia.

Clinical Pearl

In cases with ventricular cavity obliteration from myocardial hypertrophy, the EF may appear normal despite minuscule stroke volumes.

- *Diastolic dysfunction*: Diastolic function should be reviewed in cases of HCM and RCM. The atria should be evaluated for size and volume (i.e., degree of dilation), which can reflect chronically elevated ventricular diastolic pressure and failure. Right ventricular pressure should be estimated in addition to flow patterns in the inferior vena cava and hepatic veins, as this can help differentiate RCM from constrictive pericarditis.
- *Atrioventricular valves* can be affected by both HCM and RCM. Septal hypertrophy in HCM can disrupt the mitral valve apparatus. In cases of RCM or late-stage HCM, ventricular enlargement can affect valve coaptation, resulting in atrioventricular valve regurgitation. Similarly, valve function can be affected as a result of ischemia.
- *Left ventricular outflow tract*: In patients with HCM, the LV outflow tract should be examined for dynamic obstruction, including the mechanism and severity. Evaluation for systolic anterior motion of the mitral apparatus should be performed.
- *Rhythm disorders*: A baseline electrocardiogram should be obtained along with any history of arrhythmias, as patients with prolonged diastolic failure and atrial enlargement are prone to atrial arrhythmias. Similarly, severe septal hypertrophy may disrupt the conduction pathway either mechanically or as a result of ischemia. As noted earlier, patients with cardiomyopathy are at risk for sudden cardiac death. Patients with implantable defibrillators/pacemakers should be assessed for their underlying native rhythm. (See Chapter 23, Table 23.2 for details of preoperative assessment of implanted devices.) For those requiring temporary deactivation or those at high risk of malignant arrhythmias, defibrillation pads should be placed prior to induction of anesthesia.
- *Catheterization data*: If available, this helps inform the anesthesia provider regarding the degree of diastolic failure, degree of pulmonary hypertension, global ventricular function, coronary ischemia, and degree of LVOT obstruction.
- *Vascular access*: Cardiomyopathy patients should have intravenous (IV) access prior to induction of anesthesia. In cases of difficult IV access or lack of patient compliance premedication may be helpful, particularly in young children. Oral midazolam or intramuscular ketamine may be used.
- *Collaborative discussion*: A discussion should take place with the patient's primary cardiologist prior to anesthesia. If the patient is a candidate for cardiac surgical intervention, it should be performed prior to other elective interventions if possible. Additionally, if performing general anesthesia on patients with end-

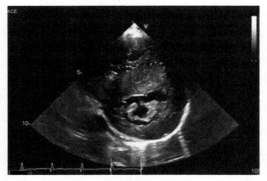

Figure 33.5 Transthoracic short axis view showing circumferential LV hypertrophy, especially in the septum, and resulting cavitary obliteration. Courtesy of Adam C. Adler, MD.

stage cardiomyopathy, a discussion regarding extracorporeal support candidacy should occur preoperatively and in conjunction with the patient's family and primary cardiologist.

What constitutes a reasonable intraoperative plan for patients with end-stage cardiomyopathy?

The anesthetic plan should be based on the severity of the patient's cardiac illness as well as the procedural needs. Generally, most pediatric cases require general anesthesia, and it is preferable to place an airway device to ensure adequate ventilation (either a laryngeal mask airway or endotracheal tube). For procedures of shorter duration with minimal expected physiologic changes (e.g., line placement), sedation may be possible. However, it is critical to ensure the absence of airway obstruction, which can result in increased ventricular afterload. In a small subset of surgical situations, including this case, a regional technique can be proposed.

What are intraoperative anesthetic goals for patients with HCM and/or RCM?

Anesthetic goals include maintenance of normovolemia, preload and afterload. For patients with severe HCM, while the EF may remain normal, their beat-to-beat stroke volume is often minimal and dependent on adequate preload; however, *care must be taken to avoid volume overload.*

With regard to heart rate, *tachycardia is generally poorly tolerated.* In patients with HCM and restrictive physiology (i.e., diastolic failure), diastolic time is vital to maintain ventricular filling. Similarly, heart rate elevations are poorly tolerated with respect to the degree of LVOT obstruction. Negative inotropy is the primary medical management, usually in the form of calcium channel and ß-blockers, and should be continued perioperatively. Negative inotropy helps decrease the gradient across the LVOT, thereby reducing obstruction and promoting forward flow.

Afterload should be maintained in patients with HCM to reduce the pressure gradient across the LVOT obstruction, as well as to maintain coronary perfusion.

Anesthetic goals are similar for patients with isolated RCM and diastolic failure. While systolic function is preserved, extreme elevation in diastolic pressure from ventricular noncompliance/nonrelaxation means that large volume loads are not well tolerated. Similarly, tachycardia reduces diastolic time and ventricular filling. In the setting of significant ventricular dilation leading to mitral annular dilation and valvular regurgitation, bradycardia can also be detrimental. Ideally, the patients should be maintained at their baseline heart rate.

As mentioned earlier, dysrhythmias in cardiomyopathy patients are common and not well tolerated; for patients with a history of arrhythmia, defibrillation/pacing pads should be applied prior to induction of anesthesia.

Hypotension in HCM should be treated by augmenting preload and/or administering medication to increase afterload, while maintaining a normal heart rate. Generally, patients should undergo IV induction of anesthesia. Propofol and inhalation agents are often poorly tolerated due to the reduction in preload and afterload and compensatory tachycardia. Ketamine is a suitable induction agent, especially in the presence of opioids to reduce sympathetic activity. Similarly, an opioid-based anesthetic is generally well tolerated while preserving systemic vascular resistance (SVR).

Dilute phenylephrine should be available as a first-line therapy for hypotension. Response to inotropic drugs (epinephrine, norepinephrine) and calcium may be poorly tolerated for a variety of reasons, including increased LVOT obstruction and tachycardia. If hypotension persists, continuous infusions of phenylephrine or vasopressin should be used.

Insufflation of body cavities (thoracic or abdominal) or extremes of patient positioning (steep reverse Trendelenburg) should be performed judiciously, as they are poorly tolerated. When required, insufflation pressure should be increased gradually to allow time to assess the hemodynamic response.

When appropriate, regional or neuraxial anesthesia should be considered to blunt hemodynamic responses and potentially reduce anesthetic requirements. The use of an epidural catheter is preferable to spinal anesthesia to avoid drops in both SVR and preload. However, when using an epidural, initial bolus dosing of local anesthetic should be avoided. (See Table 33.1.)

Table 33.1 Pathophysiology Characteristics of Cardiomyopathies

	Dilated Cardiomyopathy (Ischemic and Nonischemic)	Hypertrophic Cardiomyopathy (Obstructive and Nonobstructive)	Restrictive Cardiomyopathy
Diastolic function and atrial transport function	• Biventricular diastolic dysfunction • Reduced biventricular compliance • Biatrial enlargement • Increased atrial pressures	• LV diastolic dysfunction • Reduced LV compliance • Left atrial enlargement • Increased left atrial pressure	• Severe biventricular diastolic dysfunction • Severely reduced biventricular compliance • Biatrial enlargement • Increased atrial pressures
Ventricular systolic function	• Decreased biventricular contractility; usually limited to LV in ischemic form • Exhausted preload reserve • Afterload mismatch	• Preserved or hyperdynamic LV contractility • Normal RV contractility	• Preserved biventricular contractility
Pulmonary vasculature	• Elevated LAP initially leads to passive elevation of PAP • Chronic elevation of LAP leads to reversible then irreversible elevation of PVR	• Elevated LAP initially leads to passive elevation of PAP • Chronic elevation of LAP leads to reversible then irreversible elevation of PVR	• Elevated LAP initially leads to passive elevation of PAP • Chronic elevation of LAP leads to reversible, then irreversible elevation of PVR
Effect of preload alterations on hemodynamics	• Exhausted preload reserve; little or no ability to recruit SV with preload augmentation	• Retained preload reserve but reduced LV compliance results in elevated LAP with preload augmentation • In obstructive form reduced LV volumes will worsen obstruction	• Baseline LV and RV EDV are low • Severely reduced biventricular compliance results in markedly elevated atrial pressures with minimal preload augmentation
Effect of heart rate alterations on hemodynamics	• Avoid bradycardia; fixed SV due to exhausted preload reserve • Tachycardia unlikely to reduce LV filling but subendocardial perfusion may be compromised in ischemic form	• Avoid tachycardia; with retained preload reserve, LV filling will be compromised, subendocardial perfusion may be compromised • Bradycardia is well tolerated	• Avoid bradycardia; fixed SV due to severely reduced LV compliance • Tachycardia may reduce LV filling resulting in reduced SV
Effect of afterload alterations on hemodynamics	• Avoid increases in SVR; large reduction in SV will occur due to reduced contractility • SVR reduction is mainstay of medical management	• Avoid decreases in SVR particularly in obstructive form; reduced LVESV will worsen obstruction • Increases in SVR well tolerated	• Avoid decreases in SVR; with fixed SV, hypotension will result • Increases in SVR well tolerated

From V. G. Nasr and J. A. DiNardo. *The Pediatric Cardiac Anesthesia Handbook*, 1st ed. John Wiley & Sons; 2017, 199–215. With permission.
EDV, end-diastolic volume; LAP, left atrial pressure; LV, left ventricle; LVESV, left ventricular end-systolic volume; PAP, pulmonary artery pressure; PVR, pulmonary vascular resistance; SV, stroke volume; SVR, systemic vascular resistance; RV, right ventricle.

What is distraction and how can it be used?

Distraction is a technique that can replace, reduce, or augment procedural sedation for painful or anxiety-provoking procedures. Distraction works on the theory that the brain has limited ability to process sensory input and using deliberate stimuli to bombard the brain results in lesser ability for the brain to process other incoming stimuli.

Distraction can be passive or active and has been proven effective at allaying anxiety, fear, and pain in procedures ranging from small (IV placement) to more invasive (as done for this case when a neuraxial technique is offered). (See Table 33.1.) In younger children, a degree of IV sedation may also be required, while older children may tolerate procedures with distraction alone. For select procedures, adjuncts like topical or subcutaneous local anesthetic combined with distraction may be suitable and allow for avoidance of general anesthesia in challenging cardiac patients.

Clinical Pearl

Distraction techniques are designed to block the brain's input of sensory stimuli and can significantly help with painful procedures such as IV placement. Audiovisual distractors (video games, iPads, etc.) work well in children and adolescents.

Table 33.2 Commonly Employed Forms of Procedural Distraction by Patient Age

	Cognitive Distraction		Behavioral Distraction	
	Active	**Passive**	**Active**	**Passive**
Young children	Audiovisual devices Interactive games	Music		
Adolescents	Singing Counting aloud Audiovisual devices	Music	Breathing	Reimagination of pain Emotive imagery

From A. C. Adler. With permission.

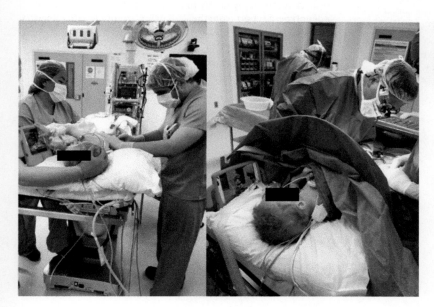

Figure 33.6 (Left) Preoperative placement of caudal block using patient audiovisual distraction and (right) intraoperative patient positioning, proving patient comfort and continued use of audiovisual distraction during surgery. Courtesy of Adam C. Adler, MD, MS.

What is the recovery plan for patients with cardiomyopathy following anesthesia?

Patients with end-stage cardiomyopathy have a high perioperative rate of cardiovascular complications. For minimally invasive procedures in relatively stable patients, anesthetic recovery should occur in a post-anesthesia care unit (PACU) that is familiar with pediatric and pediatric cardiovascular patients. When post-anesthesia admission is required, admission to the cardiology floor should be considered. Similarly, for more invasive surgeries and/or patients who are less stable, the ideal place for recovery is the cardiovascular intensive care unit. In situations in which the patient is admitted to the surgical floor or pediatric intensive care unit, the cardiology or heart failure team should be consulted for optimization of medical management.

Pain control in the immediate postoperative period is vital to minimize or reduce the incidence of heart failure and/or ischemia. Pain management with continuous infusion or patient-controlled analgesia pumps or via continuous regional or neuraxial techniques should be considered. Consultation with the pain management team can provide recommendations for analgesic adjuncts, as well as bridging to oral pain medications.

Case Completion

After discussion with the primary cardiologist and surgeon, it was decided that while the surgery should be done due to the near certain risk of reincarceration, it was felt that the risk of general anesthesia was unacceptably high. Unfortunately, the patient was not a cardiac surgical candidate for myectomy, transplantation, or extracorporeal support. The decision was made to proceed with a caudal block and audiovisual distraction using the patient's iPad device. The parents consented to give very light sedation if necessary but preferred to abort the procedure if this plan failed rather than convert to general anesthesia. Topical anesthetic was placed over the sacrum and a dense caudal block was performed using 0.25% bupivacaine. The patient was placed supine with cushions under his back in a position allowing him to watch the audiovisual device. (See Figure 33.6.) He received IV dexmedetomidine in 2-mcg aliquots for restlessness toward the end of the procedure. After PACU recovery, he was monitored by the cardiology service until discharge.

Suggested Reading

Adler A. C., Elattary T., and Chandrakantan A. Anesthesia in the form of audiovisual distraction for a child requiring surgery with end-stage cardiomyopathy: a case report. *A A Pract* 2019; **13**: 346–9.

Adler A. C., Schwartz E. R., Waters J. M., et al. Anesthetizing a child for a large compressive mediastinal mass with distraction techniques and music therapies as the sole agents. *J Clin Anesth* 2016; **35**: 392–7.

Arghami A., Dearani J. A., Said S. M., et al. Hypertrophic cardiomyopathy in children. *Ann Cardiothorac Surg* 2017; **6**: 376–85.

Birnie K. A., Noel M., Chambers C. T., et al. Psychological interventions for needle-related procedural pain and distress in children and adolescents. *Cochrane Database Syst Rev* 2018; **10**: CD005179.

Hensley N., Dietrich J., Nyhan D., et al. Hypertrophic cardiomyopathy: a review. *Anesth Analg* 2015; **120**: 554–69.

Webber S. A., Lipshultz S. E., Sleeper L. A., et al. Outcomes of restrictive cardiomyopathy in childhood and the influence of phenotype: a report from the Pediatric Cardiomyopathy Registry. *Circulation* 2012; **126**: 1237–44.

Wilkinson J. D., Landy D. C., Colan S. D., et al. The Pediatric Cardiomyopathy Registry and heart failure: key results from the first 15 years. *Heart Fail Clin* 2010; **6**: 401–13.

Chapter 34

Extracorporeal Membrane Oxygenation

Rita Saynhalath and M. Iqbal Ahmed

Case Scenario

A full-term infant boy weighing 3.5 kg with a prenatal diagnosis of left-sided congenital diaphragmatic hernia with bowels and stomach in the left chest was transferred on day of life 1 for escalation of care. A restrictive patent ductus arteriosus was suspected, so an alprostadil infusion at 0.01 mcg/kg/minute was initiated, along with inhaled nitric oxide at 20 parts per million. Persistent hypercapnia and hypoxemia prompted a transition from conventional ventilation to high-frequency oscillatory ventilation on day of life 3. Due to persistent hypotension and worsening ventricular function, epinephrine 0.05 mcg/kg/minute was started. With no clinical improvement noted the decision was made to initiate veno-arterial extracorporeal membrane oxygenation on day of life 5. Current infusions include fentanyl 1 mcg/kg/hour, midazolam 0.1 mg/kg/hour, dexmedetomidine 0.5 mcg/kg/hour, and heparin 28 units/kg/hour. An epinephrine infusion has been weaned to 0.03 mcg/kg/hour. Now, on day of life 10, after discussion among the multidisciplinary teams, the patient is scheduled for repair of his diaphragmatic hernia in the neonatal intensive care unit.

Echocardiography revealed the following:

- *Large patent ductus arteriosus*
- *Severely hypoplastic left pulmonary artery*
- *Right ventricular hypertrophy*
- *Normal biventricular function*

Key Objectives

- Discuss the intraoperative management of congenital diaphragmatic hernia repair.
- Review the main components of an extracorporeal membrane oxygenation circuit.
- Delineate the differences between veno-venous and veno-arterial extracorporeal membrane oxygenation.
- Identify the anesthetic considerations when caring for a patient on extracorporeal membrane oxygenation support.

Pathophysiology

What is a congenital diaphragmatic hernia and what are the physiologic implications? What are the prognostic indicators?

A congenital diaphragmatic hernia (CDH) is a rare birth defect that occurs in approximately 0.8–5 out of 10,000 births. It is characterized by a diaphragmatic defect allowing herniation of abdominal contents into the chest and subsequently impeding normal lung development. This results in structural and functional changes to lung structure, pulmonary circulation, and the heart. Classification of CDH is based on the location of the defect: posterolateral (Bochdalek), anterior (Morgagni), and central. Posterolateral hernias are by far the most common, with the majority occurring on the left side. The size of the defect can significantly affect the prognosis, as the severity of this condition is proportional to the severity of lung hypoplasia and pulmonary hypertension (PH). Vascular remodeling with hypertrophied muscular arterial extension more peripherally results in a "fixed, irreversible" component of PH, while an imbalance in vasoreactive mediators and autonomic innervation contribute to a "reversible" component. From a cardiac function perspective, PH results in right ventricular dysfunction that manifests after birth. Additionally, abnormalities of the left ventricle have been observed, especially in infants with left-sided CDH.

Several factors are associated with an adverse outcome, including the presence of associated anomalies, significant liver herniation into the thorax, severe pulmonary hypoplasia, and right-sided CDH. Additionally, liver herniation is predictive of the need for extracorporeal membrane oxygenation (ECMO)[1] and places the patient at a higher risk for mortality [2]. Gestational age at the time of diagnosis is significant, as an early diagnosis usually correlates with a large defect and possible complete absence of diaphragm.

Do other anomalies frequently coexist with CDH?

Congenital diaphragmatic hernia occurs as an isolated defect in 50%–70% of cases. The remaining cases are associated with major structural abnormalities and/or chromosomal anomalies. Therefore, a diagnosis of CDH should trigger an evaluation for associated conditions. The most commonly affected organ system is the cardiovascular system, followed by the genitourinary, musculoskeletal, and central nervous systems. A postnatal echocardiogram is imperative to rule out associated congenital heart defects. Echocardiography is also helpful in evaluating biventricular function in the face of pulmonary hypertension, as well as flow direction across the patent ductus arteriosus (PDA) and patent foramen ovale.

Is there a preferred ventilation strategy for a CDH patient?

Ventilation strategies have evolved from historically aggressive (to reduce pulmonary hypertension via hypocapnia and alkalosis) to gentler ventilation, attempting to protect already damaged lung parenchyma from further injury related to mechanical ventilation. The CDH EURO Consortium has published recommendations on ventilator parameters should the patient require mechanical ventilation after birth: target $PaCO_2$ between 50 and 70 mm Hg, peak inspiratory pressures (PIP) <25 cm H_2O, and positive end-expiratory pressure (PEEP) limited to 3–5 cm H_2O [3]. This "gentle ventilation" strategy should target a preductal oxygen saturation between 80% and 95% and a postductal oxygen saturation >70%. Unfortunately, in the most severe cases of CDH, conventional ventilation is not sufficient to prevent hypoxia and severe hypercapnea. High-frequency oscillatory ventilation can be used as a rescue strategy but has not been shown to decrease mortality.

What is the role of extracorporeal membrane oxygenation in the management of CDH patients?

Extracorporeal membrane oxygenation is considered a last resort, life-preserving option for neonates with CDH who have failed all other medical therapies. Support of infants with CDH is the most common indication for neonatal ECMO utilization, but prognosis is guarded, as survival rates remain only 50% in this high-risk population. Most agree that ECMO does confer a survival advantage in the most severe cases of CDH, meaning those patients with a predicted mortality >80%.

Selection criteria for ECMO use in CDH patients varies among institutions, but according to the CDH EURO Consortium Consensus, ECMO should be considered in the following circumstances [3]:

- Inability to maintain preductal saturation >85% or postductal saturation >70%
- Increased $PaCO_2$ and respiratory acidosis with pH <7.15 despite optimal ventilator management
- Peak inspiratory pressure >28 cm H_2O or mean airway pressure >17 cm H_2O to achieve SpO_2 >85%
- Inadequate oxygen delivery with metabolic acidosis as measured by elevated lactate ≥5 mmol/L and pH <7.15
- Systemic hypotension resistant to fluid and pressor therapy, resulting in decreased urine output <0.5 mL/kg/hour for 12–24 hours
- Oxygenation index ≥40 for at least 3 hours

Should repair be delayed until the patient is weaned off ECMO?

The surgical repair of a CDH is not an emergency. The patient should meet the following criteria set by the CDH EURO Consortium: (1) appropriate mean arterial pressure for gestational age; (2) appropriate preductal saturations with FiO_2 <50%; and (3) adequate organ perfusion with lactate <3 mmol/L and urine output >1 mL/kg/hour [3].

Provided the patient has shown signs of stabilization since ECMO was initiated, repair would generally not be delayed until after the patient was weaned from ECMO. The increased risk of bleeding when performing surgery while on ECMO must be taken into account, however. The timing of surgery for an ECMO-dependent patient remains controversial, as studies provide conflicting results. Three approaches have been described: early repair <72 hours after ECMO initiation, delayed repair as a last resort operation when patient has been unable to wean from ECMO, and after decannulation. While some studies have shown improved outcomes if the surgery occurs after decannulation from ECMO [4], others have found a higher likelihood of survival and shorter duration on ECMO if the CDH is repaired within 72 hours of initiation of ECMO [5, 6].

What is ECMO and how does it work?

Extracorporeal membrane oxygenation is essentially a modified cardiopulmonary bypass (CPB) system, providing support when the cardiac and/or pulmonary systems are failing. Venous blood is drained from the patient and passed through a lung membrane for gas exchange and oxygenation. It is then returned to the patient via a large vein (veno-venous ECMO) or artery (veno-arterial ECMO).

What are the components of an ECMO circuit?

A standard ECMO circuit consists of a venous access cannula draining blood from the patient to a mechanical blood pump that moves blood through an oxygenator and a heat exchanger before returning blood to the patient through either the arterial (VA) or venous (VV) infusion cannula. Variability in the circuit arises from the number of monitors and circuit access points and presence of a bridge between venous access and arterial infusion limbs. Circuit pressures are monitored at different points on the circuit to identify complications: pressure difference across the oxygenator, inlet/suction pressure applied to the patient, and outlet/line pressure delivering flow to the patient. Flow monitors use ultrasound technology to estimate flow within the circuit and are commonly located at the pump outlet to measure flow generated by the pump and beyond the oxygenator to determine the flow actually delivered to the patient.

The goal of an ECMO pump is to provide appropriate blood flow for the patient at a safe pressure that avoids hemolysis. There are two main types of ECMO pumps. For decades, the *roller pump* has been the standard of care. It consists of a positive displacement pump that uses a roller head to sequentially compress the tubing, thereby displacing the column of blood forward. A collapsible bladder exists on the venous line to prevent direct suction on the venous catheter, which could lead to suction on the right atrium at low filling pressures. Disadvantages of a roller pump include the need for a large and heavy motor, possible wear or rupture of the tubing in the pump head, and risk of blowout from high infusion pressures. More centers currently use a *centrifugal pump*, where a spinning rotor generates flow and pressure. The inflow to the pump can connect directly to the venous cannula. Disadvantages of a centrifugal pump include possible thrombus formation at low flows or with occlusion of the outlet line. Occlusion of the venous inlet line can lead to cavitation and hemolysis.

The gas exchange device or "lung" in the ECMO circuit is a *membrane oxygenator*. Gas and blood flow in countercurrent directions on opposite sides of the membrane, and gas exchange occurs via diffusion. The gas flow or "sweep" rate via an oxygen/nitrogen blender can be adjusted to maintain the desired arterial PaO_2 and $PaCO_2$. The *heat exchanger* warms the blood to the appropriate temperature before it is returned to the patient. Commonly used hollow-fiber oxygenators incorporate a heat exchanger into the oxygenator.

The *vascular access cannulas* used for ECMO are made of biocompatible polyurethane material and come in a variety of sizes with different features. The body is wire reinforced in most cannulas to prevent collapse and internally coated to prevent thrombus formation. Various cannula tip configurations are available; examples include single-end-hole, multifenestrated flexible tip, and short fenestrated tip. Single-lumen cannulas are used for venous and arterial access for patients on veno-arterial (VA) ECMO or multiple site venous access for veno-venous (VV) ECMO patients. Dual-lumen cannulas can provide VV-ECMO via a single jugular venous access site, as blood is removed from the patient through one lumen and returned to the patient by the smaller lumen. (See Figure 34.1.)

What is the difference between veno-venous and veno-arterial ECMO?

Veno-venous ECMO provides respiratory support in a patient with stable cardiac function. Pulmonary blood flow is maintained, and an advantage is that with oxygenated flow through the pulmonary circulation, there is a decrease in hypoxia-induced vasoconstriction. Adequate support is defined as arterial saturation >80%. Neonatal and pediatric patients are most commonly cannulated in the right internal jugular vein, using a multiport double-lumen cannula that has outflow ports situated in the superior vena cava (SVC) and inferior vena cava (IVC) positions and the return port for oxygenated blood in the right atrium. Optimal positioning of the ports is crucial for proper functioning. Malposition of cannulae in VV-ECMO can cause significant recirculation of oxygenated blood resulting in inefficient oxygenation. Examples of situations where only respiratory support might be required include acute respiratory distress syndrome, status asthmaticus, pulmonary hemorrhage, congenital diaphragmatic hernia with good cardiac function, and situations in which the lungs need to "rest" such as pulmonary contusion or smoke inhalation.

On the other hand, *veno-arterial ECMO* bypasses both the heart and the lungs and provides complete cardiac and pulmonary support. The venous cannula takes blood from the right atrium or vena cavae and the arterial cannula returns the oxygenated blood to a peripheral or central artery; there is no recirculation. Veno-arterial support provides the most oxygen delivery to the patient. Typically neonatal cannulas are surgically placed in the right internal jugular vein and right carotid artery. (See Figure 34.2.) Patients must be larger for their femoral vessels to be of adequate size to accommodate ECMO cannulas. Central cannulation is used when patients are unable to wean from CPB intraoperatively. Other indications for VA-ECMO include cardiogenic shock, bridge therapy for chronic cardiomyopathy, and intraoperative use in high-risk percutaneous cardiac interventions.

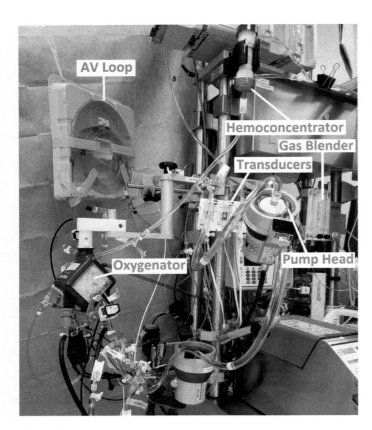

Figure 34.1 Extracorporeal membrane oxygenation pump. Courtesy of Mr. James Reagor.

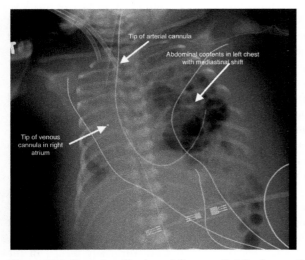

Figure 34.2 Neonate with a large left congenital diaphragmatic hernia on VA-ECMO, cannulated through the right neck. The distal part of the venous cannula is radiolucent except the tip.

Clinical Pearl

Veno-venous ECMO provides only respiratory support, while veno-arterial ECMO provides both respiratory and cardiac

support. Cannulation in the neonatal and pediatric population up to 15 kg or approximately 2 years of age is exclusively through neck vessels (right internal jugular vein and right carotid artery) or centrally in cases of post-CPB heart failure.

How does ECMO differ from a ventricular assist device?

Extracorporeal membrane oxygenation differs from a ventricular assist device (VAD) in that it has an oxygenator and can therefore provide pulmonary support. By contrast, a VAD can only support cardiac function, and can be oriented to support either right ventricle, left ventricle, or both ventricles. (See Chapters 35 and 36.)

What ventilator settings are recommended for a patient on ECMO?

Utilization of ECMO should allow damaged lungs to recover, so ventilator settings should avoid inducing further injury. Minimal "rest" settings focus on tidal volumes <6 mL/kg with long inspiratory time, low plateau pressure <25 cm H_2O, FiO_2 <30%, and PEEP <10 cm H_2O. Some advocate a low respiratory rate of 3–5 breaths per minute to minimize movement of the lungs. Inspired oxygen is maintained at 0.21–0.3. It is essential to remember that during VV-ECMO, a significant amount of blood still circulates through the native lung. Therefore, the lungs need to be adequately ventilated, as complete collapse of the lungs would actually delay recovery.

> **Clinical Pearl**
>
> *Issues with gas exchange and oxygenation are addressed through adjustments of ECMO settings and optimizing patient hemoglobin level and not by ventilator management.*

Anesthetic Implications

What ECMO-related factors should be considered during preoperative assessment?

The anesthesiologist should have a clear idea of the current ECMO settings and flow rates. An assessment of coagulation status is necessary and should include both a review of laboratory values and evaluation of any clinical evidence of either bleeding or thrombosis. This includes a review of neuroimaging studies (cranial ultrasound and/or portable head computed tomography follow-up scans of abnormal head ultrasounds), evaluation of cannulation sites, and determination of whether gastrointestinal bleeding is present. The ECMO circuit should similarly be inspected for the presence of thrombus. If possible, the heparin infusion should be decreased or even stopped to minimize surgical bleeding; this decision, however, must be made jointly by the multidisciplinary team, given the risk of circuit thrombosis. The patient's hemoglobin level, platelet count, and fibrinogen levels should be optimized. Blood products should be crossmatched and available at bedside. Resting ventilator settings should be reviewed and continued.

How should an ECMO patient be monitored intraoperatively?

A patient on ECMO will likely have all necessary lines and monitors for a surgical procedure, as they are requisite for patient stabilization, initiation of ECMO, and ongoing monitoring. Arrhythmia monitoring by continuous electrocardiogram (ECG) is especially important for VV-ECMO patients who are dependent on their native cardiac function. Central venous access is typically present, as most of these patients will have required inotropic support prior to initiation of ECMO. Similarly, peripheral vascular access is often already in place. An arterial line is mandatory for following the mean arterial pressure (MAP) as well as

blood gas monitoring. Mixed venous saturation is the best measurement of systemic perfusion, with a venous saturation >65% indicative of adequate systemic oxygen delivery. Urine output is another surrogate indicator of perfusion and should be monitored closely. Measurement of lactate levels at regular intervals can also signal possible organ hypoperfusion. Echocardiographic evaluation is useful should issues with cannula positioning arise.

Ideally, the anesthesiologist should have a dedicated vascular line for administration of anesthetic medications. Use of a dedicated line prevents inadvertent boluses of anticoagulants or vasoactive agents currently being administered. Medications and volume can also be delivered by the perfusionist directly into the ECMO circuit.

> **Clinical Pearl**
>
> *Patients on ECMO support typically already have necessary monitors and lines in place, including ECG monitoring, arterial line, central venous line for inotropic medication infusion, peripheral vascular access, Foley catheter, and temperature monitor. Dedicate a vascular line for anesthetic medications to avoid bolusing anticoagulants or vasoactive agents.*

What is an appropriate anesthetic plan for this patient?

A total intravenous anesthetic (TIVA) based primarily on narcotics and benzodiazepines is the most practical method of anesthetizing a patient on ECMO. All preoperative sedative infusions should be continued. Depending on the level of current sedation and the planned procedure, the patient may require only a small amount of additional anesthetic. The bedside nurse can provide information on the patient's sedation status and whether he has required any intermittent bolus dosing in addition to his fentanyl, midazolam and dexmedetomidine infusions. Prior to incision, an additional bolus of fentanyl along with neuromuscular blocking agent can be administered. The limitation with TIVA is drug sequestration by the ECMO circuit, especially for lipophilic drugs, and medications should therefore be titrated to effect.

> **Clinical Pearl**
>
> *A narcotic- and benzodiazepine-based intravenous anesthetic is most reliable in ECMO-dependent patients. However, dose requirements may be increased due to medication sequestration by ECMO circuitry.*

How should coagulopathy, bleeding, and anticoagulation be managed in the perioperative period?

Exposure of blood to the artificial, nonnatural surfaces of the ECMO circuit triggers an inflammatory response and the coagulation pathway, leading to both procoagulant activity and fibrinolysis. The balance between preventing circuit thrombosis and patient hemorrhage is challenging. When a patient is dependent on ECMO for survival, a clot in the circuit due to inadequate anticoagulation can be devastating, as it can lead to inadequate oxygenation, consumption coagulopathy, and emboli throughout the body. *Unfractionated heparin is the most commonly used anticoagulant in ECMO patients.* A bolus dose is typically given during ECMO cannulation, and levels are then maintained at therapeutic levels with a continuous infusion. Neonates may require higher infusion rates due to low plasma antithrombin III (ATIII) levels. Low ATIII levels can contribute to heparin resistance, which can be treated with either fresh frozen plasma or recombinant ATIII. While heparin-induced thrombocytopenia is extremely rare in neonates, possible alternatives to the use of heparin include the direct thrombin inhibitors bivalirudin and argatroban.

Activated coagulation time (ACT) is the most commonly used measure of anticoagulation for ECMO patients, as it is a simple and quick test that can be performed at the bedside, making it ideal for intraoperative monitoring. The goal ACT for ECMO patients generally ranges from 180 to 220 and should be checked every 1–2 hours (depending on hospital protocol) and as needed. In addition to ACT monitoring, the ECMO team often uses an expanded array of coagulation parameters including anti-Xa assay, partial thromboplastin time, fibrinogen, prothrombin time, thromboelastography, and ATIII levels to monitor coagulation status and guide therapeutic decision-making.

The benefit of withholding systemic anticoagulation preoperatively is to reduce the risk of perioperative bleeding. This may not be possible in patients who are known to have clot burden in their circuit or have other ongoing thrombotic complications. For CDH repair, there are institution-specific perioperative protocols that reduce the systemic anticoagulation goal ACT to 140–160 (compared to the aforementioned 180–220) in combination with the use of aminocaproic acid, but bleeding complications remain significant in this population [5, 6]. Although cannula site bleeding, surgical site bleeding, and gastrointestinal hemorrhage can all occur, cerebral hemorrhage is perhaps the most feared complication. Neonates are at higher risk for intracranial bleeding. Seizures may be a presenting symptom, although some patients present with subclinical findings determined only by electroencephalogram.

In light of the bleeding risk, ample blood products should be available to optimize conditions. Patients should be transfused to maintain platelet levels ≥100,000, recognizing that even though the platelet level may be above the transfusion threshold, platelet function may still be impaired. The fibrinogen level should be maintained within the normal range of >150 mg/dL by transfusion of cryoprecipitate if necessary. Packed red blood cells should be given to maintain at least a hematocrit ≥30%, although ELSO Guidelines for Neonatal Respiratory Failure suggest maintaining a hemoglobin level of 13–14 g/dL to optimize oxygen carrying capacity [7].

> **Clinical Pearl**
>
> *Bleeding risk is significant in ECMO-dependent surgical patients. Decisions regarding decreasing or withholding anticoagulant infusions should be made by a multidisciplinary team. Hemoglobin, platelet, and fibrinogen levels should be optimized preoperatively. Monitoring of anticoagulation status should be continued intraoperatively. Adequate blood products should be available to replace intraoperative losses.*

Aside from balancing hemorrhage and thrombosis, what other ECMO-related complications can arise?

Mechanical pump malfunction is uncommon but possible. An integrated battery exists as backup support during transport or electrical failure, with an audible alert signaling loss of power and transition to battery power. Additionally, a hand pump system exists as a secondary backup. Oxygenator failure can present over time as a result of clot buildup in the membrane lung; an inability to oxygenate and exchange CO_2 and a widening pressure gradient across the oxygenator with increased resistance to flow would be noted. Tubing rupture is less common in the era of centrifugal pumps. Air in the circuit, especially post-oxygenator, can enter the patient and requires immediate response. Accidental decannulation is life threatening and is more likely during patient transport and positioning.

How should intraoperative hemodynamic instability be managed in a VA-ECMO–dependent patient?

Unlike the VV-ECMO patient who is solely dependent on his native cardiac function, the VA-ECMO patient's hemodynamics are driven by blood flow generated by both the pump and native cardiac output as well as vascular resistance. An appropriate MAP for this neonate would be 40–50 mm Hg. Hypotension intraoperatively is commonly due to inadequate circulating volume. The ECMO personnel may notice "chattering" of the venous cannula and fluctuating flow rates. Intravascular volume depletion can be managed with fluid and/or blood administration. Vasopressor infusions may be needed in cases of vasodilatation from infection. In the setting of septic shock, higher ECMO flow rates may be also necessary. Hypertensive episodes impede perfusion, so high systemic vascular resistance should be avoided and promptly treated. Once certain that the patient is adequately anesthetized, judicious use of a vasodilator may be considered if signs of high systemic vascular resistance persist. If any acute changes in pressure occur, circuit factors (pump issues, oxygenator failure, tubing kink, or malpositioned/obstructed cannulas) should be eliminated from the differential.

Who should manage ECMO circuitry and transfusion of blood products?

During the surgery, there should be dedicated personnel to monitor the ECMO machine, its parameters and function; often this is a perfusionist or specially trained ECMO nurse who manages ECMO during the day under the supervision of the intensivist. Any changes in the ECMO system should be communicated to the anesthesiologist immediately. Closed-loop communication is essential. Intraoperative transfusion will ultimately be at the discretion of the anesthesiologist; however, input from the surgeon and intensivist may be helpful to delineate surgical bleeding and ongoing medical bleeding or thrombotic concerns. Products can be directly infused directly into the ECMO circuit or through other available vascular access.

What considerations are important when surgical cases are performed in the intensive care unit?

The primary benefit of doing this particular case at bedside is the avoidance of transporting an ECMO-dependent neonate through the hospital. Physical space constraints can exist at the bedside however, given the abundance of equipment necessary to maintain a patient on ECMO. The anesthesiologist must ensure unfettered access to the patient, in particular the airway, infusion pumps, and vascular access sites. Availability of all required medications and equipment should be verified for both anesthesia and surgical services. Personnel to manage less familiar equipment, such as the ICU ventilator, should be immediately available. The bedside nurse or a surrogate should remain on the unit as an extra resource person. The physical room or space should be decluttered by removal of nonessential equipment and furniture and the pod should be closed to visitors.

References

1. H. L. Hedrick, E. Danzer, A. M. Merchant, et al. Liver position and lung-to-head ratio for prediction of extracorporeal membrane oxygenation and survival in isolated left congenital diaphragmatic hernia. *Am J Obstet Gynecol* 2007; **197**: 422.e1–4.

2. D. Mullassery, M. E. Ba'ath, E. C. Jesudason, et al. Value of liver herniation in prediction of outcome in fetal congenital diaphragmatic hernia: a systematic review and meta-analysis. *Ultrasound Obstet Gynecol* 2010; **35**: 609–14.

3. K. G. Snoek, I. K. M. Reiss, A. Greenough, et al. Standardized postnatal management of infants with congenital diaphragmatic hernia in Europe: The CDH EURO Consortium Consensus – 2015 Update. *Neonatology* 2016; **110**: 66–74.

4. E. A. Partridge, W. H. Peranteau, N. E. Rintoul, et al. Timing of repair of congenital diaphragmatic hernia in patients supported by extracorporeal membrane oxygenation (ECMO). *J Pediatr Surg* 2015; **50**: 260–2.

5. M. S. Dassinger, D. R. Copeland, J. Gossett, et al. Early repair of congenital diaphragmatic hernia on extracorporeal membrane oxygenation. *J Pediatr Surg* 2010; **45**: 693–7.

6. S. C. Fallon, D. L. Cass, O. O. Olutoye, et al. Repair of congenital diaphragmatic hernias on extracorporeal membrane oxygenation (ECMO): does early repair improve patient survival? *J Pediatr Surg* 2013; **48**: 1172–6.

7. B. Gray, N. Rintoul. Extracorporeal life support organization (ELSO) guidelines for neonatal respiratory failure supplement to the ELSO General Guidelines, Version 1. December 4, 2017, Ann Arbor, MI.

Suggested Reading

Chatterjee D., Ing R. J., and Gien J. Update on congenital diaphragmatic hernia. *Anesth Analg* 2020 Sep; 131(3): 808–821. doi: 10.1213/ANE.0000000000004324

Jenks C. L., Raman L., and Dalton H. J. Pediatric extracorporeal membrane oxygenation. *Crit Care Clin* 2017; 33: 825–41.

Lequier L. L., Horton S. B., McMullan D. M., et al. Extracorporeal membrane oxygenation circuitry. *Pediatr Crit Care Med* 2013; 14: S7–12.

Chapter 35

Left Heart Ventricular Assist Device

J. Nick Pratap

Case Scenario

A 5-year-old male weighing 17 kg presents from the cardiac step-down floor with melena and a drop in hematocrit from 33% to 26% over 72 hours. The patient is to undergo an upper endoscopy in the operating room.

He has a history of dilated cardiomyopathy and underwent placement of a Berlin Heart left ventricular assist device 2 months earlier. His current vital signs are pulse rate 98 beats/minute, respiratory rate 20 breaths/minute, blood pressure 124/94, temperature 36.6°C, and SpO$_2$ 100% on room air.

Current Berlin Heart settings are left systole 205 mm Hg; left diastole 25 mm Hg; left rate 98 beats/minute; 40% left systole. Monitoring parameters: fill: partial to full; emptying: 100%.

Key Objectives

- Understand the mechanics of the Berlin Heart.
- Describe indications for placement of a Berlin Heart.
- Discuss comorbidities experienced by Berlin Heart patients.
- Describe specific considerations in providing anesthesia for a patient with a Berlin Heart.

Pathophysiology

What is a ventricular assist device?

A ventricular assist device (VAD) is a mechanical pump used to support failing heart function when medical therapies have been exhausted.

Ventricular assist devices are most often classified according to the mode of blood flow generated by the pump:

- *Pulsatile pumps* mimic the natural pumping action of the heart. The Berlin Heart EXCOR (which this patient has implanted) is a paracorporeal pulsatile system. The 50cc Total Artificial Heart (SynCardia Systems, Inc.) is another pulsatile system, albeit a biventricular system,

that is currently in clinical trial. It may be suitable for pediatric patients aged 10–18 years with a body surface area (BSA) down to 1.2 m^2, and possibly even smaller patients with virtual implantation.

- *Continuous flow pumps* are further characterized by the type of mechanical pump utilized. An *axial pump* generates flow by rotating an impeller and causing blood to be accelerated in the direction of the rotor's axis. The HeartMate II (Thoratec Corporation) device is an example of an axial continuous flow pump.
A *centrifugal pump* draws blood in along a central axis and expels it tangentially by the impeller blades of the rotor. Centrimag (Thoratec Corporation), HeartMate 3 (Thoratec Corporation), and HeartWare (HeartWare Systems) devices utilize centrifugal pumps.

All VADs share the following components:

- Inflow and outflow cannulas
- Pump
- Power source with driveline
- System controller
- Clinical monitor console that can be attached to the controller to interrogate the device

How is the type of VAD selected for a child?

Device selection factors include the following:

- Underlying disease and cause of heart failure
- Duration of need for circulatory support
- Type of ventricular support needed (left, right, or biventricular)
- Patient's weight and body surface area
- Discharge potential

What is unique about the Berlin Heart EXCOR VAD?

The Berlin Heart EXCOR (Berlin Heart GmbH) is the only Food and Drug Administration (FDA)-approved VAD for long-term support of younger children with low cardiac output syndrome. It is a paracorporeal system that consists of a pulsatile blood pump with an electropneumatic drive system. It can be used for right (RVAD), left (LVAD), or biventricular (BiVAD) support. (See Figure 35.1.) The pump is available in a range of sizes with different stroke volumes suitable for neonates through adolescence. (See Figure 35.2.) Inlet and outlet connectors with tri-leaflet, one-way valves (Sorin-type tilting metal disks in larger devices) ensure unidirectional blood flow into and out of the heparin-coated blood chamber that is separated from an air chamber by a flexible, triple-layered membrane diaphragm. This curved diaphragm is driven by alternating pressures generated via the single driveline to the driving system unit: positive pressure applied essentially ejects blood out of the blood chamber into the patient's circulation, while negative pull entrains blood into the chamber during a fill cycle. The pump rate setting determines how often the membrane moves in 1 minute. The rate should be chosen such that the resulting blood flow meets the patient's requirements.

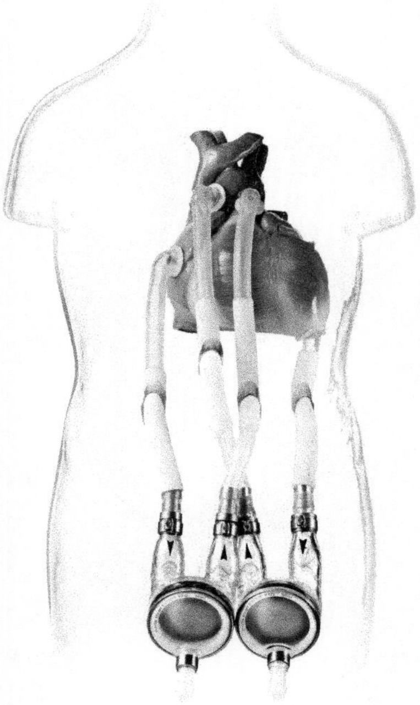

Cannulas are an important part of the Berlin Heart (BH) system and are constructed of noncoated reinforced silicone with a suture ring to facilitate anastomosis. The Dacron-velour mid-portion that exits the skin supports tissue ingrowth and thus protects against tracking infection. The availability of varied types and sizes of BH cannulas with differing lengths, angles, and tip styles has enabled a broader application for these cannulas compared with other devices. (See Figure 35.3.) Berlin Heart cannulas have been used for transthoracic extracorporeal life support with a temporary device when the outlook for native cardiac recovery is poor, thus allowing conversion to a BH pump without reopening the chest.

> **Clinical Pearl**
>
> *The Berlin Heart EXCOR is the only FDA-approved VAD for long-term support of younger children with low cardiac output syndrome. It can be used for right, left, or biventricular support.*

Figure 35.1 Biventricular support with two Berlin Heart devices.
LVAD configuration has inflow cannula in the LV apex, with outflow to the aorta. RVAD configuration has inflow from the right atrium, with outflow to the pulmonary artery. Reproduced with permission of Berlin Heart Inc.

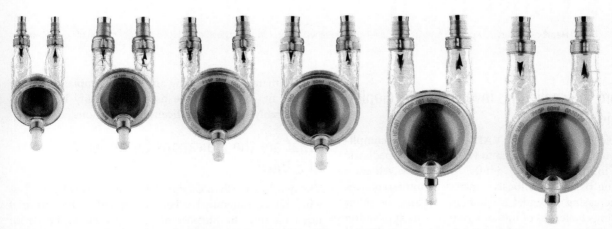

Figure 35.2 The wide range of pump sizes broadens the applicability of the Berlin Heart EXCOR to all pediatric ages from neonates to adolescence. Reproduced with permission of Berlin Heart Inc.

(a) (b)

(c)

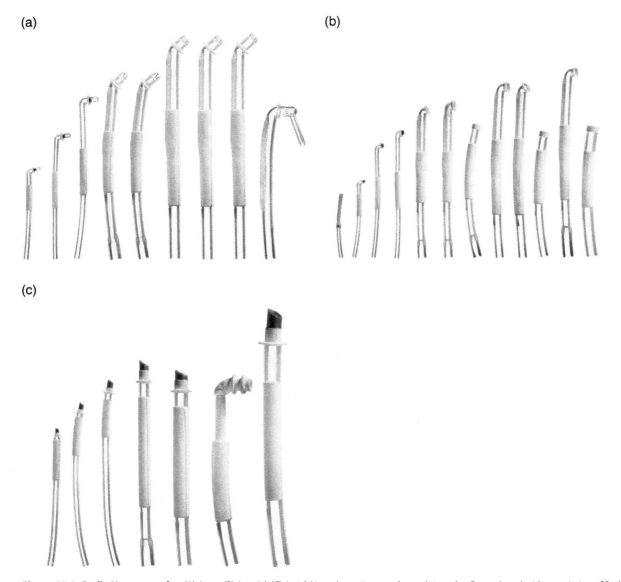

Figure 35.3 Berlin Heart cannulas. (A) Apex. (B) Arterial. (C) Atrial. Note the various angles and tip styles. Reproduced with permission of Berlin Heart Inc.

What are the challenges involved in developing pediatric VADs?

The development of suitable VADs for children is complicated by the large surface area to volume ratio of pediatric patients in comparison to adults, lower flow velocities (increasing risk of thrombosis), narrow cannulas/connections (increasing potential for hemolysis), and the other engineering challenges of miniaturization. The application of adult-sized devices to children is inherently complicated by size mismatch, especially with smaller patients. With three-dimensional modeling and "virtual implantation" to test for fit, devices can be used successfully in patients considerably smaller than licensed indications.

What are the indications for placement of a VAD?

The need for mechanical circulatory support (MCS) arises when medical therapy has been exhausted in the setting of heart failure. The purpose of a VAD such as the Berlin Heart EXCOR is to assume or augment ventricular function and restore cardiac output and adequate perfusion to end-organs. The device unloads the ventricle, thereby decreasing wall stress and optimizing chances for myocardial recovery and remodeling. Ventricular assist devices have been placed in children with myocardial disease (e.g., cardiomyopathy, myocarditis) or after failed palliation of congenital heart disease. They have also been implanted when it has not been possible to separate from temporary MCS such as cardiopulmonary bypass or extracorporeal membrane oxygenation (ECMO). Generally, especially in younger pediatric patients, the VAD serves as a bridge therapy, either to transplantation or to recovery. Rarely is destination therapy an aim in this patient population, although with certain devices, it is possible for patients to be discharged home to await transplantation.

What are the outcomes for children after placement of a BH?

In the early years after introduction of the BH, higher mortality was reported in patients weighing <5 kg, with congenital heart disease, transitioned from ECMO, or requiring biventricular support. Recent outcome studies now suggest that these are no longer risk factors. This device is most commonly placed as a bridge-to-transplantation. Following transplantation, contemporary series show that children bridged with a BH have similar survival, infection, and rejection rates compared to those not requiring MCS. Although earlier patients fared less well, since 2013 children in the BH prospective registry have enjoyed survival rates in excess of 70%.

> **Clinical Pearl**
>
> *Following transplantation, contemporary series show that children bridged with a BH have similar survival, infection, and rejection rates compared to those not requiring mechanical circulatory support.*

Anesthetic Implications

What is the likely health status of a child with a BH?

In the early period after BH placement, children still experience the typical sequelae of their preceding advanced heart failure. These sequelae include chronically increased catecholamine release, down-regulation of β- and α$_2$-adrenoreceptors, increased pulmonary vascular resistance (PVR), poor nutritional status, renal and hepatic impairment, and fluid overload. There can also be consequences of prolonged critical care support such as ventilator-associated lung injury, challenging vascular access, line-

associated thrombi or infections, dependence on or tolerance to opioids and other sedative/analgesic agents, or even stroke (particularly following ECMO). Over time, restitution of excellent tissue perfusion will hopefully ameliorate many of these issues.

Arterial thromboembolism is the most feared complication of the BH. Implantation has been associated with a 28% incidence of neurologic complications (notably ischemic stroke) and major bleeding occurs in 50% of patients. Although infectious complications, including fungal infection of the BH itself, have been reported in 86.7% of BH patients, they are not believed to contribute to mortality. Also, for patients supported only with a BH LVAD, it is very common for a degree of pulmonary hypertension to develop as a result of left atrial hypertension, even if the underlying cardiac pathology is predominantly left-sided.

> **Clinical Pearl**
>
> *For patients supported only with a BH LVAD, it is very common for a degree of pulmonary hypertension to develop as a result of left atrial hypertension, even if the underlying cardiac pathology is predominantly left-sided.*

What medications are typically taken by children with a BH?

Anticoagulation is invariably required by BH patients. Clinicians are challenged by the proverbial "tightrope" between bleeding and clotting risks. The Edmonton Anticoagulation and Platelet Inhibition Protocol was developed from early European experience with the device and forms the basis of most protocols in use. Protocols are typically institution specific and modified based on each center's own experiences. Standardly utilized drugs include an unfractionated heparin infusion initiated early postoperatively after bleeding has settled, followed by aspirin, enoxaparin or warfarin, and dipyridamole. The use of the newer direct thrombin inhibitor bivalirudin, instead of heparin, in the early postimplantation period is increasing. Clopidogrel is often added as well. High-dose steroids may be administered, particularly for the prothrombotic state that accompanies an inflammatory response in the absence of infection.

Anticoagulant effectiveness is generally monitored using laboratory testing of anti-Xa activity, often along with prothrombin time, thromboelastography (TEG), platelet mapping, and similar tests. Higher doses of anticoagulants are occasionally required compared to dosages typically employed for other indications. In many centers, either a multidisciplinary group or one or two designated physicians manage anticoagulation for BH patients. It is imperative that

271

these individuals are involved in perioperative decision making. A hematologist may additionally be consulted.

Berlin Heart patients with long intensive care unit (ICU) courses are also frequently on weaning regimens of methadone, benzodiazepines, clonidine, and other similar sedatives.

Clinical Pearl

In many centers, either a multidisciplinary group or designated physicians manage anticoagulation for BH patients. It is imperative that these individuals are involved in perioperative decision making.

For which procedures are children with a BH most likely to need anesthesia care?

Given the poor chronic health of many BH recipients, along with the need for early anticoagulation, the need to provide anesthesia for surgical control of early postoperative bleeding is only to be expected. In these situations, patients are likely to still be mechanically ventilated. Surgical reexploration is often performed at bedside in the ICU, thus avoiding the hazards of transport.

The BH pumping chamber may need to be changed out for traumatic damage or clot burden. As this procedure can be performed within a matter of seconds, a single bolus of a sedative agent will likely suffice, unless high urgency and a full stomach necessitate protection of the airway with rapid sequence intubation.

In view of the need for administration of multiple medications and frequent blood draws, vascular access placement is one of the most commonly performed procedures in children with a BH. Peripherally inserted central catheter (PICC) line insertion typically requires a relatively cooperative child, but the use of anxiolytic medications and local anesthesia often suffice as there is minimal pain or hemodynamic disturbance. Insertion of a tunneled central line, however, usually requires general anesthesia.

Diagnostic imaging may also require sedation or anesthesia. Procedures may be brief (such as a brain computed tomography [CT] scan for workup of stroke) or more involved, such as a cardiac catheterization for pretransplant evaluation or evaluation of PVR.

A thorough analysis must be conducted of the potential risks and benefits when any procedure is proposed for a BH patient. In some cases, procedures are better deferred until after device explantation. At other times, indications are so overwhelming that surgery must proceed. These cases often include diagnostic or therapeutic endoscopy, interventional radiology procedures for gastrointestinal bleeding, surgical airway evaluation, and laparotomy for ischemic bowel.

In the adult VAD literature, laparoscopic cholecystectomy has been reported, as VAD-associated chronic hemolysis may lead to cholelithiasis. This seems unlikely in children for whom the BH is used as a bridge to transplantation but may be relevant for any child with a different type of VAD being utilized for long-term or "destination" therapy.

Orthotopic cardiac transplantation is the expected outcome for most BH patients. Anesthesia considerations are standard as utilized for re-do median sternotomy, and heavy blood loss is expected in view of the therapeutic coagulopathy.

What anesthetic considerations exist for this patient and how do they impact the anesthesia plan?

Given the patient's low hematocrit, he should be transfused prior to the procedure with 15–20 mL/kg of packed red blood cells. This is important in restoring preload for this patient. An intravenous induction with either etomidate (0.2–0.3 mg/kg) or ketamine (1–2 mg/kg) and rocuronium (0.6–1.2 mg/kg) should provide good conditions for endotracheal intubation. Maintenance with sevoflurane should be well tolerated, but volatile agents should be titrated to account for loss of systemic vascular tone and possible resulting hypotension. In the event of hypotension, a fluid bolus of 10 mL/kg is a reasonable first-line therapeutic intervention, followed by phenylephrine boluses (1 mcg/kg initially) to address vascular tone issues.

Finally, in view of their often complicated preceding ICU course, long-term inpatient status, and the challenges of living on a VAD, these patients often have high anxiety about any procedure, especially those requiring anesthesia. Furthermore, many of these patients have developed a significant tolerance to sedatives and analgesics.

Clinical Pearl

Berlin Heart pre-anesthesia check:

- *Hematologic plan discussed and understood by surgeon/ proceduralist, VAD team +/– hematology, blood bank, intensivist, and anesthesiologist*
- *Current hemoglobin/hematocrit, coagulation panel, TEG, and other relevant labs reviewed*
- *Protamine, heparin, and mirror (for observing filling and ejection of the BH chamber) available*
- *Anti-siphon valves on any existing central vascular access lines (and precautions if placing new lines)*
- *VAD team/perfusionist contact details readily available*

What complications might be anticipated during anesthesia for a child with a BH?

Malignant dysrhythmias

In the event of "cardiac arrest" rhythms (such as ventricular fibrillation or tachycardia), the continuous pumping of the BH should ensure that cardiac output is maintained. Indeed, even if the right heart is unsupported, passive pulmonary perfusion should be sufficient in the short term. The manufacturer cautions that external cardiac compressions should not be performed as they risk trauma to the cannulas or their anastomoses. However, there are case reports of prolonged chest compressions without damage. In general, dysrhythmias should receive standard therapy including electrical cardioversion if necessary, although this may require anesthesia rather than sedation, as cerebral perfusion is maintained by the VAD and thus consciousness is maintained during malignant dysrhythmias.

Sudden loss of VAD output

Loss of device output may be heralded by loss of consciousness in the awake patient, interruption to the normal sounds emitted by the BH device, or an alarm signal from the driver unit. In parallel with checking the status of the patient, it is essential to ensure that the compressor hose has not become kinked, which is a common problem in the mobile child. It can also result from the movements of the operating table or personnel. Air leak is also possible and certainly should be considered after resolution of a kinked hose. Although the BH drive unit has a battery backup, prolonged loss of electricity can lead to loss of VAD output. A hand pump is kept with the drive unit for this type of emergency and for catastrophic mechanical failure of the drive unit itself.

Inadvertent cannula disconnection or brisk leakage of blood from a cannula necessitates clamping of the cannulas, disconnection of the compressor hose, and urgent summoning of both cardiac surgeon and perfusionist. Actual or impending embolism of a large clot or the appearance of air in the chamber (air embolism) requires a similar approach.

Sudden cyanosis

In addition to the usual causes of cyanosis, pulmonary embolism must be considered in patients with either an RVAD or poor native right heart contractility. Cyanosis may also result from right-to-left shunt through a previously unrecognized patent foramen ovale or atrial septal defect, which can occur when VAD-assisted left heart output exceeds pulmonary venous return. Echocardiography will reveal this complication. A change in VAD programming to raise left atrial pressure above right atrial pressure should eliminate the shunt. Intravenous fluid boluses may be required.

> **Clinical Pearl**
>
> *Loss of device output may be heralded by loss of consciousness in the awake patient, interruption to the normal sounds emitted by the BH device, or an alarm signal from the driver unit.*

What special precautions are necessary for a child with a BH?

In view of the complexity in dealing with BH patients, and the substantial individual history associated with each patient, the importance of having the appropriate VAD physician and a perfusionist both fully informed in advance of any procedure and immediately available cannot be overemphasized. In times of crisis, the ICU team is a valuable resource. When not emergent, cases should be scheduled at times when personnel and resources are immediately available.

Management of the BH device

The presence of a BH-trained nurse or perfusionist throughout the perioperative period is necessary. Although some institutions do not insist on the immediate presence of a perfusionist, it is desirable that such an individual be available within the facility for immediate consultation. Transfer of the patient and associated equipment to the operating room must be organized and efficient, as the driver battery has a finite capacity.

Great care must be taken during manual handling, such as transferring the patient to the operating table. Damage to or disconnection of components is possible and life threatening. Clear sterile drapes should be placed over all paracorporeal BH components during surgery so that visual confirmation of function and filling remains possible. Alcohol-based antiseptic solutions and radiant heaters may damage the chamber.

> **Clinical Pearl**
>
> ***Monitoring BH chamber status:*** *Clear sterile drapes should be placed over all paracorporeal BH components during surgery so that visual confirmation of function and filling remains possible. Filling and ejection of the BH chamber is best observed using a mirror to view the undersurface of the chamber. Look for irregularities in the smooth surface of the membrane at the end of filling or ejection to show that the preceding phase has not been fully completed. A little less than full filling is ideal, signifying that the upstream venous*

pool is adequately decompressed. Specifically, in the case of an LVAD, this reflects an absence of pulmonary venous congestion. In the case of ejection, however, it is desirable that all of the blood in the chamber is expelled, as incomplete emptying risks thrombosis.

Hematologic Considerations

The effects of multimodal anticoagulation and the necessity for its continuation must be appreciated. A TEG may be useful to demonstrate the effects of therapy. For some surgeries, temporary conversion from warfarin or low molecular weight heparin to an unfractionated heparin infusion is indicated. This would allow anticoagulation to be withheld for a short time perioperatively. A typical approach would be to stop the heparin drip 2 hours before surgery, and then to resume it an hour after hemostasis is achieved. Any use of vitamin K must be discussed with the VAD team and hematology colleagues, as it may prevent the immediate effective postprocedural use of warfarin. Both heparin and protamine should be available in the operating room. Packed red blood cell and platelet transfusions may be necessary, and it should be anticipated that significant coagulopathy can exist. Regional anesthesia is generally contraindicated due to anticoagulation.

Hemodynamic Considerations

Either intravenous or volatile induction agents are generally well tolerated as the supported ventricle is not susceptible to their negative inotropic effects, but since the BH system offers no compensation for any drop in systemic vascular resistance (SVR), fluid boluses or α-receptor agonists may be required for treatment of hypotension, especially during induction. A lower incidence of hypotension has been reported with ketamine compared to other induction agents. If substantial fluid shifts are likely, invasive hemodynamic monitoring is appropriate. Transesophageal echocardiogram (TEE) is useful if major cardiovascular instability is encountered. Principles for hemodynamic management are listed below.

- As fixed VAD output is the major hemodynamic concern, maintaining circulating volume is of prime importance.
- Minimize PVR, especially if the right heart is not supported by a device.
- Spontaneous ventilation may maintain better systemic venous return than positive pressure ventilation but risks pulmonary hypertensive crisis in susceptible patients when considering the respiratory depressive effects of the vast majority of sedatives/anesthetics.

- In patients with only LVAD support, if the procedure is major or the patient is unstable, right heart support may be necessary, so inhaled nitric oxide (iNO) and an epinephrine infusion (beginning at a low dose of 0.02–0.04 mcg/kg/minute) should be available.

Elevations in SVR risk stasis and thrombosis, so excellent analgesia should be provided. Although remifentanil has been used in adult VAD patients undergoing surgery, its use has not been reported in children with a BH; it can lead to bradycardia and hence insufficient venous return in cases where the left but not the right heart is being supported.

Infection Control

Antibacterial prophylaxis should be agreed upon in advance and should include antistaphylococcal coverage where appropriate, although published guidance on this aspect of care is not readily available.

> **Clinical Pearl**
>
> *Occasionally, for LVAD patients, if the procedure is major or the patient is unstable, right heart support may be necessary. Inhaled nitric oxide and an epinephrine infusion (start at low dose 0.02–0.04 mcg/kg/minute) should be available.*

What considerations exist when placing invasive lines in a patient with a BH?

In the case of right heart support with a BH, there is considerable risk of air entrainment during attempted central line placement, as the VAD generates negative pressure to fill its chamber. During puncture of great veins, some centers change the programming to decrease suction on the RVAD until the inserted catheter is closed to the atmosphere, at which point VAD settings are restored.

Furthermore, when placing a central venous line in any patient with BH RVAD, great care must be taken to avoid damage to the chamber inlet valve, embolism, or thrombus. Anti-siphon valves are advisable on infusions running through central lines in cases of RVAD or BiVAD support, as the BH may generate back pressure.

> **Clinical Pearl**
>
> *In the case of right heart support with a BH, there is considerable risk of air entrainment during attempted central line placement, as the VAD generates negative pressure to fill its chamber. Anti-siphon valves are advisable on infusions running through central lines in cases of right- or biventricular support, as the Berlin Heart may generate back pressure.*

What is the appropriate disposition for a BH patient after anesthesia?

Due to the complexity of anticoagulation management for BH patients, these patients must remain in the hospital. Postimplantation, patients are recovered in the ICU, but as their overall health status improves, they can be transitioned to stepdown or floor status, depending on the institutionally driven comfort level of the staff. Following major surgery, the patient should return to the ICU. For minor procedures, return from the post-anesthesia care unit to a high-dependency environment is reasonable. In this patient's case, provided the procedure is uneventful, return to the cardiac stepdown unit would be appropriate.

Suggested Reading

Cave D. A., Fry K. M., and Buchholz H. Anesthesia for noncardiac procedures for children with a Berlin Heart EXCOR Pediatric Ventricular Assist Device: a case series. *Paediatr Anaesth* 2010; **20**: 647–59.

May L. J., Lorts A., VanderPluym C., et al. Marked practice variation in antithrombotic care with the Berlin Heart EXCOR pediatric ventricular assist device. *ASAIO J* 2019; **65**: 731–37.

Miera O., Morales D. L. S., Thul J., et al. Improvement of survival in low-weight children on the Berlin Heart EXCOR ventricular assist device support. *Eur J Cardiothorac Surg* 2019; **55**: 913–19.

Right Ventricular Assist Device

Chapter 36

Rajeev Wadia and Jamie McElrath Schwartz

Case Scenario

A 14-year-old male with acute decompensated heart failure secondary to viral myocarditis underwent placement of a HeartWare™ left ventricular assist device. Prior to separation from cardiopulmonary bypass (CPB), transesophageal echocardiography showed moderate right ventricular (RV) dysfunction despite adequate right heart filling, and infusions of milrinone 0.5 mcg/kg/minute and epinephrine 0.03 mcg/kg/minute were initiated, along with inhaled nitric oxide at 20 ppm. As CPB was weaned, echocardiography was utilized to determine optimal HeartWare™ speed by ensuring maintenance of appropriate midline intraventricular septal position and aortic valve closure. After separating from CPB, RV function further declined, and central venous pressures >18 mm Hg were noted along with a low pulsatility index and calculated flow output on the HeartWare™ monitor. Transesophageal echocardiography showed a hypocontractile and dilated RV with moderate-to-severe tricuspid regurgitation, a dilated inferior vena cava, and no tamponade. Therefore, CPB was reinitiated and a CentriMag® continuous flow right ventricular assist device was implanted. The patient remained intubated and sedated at the completion of the surgery, with his initial postoperative course characterized by significant bleeding requiring aggressive fluid and blood product resuscitation. By postoperative day 5 bleeding had subsided, and he was started on systemic anticoagulation with heparin. On postoperative day 6, as the patient appeared ready to extubate, a large, rapidly expanding hematoma within the abdominal wall adjacent to the HeartWare™ driveline exit site was noted, requiring urgent evacuation.

Key Objectives

- Describe the different types of ventricular assist devices.
- Understand why right heart function is important for proper functioning of a left ventricular assist device.
- Understand why patients with a left ventricular assist device may develop right heart failure.
- List medical interventions that can augment right heart function in patients with a left ventricular assist device.
- Discuss intraoperative strategies that can be used to minimize right ventricular afterload.

Pathophysiology

What types of mechanical circulatory support are available for children?

Mechanical circulatory support (MCS) for children includes extracorporeal membrane oxygenation (ECMO) and ventricular assist devices (VADs). While ECMO provides both cardiac and respiratory support, VADs support only cardiac function. The device chosen for MCS depends on the individual patient's acuity and comorbidities as well as the anticipated length of required support and potential for recovery. Extracorporeal membrane oxygenation can be rapidly instituted in an emergent situation via peripheral vessel cannulation, even during cardiopulmonary resuscitation. This is not true for VAD placement, as it requires a sternotomy and the use of cardiopulmonary bypass (CPB). Furthermore, there is a tremendous amount of experience with ECMO in the pediatric population; it has been used for cardiorespiratory failure in children since the early 1980s. In contrast, the routine use of VADs in adults began in the late 1980s, while in pediatric patients widespread use did not begin until more than a decade later due to the need for technological improvements and device "miniaturization." In pediatric heart failure, implantation of a VAD is most often used as a bridge to transplant or recovery.

Clinical Pearl

Extracorporeal membrane oxygenation provides both cardiac and respiratory support, whereas a VAD only supports cardiac function.

276

What types of VADs are commonly used for pediatric heart failure?

There are two broad categories of VADs: those utilized for short-term support (<2 weeks) and those designed for long-term use (>2 weeks).

1. **Short-term** devices are **extracorporeal** (external to the body) centrifugal pumps. The most commonly utilized devices are RotaFlow® (Maquet, Wayne, NJ); TandemHeart® (CardiacAssist, Pittsburgh, PA); and CentriMag® and PediMag® (Thoratec, Pleasanton, CA).

2. **Long-term** devices can be either **extracorporeal** or **intracorporeal** (within the body), and pumps may provide either pulsatile or continuous flow.

   a. The **pulsatile flow** Berlin Heart EXCOR® (BH) device (see Chapter 35) is currently the only US Food and Drug Administration (FDA)-approved pediatric VAD. This pulsatile, extracorporeal VAD has been the most frequently implanted device in pediatric patients and can be used for both LV and biventricular support.

   b. Newer generation **continuous flow** pumps have supplanted pulsatile-flow pumps in appropriately-sized patients due to improved safety and the option for hospital discharge. These newer continuous flow devices are intracorporeal and utilize either **axial or centrifugal** pumps. Continuous flow devices are almost exclusively used for left heart support in children; however, biventricular support can also be

accomplished using two separate pumps. The major drawback with a continuous flow pump is its size, which often precludes use in younger children and instead requires placement of an extracorporeal pulsatile pump. (See Figure 36.1.) The most commonly implanted axial device is the HeartMate II™ (Thoratec), while the most commonly implanted centrifugal pump is the HeartWare™ HVAD™ (HeartWare™ ventricular assist device) (HeartWare, Framingham, MA).

Why is a LV assist device dependent on adequate RV function to work?

Right ventricular output has to increase to match the work of the implanted left ventricular assist device (LVAD). The RV must provide enough flow across the pulmonary vascular bed to provide adequate preload to the LVAD. Therefore, when weaning from CPB after LVAD placement, RV afterload reduction with pulmonary vasodilators such as inhaled nitric oxide (iNO) and milrinone is often utilized and factors that can increase pulmonary vascular resistance (PVR) are avoided. The temporary use of inotropic agents, such as epinephrine, may be required in the immediate postoperative period to improve RV performance and forward blood flow from the right heart to the left. Without adequate filling of the LV, there is collapse of the walls of the LV, restricted inflow into the LVAD, and a reduction in LVAD flow.

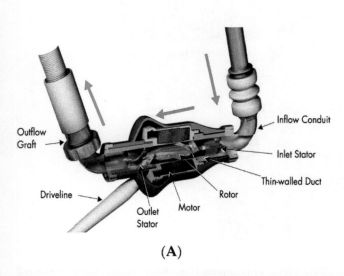

(A)

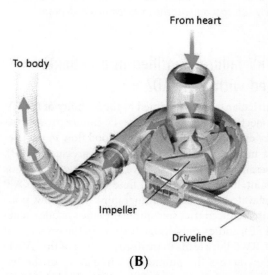

(B)

Figure 36.1 Extracorporeal continuous flow left ventricular assist device systems. (A) Axial-flow pump. (B) Centrifugal-flow pump. Figure from Singhvi A. and Trachtenberg B. Left ventricular assist devices 101: Shared care for general cardiologists and primary care. *J Clin Med* 2019; **8**(10): E1720 (PMID 31635239).

How does RV failure occur in patients supported with an LVAD?

It has been suggested that systolic pressure and stroke volume in the RV are generated by the ability of the RV free wall to contract against the intraventricular septum. Thus, RV failure following LVAD implantation is thought to result from the leftward shift of the intraventricular septum that occurs with excessive unloading of the LV. This shift then causes a decline in RV performance by inhibiting the ability of the RV free wall to effectively contract against the intraventricular septum. Furthermore, with high LVAD flows, the tricuspid annulus may be distorted, which can increase the amount of tricuspid regurgitation. Finally, the augmentation of cardiac output from the LVAD results in increased systemic venous return to the right heart, which can further hinder the performance of an already failing RV, especially if RV afterload is not effectively reduced. Fortunately, this constellation of findings does not happen every time an LVAD is placed. In most cases, the leftward shift of the septum is not excessive and actually improves RV diastolic compliance. In fact, in the absence of pulmonary vascular disease, the off-loading of the LV typically reduces RV afterload and prevents further decline of RV function.

> **Clinical Pearl**
>
> *Right ventricular failure following LVAD implantation is thought to result from the leftward shift of the intraventricular septum that occurs with excessive unloading of the LV. This shift then causes a decline in RV performance by inhibiting the ability of the RV free wall to effectively contract against the intraventricular septum.*

How is RV failure identified in a patient supported with an LVAD?

Right ventricular failure is defined as the inability of the RV to fill and eject normally, or when the RV cannot provide the pulmonary circulation with adequate blood flow in the presence of a normal preload/central venous pressure (CVP). When present, patients may have symptoms of venous engorgement, hepatomegaly, and fluid retention. The CVP is often elevated and echocardiography may show poor contractility, reduced tricuspid annular plane systolic excursion (TAPSE), and/or right heart dilation. In the presence of an LVAD, RV failure leads to ineffective filling of the LVAD because flow across the pulmonary circulation to the left heart is suboptimal. Inadequate filling of the LVAD is identified by reduced pulsatility and low flow on the HeartWare™ HVAD™ system. This decreased systemic flow reduces end-organ perfusion and can be identified by findings of increased bilirubin, elevated liver function tests, and decreased renal function.

What is a RV assist device?

A right ventricular assist device (RVAD) is a mechanical circulatory device, usually continuous flow, that provides antegrade flow of systemic venous return blood to the pulmonary artery without performing gas exchange. Devices may either be intracorporeal or extracorporeal. Most commonly, MCS for the RV is only required for a short time until RV function can recover. In these situations, an extracorporeal device such as the CentriMag® is commonly inserted. (See Figure 36.2.) The CentriMag® (see Figure 36.3) is a continuous flow device with two cannulas, one draining the right heart and a second returning blood to the pulmonary artery. Similarly to a continuous flow LVAD, the speed of the RVAD is programmed to achieve the desired amount of flow. Adequate decompression of the right heart is best evaluated with echocardiographic imaging and assessment of LVAD performance.

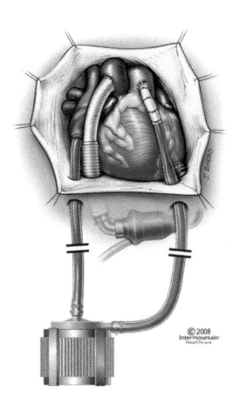

Figure 36.2 Extracorporeal CentriMag® RVAD is shown connected to cannulas that enter the body and are connected to the heart and great vessels. A continuous flow HeartMate II™ LVAD is also depicted. Figure used with permission from Intermountain® Healthcare.

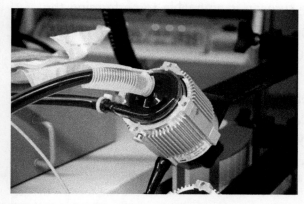

Figure 36.3 CentriMag® extracorporeal continuous flow pump used to support the RV. Image from www.flickr.com/photos/ec-jpr/9243359624

Why is an RVAD not always placed at the same time as an LVAD in children with heart failure requiring MCS?

Patients with heart failure who are candidates for an LVAD can have a broad range of RV dysfunction. Right ventricular function typically improves in many patients after placement of an LVAD. However, in some patients RV failure may persist. Many of these patients improve with medical management alone, but those who do not can be mechanically supported with an RVAD. An RVAD can be placed either at the time of LVAD placement or soon thereafter. Patients requiring biventricular mechanical support (BiVAD) have higher mortality, irrespective of the timing of RVAD placement. It remains unclear how much of the reduced survival associated with BiVAD support is due to the morbidity of having a second device, or if it is secondary to the severity of the underlying heart failure necessitating BiVAD support. Because there are no established criteria for RVAD implementation in children, centers often prefer aggressive medical therapy for RV dysfunction as first-line management. However, if mechanical support seems unavoidable, early RVAD implantation is recommended.

Anesthetic Implications

The patient is receiving systemic anticoagulation with a heparin infusion to prevent device-associated thrombus formation. How should anticoagulation be managed for the upcoming procedure?

Anticoagulation management for patients on MCS is complex. The risk for thrombus formation due to foreign material is not trivial and must be balanced against the risk of hemorrhage. Initiation of systemic anticoagulation does not generally occur until postoperative bleeding has subsided, typically on postoperative day 2 or 3. This patient has a hematoma that likely formed following surgery and then acutely worsened with the initiation of anticoagulation. Monitoring of anticoagulation parameters (activated partial thromboplastin time [aPTT], prothrombin time/international normalized ratio [PT/INR], antifactor Xa, and thromboelastogram) helps guide therapies. While minor surgeries may not require anticoagulation to be discontinued, major surgeries or surgeries with a high risk of bleeding (i.e., neurosurgical) may require adjustments. Therefore, a consensus among providers (intensivist, cardiologist, surgeon, anesthesiologist) or the team managing anticoagulation must be reached regarding the risk/benefit ratio of continuing, discontinuing, or modifying management of anticoagulation in the perioperative period prior to every surgical intervention. The surgical evacuation of a hematoma is a relatively minor surgery and anticoagulation could most likely be discontinued for a brief period. However, if there is concern for thrombus formation in either device (which would be unusual at this early stage in the postimplantation period), the risk of even briefly discontinuing anticoagulation may outweigh the risk of continuing it through the perioperative period.

> **Clinical Pearl**
>
> *A consensus among providers (intensivist, cardiologist, surgeon, and anesthesiologist) must be reached regarding the risk-benefit ratio of continuing, discontinuing, or modifying anticoagulation in the perioperative period prior to every surgical intervention.*

The surgeon requests that the procedure be performed in the operating room. Is this reasonable and if so, which additional staff can provide valuable assistance with this procedure?

Transporting any patient on life-sustaining technology presents unique challenges and risks. This patient has two mechanical devices supporting his heart. The CentriMag® RVAD system is an extracorporeal device residing outside of the body and connected to a control unit. (See Figure 36.4.) The implanted HVAD™ also has a dedicated control console. Both of these devices require trained personnel (either VAD specialist and/or perfusionist) to be immediately present. Any movement of the patient

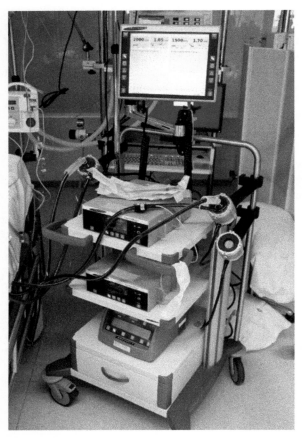

Figure 36.4 Example of a control unit for an extracorporeal, continuous-flow mechanical circulatory system. Image from www .flickr.com/photos/ec-jpr/9243362372/in/photostream/

requires meticulous attention to cannula position and integrity to maintain optimal pump flow and prevent catastrophic disconnections. If transportation of the patient is absolutely required, then all appropriate personnel must accompany the patient.

Given the risks associated with transport and the scope of the proposed surgery, it is reasonable to discuss with the surgeon whether the hematoma evacuation can be safely performed in the intensive care unit (ICU) at the bedside.

Clinical Pearl

Transporting a patient on extracorporeal mechanical support requires thoughtful planning, and every effort to perform tests and procedures at the patient's bedside should be made when appropriate. Any movement of the patient requires meticulous attention to cannula position and integrity to maintain optimal pump flow and prevent catastrophic disconnections.

The surgeon is amenable to performing the procedure in the ICU, but requests that the patient receive a general anesthetic provided by an anesthesiologist. Currently the patient is receiving morphine and dexmedetomidine infusions for sedation while mechanically ventilated. How should an anesthetic be planned?

Since the procedure is being performed in the ICU, there is no anesthesia machine to administer inhalational volatile agents. Therefore, a total intravenous anesthetic is the best choice. Because chronically ill patients who are mechanically ventilated in the ICU often require high doses of sedative infusions over prolonged periods, they often develop significant tolerance. Therefore, simply increasing the background sedative infusions may not be adequate to provide a surgical depth of anesthesia. Additional amnestic and analgesic drugs (i.e., propofol, ketamine, midazolam, or a combination) are necessary. It can be helpful to use bispectral index monitoring in this situation to assess the depth of anesthesia.

What important preparation is necessary for this patient when performing a general anesthetic in the ICU?

The presence of a VAD with the subsequent administration of anticoagulant and antiplatelet agents places patients at increased risk for bleeding during surgical procedures. Therefore, it is prudent to have appropriate cross-matched blood products immediately available along with all proper equipment (i.e., blood warmer with filter and tubing) required to rapidly administer blood products. In addition, all medications (emergency and anesthetic) and airway equipment normally available in the OR should be brought to the patient's bedside in the ICU. The anesthesia team should also familiarize themselves with the ICU ventilator, and a respiratory therapist should be available for ventilator adjustments or troubleshooting if required. Finally, bedside monitors should be positioned so that both the anesthesia team and surgeons can easily observe intraoperative hemodynamics.

Clinical Pearl

The presence of a VAD and the ongoing administration of anticoagulant and antiplatelet agents places patients at increased risk for bleeding during surgical procedures. Therefore, it is prudent to have appropriate cross-matched blood products immediately available.

How should the intraoperative plan be designed to maintain low PVR and ensure adequate HVAD™ filling and flow?

As an LVAD is preload dependent, LV filling must be maintained to ensure adequate systemic flow. Systemic venous return to the right heart must be pumped across the pulmonary vascular bed before it reaches the left heart. Any pathology that inhibits this forward flow of blood can lead to inadequate HVAD™ filling, therefore limiting the systemic flow that can be generated. Right heart pathology (i.e., tricuspid regurgitation, ventricular dysfunction, pulmonary valve insufficiency) disrupts flow of blood into the pulmonary vasculature. Downstream from the RV, pulmonary vascular pathology (i.e., pulmonary hypertension, pulmonary artery stenosis, pulmonary vein stenosis) and mitral valve disease (i.e., mitral stenosis and mitral regurgitation) can also contribute to poor LV filling. While some of these factors may not be amenable to manipulation, those that can be optimized are important in the intraoperative management of these patients. The primary goal is to avoid elevations in RV afterload by maintaining low PVR. Avoiding triggers that elevate PVR, such as hypercarbia, acidosis, hypoxemia, hypothermia, and sympathetic stimulation, is of the utmost importance. Pulmonary vasodilators such as iNO or prostacyclin analogues may be considered to reduce PVR.

Reviewing the most recent chest radiograph and blood gas prior to the start of surgery is important to gain a qualitative estimation of current pulmonary pathology. Periodic monitoring of blood gases and continuous end-tidal CO_2 monitoring throughout the case aids in guiding ventilator manipulations. Care must be taken to avoid extremes of mean airway pressure, as both overdistention and underinflation of the lungs can lead to elevations in PVR. Ensuring an adequate depth of anesthesia/analgesia can prevent increases in PVR that can occur with sympathetic stimulation from painful procedures. Should a sudden increase in RV afterload occur, a chest radiograph or point-of-care ultrasound of the lungs should be performed to rule out intrathoracic pathology (i.e., pneumothorax or hemothorax).

Clinical Pearl

The primary goal is to avoid elevations in RV afterload by maintaining low PVR. Avoiding triggers that elevate PVR, such as hypercarbia, acidosis, hypoxemia, hypothermia, and sympathetic stimulation, is of the utmost importance.

In patients with an RVAD, what considerations are important to ensure adequate blood flow into the pulmonary circulation?

In patients with an RVAD, the forward flow of blood from the right heart to the pulmonary circulation is largely dependent on RVAD flow, and to a lesser degree, RV function. If a decrease in RVAD flow occurs, the etiology should be determined, and appropriate measures undertaken.

A decrease in RVAD flow can occur from any of the following:

- Decreased inflow (i.e., hypovolemia, inflow cannula obstruction)
- Pump failure (i.e., thrombosis)
- Increase in afterload (i.e., outflow cannula obstruction, increased PVR)

Information obtained from the perfusionist's assessment of the pump and circuit can often help narrow the possible etiologies. Echocardiographic images can also be extremely useful; therefore, placement of a transesophageal probe should strongly be considered during surgical procedures, especially if large fluid shifts are expected. Transesophageal echocardiography can evaluate device cannula position, ventricular filling, and ventricular function, all of which can help guide intraoperative therapy. With satisfactory echocardiographic imaging, if the patient is not hypovolemic and there is no concern for pump thrombosis or elevated PVR, increasing the RVAD speed to increase flow should be considered. However, the ability to increase RVAD speed may be limited by cannula size. If increasing RVAD speed cannot safely be performed, use of an inotropic agent to promote RV contractility while under anesthesia should be considered.

Clinical Pearl

It is important to consider the RVAD and RV as two separate components contributing to right ventricular stroke work. In the majority of patients with an RVAD, the RV function is usually limited; however, as the RV recovers, the overall amount of work the RVAD contributes to RV stroke work decreases. This then allows the RVAD speed to be incrementally decreased until it is low enough that it can be eventually explanted/removed. In situations in which right heart stroke work needs to increase, either the RVAD speed or RV contractility can be augmented.

Does an RVAD provide respiratory support?

An RVAD does not provide respiratory support. An RVAD system is slightly different from a veno-venous (VV) ECMO circuit. In VV-ECMO, systemic venous blood is removed and returned to the right heart after traveling through an oxygenator. The purpose of VV-ECMO is to support patients with lung injury by providing gas exchange (adding oxygen and removing carbon dioxide). It requires adequate RV function to operate properly. In contrast, an RVAD system is intended to only support depressed RV function. It is possible to place an oxygenator in the extracorporeal RVAD circuit to support gas exchange, but this is not common. Of note, an RVAD can indirectly improve oxygenation and ventilation by improving pulmonary blood flow, thereby reducing dead space.

Clinical Pearl

Veno-venous ECMO can support patients with lung injury by providing gas exchange (adding oxygen and removing carbon dioxide). It requires adequate RV function to operate properly. In contrast, an RVAD system is intended to only support depressed RV function.

Suggested Reading

Adler A., Grogan K., and Berenstain L. Mechanical circulatory support. In Coté C., Lerman J., and Anderson B., eds. *A Practice of Anesthesia for Infants and Children*, 6th ed. Philadelphia, Elsevier, 2018; 500–19.

Argiriou M., Kolokotron S., Sakellaridis T., et al. Right heart failure post left ventricular assist device implantation. *J Thorac Dis* 2014; **6**: S52–59.

Hehir D. A., Niebler R. A., Brabant C. C., et al. Intensive care of the pediatric ventricular assist device patient. *World J Pediatr Congenit Heart Surg* 2012; **3**: 58–66.

Karimov J. H., Sunagawa G., Horvath D., et al. Limitations of chronic right ventricular assist device support. *Ann Thorac Surg* 2016; **102**: 651–8.

Karimova A., Pockett C. R., Lasuen N., et al. Right ventricular dysfunction in children supported with pulsatile ventricular assist devices. *J Thorac Cardiovasc Surg* 2014; **147**: 1691–7.

Miller J. R., Epstein D. J., Henn M. C., et al. Early biventricular assist device use in children: a single-center review of 31 patients. *ASAIO J* 2015; **61**: 688–94.

Nelson McMillan K., Hibino N., Brown E. E., et al. HeartWare ventricular assist device implantation for pediatric heart failure–a single center approach. *Artif Organs* 2019; **43**: 21–9.

Stein M., Yeh J., Reinhartz O., et al. HeartWare HVAD for biventricular support in children and adolescents: the Stanford experience. *ASAIO J* 2016; **62**: e46-51.

Lung Transplantation

Arpa Chutipongtanate and Erica P. Lin

Case Scenario

A 14-year-old girl, weighing 43 kg, presents to the general operating room for routine surveillance bronchoscopy with lavage and biopsies. She has a history of cystic fibrosis and underwent double-lung transplantation 18 months ago. Her postoperative course was complicated by primary graft dysfunction and bacteremia. Today she is actively coughing during her preoperative assessment; she says that it is her "normal" cough and has been present for more than a month. She also states that she has missed several doses of tacrolimus over the past weeks. Current vital signs are temperature 38.1°C, heart rate 92 beats/minute, respiratory rate 27 breaths/minute, hemoglobin-oxygen saturation on room air 97%. Breath sounds are clear, without wheezing or rhonchi, and she does not appear to be in respiratory distress. A review of the results of her pulmonary function tests performed on the previous day shows no significant change. The chest radiograph shows questionable consolidation versus atelectasis in the right lower lobe.

Key Objectives

- Understand the anatomy and physiology of transplanted lungs.
- Describe the preoperative assessment of post–lung transplant patients.
- Review important considerations for the anesthetic management of post–lung transplant patients.
- Discuss postoperative expectations for these patients.

Pathophysiology

What are the indications for lung transplantation?

Pediatric lung transplantation is the most aggressive therapeutic option for children with end-stage pulmonary disease, but it remains a relatively rare operation. Major diagnoses necessitating transplant vary according to recipient age group. Cystic fibrosis (CF) is the most common indication in children ≥6 years, while pulmonary hypertension and surfactant disorders account for the majority of cases in infants < 1 year of age. Other indications include interstitial lung disease, bronchopulmonary dysplasia, obliterative bronchiolitis, and re-transplantation/graft failure.

What is the expected course for patients post lung transplantation?

Lung transplants have the lowest survival rate of all solid organ pediatric transplants. Lungs are unique in that they remain directly exposed to the external environment, with its infective and immunologic challenges, and therefore high levels of immunosuppression are required. The most recent report from the International Society for Heart and Lung Transplantation registry for patients transplanted between January 1990 and June 2016 disclosed a median survival of 5.5 years after pediatric lung transplantation. In patients surviving past year 1, median survival is 8.9 years [1]. The most common causes of death in the first 30 days are multiorgan failure, cardiovascular complications, graft failure, and infection. From 30 days to 1 year, infection and graft failure are the primary causes of death. Beyond 1 year, chronic allograft dysfunction and graft failure are leading causes of mortality. Bronchiolitis obliterans syndrome (BOS) is the most common form of chronic allograft dysfunction and is present in more than 50% of recipients by 5 years post-transplant [1].

Adolescents have lower survival rates compared to young children; this may be partly due to nonadherence with medical therapy leading to graft failure, compounded by transitioning from pediatric to adult care providers. Center volume and pediatric-specific expertise also affect outcome, with better survival in patients transplanted in pediatric centers with higher clinical volume [2]. Furthermore, in CF patients, lung transplantation does not confer any significant survival benefit [3].

Table 37.1 Complications of Lung Transplantation

Immediate (First Week)	Early Phase (1–3 Months)	Late Phase (Beyond 3 Months)
Surgical complications • *Bleeding* • *Anastomotic issues* • *Airway dehiscence* Hyperacute rejection Primary graft dysfunction Infection	Acute rejection Humoral rejection Poor airway clearance Infection Medication side effects	Bronchiolitis obliterans Malignancy Medication side effects

Clinical Pearl

Lung transplants have the lowest survival rates of all solid organ transplants, and adolescents have lower survival rates compared to young children. Lung transplantation confers no significant survival benefit to cystic fibrosis patients.

What complications are commonly associated with lung transplantation?

Complications can be divided into three phases as outlined in Table 37.1.

How does acute rejection present?

Acute rejection affects the majority of lung transplant recipients and typically is seen during the first 3 months post-transplantation. It may be asymptomatic or present with nonspecific symptoms mimicking infection, including cough, fever, hypoxemia, tachypnea, or dyspnea. Many centers advocate a strict surveillance schedule including scheduled bronchoscopy, bronchoalveolar lavage, and transbronchial biopsy at multiple intervals during the first 3 months to screen for acute rejection and infection.

What is the difference between primary graft dysfunction and chronic allograft dysfunction?

Primary graft dysfunction (PGD) refers to a syndrome of acute lung injury that develops in the first 72 hours after lung transplantation. It is characterized by hypoxemia and the radiographic appearance of diffuse pulmonary opacities and represents a multifactorial injury to the transplanted lung rather than immunologic rejection. Diagnosis is made by excluding other conditions such as volume overload, acute rejection, infection, aspiration, and pulmonary thromboembolism. The severity of PGD is based on the ratio of arterial fraction of oxygen (PaO_2)/fraction of inspired oxygen (FiO_2)[4]. (See Table 37.2.)

Table 37.2 Grading Scale for Primary Graft Dysfunction

PGD Grade	Pulmonary Edema on Chest Radiograph	PaO_2/FiO_2 ratio
PGD grade 0	No	Any
PGD grade 1	Yes	>300
PGD grade 2	Yes	200–300
PGD grade 3	Yes	<200

From Christie J. D., Carby M., and Bag R. Report of the ISHLT Working Group on Primary Lung Graft Dysfunction Part II: Definition. A Consensus Statement of the International Society for Heart and Lung Transplantation. *J Heart Lung Transplant* 2005; **24**: 1454–9.

Primary graft dysfunction is associated with a significantly higher mortality and has been correlated with bronchiolitis obliterans. Management is primarily supportive and includes fluid restriction and avoidance of barotrauma. In severe cases, patients may require support with extracorporeal membrane oxygenation (ECMO).

Chronic allograft dysfunction (CLAD) is a term encompassing all chronic lung dysfunction after lung transplantation. Chronic allograft dysfunction is a major limitation to long-term survival post-transplantation. There are two predominant phenotypes of CLAD:

*   ***Bronchiolitis obliterans syndrome*, or obliterative bronchiolitis**, is the most common form of chronic allograft dysfunction and manifests clinically as obstructive lung disease. It is detected clinically as a decline in forced expiratory volume in 1 second (FEV_1)>20% from baseline and pathologically as dense fibrous tissue affecting the small airway. It is the leading cause of death after the first year of transplant and 50% of surviving children develop BOS within 5 years after transplant [1].
*   ***Restrictive allograft syndrome* (RAS)** accounts for 30% of CLAD and manifests clinically as restrictive lung disease, with a persistent decrease in forced vital

capacity (FVC) or total lung capacity with chronic pulmonary infiltrates. Patients with RAS have decreased survival (6–18 months) compared with 3- to 5-year survival for patients with BOS [5].

Do transplanted lungs function like native lungs?

Overall, lung transplant recipients display marked improvement in respiratory function, gas exchange, and exercise tolerance. Respiratory rate and rhythm are typically unchanged. However, transplanted lungs do have an altered physiology compared to native lungs because of the disruption to vagal and autonomic nerves, as well as pulmonary, bronchial, and lymphatic vessels that occurs during explantation of the donor lungs. The level of preservation of the cough reflex is dependent on the surgical strategy, as coughing is stimulated from remaining native lung or from sites proximal to the airway anastomosis. (See Figure 37.1.) Impaired mucociliary clearance is especially pronounced in the early post-transplant period, but remains problematic in long-term survivors, possibly due to abnormal mucus production and diminished ciliary beat frequency. The disruption of the cough reflex and

mucociliary clearance, combined with chronic immunosuppression, increases susceptibility to infection. Lymphatic interruption predisposes transplanted lungs to pulmonary edema from fluid overload, especially in the early post-transplant period, and lung compliance is reduced. Single lung transplant recipients can have differential ventilation and perfusion, dependent on compliance differences between native and implanted lung and the pulmonary circulation. The hypoxic pulmonary vasoconstriction reflex remains intact, as does airway response to β_2-agonists.

Clinical Pearl

Transplanted lungs have diminished cough reflex and mucociliary clearance and are predisposed to pulmonary edema due to interruption of lymphatic drainage.

What common coexisting medical issues are frequently seen in lung transplant recipients?

Roughly half of early post-transplant patients exhibit some degree of gastrointestinal dysmotility, gastroparesis, and/or gastroesophageal reflux. Arrhythmias (e.g., supraventricular

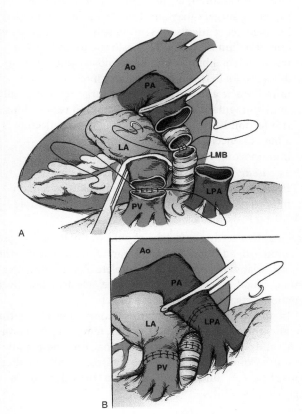

Figure 37.1 (A) Lung implantation. Typically, the bronchus is anastomosed first, followed by the left atrial/pulmonary venous connection. **(B)The implantation is completed with the left pulmonary artery anastomosis.** Ao, aorta; LA left atrium; LMB, left mainstem bronchus; LPA, left pulmonary artery; PA, pulmonary artery; PV, pulmonary vein. From Ryan T. D., Chin C., and Bryant R. III. Heart and Lung Transplantation. In Ungerleider R. M., Meliones J. N., McMillan K. N., et al., eds. *Critical Heart Disease in Infants and Children*, 3rd ed. Elsevier, 2019; 868–84. With permission.

tachycardia, atrial flutter, atrial fibrillation) related to the left atrial cuff suture line may also be present but can be treated with conventional therapies and are often self-limited.

A host of medical issues can be attributed to chronic immunosuppression therapy.

- **Cardiovascular**: Hypertension may develop due to the pressor effects of corticosteroids and calcineurin inhibitors and affects approximately 70% of patients within 5 years. Hyperlipidemia is also common, developing in 18% of survivors by 5 years [6].
- **Renal**: Long-term use of calcineurin inhibitors can also result in renal dysfunction, with almost one-third of patients affected within 5 years post-transplant [6]. Early postoperative renal insufficiency, however, is more likely related to preexisting renal dysfunction.
- **Neurologic**: Calcineurin inhibitors can cause neurologic symptoms including seizures.
- **Endocrine**: Diabetes may result from immunosuppression with steroids and calcineurin inhibitors and is more common in CF patients with pancreatic disease. Prevalence ranges from 18.8% within 1 year to 28.6% at 5 years [1].
- **Orthopedic**: Steroid-induced osteoporosis markedly increases the risk of fractures, and avascular necrosis is most commonly seen in the lumbar spine, ribs, and femoral heads.
- **Oncologic**: Ten percent of transplant survivors develop malignancy by 5–7 years, most commonly a lymphoma variant termed post-transplant lymphoproliferative disease [1].

Clinical Pearl

Lung transplant recipients develop comorbidities related to chronic immunosuppression. Hypertension, renal dysfunction, diabetes, hyperlipidemia, and osteoporosis are frequently seen. Chronic steroid use also leads to osteoporosis and avascular necrosis.

Anesthetic Implications

What special considerations exist when assessing a post–lung transplant patient preoperatively?

The patient's transplant team is an excellent point of contact during the preoperative evaluation, as they will have detailed knowledge of their patient's history, current status, ongoing morbidity, medication regimen, and medical compliance.

The following factors should be considered in the preoperative evaluation of patients with transplanted lungs:

- **Assessment of pulmonary graft function** and possible rejection/infection is crucial. Red flag signs such as increasing dyspnea or the need for supplemental oxygen, fever, cough, infiltration on chest radiograph, and deterioration of pulmonary function should be noted. If any of those are present, discussion with the patient's multidisciplinary team, particularly the patient's pulmonologist, should take place prior to surgery.
- **Immunosuppressive medications** should be continued throughout the perioperative period. Triple-drug immunosuppression is standard and typically consists of a calcineurin inhibitor (e.g., tacrolimus, cyclosporine), a cell cycle inhibitor (e.g., mycophenolate mofetil, azathioprine), and corticosteroids, with the International Pediatric Lung Transplant Collaborative advocating tacrolimus, mycophenolate mofetil, and prednisolone as the predominant regimen [7]. It is important to appreciate side effects and potential toxicities of commonly used immunosuppressive agents. (See Table 37.3.)
- The **indication for the surgical procedure** should be taken into account, as the nature of the condition requiring surgery may affect the transplanted lungs. For instance, patients presenting with acute changes in lung function may require anesthesia to undergo transbronchial biopsy and bronchioalveolar lavage to differentiate between rejection and infection. Both intrathoracic and intraabdominal surgeries may result in diaphragmatic splinting and impaired respirations. If infection is the indication for surgery, septicemia is a major concern given the patient's immunocompromised status.
- The **underlying disease process necessitating transplant** and the associated comorbidities remain important, especially in CF patients where multiple "distant" organs are involved.

Preoperative testing and labs should evaluate end-organ function. In addition to pulmonary function tests, the following labs are appropriate: complete blood count, creatinine, blood urea nitrogen, glucose, electrolytes, liver function tests, and a coagulation panel.

In this patient, one should be concerned about the cough with mild tachypnea, mild temperature elevation, and questionable consolidation on chest radiograph. Combined with the history of medical nonadherence, underlying rejection or infection is a distinct possibility.

Table 37.3 Side Effects and Toxicity of Commonly Used Immunosuppressive Agents

Agent	Side Effect/Toxicity
Tacrolimus (calcineurin inhibitor)	Nephrotoxicity Hypertension Neurotoxicity (headache, tremor, paresthesia, seizure) Glucose intolerance Thrombocytopenia
Mycophenolate mofetil (cell cycle inhibitor)	Hypertension Hyperkalemia/hypophosphatemia Anemia Arrhythmias (tachycardia) Muscle weakness
Corticosteroids	Hypertension Fluid retention Glucose intolerance Adrenal suppression Electrolyte abnormalities Peptic ulcerations, pancreatitis Osteoporosis, myopathy, aseptic necrosis Poor wound healing Psychological disturbance, mood change
Azathioprine (cell cycle inhibitor)	Hepatotoxicity Myelosuppression (anemia, leukopenia, thrombocytopenia) Pancreatitis Nausea, vomiting Arthralgia, rash, stomatitis
Cyclosporine (calcineurin inhibitor)	Nephrotoxicity Hypertension Hepatotoxicity Neurotoxicity (tremor, paresthesias, headache, confusion, seizures) Gastric atony Hyperkalemia/hypomagnesemia

Clinical Pearl

Preoperative evaluation of lung transplant patients should include the following:

- *Ensuring that the transplant team is aware of the planned surgery*
- *Evaluation of pulmonary graft function*
- *Consideration for rejection and/or infection*
- *Effects of the immunosuppressive regimen on other organ systems*
- *Effect(s) of other organ dysfunction on transplanted lungs*
- *Medical noncompliance risk, especially in adolescent patients*
- *Indication for the surgical procedure and potential effects on the lungs*

Are there specific anesthetic management goals for a post–lung transplant patient?

- **Premedication**: As these patients are frequent visitors to the medical environment, they may experience significant anxiety preoperatively. Anxiolytic premedication is appropriate, provided the patient has adequate ventilatory function. Supplemental perioperative steroid administration should also be considered for major invasive surgeries in patients on chronic steroid therapy or those who have recently completed steroid therapy.
- **Monitoring**: The use of invasive monitors intraoperatively should be dictated by the severity of the patient's condition and the intended surgery. The risk of infection during line placement cannot be underestimated.
- **Induction**: Unless hemodynamic instability exists, all induction agents may be considered safe. In the face of compromised cardiopulmonary function, the use of etomidate or ketamine should be considered. Rapid-sequence induction is indicated for patients with severe GERD or gastroparesis.
- **Airway management**: A recognized side effect of chronic steroid treatment is the rounded Cushingoid moon face, which can adversely impact the ability to mask ventilate a patient. While a laryngeal mask airway (LMA) may be appropriate for procedures of short duration, it is not advisable for patients with active mucositis or those who are at risk of aspiration from gastric atony. Tracheal intubation is preferable for longer procedures and those performed in the nonsupine position. Positioning of the endotracheal tube with the cuff just distal to the vocal cords avoids traumatizing tracheal or bronchial anastomotic suture lines. Especially in the early post-transplant period, direct visualization with a fiberoptic scope may be desirable, and certainly if advanced lung-isolation techniques are required. Long-term airway complications such as stenosis, bronchomalacia, granulomas, and mechanical bronchial distortion can complicate lung-isolation techniques. Avoidance of reactive bronchospasm, especially during airway manipulation, is a high priority, as bronchodilators are less effective, particularly if there is underlying rejection.

Clinical Pearl

Tracheal intubation is preferable for longer procedures and those performed in the nonsupine position. Positioning of the endotracheal tube with the cuff just distal to the vocal cords avoids traumatizing tracheal or bronchial anastomotic suture lines.

- **Ventilation strategy**: Particularly in recently transplanted lungs, when utilizing positive pressure ventilation, maintenance of a low peak inspiratory pressure (PIP) is desirable to minimize stress on surgical anastomoses. Most programs suggest a "lung protective" ventilation strategy with the following limits: tidal volume <7 mL/kg body weight, PIP <30 cm H_2O, plateau pressure 20–25 cm H_2O, positive end-expiratory pressure 5–8 cm H_2O, and adjustment of respiratory rate to provide appropriate minute ventilation with $PaCO_2$ at a level similar to preoperative baseline values for each patient [8]. Infection, rejection, or bronchiolitis obliterans can cause high PIP and plateau pressures.
- **Anesthetic maintenance**: A balanced anesthetic technique utilizing volatile anesthetic or propofol along with short-acting opioids and/or neuromuscular blocking agents is usually well tolerated. The goal is rapid emergence from anesthesia with full muscular strength recovery. Opioids should be used judiciously to balance analgesic effects against the risks of respiratory depression and attenuation of cough reflex. Multimodal analgesia with local and regional/neuraxial anesthesia techniques should be considered if appropriate.
- **Fluid balance**: Transplanted lungs are susceptible to fluid overload, most notably in the early post-transplant period, so large-volume fluid resuscitation for treatment of hypotension is generally discouraged. Furthermore, patients with concomitant renal dysfunction are further predisposed to fluid retention. Vasopressors such as phenylephrine should be considered early for treatment of hypotension.
- **Weaning from mechanical ventilation**: Early postoperative extubation is always encouraged, as prolonged intubation carries a significant risk of respiratory infection. Neuromuscular blockade must be reversed to promote robust respiratory mechanics. The presence of compromised airway reflexes emphasizes the importance of having an awake patient with an effective cough prior to removing an invasive airway. Extubation to a noninvasive ventilation system to assist the patient's spontaneous efforts may be prudent.

For the patient in this scenario, who is hemodynamically stable, premedication with intravenous midazolam would be acceptable. After preoxygenation, induction with propofol 2 mg/kg and fentanyl 1 mcg/kg should be well tolerated. The patient could be maintained on either volatile anesthetic or a propofol infusion, with orotracheal intubation and controlled ventilation. Invasive monitors are not required for this procedure. If there is indeed ongoing infection or rejection, one

should anticipate the possibility of the need for admission and temporary oxygen requirement post-procedure.

What complications can occur with bronchoscopic procedures?

Bronchoscopy remains the gold standard for evaluating lung allograft in post–lung transplant management programs. While generally safe, complications do occasionally occur and can be divided into three categories as set forth in Table 37.4. Hypoxia and hypercapnia are a direct result of ineffective oxygenation and ventilation occurring when the bronchoscope occludes the airway device. Repeated lavage and excessive suctioning can also contribute. Significant hypoxia may result in bradycardia. The most effective management involves temporary cessation of the procedure, withdrawal of the bronchoscope, and administration of alveolar recruitment breaths with applied positive pressure. Laryngospasm and bronchospasm can arise in the setting of light anesthesia or inadequate topical anesthesia.

Thankfully, serious complications like pneumothorax and hemorrhage are rare, with an incidence of 0.8%–3.4% and 1%–5% respectively [9]. Biopsies should be restricted to a single side to avoid bilateral pneumothoraces or hemorrhage. Uremia and thrombocytopenia have both been identified as risk factors for bleeding and should be addressed prior to lung biopsy.

Can this procedure be performed as an outpatient procedure?

Generally, bronchoscopy with lavage and biopsies can be done as an outpatient procedure. However, the patient should be admitted if there is refractory hypoxemia requiring prolonged oxygen supplementation, persistent ineffective ventilation with hypercapnia, hemodynamic instability, or severe complications associated with the procedure such as pneumothorax or significant bleeding.

Table 37.4 Complications of Bronchoscopic Procedures

Physiologic	Mechanical	Bacteriologic
Hypoxia	Pneumothorax	Iatrogenic infection
Hypercapnia	Hemorrhage	Fever
Arrhythmia, hypotension	Mucosal edema	
Laryngospasm/ bronchospasm		

References

1. S. B. Goldfarb, D. Hayes Jr., B. J. Levvey, et al. The International Thoracic Organ Transplant Registry of the International Society for Heart and Lung Transplantation: twenty-first Pediatric Lung and Heart-Lung Transplantation Report-2018; focus theme: Multiorgan Transplantation. *J Heart Lung Transplant* 2018; **37**: 1196–206.

2. M. S. Khan, W. Zhang, R. A. Taylor, et al. Survival in pediatric lung transplantation: the effect of center volume and expertise. *J Heart Lung Transplant* 2015; **34**: 1073–81.

3. T. G. Liou, F. R. Adler, D. R. Cox, et al. Lung transplantation and survival in children with cystic fibrosis. *N Engl J Med* 2007; **357**: 2143–52.

4. J.D. Christie, M. Carby, R. Bag, et al. Report of the ISHLT Working Group on Primary Lung Graft Dysfunction Part II: Definition. A Consensus Statement of the International Society for Heart and Lung Transplantation. *J Heart Lung Transplant* 2005; **24**: 1454–9.

5. S. C. Sweet. Pediatric lung transplantation. *Respir Care* 2017; **62**: 776–98.

6. S. B. Goldfarb, B. J. Levvey, L. B. Edwards, et al. The Registry of the International Society for Heart and Lung Transplantation: nineteenth Pediatric Lung and Heart-Lung Transplantation Report-2016; focus theme: primary diagnostic indications for transplant. *J Heart Lung Transplant* 2016; **35**: 1196–205.

7. C. Benden. Pediatric lung transplantation. *J Thorac Dis* 2017; **9**: 2675–83.

8. A. Beer, R. M. Reed, S. Bölökbas, et al. Mechanical ventilation after lung transplantation. *Ann Am Thorac Soc* 2014; **11**: 546–53.

9. J. Y. Wong, G. P. Westall, G. I. Snell. Bronchoscopic procedures and lung biopsies in pediatric lung transplant recipients. *Pediatr Pulmonol* 2015; **50**: 1405–19.

Suggested Reading

Bryant R. III, Morales D., Schecter M. Pediatric lung transplantation. *Semin Pediatr Surg* 2017; **26**: 213–16.

Feltracco P., Falasco G., Barbieri S., et al. Anesthetic considerations for nontransplant procedures in lung transplant patients. *J Clin Anesth* 2011; **23**: 508–16.

LaRosa C., Glah C., Baluarte H. J., et al. Solid-organ transplantation in childhood: transitioning to adult health care. *Pediatrics* 2011; **127**: 742–53.

Post Orthotopic Cardiac Transplantation

Zachary Kleiman and Luis M. Zabala

Case Scenario

A 3-year-old male, weighing 14 kg, presents for elective tonsillectomy and adenoidectomy. He has a history of hypoplastic left heart syndrome and underwent a Norwood procedure with a Sano modification soon after birth, which was followed by a bidirectional Glenn procedure at 4 months of age. Shortly after his second-stage surgery he required an orthotopic heart transplant due to severe tricuspid valve regurgitation and moderate-to-severe ventricular dysfunction and the inability to wean from milrinone. Today, his mother states that he is very active and growing well. His cardiologist sees him regularly and his last surveillance annual catheterization 1 month ago revealed good hemodynamics and no evidence of rejection.

Table 38.1 Common Indications for Heart Transplantation in Children

Congenital heart disease	*Most common*: Hypoplastic left heart syndrome, pulmonary atresia with intact ventricular septum and right ventricular dependent coronary circulation, truncus arteriosus, Ebstein's anomaly, unbalanced atrioventricular septal defect
Cardiomyopathy	Dilated cardiomyopathy (idiopathic and familial), idiopathic restrictive cardiomyopathy, and myocarditis
Unresectable cardiac tumors	Sarcoma, lymphoma, fibroma, pheochromocytoma
Chemotherapy-induced myocardial dysfunction	Anthracyclines (doxorubicin, daunorubicin, epirubicin, and idarubicin); trastuzumab (transient cardiomyopathy)

Key Objectives

- Understand common causes of heart transplantation in pediatric patients.
- Describe biatrial versus bicaval surgical implantation techniques.
- Understand the physiology of the transplanted heart.
- Describe the perioperative assessment for a heart transplant patient undergoing noncardiac surgery.
- List common immunosuppressant medications, their side effects, and anesthetic considerations.
- Describe the appropriate perioperative management of this patient.

Pathophysiology

What are the most common indications for heart transplantation in children?

The most common indications for pediatric heart transplantation are listed in Table 38.1. Approximately 55% of infants <1 year of age listed for heart transplantation have complex congenital heart disease (CHD). In contrast, 44%–54% of older children listed for transplantation have cardiomyopathy,

with the percentage of patients transplanted for CHD decreasing steadily with increasing patient age [1].

What are the two most common surgical implantation techniques for orthotopic heart transplants?

Transplantation is usually performed using either a biatrial or bicaval technique. (See Figures 38.1–38.3.) In the early days of orthotopic heart transplantation, the biatrial technique was more commonly used. This technique involved excision of the posterior portion of donor left and right atrium, from the inferior vena cava (IVC) to the right atrial appendage, with the intent of preserving the sinoatrial node. The resultant figure-of-eight orientation of both atria, however, actually interfered with atrial contraction and electrical conduction, leading to acute atrial enlargement and atrioventricular (AV) valve regurgitation. Thus, in the late 1980s, the bicaval technique became popular because it preserved the integrity of donor atria by separating the anastomosis of the pulmonary vein confluence from the caval anastomosis. A meta-analysis reported the bicaval technique's superiority in regard to decreased right

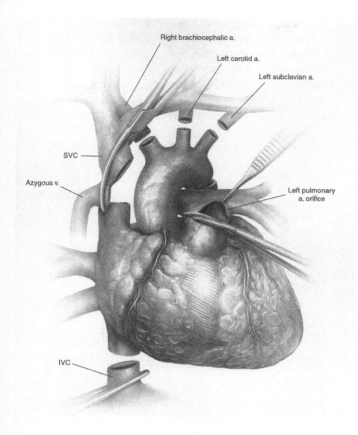

Right brachiocephalic a.

Left carotid a.

Left subclavian a.

SVC

Azygous v.

Left pulmonary
a. orifice

IVC

Figure 38.1 Once the heart and lung perfusion is complete, the donor cardiectomy is completed next. From Camp P. C. Heart transplantation: donor operation for heart and lung transplantation. *Oper Tech Thorac Cardiovasc Surg* 2010; **15**: 125–37. With permission.

atrial pressure, perioperative mortality, tricuspid regurgitation, and higher likelihood of sinus rhythm. However, in smaller recipients, the bicaval technique has a higher risk of both superior vena cava (SVC) and IVC stenosis. The biatrial implantation is the preferred technique in cases of caval size mismatch, reoperation, or complex anatomy [2, 3].

Clinical Pearl

The bicaval technique preserves the integrity of donor atria by separating the anastomosis of the pulmonary vein confluence from the caval anastomosis. However, in smaller recipients, the bicaval technique has a higher risk of both SVC and IVC stenosis. The biatrial implantation is the preferred technique in cases of caval size mismatch, reoperation, or complex anatomy.

What is the life expectancy for a heart transplant recipient?

There is an indirect correlation between age at transplant and survival. Those who receive a heart at 1 year of age or earlier have an average life expectancy of 22.3 years. Those

transplanted at age 1–5 years, 6–10 years, and >11 years can expect to have an average life expectancy of 18.4, 14.4, and 13.1 years post-transplant, respectively. The indication for heart transplantation also impacts mortality. Patients with CHD experience higher mortality than patients with cardiomyopathies (79% survival vs. 88% at 5 years). By 10 years post-transplant, both groups have similar long-term mortalities. Single-ventricle patients have a 53% 10-year survival. The need for extracorporeal membrane oxygenation (ECMO), end-organ damage prior to transplant (need for dialysis or mechanical ventilation), recipient's body mass index, ischemic time, and transplant center volume/experience all influence 1-year mortality rates [4, 5].

What are the causes of death after a cardiac transplant?

Graft failure, rejection, infection, and coronary allograft vasculopathy (CAV) are all major causes of death within the first 5 years post-transplant. Graft failure is the most common cause of death following transplantation. Coronary allograft vasculopathy becomes more common after 3 years, with an incidence of 10% per year post-transplant [6].

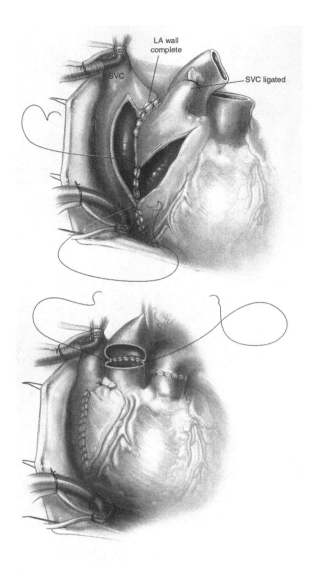

Figure 38.2 Orthotopic heart transplantation: biatrial anastomosis technique. From John R. and Liao K. Orthotopic heart transplantation. *Oper Tech Thorac Cardiovasc Surg* 2010; **15**: 138–46. With permission.

What are the most common complications following heart transplantation?

Rejection is most common in the first year post-transplant. Older donor age, older recipient age, lack of induction therapy, retransplantation, and repeated cellular rejection are all risk factors for new-onset rejection. Endomyocardial biopsy remains the gold standard for diagnosing acute or chronic rejection. Coronary allograft vasculopathy is the leading cause of mortality after 3 years post-transplant. Once CAV is angiographically present, short-term mortality

risk is high. Classic signs and symptoms of pediatric heart failure will be evident, with tachypnea, tachycardia, diaphoresis, dyspnea on exertion, lack of appropriate growth, and grunting being the most common. In the setting of CAV, ejection fraction <45%, right atrial pressure >12 mm Hg, and/or pulmonary capillary wedge pressure >15 mm Hg are all risk factors for graft failure. Due to the diffuse nature of CAV, coronary interventions are rarely effective, and retransplantation is usually the only viable option [6, 7].

> **Clinical Pearl**
>
> *Coronary allograft vasculopathy is the leading cause of mortality after 3 years post-transplant. Once CAV is angiographically present, short-term mortality risk is high. Classic signs and symptoms of pediatric heart failure will be evident, with tachypnea, tachycardia, diaphoresis, dyspnea on exertion, lack of appropriate growth, and grunting being the most common.*

What iatrogenic transplant complications should be considered prior to any elective surgery?

If the patient required ECMO support prior to transplantation, this can create future issues if central access is required. Neck and groin vessels are commonly thrombosed or have been sacrificed for ECMO cannulation. The need for multiple indwelling catheters during the perioperative transplant period can also complicate future catheterizations. In addition, some patients are colonized with drug-resistant organisms from their indwelling catheters; in this event communication between the proceduralist and infectious disease specialist (especially if the transplanted heart has valvular issues) is warranted [6].

Is it important to distinguish between an ABO-compatible and an ABO-incompatible heart transplant patient?

Over the past two decades, pediatric ABO-incompatible (ABOi) heart transplantation has become more common in an effort to broaden organ availability and overcome the restriction placed by the need for ABO compatibility. The majority of ABOi recipients are children <2 years of age who have not yet developed or have low levels of ABO isohemagglutinin; they have low levels of anti-A and anti-B titers. The ABO structures continue to be expressed in the heart graft years after the transplant. Thus, following the transplant, select ABOi recipients could encounter ABO isohemagglutinins directed toward their donor blood structures on the transplanted heart. As a consequence, transfusing blood products containing donor-directed ABO isohemagglutinins could be risky for inciting future organ rejection [8]. Table 38.2 outlines suggested transfusion guidelines for ABOi recipients.

How does the physiology of the transplanted heart compare to that of a normal heart?

Due to the interruption of the cardiac plexus and the inability for conduction to cross suture lines, the efferent limbs of the autonomic nervous system are compromised. As a result, the normal response to baroreceptor activation is altered. Response to baroreceptor activation is dependent on the generation of circulating endogenous catecholamines for chronotropic and inotropic effect. The resting heart rate of a transplanted patient is generally higher compared to the normally innervated heart but maintains similar minimum and maximum rates. The normal response to exercise and stress occurs at a delay, compared to the innervated heart, as it follows the gradual increase in serum catecholamines, which takes several minutes to generate [9]. Cardiac output is primarily reliant on preload; therefore, adequate hydration is paramount in maintaining adequate end-organ perfusion. In addition, systemic response to atrial

and ventricular filling is also impaired; therefore, hypovolemia will not cause the normal reflex compensatory tachycardia and is poorly tolerated. Due to the absence of sensory efferent pathways, chest pain is also an unreliable symptom of ischemia [5, 10].

Clinical Pearl

Due to interruption of the cardiac plexus the efferent limbs of the autonomic nervous system are compromised, removing sympathetic and parasympathetic innervation to the transplanted heart. Inotropic and chronotropic responses are therefore dependent on endogenous circulating catecholamines. Hypovolemia does not result in the normal compensatory tachycardia.

Table 38.2 Transfusion Guidelines for ABO-Incompatible Heart Transplant Patients Receiving Transfusion

Recipient	RBC	FFP, Platelets or Cryoprecipitate
Group O (donor A, B, AB)	O	AB or donor type
Group A (donor B, AB)	A or O	AB
Group B (donor A, AB)	B or O	AB

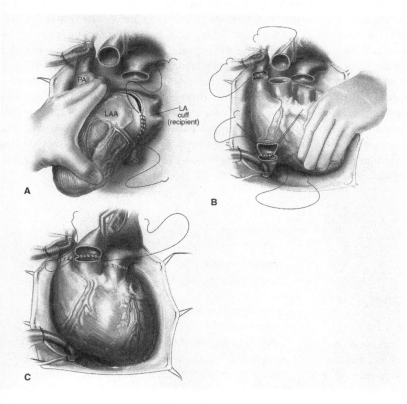

Figure 38.3 Orthotopic heart transplantation: bicaval anastomosis technique. From John R. and Liao K. Orthotopic heart transplantation. *Oper Tech Thorac Cardiovasc Surg* 2010; **15**: 138–46. With permission.

What are common symptoms of heart failure in children and can they occur after heart transplantation?

Depending on the age of the child, heart failure symptoms can include failure to thrive, feeding dysfunction, lack of appropriate weight gain, nausea and vomiting, chest pain, abdominal pain, palpitations, increased daytime sleepiness, reduced exercise tolerance, and problems sleeping while supine [5]. Symptoms of ongoing rejection mimic those of heart failure prior to transplantation. The ability of transplant patients to experience chest pain is dependent on sympathetic afferent reinnervation and is not a reliable symptom. An abnormally high heart rate (tachycardia) may be present and representative of ongoing rejection, thereby warranting further evaluation.

Anesthetic Implications

What findings on physical examination warrant additional workup prior to an elective anesthetic?

Carefully worded, open-ended questions are necessary to elucidate accurate information regarding activity level, rest requirements after activity, and increased daytime sleepiness. Any significant change in physical activity level is worrisome and should be investigated further. The integrity of pacemakers and/or defibrillators should be queried, including last interrogation date and any patient-triggered discharges. Signs and symptoms of heart failure specific to children should be noted, including feeding dysfunction, early satiety, poor weight gain, nausea/vomiting, and dyspnea. Dependent edema, hepatomegaly, and jugular venous distension may be present as well. Unexplained tachycardia in the preoperative setting may be the only sign of subclinical rejection and warrants consultation with the transplant cardiologist.

> **Clinical Pearl**
>
> *Unexplained tachycardia may be a sign of subclinical rejection and should be investigated.*

What imaging is important to order and/or review prior to an anesthetic?

A chest radiograph may show evidence of cardiomegaly, increased pulmonary vascular markings due to left heart failure, and fluid overload, all of which are highly suggestive of ongoing rejection. Reviewing computed tomography scans and/or cardiac magnetic resonance imaging can be helpful in evaluating the patency of systemic veins and arteries. Of note, if the patient previously required ECMO prior to transplantation, neck and/or groin vessels may have been sacrificed and would therefore be inaccessible for future cannulation. Previous cardiac catheterization data, including filling pressures and vascular resistance calculations are important to note, with special attention paid to any trends. An electrocardiogram (ECG) may reveal arrhythmias and should be obtained prior to an anesthetic. Additionally, after induction of anesthesia it is important to be vigilant for any ST segment and/or rhythm changes. The most important imaging modality to review is the patient's most recent echocardiogram. An echocardiogram within the last 6–12 months is acceptable, unless new onset or worsening symptoms of heart failure are present, in which case a more recent study is warranted. Contractility, valvular function, and patency of anastomosed structures should be assessed.

What preoperative labs should be ordered prior to this patient's anesthetic?

In addition to a thorough physical exam, basic preoperative labs should be obtained to evaluate for anemia, thrombocytopenia, and pre-tonsillectomy, any possible coagulopathies due to either medications or impaired liver synthetic function. Additionally, labs reflecting end-organ function such as blood urea nitrogen/creatinine, liver function tests, and brain natriuretic peptide or B-type natriuretic peptide are also important. Looking for trends in a patient's laboratory results can aid in differentiating between a stable or an acutely or chronically decompensating patient. B-type natriuretic peptide levels have a high sensitivity for evaluation of acute rejection in pediatric heart transplant patients. Some institutions will also order immunosuppressive drug levels to assess patient medication compliance, as rejection will increase morbidity and mortality.

> **Clinical Pearl**
>
> *Basic preoperative workup for elective nonthoracic or abdominal surgery should include:*
>
> - *Noting changes in activity level or medication compliance*
> - *Chest radiograph (day of surgery, if recent changes noted in clinical status)*
> - *Echocardiogram (within 6 months) unless worsening symptoms present*
> - *Cardiology/transplant clinic visit (within 6 months)*
> - *Basic labs (coagulation panel, hemoglobin/hematocrit, platelet count, electrolytes, BUN/creatinine, and liver enzymes)*

Which commonly utilized anesthetic medications are effective and ineffective in a transplanted heart?

Due to a lack of parasympathetic innervation, anticholinergic therapies are ineffective and treatment for symptomatic bradycardia should rely on drugs with direct ß-stimulation (isoproterenol) or electrical pacing. Cardiac medications with direct effect on ß-receptors (agonist or antagonist) and calcium channel blockers will elicit their appropriate response. Another important consideration is the bradycardic effect of acetylcholinesterase inhibitors; advanced heart block has been reported in some transplant recipients with administration of anticholinesterase inhibitors.

Clinical Pearl

Due to a lack of parasympathetic innervation, anticholinergic therapies are ineffective and the best treatment for symptomatic bradycardia should rely on drugs with direct ß-stimulation (isoproterenol) or electrical pacing.

What cardiac dysrhythmias are common in the transplanted heart?

There is a propensity to develop heart block after transplant because of an increased refractory period at the sinus node. Any implanted pacemaker should be interrogated before and after any operation (asynchronous mode should be programmed during the operation). Ectopic beats are more common than atrial or ventricular arrhythmias. The presence of ventricular dysrhythmias should be concerning for acute rejection due to CAV. Carotid massage and Valsalva maneuvers have no effect on heart rate in transplant patients due to vagal denervation [7].

What ECG findings would be considered normal?

The ECG may show two separate P-waves due to recipient and donor atrial focus. Pacing spikes, if present, should be consistent with the programming of the pacemaker and/or implantable cardioverter-defibrillator.

What should parents be told about anesthetic risk for elective surgery following heart transplantation?

Local, regional, or general anesthesia can be safely administered to pediatric heart transplant recipients. Little data are available with regard to morbidity and mortality of surgical procedures after pediatric heart transplantation. However, data from adult heart transplant patients suggest a 15% rate of surgical complications, the most common categories being major bleeding (26%), impaired wound healing (22%), and local infections (22%) [11].

What fasting considerations exist?

The American Society of Anesthesiologists (ASA) fasting guidelines of 8 hours for solids, 6 hours for formula, 4 hours for breast milk, and 2 hours for clear liquids should be followed. No special considerations are necessary for heart transplant patients undergoing elective noncardiac surgery.

Is bacterial endocarditis prophylaxis indicated?

According to the American Heart Association subacute bacterial endocarditis prophylaxis guidelines [12], a cardiac transplant patient *with valvulopathy* is considered high risk for adverse outcome from endocarditis and should receive antibiotics, even if the specific operation does not require their use.

Clinical Pearl

According to the American Heart Association, a cardiac transplant patient with valvulopathy is considered high risk for adverse outcome from endocarditis and should receive antibiotics.

What anesthetic considerations exist with commonly utilized immunosuppressant medications in heart transplant patients?

Commonly utilized immunosuppressive agents include cyclosporine, azathioprine, antilymphocyte globulin, monoclonal antibodies, and corticosteroids.

Immunosuppressive agents may be divided into six groups according to their mechanism of action:

- *Broad-spectrum immunosuppressants*: corticosteroids
- *Calcineurin inhibitors*: cyclosporine and tacrolimus
- *Antiproliferative agents*: mycophenolate (MMF) and azathioprine
- *Antibodies against interleukin-2*: basiliximab and daclizumab
- *Mammalian target of rapamycin protein (mTOR) inhibitors*: sirolimus and everolimus
- *Mono- and polyclonal T-cell antibodies*: OKT3, antithymocyte globulin (ATG), antilymphocyte globulin

295

Patients may be treated with a combination of any of these agents in the perioperative period. The specific combination is largely dictated by institutional experience, new or recent episode of rejections, other comorbid conditions, and time since transplantation [13].

Individual agents deserve special considerations. The blood level of both cyclosporine and tacrolimus must be kept within a certain level to achieve the desired therapeutic effect. Both of these drugs are metabolized by the cytochrome P450 system of the liver, and therefore many drugs administered perioperatively can affect their plasma levels. In addition, the two mTOR inhibitors used in cardiac transplantation, sirolimus and everolimus, have been associated with impaired wound healing that results in higher rates of wound complications. In transplant patients undergoing elective noncardiac surgery, mTOR inhibitors should generally be stopped at least 1 week prior to surgery, with resumption approximately 10–15 days after surgery once adequate wound healing has been achieved [14]. However, any adjustments to immunosuppression regimens should be discussed with the primary transplant team.

Arterial hypertension is relatively common after transplantation; it is present in 75% of patients in long term follow-up. Early risk factors include the administration of calcineurin inhibitors and corticosteroids, especially when administered in high doses. Renal dysfunction, although uncommon, is also another complication after early initiation of calcineurin inhibitors, especially when drug levels are elevated.

Another important consideration is the interaction of grapefruit juice with the metabolism of specific immunosuppressant medications. Grapefruit juice is an inhibitor of the intestinal cytochrome P450 3A4 system, which is responsible for the first-pass metabolism of many medications. As such, grapefruit has marked effects on blood levels of cyclosporine, 1,4-dihydropyridine calcium antagonists, and some 3-hydroxy-3methylglutaryl coenzyme A reductase inhibitors.

Is there a need for stress dose steroids?

Corticosteroids were widely used in the pre-cyclosporine era. More recently, steroids have been used during the induction phase of immunosuppression (pulse dose steroids tapered for 7 days in combination with thymoglobulin) or during episodes of acute rejection. Many institutions attempt to minimize the use of corticosteroids due to their extensive list of known side effects. Some studies suggest steroids may be withdrawn soon after transplantation in low-risk patients without circulating anti-HLA antibodies and in those without a history of rejection. However, patients receiving more than 20 mg/kg of prednisone or its equivalent for more than 3 weeks should be considered to have a suppressed hypothalamic-adrenal axis (HAA) and are at risk of adrenal insufficiency with the stress of surgery. The HAA is not suppressed with doses of less than 5 mg/day of prednisone or its equivalent, whereas intermediate doses have equivocal effects on axis suppression [10]. However, even patients taking low or intermediate doses should receive stress dose steroids if unexplained intraoperative hypotension persists despite adequate resuscitation from fasting or blood loss.

> **Clinical Pearl**
>
> *Perioperative administration of stress dose steroids should be considered for patients receiving steroids as part of their immunosuppression regimen.*

Are there interactions between immunosuppressants and commonly utilized anesthetic agents?

Immunosuppression represents a unique challenge during the perioperative period of any heart transplant patient undergoing noncardiac surgery. It potentially contributes to an increased risk of infection, delayed wound healing, drug interactions, and more importantly, hemodynamic instability due to adrenal insufficiency. Evidence of major drug interactions between immunosuppressants and anesthetic agents is lacking; however, minor reactions have been reported [5, 9].

Corticosteroids

- *Prednisone* and *methylprednisolone* are known to decrease the effectiveness of nondepolarizing neuromuscular blockers, prolong muscle weakness, and promote steroid-related myopathy. If succinylcholine is used, expect prolonged neuromuscular blockade.

Calcineurin Inhibitors

- *Tacrolimus*: Sevoflurane and ondansetron are associated with QT-prolongation. Furosemide and bumetanide may precipitate acute renal failure. Diltiazem, verapamil, and amiodarone may increase the risk of QT-prolongation and increase tacrolimus levels.
- *Cyclosporine*: Midazolam clearance is decreased in the presence of cyclosporine. Cyclosporine is a weak CYP3A4 inhibitor, and thus the potential of increased opioid toxicity exists.

Nonsteroidal antiinflammatory agents are generally contraindicated in heart transplant patients due to the risk of renal failure when combined with some immunosuppression agents.

Chronic immunosuppressive therapy has multiple adverse effects, including diabetes, hyperlipoproteinemia, hypertension, lowered seizure threshold, hyperkalemia, hypomagnesemia, increased risk of wound infections, pancytopenia, and poor wound healing [15].

Is invasive monitoring indicated?

The degree of intraoperative monitoring will depend on the type of surgery as well as the availability of monitoring. In the case of elective major surgery (intrathoracic or abdominal) or emergent surgery, monitoring of invasive arterial blood pressure and central venous pressures may be indicated. Perioperative invasive monitoring requires special attention to aseptic technique to minimize the risk of infection and should be discussed in terms of the risk/benefit ratio. For minor surgery such as a tonsillectomy and adenoidectomy, the use of recommended ASA standard monitoring with 5-lead ECG is acceptable.

What methods are appropriate for induction of anesthesia?

Either intravenous (IV) or inhalation induction is safe for heart transplant recipients who remain healthy. Age, cognition, weight, comorbidities, and cardiac reserve are factors that should be considered when planning an induction. If concern for rejection exists, a carefully titrated IV induction is safer. Transplanted patients have increased systemic vascular resistance (SVR) and are dependent on venous return for cardiac output. The use of any technique that may suddenly reduce either venous return or SVR necessitates careful monitoring. When considering general endotracheal anesthesia, oral endotracheal intubation is preferred over nasal intubation because of potential infection caused by nasal flora and blood loss from friable nasal mucosa. The use of a laryngeal mask airway is acceptable in appropriate situations.

What is an appropriate anesthetic maintenance strategy for patients post-transplantation?

The ability of post-transplant patients to tolerate premedication is similar to patients without transplant. The intraoperative anesthetic strategy is dictated by the underlying surgical diagnosis and any other complicating factor that may be present. Following safe and uneventful induction of anesthesia, maintenance of anesthesia can be provided with a combination of IV and inhaled anesthetics. Most forms of anesthesia and sedation are well tolerated in cardiac transplant patients with stable graft function.

Any there any special drug or equipment considerations based on the physiology of the transplanted heart?

The occurrence of advanced heart block and cardiac arrest have been reported after the use of either pyridostigmine or neostigmine to reverse neuromuscular blockade. Bradycardia has also been reported after reversal with sugammadex, so it is unclear whether this drug is a safe alternative in this population. Careful attention to intraoperative volume status is warranted to avoid hypotension. Because of the absence of reflex sympathetic tachycardia due to autonomic denervation, heart transplant patients may be very sensitive to the vasodilating properties of anesthetics such as propofol and volatile agents. Additionally, knowledge of the mechanisms of metabolism and excretion for anesthetic drugs is imperative. The presence of chronic kidney disease may diminish the ability to excrete various anesthetics. In the absence of any hepatic or renal insufficiency, there are no strict contraindications to using an IV versus inhaled anesthetic technique.

Clinical Pearl

The occurrence of advanced heart block and cardiac arrest have been reported after the use of either pyridostigmine or neostigmine to reverse neuromuscular blockade.

Can patients post–heart transplant undergo same-day surgery?

Post–heart transplant patients who have stable graft function, are on stable maintenance immunosuppressive therapy, and have recently undergone evaluation by their transplant cardiologist can be appropriate candidates for same-day surgery for low-risk procedures when minimal concern exists for postoperative pain or limited functional capacity. Nevertheless, planned outpatient procedures (annual catheterization, endoscopy, or magnetic resonance imaging) should still be performed at a hospital with in-house cardiology consultants, heart transplant team, and admission capability should any complication arise. This patient would be suitable to undergo same-day surgery with recovery in the post-anesthesia care unit and discharge home after meeting appropriate discharge criteria. If the patient experienced postoperative nausea and/or vomiting resulting in limited oral intake, it would be prudent to plan overnight hospital admission.

Do specific postoperative concerns exist?

Early extubation is desirable to minimize the risk of ventilator-associated pneumonia. Depending on the surgical procedure, the function of other organs (kidney and liver) should be closely monitored by laboratory testing. The kidneys are at risk for acute kidney injury in the presence of large volume loss and hypotension. Also, the ECG should be monitored in the immediate postoperative period for signs of silent ischemia due to high demand states, such as shivering, uncontrolled pain, and fever.

References

1. T. D. Ryan, C. Chin, R. Bryant III. Heart and lung transplantation. In Ungerleider R. M., Meliones J. N., McMillan K. N., et al., eds. *Critical Heart Disease in Infants and Children*, 3rd ed. Philadelphia, Mosby Elsevier, 2019; 868–84.

2. M. Schnoor, T. Schäfer, D. Lühmann, et al. Bicaval versus standard technique in orthotopic heart transplantation: a systematic review and meta-analysis. *J Thorac Cardiovasc Surg* 2007; **134**: 1322–31. e7.

3. O. Coskun, A. Parsa, T. Coskun, et al. Outcome of heart transplantation in pediatric recipients. *ASAIO J* 2007; **53**: 107–10.

4. A. I. Dipchand. Current state of pediatric cardiac transplantation. *Ann Cardiothorac Surg* 2018; **7**: 31–55.

5. M. Choudhury. Post-cardiac transplant recipient: implications for anaesthesia. *Indian J Anaesth* 2017; **61**: 768–74.

6. D. Ramzy, V. Rao, J. Brahm, et al. Cardiac allograft vasculopathy: a review. *Can J Surg* 2005; **48**: 319–27.

7. J. Conway, A. Dipchand. Heart transplantation in children. *Pediatr Clin North Am* 2010; **57**: 353–73.

8. C. L. Dean, H. C. Sullivan, S. R. Stowell, et al. Current state of transfusion practices for ABO-incompatible pediatric heart transplant patients in the United States and Canada. *Transfusion* 2018; **58**: 2243–49.

9. V. G. Nasr, J. A. DiNardo. Heart transplantation. In Nasr V. G., DiNardo J. A., eds., *The Pediatric Cardiac Anesthesia Handbook*. Hoboken, NJ: John Wiley & Sons, 2017; 199–216.

10. P. Jurgens, C. Aquilante, R. Page, et al. Perioperative management of cardiac transplant recipients undergoing noncardiac surgery: unique challenges created by advancements in care. *Semin Cardiothorac Vasc Anesth* 2017; **21**: 235–44.

11. P. Jurgens, A. Ambardekar. Non-cardiac surgery is common in cardiac transplanted recipients and has a similar complication rate as the general population. *J Card Fail* 2017; **23**: S126–7.

12. Committee on Rheumatic Fever, Endocarditis, and Kawasaki Disease. Prevention of infective endocarditis: Guidelines from the American Heart Association. *Circulation* 2007; **116**: 1736–54.

13. G. D. Williams, C. Ramamoorthy, A. Sarma. Anesthesia for cardiac and pulmonary transplantation. In Andropoulos D. B., Stayer S., Mossad E. B., et al., eds., *Anesthesia for Congenital Heart Disease*, 3rd ed. Hoboken, NJ: John Wiley & Sons, 2015; 636–60.

14. N. Manito, J. F. Delgado, M. G. Crespo-Leiro, et al. Clinical recommendations for the use of everolimus in heart transplantation. *Transplant Rev (Orlando)* 2010; **24**: 129–42.

15. V. E. Papalois, N. S. Hakim. New immunosuppressive drugs in organ transplantation. In Hakim N. S., ed., *Introduction to Organ Transplantation*. London: Imperial College Press, 1997; 225–36.

Suggested Reading

Dipchand A. I. Current state of pediatric cardiac transplantation. *Ann Cardiothorac Surg* 2018; **7**: 31–55.

Jurgens P. and Ambardekar A. Non-cardiac surgery is common in cardiac transplanted recipients and has a similar complication rate as the general population. *J Card Fail* 2017; **23**: S126–7.

Jurgens P., Aquilante C., Page R., et al. Perioperative management of cardiac transplant recipients undergoing noncardiac surgery: unique challenges created by advancements in care. *Semin Cardiothorac Vasc Anesth* 2017; **21**: 235–44.

Williams G. D., Ramamoorthy C., and Sarma A. Anesthesia for cardiac and pulmonary transplantation. In Andropoulos D. B., Stayer S., Mossad E. B., et al., eds. *Anesthesia for Congenital Heart Disease*, 3rd ed. Hoboken, NJ, John Wiley & Sons, 2015; 636–60.

Failing Cardiac Transplant

Kelly Chilson and James Fehr

Case Scenario

A 12-year-old male weighing 40 kg with a history of congenital aortic stenosis for which he underwent cardiac transplantation in infancy has been posted for cardiac catheterization to assess hemodynamics, obtain myocardial biopsies, and perform coronary angiography. He was clinically well until the previous several weeks but has recently developed decreased exercise tolerance and is no longer keeping up with his peers. At his last cardiology visit 6 months ago there were no concerns, and an echocardiogram at that time showed normal biventricular function. In the holding area, he is quiet and reserved. He is tachypneic and has a heart rate of 130 beats/minute.

Key Objectives

- Understand preoperative assessment goals for cardiac transplant patients.
- Describe the risks and benefits of anesthesia for cardiac transplant patients.
- Describe team preparation for patient management to optimize patient outcomes.
- Discuss commonly seen complications in patients with heart failure undergoing an anesthetic.

Pathophysiology

What is the epidemiology of pediatric cardiac transplantation?

Cardiac transplantation is a life-saving procedure for children with heart failure unresponsive to medical management. In 2015 alone 684 pediatric heart transplants were performed, representing approximately 12% of all heart transplants [1]. Congenital heart disease (CHD) remains the most common indication for recipients under 1 year of age. Dilated cardiomyopathy, the most common etiology for transplantation in older children, is increasingly a reason for heart transplantation in patients less than 1 year of age.

What are the outcomes for patients who undergo pediatric cardiac transplantation?

Recent data from the International Society of Heart and Lung Transplant (ISHLT) registry demonstrate an impressive 1-year survival of 83% for all pediatric age groups. The best outcomes occur in the youngest patients, with a median survival of 22.3 years for patients <1 year of age compared to 13.1 years for those transplanted at >11 years of age [1]. From a survival standpoint, cardiomyopathy patients fare better in the early post-transplant years compared to their CHD counterparts. In the subgroup of patients with CHD, patients with single ventricle physiology who have undergone surgical palliation(s) have the least favorable outcomes. Not surprisingly, patients requiring extracorporeal membrane oxygenation (ECMO) support who undergo transplantation do less well than those who do not require mechanical support. Patients supported with ECMO also do less well than those supported by a ventricular assist device (VAD) prior to transplantation.

> **Clinical Pearl**
>
> *Patients transplanted for cardiomyopathy have lower early mortality than patients transplanted for CHD, but the long-term transplant survival is comparable for both groups.*

What are the early and late complications of cardiac transplantation?

In the early post-transplant period complications of cardiac transplantation include acute rejection, anastomotic related issues with the transplanted heart, and postoperative infection. Given the interval of time that has passed since this patient's heart transplant (>10 years), chronic complications are the more likely cause of his new symptoms; these include rejection, infection, and cardiac allograft vasculopathy. Graft survival is also compromised by poor compliance with immunosuppressant and other post-transplant medications.

Post-transplant lymphoproliferative disease is the most frequent malignancy in heart transplant patients.

Anesthetic Implications

What questions should the family be asked to better understand the patient's condition?

Patients and their guardians should be asked the baseline preoperative questions germane to all patients undergoing an anesthetic. These include medication regimen and adherence, allergy history, fasting status, the presence of coexisting illnesses or organ dysfunction, and any history of recent acute illnesses or problems with previous anesthetics. In post-menarche patients pregnancy status should be ascertained. As these patients and their families have great experience and frequent contact with the medical system, reviewing the chart prior to the preoperative interview can save the family from the frustration of repeating what is already documented and spare the interviewer from appearing unprepared. Any new symptoms, such as exercise intolerance, should be explored for duration and rapidity of onset. Often patients will deny exercise intolerance or significantly underestimate their actual disability if specific questions are not asked.

Clinical Pearl

During the preoperative patient and family interview, it is imperative to explicitly ask if new symptoms have arisen. Bear in mind that patients may underestimate changes in functional status or exercise tolerance.

What information should be gathered from the medical record?

At a minimum, the results of recent electrocardiograms (ECG) and echocardiograms should be reviewed in the medical record; ideally, the actual studies should be reviewed. Changes from previous exams should be noted. Is there an arrhythmia, prolonged QT interval, or a new bundle branch block? Has there been a change in the qualitative cardiac function? Is there any new valvular insufficiency or stenosis? The most recent chest radiograph should be reviewed for pulmonary edema, pleural effusions, and/or cardiomegaly. Previous anesthesia records should be examined for notes regarding airway management, any vital sign instability, and/or use of emergency medications. Laboratory data may give clues to the patient's volume status, overall nutritional status, and degree of heart failure.

What physical examination findings are important?

Prior to any patient receiving an anesthetic, a focused physical examination should assess the patient's general physical status, the airway, cardiac and pulmonary systems, and general cognitive state. In addition, for this previously transplanted child with heart failure, his cardiac examination should investigate whether he has any jugular venous distension, a murmur, gallop, or dysrhythmia. On pulmonary examination, does he have tachypnea, dyspnea, rales, or wheezing? Is there any hepatosplenomegaly, abdominal distension, or abdominal tenderness? How is the perfusion to his extremities? Does he have dependent edema? Is his mentation normal or is he lethargic? And does he appear ill or is he otherwise well appearing? Children with heart failure do not always appear ill despite compromised cardiac function, and supportive data such as the echocardiogram should be incorporated to provide a global assessment.

Clinical Pearl

Children in heart failure do not always appear ill. Therefore, it is important to factor in supportive data such as echocardiographic findings into the patient assessment.

What preoperative tests should be ordered prior to anesthetizing this patient?

Routine bloodwork is generally not necessary prior to cardiac catheterization, even in children with poor cardiac function. However, the impact of this patient's chronic immunosuppression and chronically decreased cardiac output would render some lab studies useful. A basic metabolic panel will provide information regarding electrolytes, blood urea nitrogen, and creatinine; this will be useful as the patient is likely to receive a contrast load if he undergoes coronary angiography and has a ventriculogram performed. Although not absolutely necessary to guide anesthetic management, a blood natriuretic peptide level would provide some insight into the degree of his heart failure. A recent echocardiogram, as mentioned earlier, will provide useful information about overall cardiac function. This patient is undergoing a diagnostic catheterization procedure; however, if interventions were proposed, a baseline hemoglobin and hematocrit as well as a type and crossmatch of red blood cells might be indicated.

Given this patient's recent change in functional status, a new echocardiogram should be completed and read by a cardiologist prior to induction of anesthesia. In this structurally normal heart, the most important considerations are biventricular systolic and diastolic function.

Can anything be done to optimize this patient prior to his procedure?

This case is time sensitive. Obtaining myocardial biopsies for evaluation is crucial for initiation of appropriate therapy. Based on clinical examination, a gentle bolus (5–10 mL/kg) of a balanced salt solution may combat potential hypotension caused by anesthetic agents; however, a patient with a failing heart may not tolerate a fluid load. If the patient is ill appearing, or supportive data indicates markedly depressed cardiac function, one should consider either initiating a low dose inotropic infusion (epinephrine 0.03 mcg/kg/minute) prior to anesthesia induction, or having such an infusion readily available.

Why and when should ECMO be considered in such a patient?

Extracorporeal membrane oxygenation is a lifesaving therapy that can stabilize a decompensating patient and provide an opportunity for further evaluation and management. It does not guarantee an excellent outcome; indeed, a large percentage of such patients will succumb to their disease despite ECMO support. One of the key concepts of successfully utilizing ECMO as rescue from cardiac decompensation or cardiopulmonary resuscitation is early activation, which typically cannot occur unless there have been discussions with the ECMO team beforehand. This includes the surgeon who will place the cannulae, the nurses who will assist the surgeon, the perfusionist who will prime and manage the pump, and intensivists who will receive the patient should they survive. If ECMO is being contemplated as a possible therapeutic intervention option, this should be discussed with the family, ideally prior to the procedure.

What risks should be discussed with the family before proceeding to the catheterization lab?

The child with a remote heart transplant presenting with acute heart failure for cardiac catherization has a high risk of cardiac arrest. This patient should be considered high-risk, given his new complaint of poor exercise tolerance and the clinical presentation of tachycardia and tachypnea. Physical exam findings of jugular venous distension, poor peripheral perfusion, abdominal distension from ascites, hepatomegaly, and hypotension would add to the level of concern.

Hemodynamic decompensation can occur upon anesthetic induction or during the catheterization procedure itself. In addition to the routine discussion regarding the anesthetic risks, the parents or guardian should be made aware of this reality. The potential need for ECMO support should be discussed and the family's wishes documented. As these patients span the age range of infants to young adults, the amount of information discussed with them should be guided by their developmental stage and their ability to provide assent or consent to the anesthetic.

What monitoring should be utilized?

Standard recommended American Society of Anesthesiologists monitoring, including 5-lead ECG, should be used, even for cases where no sedation is planned. End-tidal carbon dioxide should be monitored for all cases. The placement of an arterial line should be considered, depending on the hemodynamic status of the patient. During many cases, a femoral arterial line is placed by the interventional cardiologist and can be used for monitoring during the majority of the procedure. For this patient, while a preinduction arterial line might not be placed it would be a consideration post-procedure if continued inotropic support was required.

How should a safe and appropriate anesthetic for this patient be provided?

Depending on the age of the patient and his or her ability to cooperate, numerous sedative and anesthetic options exist for patients undergoing cardiac catheterization. Many mature patients can be managed like adults with sedation alone. In cases where the risk of hemodynamic complications outweighs the benefits of being anesthetized, the best option is generally monitored anesthesia care, reassurance, and no medications. Clearly these are not options for very young, uncooperative, or developmentally delayed patients who would not tolerate light sedation alone.

Conscious sedation can be achieved with many different agents and in many different combinations. Propofol, ketamine, midazolam, fentanyl, and dexmedetomidine have all been used for procedural sedation in this patient population. Judicious dosing of propofol is necessary to account for the potential for both respiratory depression and hypotension related to the decrease in systemic vascular resistance (SVR). While the sympathomimetic effects of ketamine are favored for maintaining cardiovascular stability, in patients who have exhausted their catecholamine reserve the negative inotropic effects of ketamine become unopposed and can precipitate cardiovascular collapse. The risk of respiratory depression is higher when midazolam, fentanyl, and/or propofol are used in combination. Although dexmedetomidine is generally well-tolerated in transplant patients [2]. it should be used with caution in patients with acute cellular rejection as there is a potential risk for cardiac arrest [3].

For this patient, the option for procedural sedation would depend on the maturity level of the patient and skill of the interventional cardiologist. A 12-year-old patient who underwent transplantation in infancy will be very familiar with catheterization procedures from annual surveillance catheterizations. His feelings could range from being well adjusted, even familiar with undergoing the procedure with light sedation, to having high anxiety as a chronic medical patient. It is also important to know if the patient can lie flat for the procedure. Mentation must be intact. If proceeding with sedation, midazolam, fentanyl, and/or very low dose propofol (20 mcg/kg/minute) could be utilized if required. The drawback to this method is that if the patient becomes unstable, the airway must first be secured. In this particular scenario, the initiation of preemptive inotropes is likely not necessary, unless of course the baseline blood pressures are already very low.

Do pediatric patients undergoing anesthesia for cardiac catheterization require endotracheal intubation?

As noted previously, cardiac catheterization procedures do not require general anesthesia (GA) for all patients, so a natural away with supplemental oxygen provided by nasal cannula is adequate for patients undergoing sedation. A laryngeal mask airway (LMA) is acceptable for patients undergoing GA, although if one is concerned that a significant risk of cardiac arrest exists, securing the airway with an endotracheal tube is prudent.

How should anesthetic induction proceed?

Induction of anesthesia is the period of greatest risk for patients with decreased cardiac function. With severe cardiac dysfunction, one must be optimally prepared and maximally vigilant. When cardiac function is compromised, the rate of intravenous (IV) administration of drugs for induction should be slow to account for delayed onset of medications. In this 12-year-old patient, an IV induction is strongly preferred; the risk of an inhalation induction with no IV access in a patient with symptoms of heart failure is simply excessive and has the

potential to quickly result in deterioration. Inhalation or mask induction should be considered only infrequently for routine diagnostic studies in nonfailing patients. Having emergency medications immediately available is a must and these should include epinephrine, phenylephrine, and calcium. As mentioned previously, initiation of a low-dose inotropic infusion prior to induction may help to minimize the potential hypotension experienced with anesthetics. The ideal induction agent would maintain SVR and have no effect on cardiac function. Judicious use of induction agents is required.

For this patient, etomidate, along with a small amount of fentanyl (less than 1 mcg/kg) and rocuronium are good induction choices. Prior to induction, an epinephrine infusion at 0.03–0.05 mcg/kg/minute could be initiated. Since this patient is at higher risk for clinical decompensation, use of an endotracheal tube would be preferred over an LMA. There is a greater likelihood of hypotension with a general anesthetic, so one must be prepared to readily treat this; both epinephrine boluses (both 1 mcg/kg spritzers and 10 mcg/kg code doses), volume, phenylephrine (bolus dose 1 mcg/kg), and calcium (chloride formulation dose 10 mg/kg, gluconate formulation dose 30 mg/kg) should be available to administer if needed.

Clinical Pearl

Inhalation or mask induction should be considered only for routine diagnostic studies in nonfailing patients. Having emergency medications immediately available is a must and these should include epinephrine, phenylephrine, and calcium.

What complications can occur and how should one be ready to treat them?

Hypotension, arrhythmias, low cardiac output syndrome, and coronary vasospasm are potential complications. As discussed previously, hypotension is very common after the induction of anesthesia, more so with GA than with monitored sedation. A decline in ventricular function of 6%–10% can be expected in patients with transplanted hearts undergoing GA [4]. Phenylephrine and epinephrine should be ready to administer. Antiarrhythmic medications such as adenosine and lidocaine should be available, and most importantly, a defibrillator with appropriately sized paddles and settings should be present in the room. Low cardiac output syndrome can be treated with a variety of inotropes. Typically, epinephrine is selected, as it provides both chronotropic and inotropic support. Coronary vasospasm can be induced during selective coronary angiography and is often first noticed by the interventional cardiologist when the contrast does not clear normally from the coronary artery. A quick response with nitroglycerin injected into the coronary artery catheter may prevent cardiovascular collapse.

> **Clinical Pearl**
>
> *Hypotension is the most common complication, but be wary of arrhythmias, low cardiac output syndrome, and coronary vasospasm in the catheterization laboratory. Vasospasm can occur during selective coronary angiography and may first be noticed by the cardiologist when the contrast does not clear normally.*

Where should the patient recover after this procedure?

A patient with an uncomplicated anesthetic course can safely be recovered in the post-anesthesia care unit (PACU). Even patients who required a low dose inotropic infusion during the case may often be weaned successfully at the end of the procedure and be taken to the PACU. Intensive care unit (ICU) admission is required for patients with an ongoing need for inotropic support; a change in neurologic status; cardiac, respiratory, or airway concerns that require advanced care and continuous monitoring; and newly diagnosed arrhythmias.

When should intensive care unit admission be considered necessary?

The ICU should be notified that this patient is being anesthetized and they should be prepared to accept him post-procedure. If there are no available ICU beds, that would be an indication to delay the procedure until a bed is available. If the procedure occurs uneventfully, and the catheterization did not reveal new information mandating ICU admission, it is possible to manage such a patient on the pediatric cardiac floor post-procedure.

References

1. A. I. Dipchand. Current state of pediatric cardiac transplantation. *Ann Cardiothorac Surg* 2018; **7**: 31–55.

2. E. H. Jooste, W. T. Muhly, J. W. Ibinson, et al. Acute hemodynamic changes after rapid intravenous bolus dosing of dexmedetomidine in pediatric heart transplant patients undergoing routine cardiac catheterization. *Anesth Analg* 2010; **111**: 1490–6.

3. L. I. Schwartz, S. D. Miyamoto, S. Stenquist, et al. Cardiac arrest in a heart transplant patient receiving dexmedetomidine during cardiac catheterization. *Semin Cardiothorac Vasc Anesth* 2016; **20**: 175–8.

4. J. J. Elhoff, S. M. Chowdhury, C. L. Taylor, et al. Decline in ventricular function as a result of general anesthesia in pediatric heart transplant recipients. *Pediatr Transplant* 2016; **20**: 1106–10.

Suggested Reading

Conway J., Manlhiot C., Kirk R., et al. Mortality and morbidity after retransplantation after primary heart transplant in childhood: an analysis from the registry of the International Society for Heart and Lung Transplantation. *J Heart Lung Transplant* 2014; **33**: 241–51.

Chapter

40 Idiopathic Pulmonary Hypertension

Jaime Bozentka and Jennifer E. Lam

Case Scenario

A 10-year-old female with newly diagnosed idiopathic pulmonary hypertension is scheduled for placement of a peripherally inserted central catheter in Interventional Radiology. Two weeks prior she presented to the emergency department after a syncopal episode, and her parents reported a history of progressive dyspnea on exertion with even minimal activity. Her SpO_2 on room air was 89%.

Transthoracic echocardiography at that time revealed:

- *Right ventricular hypertrophy with suprasystemic right ventricular pressures*
- *Mild right ventricular dysfunction*

Cardiac catheterization the following day confirmed the diagnosis of pulmonary hypertension, demonstrating pulmonary artery pressures 20 mm Hg greater than systemic, a pulmonary vascular resistance of 15 indexed Wood units and no response to nitric oxide administration. She was started on oral bosentan and sildenafil, intravenous treprostinil, and oxygen via nasal cannula. She remained in the intensive care unit as her medications were titrated to effective doses. She now requires long-term central access for continuous intravenous treprostinil therapy prior to discharge home. She has extreme anxiety and is very fearful about the proposed procedure.

Key Objectives

- Discuss clinical signs and symptoms leading to a diagnosis of idiopathic pulmonary hypertension.
- Describe the classes of medications available for treatment of these patients.
- Discuss anesthetic risk for these patients and discussion of risk with the family.
- Describe perioperative care and airway management strategies for this patient.

Pathophysiology

What is the definition of pulmonary hypertension? How does it differ from pulmonary arterial hypertension?

According to the Paediatric Task Force of the 6th World Symposium on Pulmonary Hypertension in 2018, pulmonary hypertension is defined in adults and children as a mean pulmonary artery pressure (mPAP) >20 mm Hg at rest. Normal mPAP at rest is 15 mm Hg.

Pulmonary arterial hypertension (PAH) is a subset of PH and is defined as PH due to pulmonary vascular disease, with elevated pulmonary vascular resistance (PVR) >3 indexed Wood units (iWU or WU/m^2) alongside a normal pulmonary capillary wedge pressure (PCWP) <15 mm Hg.

Clinical Pearl

Pulmonary arterial hypertension is a subset of PH due to pulmonary vascular disease and is defined by a mean PAP >20 mm Hg at rest and PVR >3 iWU with normal PCWP.

What is the pathophysiology of PAH?

Pulmonary arterial hypertension is a structural pulmonary vascular disease in which smooth muscle cell proliferation and endothelial cell dysfunction lead to a progressive narrowing of the pulmonary vasculature. Additionally, patients with PAH have an imbalance of vasoactive mediators. The production of normally abundant vasodilators, such as nitric oxide and prostacyclin, is decreased, while pulmonary vasoconstrictors, such as endothelin-1 and serotonin, are increased. Both processes combine to cause intravascular thrombosis, vascular remodeling, and eventual destruction of the pulmonary arterioles leading to pulmonary precapillary restriction to blood flow and an increase in the PVR. Initially, vasoconstriction is the major contributor and the changes are reversible. However, as the remodeling continues, the vessels reach an irreversible point where they are no longer able to respond to physiologic signals to vasodilate. This results in right ventricular (RV) pressure overload leading to RV failure, and ultimately if untreated, death.

How is PH classified in children?

According to the 5th World Symposium on Pulmonary Hypertension, PH can be grouped into one of five categories based on etiology:

1. **Pulmonary arterial hypertension (PAH)**

   1.1. Idiopathic
   1.2. Heritable
   1.3. Drug and toxin induced
   1.4. Congenital heart disease associated

1'. Pulmonary veno-occlusive disease
1". Persistent pulmonary hypertension of the newborn (PPHN) (see Chapter 46)
2. **Pulmonary hypertension due to left heart disease**
3. **Pulmonary hypertension due to lung diseases and/or hypoxia**
4. **Chronic thromboembolic pulmonary hypertension**
5. **Pulmonary hypertension with multifactorial mechanisms**

What is the World Health Organization Functional Classification for PH and why is it important?

The World Health Organization (WHO) Functional Classification describes the level of physical disability (dyspnea, fatigue, chest pain) caused by a patient's PH. It is predictive of mortality and is used when choosing a treatment plan. Levels III (symptoms at minimal activity) and IV (symptoms at rest and symptoms of right heart failure) are considered to be significant negative prognostic factors. (See Table 40.1.)

Clinical Pearl

World Health Organization Functional Class III (symptoms at minimal activity) and level IV (symptoms at rest and symptoms of right heart failure) are significant negative prognostic factors in PH patients.

What is idiopathic pulmonary arterial hypertension?

Idiopathic pulmonary arterial hypertension (IPAH) is the most common cause of pediatric PAH and has no known

Table 40.1 WHO Functional Classification for Pulmonary Hypertension

Functional Class	Symptoms
I	No limitation of physical activity
II	Comfortable at rest. Ordinary activity causes dyspnea, fatigue, chest pain, or syncope
III	Comfortable at rest. Less than ordinary activity causes dyspnea, fatigue, chest pain, or syncope
IV	Dyspnea, fatigue, or chest pain at rest that is increased with any activity. Symptoms of right heart failure

underlying cause, and thus is a diagnosis of exclusion. Presenting symptoms of IPAH are vague and nonspecific, which often leads to a delay between onset and diagnosis. Infants and younger children may present with feeding difficulties, failure to thrive, tachypnea, and irritability due to low cardiac output. The most common complaint in older children is a gradual reduction in exercise capacity, associated with fatigue and dyspnea. Other less common presenting signs include chest pain, cyanosis, cough, or syncope. Syncope as a presenting symptom of IPAH is more common in pediatric patients than in the adult population.

How is PAH diagnosed?

Echocardiography is often used as a noninvasive screening tool for the diagnosis of PAH. It can provide direct and indirect evidence of elevated PAP, evaluate RV function, and may offer information regarding etiology to aid in prognosis.

Important echocardiographic indices include the following:

- The **velocity of a tricuspid regurgitant jet** (TR) can be used to give a quantitative estimate of RV pressure, with values greater than 2.8 m/second suggestive of RV hypertension. However, a trivial or inconsistent TR jet may lead to underestimation of disease severity.
- **Flattening of the interventricular septum** is indicative of systemic RV pressures, whereas bowing of the septum to the left indicates suprasystemic RV pressures.
- **Bidirectional or reverse flow of intra- or extracardiac shunts** also indicates elevated RV pressure.

Cardiac catheterization is the gold standard for the diagnosis of PAH and is necessary for the assessment of disease severity and treatment stratification. A right heart catheterization can be performed to evaluate intra- or extracardiac shunts, to measure mPAP, PVR, and PCWP for diagnosis, and to perform acute vasoreactivity testing (AVT) to guide therapy. Cardiac catheterization is also recommended prior to the initiation of medical therapy, to evaluate the effectiveness of medical therapy, and for assessment during times of clinical deterioration.

What is acute vasoreactivity testing?

During cardiac catheterization, a pulmonary vasodilator, usually inhaled nitric oxide (iNO), is administered to determine whether it will acutely lower PVR. A positive test is defined as a >20% fall in mPAP with either no change or a decrease in the ratio of pulmonary vascular resistance to systemic vascular resistance (PVR/SVR) without a decrease in cardiac output (CO). A positive AVT result indicates a better prognosis because it reflects preserved vascular reactivity, suggesting a reversible component to the elevated PVR. It also identifies those patients who will benefit from targeted PAH therapy.

> **Clinical Pearl**
>
> *A positive AVT test is defined as a >20% fall in mPAP and either no change or a decrease in PVR/SVR without a decrease in cardiac output. A positive AVT result indicates a better prognosis because it reflects preserved vascular reactivity, suggesting a reversible component to the elevated PVR.*

What are the goals of medical therapy for PAH?

The advent of targeted therapies for PAH has significantly improved the outcomes of children living with this diagnosis, yet despite these advances, PAH remains an incurable disease. The goals of therapy, therefore, are to optimize quality of life and enhance survival by halting disease progression. Medications are used to target reversible changes by promoting pulmonary arterial vasodilation and improving RV function. Therapeutic decisions are based on the results of AVT testing as well as risk stratification.

What are the initial treatment options after diagnosis of PAH?

The American Heart Association and American Thoracic Society have established an algorithm for the treatment of PAH. Supportive therapies are first initiated at diagnosis to help minimize morbidity and control the symptoms related to PAH.

- **Oxygen supplementation** is often utilized for saturations <92% to mitigate hypoxic-induced pulmonary vasoconstriction.

- **Medical therapies** are directed toward the treatment of RV failure.
  - *Diuretics* help offload the RV but should be used with caution, as PAH patients can be dependent on preload to maintain CO.
  - *Digoxin* may also be used to improve RV function.
- **Anticoagulation** is sometimes employed due to the increased risk of thrombosis that contributes to the rise in PVR.

  Once supportive medications are started, AVT is performed and used to guide further therapy.
- **Positive AVT**: Patients who are >1 year of age without RV failure are started on oral calcium channel blockers such as nifedipine, diltiazem, or amlodipine.
- **Negative AVT** or **failure to respond to CCB**: Patients are started on targeted therapy.

What are targeted therapies for PAH?

Current treatment strategies are aimed at improving the balance between vasodilation and vasoconstriction, preventing thrombosis from forming in narrow vessels, and attenuating vascular remodeling using antiproliferative drugs.

Three primary pathways are targeted to treat PAH: the endothelin pathway, the nitric oxide pathway, and the prostacyclin pathway.

- **Endothelin receptor antagonists (ERA)** block the action of endothelin, a pulmonary vasoconstrictor that is overexpressed in PAH. Medications in this class include bosentan, ambrisentan, and macitentan, all of which are administered orally. They can cause hepatotoxicity; therefore, liver function tests should be monitored closely.
- **Phosphodiesterase type 5 inhibitors (PDE5i)** reduce the breakdown of cGMP resulting in pulmonary vasodilation. They may also possess some antiproliferative properties. Phosphodiesterase inhibitors include sildenafil and tadalafil, which are both oral medications. Side effects include headache, flushing, and nasal congestion, necessitating slow titration.
- **Prostacyclin analogs (prostanoids)** provide an exogenous source of this potent pulmonary vasodilator, which is underexpressed in patients with PAH. This class of medications has also been shown to have antiplatelet, antithrombotic, antiproliferative, and anti-inflammatory properties. There are oral (treprostinil, beraprost), inhaled (treprostinil, iloprost), intravenous (IV) (epoprostenol, treprostinil), and subcutaneous (treprostinil) formulations available. *It is important to*

307

recognize the short half-life of IV forms. Intravenous epoprostenol has a half-life of 2–5 minutes and must be continuously infused 24 hours a day via a central venous line (CVL). Discontinuation puts the patient at risk for an acute PH crisis. Intravenous treprostinil (which also requires central administration) has a longer half-life of 2–4 hours, allowing more time if medication is discontinued until an acute PH crisis ensues. Similar to PDE5i, prostanoids may cause headaches, flushing, and nasal congestion, as well as abdominal pain.

How is appropriate targeted therapy chosen?

Patients who do not have a positive response to AVT or who fail CCB therapy are placed on targeted therapy after risk stratification.

- *WHO functional class I and II* (lower risk patients) are started on oral therapy with ERA or PDE5i with or without the addition of an inhaled prostacyclin.
- *WHO functional class III and IV* (higher risk patients) or those with deterioration on oral therapy are started on aggressive combination therapy (commonly referred to as *triple therapy*) using a medication from each of the receptor pathways.

Clinical Pearl

"Triple therapy" utilizes one medication from each of the three pulmonary vasodilator pathways: an endothelin receptor antagonist, a phosphodiesterase inhibitor, and a prostanoid. Both triple therapy and the need for intravenous PH therapy are indicative of severe PH.

What are the procedural options for the treatment of PAH?

Procedural interventions are reserved for patients who are still decompensating despite maximal medical therapy.

- An *atrial septostomy* can be created in the catheterization lab to augment left ventricular (LV) preload by serving as a "pop-off" valve, allowing shunting of blood from R-to-L during times of high right-sided pressures.
  - The ability to shunt R-to-L can worsen hypoxia. It is not performed on patients with oxygen saturations <90% or high right atrial pressure (>20 mm Hg), as excessive R-to-L shunting can then occur.
  - Without such a shunt, during times of increased PVR, less blood is able to get through the pulmonary system to the LV and CO will decrease.

- A *Potts shunt,* a surgically created anastomosis between the left pulmonary artery and the descending aorta, is an alternative to atrial septostomy.
  - Physiologically it achieves a similar result to an atrial septostomy by unloading the RV and providing systemic blood flow.
  - Because shunted blood enters the aorta beyond the coronary and cerebral circulations, these vessels will receive oxygenated blood from the LV, possibly offering an advantage over septostomy.

These treatments are both palliative efforts. The only definitive treatment for PAH is lung transplantation, or if the RV is severely damaged, a combined heart–lung transplant. Both operations carry significant morbidity and mortality.

Anesthetic Implications

What is known about anesthetic risk in patients with PH?

Assessing anesthetic risk in children with PH is difficult due to the heterogeneity among studies, as well as heterogeneity among the children themselves. Regardless, data show children with PH have a 20-fold higher incidence of perioperative cardiac arrest compared to the general pediatric population (1%–5% vs. 0.014%, respectively). Approximately 20% will have a change in oxygen saturation, carbon dioxide (CO_2), blood pressure, or mPAP that is unrelated to the type of procedure, anesthetic, or their specific type of PH. Pulmonary hypertensive crises have been reported in 2% and the risk of perioperative death has also been reported to be as high as 1.5%.

Clinical Pearl

Children with PH have a 20-fold higher incidence of perioperative cardiac arrest compared to the general pediatric population.

How is risk stratified in PH patients?

Not all patients with PH present with the same risk; therefore, preoperative risk stratification is imperative in preparing an appropriate anesthetic plan and determining the need for cardiovascular drug preparation, advanced life support availability (including extracorporeal membrane oxygenation [ECMO] backup), and postsurgical recovery location. Risk stratification requires evaluation of available diagnostic data, patient medication and functional status, as well as contributing anesthetic and surgical factors.

Cardiac catheterization: Factors placing patients in a high-risk category include systemic or suprasystemic RV and PA pressures (ratio of mean PA pressure to mean systemic pressure >70%), elevated RA pressure (>10–15 mm Hg), and decreased cardiac index (<2.5 L/minute/m^2). A PVR greater than 15 iWU and PVR/SVR ratio >1 are also considered severe.

Echocardiography: Signs of severe PH include evidence of significant RV enlargement, dysfunction, or failure; septal flattening or bowing into the LV; systemic or suprasystemic RV pressures; and bidirectional shunting or reversal of shunting. The presence of either a surgically created pulmonary to systemic (Potts) shunt or a percutaneously created atrial septal defect for therapeutic management of elevated right-sided pressures also reflects severe PH.

Medications: The patient's current medical therapies also provide a clue to disease severity. Escalation of care, the use of multidrug therapy, IV or subcutaneous medication administration, and home oxygen use are all suggestive of significant disease.

Signs and symptoms: Other indicators of PH severity include WHO class III/IV, syncope, chest pain, fatigue, dyspnea, cyanosis, and failure to thrive.

In addition to patient factors, the type of operation and timing of surgery also have an impact on anesthetic risk, with emergency surgery, major thoracic or abdominal surgeries, and anesthetic duration >3 hours considered higher risk.

What is involved in preoperative planning?

Due to the complexity and higher perioperative risk in patients with PH, a preoperative multidisciplinary team discussion is advised to ensure a careful plan is in place to mitigate this risk. Planning should include the anesthesiologist (who preferably has experience with PH patients), cardiologist, and proceduralist, all of whom can offer unique insights into care of the patient. Specific issues to address include the urgency and timing of the procedure, patient optimization, intraoperative concerns, and postoperative disposition. Patients with PH should be cared for in a setting capable of providing advanced life support and intensive care in the event of acute decompensation or cardiac arrest.

What are the preoperative considerations for a patient with IPAH?

Optimization: Care must be taken to ensure the patient has been medically optimized and has not been experiencing acute PH exacerbations. However, in this case, placement of the peripherally inserted central catheter (PICC) line will provide access for ongoing medical therapy and will

likely be necessary despite exacerbations. The most recent imaging data, cardiac catheterization and medication regimen must be reviewed. It is imperative that the patient be under the active care of a cardiologist.

Medication: Maintain the home regimen of PH medications, as even small interruptions can result in increases in PVR. Oral medications can be taken with a small sip of water on the day of surgery. Continuously delivered PH medications via inhaled, subcutaneous, and/or IV routes must remain uninterrupted. Any indwelling catheter delivering these medications should be considered a dedicated line and never used by the anesthesiologist. The use and management of anticoagulant, antihypertensive, and diuretic medications should also be discussed with the cardiologist. The surgical team should be aware of planned strategies for management of anticoagulation therapies.

Nil per os (NPO) status: Dehydration leads to decreased preload and is poorly tolerated. Consideration should be given to scheduling the patient as the first case of the day to minimize NPO time and intake of clear fluids up to 2 hours prior to the procedure should be encouraged. Patients at higher risk may benefit from overnight preoperative admission for IV hydration or should have IV fluids started in the holding area while waiting for their procedure.

Illness: Patients with PH who present with an acute respiratory infection or reactive airway exacerbation are at increased risk for a PH crisis. Gastrointestinal illness may lead to dehydration and decreased preload. Elective cases should be cancelled under these circumstances.

Clinical Pearl

The home medication regimen should be maintained throughout the perioperative period, as even small interruptions can result in increases in PVR. Continuously delivered PH medications via inhaled, subcutaneous, and/or IV routes should remain uninterrupted. Intravenous medications should run via a dedicated line that is not used by the anesthesiologist.

What are the goals in the anesthetic management of patients with IPAH?

The primary anesthetic management goal is to avoid increases in PVR while maintaining SVR, preload, and RV contractility. Maintenance of hemodynamic stability is crucial in this population, as even small hemodynamic deviations can overwhelm compensatory mechanisms and lead to a PH crisis.

What is a PH crisis and what factors can precipitate it?

A PH crisis is a sudden and potentially lethal increase in PVR that causes an unsustainable rise in the afterload of the RV leading to RV failure. This results in decreased LV preload with a fall in both CO and coronary perfusion, which, in turn, results in biventricular failure. If the PH crisis is not rapidly and aggressively treated, this cycle can lead to cardiac arrest. (See Figure 40.1.)

Acute increases in PVR can be precipitated by hypoxia, hypercarbia, acidosis, and hypothermia. Normothermia should be maintained during the perioperative period. Care must be taken to ensure adequate ventilation and respiratory and metabolic acidosis should be promptly corrected. Sympathetic activation or noxious stimuli can also precipitate an acute increase in PVR. The most vulnerable times are during intubation, tracheal and pharyngeal suctioning, surgical stimulation, and emergence from anesthesia. Blunting sympathetic responses with sufficient anesthetic depth and the use of narcotics can help attenuate increases in PVR.

Because a PH crisis is a cycle revolving around RV failure, disturbances at any point in the cycle which contribute to RV failure can trigger a crisis. A decrease in SVR, which often accompanies anesthetic induction, can lead to hypotension and coronary ischemia. Volatile anesthetics and certain IV induction agents can also cause direct myocardial depression. While hypovolemia can contribute to inadequate preload and cardiac output, RV dysfunction from overdistension may also decrease LV preload. All of these mechanisms may contribute to or exacerbate a PH crisis.

What are the impending signs of a PH crisis?

Impending signs of a PH crisis include hypotension, hypoxemia, decreased end-tidal CO_2, and changes in heart rate. Bradycardia is often observed and is an ominous sign. Signs of RV strain, such as ST depression or T-wave inversion in the right precordial or inferior leads, may be seen on ECG. The onset of a PH crisis can be gradual, with a slow decline in blood pressure and oxygen saturation. However, a PH crisis can also be sudden, with complete cardiovascular collapse. It is important to be extremely vigilant and treat hemodynamic changes promptly because if the cycle ends in cardiac arrest the resuscitative outcomes in this population are poor.

Clinical Pearl

Signs of impending PH crisis include hypotension, hypoxemia, decreased end-tidal CO_2, and bradycardia. Signs of RV strain, such as ST depression or T-wave inversion in the right precordial or inferior leads, may be seen on ECG.

How should a PH crisis be treated?

The aims in treating a PH crisis are to support CO and coronary perfusion while taking measures to decrease PVR and augment SVR. (See Table 40.2.)

Decrease PVR

- Ensure delivery of 100% oxygen and institute mild hyperventilation.
- Make sure the patient is warm and correct metabolic or respiratory acidosis.
- Ensure adequate analgesia to decrease sympathetically mediated increases in PVR.
- Inhaled nitric oxide, administered within a range of 20–80 ppm, is the pulmonary vasodilator of choice for acute PH crisis, as it selectively and rapidly dilates the pulmonary vasculature without decreasing SVR. Abruptly stopping iNO can lead to rebound PH, so once started iNO should be slowly titrated off.

Increase SVR

- Vasopressors should be started to maintain and/or increase SVR. It is essential to preserve coronary perfusion and maximize oxygen delivery to the deteriorating RV by increasing SVR.

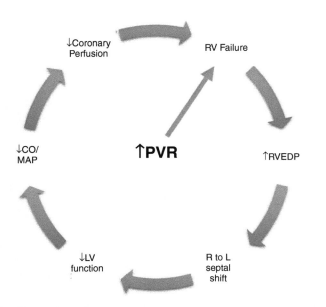

Figure 40.1 The cycle of a pulmonary hypertensive crisis. CO, cardiac output; MAP, mean arterial pressure; PVR, pulmonary vascular resistance; RVEDP, right ventricular end-diastolic pressure.

Table 40.2 Treatment of a Pulmonary Hypertensive Crisis

Goal	Therapy

Decrease PVR	100% Oxygen
	Nitric oxide
	Increase anesthetic depth
	Correct respiratory acidosis
	   Mild hyperventilation
	Correct metabolic acidosis
	   Sodium bicarbonate

Increase SVR	Vasopressors
	   Phenylephrine
	   Vasopressin
	   Norepinephrine

Support CO	Judicious fluid resuscitation
	Inotropes
	   Epinephrine
	   Dopamine
	   Dobutamine
	ECLS/ECMO

ECLS, extracorporeal life support; ECMO, extracorporeal membrane oxygenation; iNO, inhaled nitric oxide; PVR, pulmonary vascular resistance; SVR, systemic vascular resistance.

- ○ Vasopressin lowers PVR while increasing SVR, making it an attractive choice.
- ○ β-Agonist effects of norepinephrine add the advantage of inotropic support.
- ○ Phenylephrine, often more easily obtained, can also be safely used.

Support CO

- A fluid bolus can be considered to ensure adequate preload and support CO, but RV distension should be avoided, especially with severe RV failure.
- Epinephrine, dopamine, or dobutamine can all be used for support of CO, though the tachycardia caused by these agents can worsen ventricular filling and increase myocardial oxygen consumption.
- Milrinone, in addition to its inotropic and lusitropic properties, is also a pulmonary vasodilator. However, the accompanying decrease in SVR often limits its utility and this medication is best avoided during a PH crisis.
- If cardiac arrest occurs, extracorporeal life support (ECLS, ECMO) should be initiated early.

Clinical Pearl

Milrinone, in addition to its inotropic and lusitropic properties, is also a pulmonary vasodilator and can seem like an attractive choice. However, the accompanying decrease in SVR often limits its utility and this medication is best avoided during a PH crisis.

What medications should be prepared for a patient with PH?

Resuscitation medications, including epinephrine and phenylephrine, should be immediately available. For higher risk patients, inotropic and vasopressor infusions should be prepared. Immediate availability of iNO is often prudent. In the highest risk patients, instituting "ECMO standby," or having a team available to initiate ECMO should decompensation occur is advisable.

Should invasive or advanced monitors be utilized?

The decision to use invasive monitoring depends on the severity of the patient's PH as well as the complexity of the case. Arterial access is often advantageous, as it facilitates close monitoring of hypotension, hypercarbia, or acidosis, all of which can trigger a PH crisis. Central venous access may be necessary for the administration of vasoactive medications and can serve as a guide to monitor preload through observation of central venous pressure trends. Transthoracic or transesophageal echocardiography can also provide valuable real-time information about the function and filling of the RV.

Is it safe to premedicate patients with PH?

Premedication carries both risks and benefits. In an anxious child sedation can prove beneficial by alleviating the increase in PVR and myocardial oxygen consumption caused by catecholamine surges. However, oversedation can result in hypoventilation, hypercarbia, and hypoxia, which may increase PVR. Therefore, if premedication is used, the patient should be closely monitored.

Is general anesthesia indicated for PICC line placement in this patient?

Placement of a PICC line is typically not a painful procedure; therefore, general anesthesia is usually not indicated. However, if a patient proves uncooperative or unsafe for sedation or monitored anesthesia care, a deeper level of sedation or anesthesia may be indicated.

What type of anesthetic induction could be performed on this child?

While general anesthesia is unlikely to be required in a developmentally normal 10-year-old patient for PICC line placement, this patient would likely require anxiolysis during the procedure. Slow titration of an anxiolytic, such as midazolam, is indicated to ensure cooperation while maintaining adequate ventilation. Anxiolysis with other medications, such as dexmedetomidine and ketamine, may also prove effective. Caution is advised with the use of dexmedetomidine in patients with untreated PH, as concern exists for sudden increases in PVR with bolus administration in children.

How do anesthetic medications affect patients with PH?

Volatile Agents

Volatile agents cause a dose-dependent depression of myocardial contractility and SVR. On the other hand, they also attenuate hypoxic pulmonary vasoconstriction and cause a small amount of pulmonary vasodilation, lowering PVR. These agents are generally well tolerated for anesthetic maintenance in patients with PH. Though not well studied, nitrous oxide appears to have minimal effects on PVR in infants and children. Its use may be limited if the patient is unable to tolerate an FiO_2 of <100%.

Intravenous Agents

Propofol causes a significant reduction in SVR, necessitating caution with its use as a bolus medication in patients with moderate to severe PH. However, the combination of propofol and ketamine administered as an infusion has been successfully utilized in patients with PH.

Ketamine increases SVR and maintains blood pressure with minimal to no change in PVR, making it a useful medication for patients with PH. Recent studies demonstrate its use is well tolerated in children with PH and may even lower PVR.

Etomidate has a favorable cardiovascular profile with minimal to no effects on contractility, mean arterial blood pressure and SVR, making it an appropriate agent for induction in patients with PH. Studies are inconsistent regarding effects on PVR.

Dexmedetomidine can serve as a useful adjunct to an anesthetic by providing sedation, anxiolysis, and analgesia while avoiding significant respiratory depression. It has no effect on PAP or PVR and can transiently increase SVR. However, dexmedetomidine may also decrease heart rate, which may not be well tolerated in a patient with impaired ventricular function. This decrease in heart rate can be attenuated by using a bolus dose of 0.5–1 mcg/kg administered slowly over 10–15 minutes. Additional caution is advised when medications, such as digoxin, are part of the child's medication regimen, as the combination may result in profound bradycardia.

Opioids have a very stable hemodynamic profile and blunt the effects of noxious stimuli, making them a vital part of the anesthetic plan. Bradycardia may also occur with opioid administration. Care must be taken with long-acting opioids if extubation is planned, as they can lead to hypoventilation, hypercarbia, and hypoxia.

Midazolam also has minimal hemodynamic effects and can be useful in patients with PH. When used as premedication for anxiolysis patients should be carefully monitored, as hypoventilation may occur, especially in patients with upper airway disease.

How can general anesthesia be induced in patients with PH?

Slow IV titration of lower doses of several drugs can achieve adequate anesthetic depth without incurring the marked hemodynamic changes associated with high doses of a single drug. Inhalational induction of anesthesia will be tolerated only in patients with very mild forms of PH. An IV induction is recommended for patients with moderate to severe PH using medications with minimal hemodynamic effects such as etomidate and ketamine, supplemented with opioids and/or midazolam. For the highest risk patients, a slow induction with a propofol–ketamine infusion, as described earlier, may be utilized, in addition to a phenylephrine infusion to maintain SVR. In these patients, if feasible, blood pressure monitoring via an arterial line during induction is advisable.

What airway management methods are appropriate?

The incidence of anesthetic complications in this population has not been shown to correlate with the type of airway used. Sympathetic stimulation caused by insertion of an endotracheal tube (ETT) or laryngeal mask airway (LMA) must be mitigated by adequate depth of anesthesia, opioid use and/or airway topicalization. The use of muscle relaxants to avoid coughing and enhance the ability to control ventilation offers advantages in most procedures. The use of an LMA, when appropriate, is often less stimulating than an endotracheal tube. A natural airway, if appropriate, has the advantage of avoiding airway instrumentation; however, the risks of hypoventilation and hypercarbia necessitate a high level of vigilance.

What ventilatory concerns exist in patients with PH?

Ventilation strategies to decrease PVR should be employed, with avoidance of hypercarbia. Physiologic levels of positive end-expiratory pressure (PEEP) and tidal volumes at functional residual capacity should be used to prevent atelectasis, which leads to ventilation-perfusion mismatch. High PEEP and/or high peak inspiratory pressures, excessive tidal volumes, and long inspiratory times overdistend alveoli and compress alveolar capillaries. This combination leads to decreased venous return and increased PVR and should be avoided. Supplemental levels of inspired oxygen should be used as needed to avoid hypoxemia.

How should fluid management be approached in this population?

Patients with PH typically have a stiff RV that requires an elevated central venous pressure to maintain filling volumes and forward flow. However, overadministration of fluid can distend the RV, negatively impacting contractility. Resuscitative fluids should be given judiciously and slowly with time to allow equilibration while avoiding any rapid or major fluid shifts. If RV function is at all compromised, the use of inotropes and vasopressors should be initiated early to minimize the amount of fluid administered to maintain CO.

What precautions are necessary during emergence from anesthesia?

Emergence from anesthesia is perhaps even more risky than induction in patients with PH as it can be less well controlled. Increases in PVR can occur with coughing or bucking, inadequate pain control, and tracheal suctioning. Suctioning should take place during a deeper level of anesthesia and the use of opioids to limit sympathetic stimulation can also help minimize risk. In some patients extubation to noninvasive positive airway pressure or high-flow nasal cannula may be advisable.

Clinical Pearl

Emergence from anesthesia is perhaps even more risky than induction in patients with PH as it can be less well controlled. Suctioning during a deeper level of anesthesia and the use of opioids to limit sympathetic stimulation will help minimize risk.

What should the postoperative care of the patient include?

The increased risk of morbidity and mortality associated with anesthesia in the PH patient continues in the recovery room. Continuous monitoring with prompt recognition and treatment of symptoms is imperative. Either splinting due to inadequate pain control or the excessive use of narcotics can lead to hypoventilation and hypercarbia. Nausea, vomiting, and fluid underresuscitation may lead to dehydration and inadequate preload. Pain or postoperative delirium can cause a sympathetic surge. High-risk patients, or those who had any significant intraoperative events, should be admitted to the intensive care unit immediately following surgery. Outpatient surgery should be considered only for the lowest risk patients who undergo uneventful anesthetics, recover completely to baseline status, and are able to resume all preoperative medications.

Suggested Reading

Abman S. H., Hansmann G., and Archer S. L. Pediatric pulmonary hypertension: Guidelines from the American Heart Association and American Thoracic Society. *Circulation* 2015; **132**: 2037–99.

Friesen R. H., Nichols C. S., Twite M. D., et al. The hemodynamic response to dexmedetomidine loading dose in children with and without pulmonary hypertension. *Anesth Analg* 2013; **117**: 953–9.

Friesen R. H. and Williams G. D. Anesthetic management of children with pulmonary arterial hypertension. *Pediatr Anesth* 2008; **18**: 208–16. DOI: 10.1111/j.1460-9592.2008.02419.x.

Galie N. and Simonneau G. The Fifth World Symposium on Pulmonary Hypertension. *J Am Coll Cardiol* 2013; **62**: D1–D3.

Latham G. J. and Yung D. Current understanding and perioperative management of pediatric pulmonary hypertension. *Pediatr Anesth* 2019; **29**: 441–56. DOI: 10.1111/pan.13542.

Nathan A. T., Nicolson S. C., and McGowan F. X. A word of caution: dexmedetomidine and pulmonary hypertension. *Anesth Analg* 2014; **119**: 216–17.

Shah S. and Szmuszkovicz J. R. Pediatric perioperative pulmonary arterial hypertension: a case-based primer. *Children* 2017; **4**: 92. DOI: 10.3390/children4100092.

Twite M. D. and Friesen R. H. Anesthesia for pulmonary hypertension. In Andropoulos D. B., Stayer S., Mossad E. B., et al. eds., *Anesthesia for Congenital Heart Disease*, 3rd ed. Hoboken, NJ: John Wiley & Sons, 2015; 661–76.

41

Pulmonary Hypertension and Congenital Heart Disease

Premal M. Trivedi

A 7-year-old female with hearing loss is scheduled to undergo a tympanoplasty. Her past medical history is significant for repair of a complete atrioventricular septal defect at age 6 months with residual pulmonary hypertension. She additionally has Down syndrome, hypothyroidism, moderate obstructive sleep apnea, recurrent bronchitis, and gastroesophageal reflux. She is managed with continuous positive airway pressure at night, and her medications include tadalafil, ambrisentan, levothyroxine, and ranitidine. Ambrisentan was added to the tadalafil a year ago to slow the progression of her pulmonary hypertension, and a recent cardiac catheterization was performed to evaluate its effect. A review of the pulmonologist's notes shows that the child has maintained her baseline level of activity with minimal reported symptoms. She has had no syncopal episodes or complaints of angina.

Her echocardiography report from earlier this year shows:

- *Mild right atrioventricular valve regurgitation*
- *Mild to moderate left atrioventricular valve regurgitation*
- *Mild right ventricular hypertrophy and dilation*
- *No left ventricular outflow obstruction and normal biventricular systolic function*

A review of serial echocardiograms reveals that the pulmonary artery systolic and main pulmonary arterial pressures have slightly increased over time.

Key Objectives

- Describe features of Down syndrome that can contribute to development of pulmonary hypertension.
- Identify common residual lesions in patients who have undergone repair of complete atrioventricular septal defect.
- Describe how to utilize echocardiography and cardiac catheterization reports to assess the severity of pulmonary hypertension.

- Risk stratify patients with pulmonary hypertension undergoing noncardiac surgery.
- Develop a plan for management of perioperative pulmonary hypertension medications.
- Describe intraoperative management strategies and factors to consider when determining postoperative disposition in patients with pulmonary hypertension.

Pathophysiology

Is Down syndrome relevant to this patient's diagnosis of pulmonary hypertension?

Down syndrome increases the risk of developing pulmonary hypertension (PH) *even in the absence of congenital heart disease* (CHD). Contributing factors include intrinsic airway and lung abnormalities, multifactorial lung injury, and a tendency toward obesity that in combination often lead to respiratory acidosis and hypoxia. (See Table 41.1.) Patients with Down syndrome also have an increased incidence of hypothyroidism. While the relationship between thyroid dysfunction and PH is unclear, the cardiopulmonary effects of hypo- or hyperthyroidism can also have detrimental effects on pulmonary vascular resistance (PVR) and respiratory function. Due to these comorbidities and the frequent presence of CHD, the incidence of PH in children with Down syndrome may be as high as 28%. The majority of such patients are diagnosed within the first year of life, and while most experience remission over time, nearly 30% can have persistent or recurrent disease. This patient has the contributing factors of obstructive sleep apnea, recurrent bronchitis, gastroesophageal reflux, and hypothyroidism.

Table 41.1 Contributors to the Development of Pulmonary Hypertension in Down Syndrome

Anatomic or Physiologic Contributors	Clinical Manifestations	Diagnostic and Therapeutic Interventions
Airway anomalies Midface hypoplasia Macroglossia Narrow nasopharynx Adenotonsillar hypertrophy Generalized hypotonia Laryngomalacia Tracheomalacia Bronchomalacia	Obstructive sleep apnea Chronic lung disease	Continuous positive airway pressure Tonsillectomy and adenoidectomy Laryngoscopy and bronchoscopy
Pulmonary anomalies Impaired lung growth Lung immaturity Lung injury Aspiration Recurrent pneumonias Gastroesophageal reflux	Impaired lung compliance and gas exchange	Gastrostomy tube and/or Nissen fundoplication Frequent antibiotic therapy H_2 blockers
Relative immunodeficiency T- and B-cell lymphopenia Reduced antibody response to immunization Impaired neutrophil chemotaxis	Exacerbation of airway obstruction and lung injury through frequent and prolonged upper and lower respiratory infections	Frequent antibiotic therapy
Thyroid dysfunction Congenital hypothyroidism Hyperthyroidism	Potential adverse effect on pulmonary vasculature	Thyroid replacement therapy

What other risk factors for PH does this patient have?

Left-to-right (L-to-R) shunts can also affect the pulmonary vasculature. Because the shunt in complete atrioventricular septal defect (CAVSD) is generally unrestrictive and occurs at both the atrial and ventricular levels, thereby subjecting the pulmonary bed to both a volume *and* pressure load, increases in PVR can occur rapidly. To decrease this risk, surgical repair is commonly performed within the first year of life, ideally between 4 and 6 months of age. Repairs taking place late in the first year of life or beyond, particularly in a child with Down syndrome, should raise concern for the presence of PH.

Residual or newly acquired defects following surgical repair can also exacerbate existing PH. The most common residual lesion in CAVSD is left atrioventricular valve (LAVV) regurgitation. Left ventricular outflow tract obstruction (LVOTO) may also develop depending on the initial anatomy and surgical technique used for the repair. Both defects affect the pulmonary vasculature by causing an increase in left atrial pressure that is transmitted to the pulmonary veins. If severe and prolonged, these lesions can produce changes in the pulmonary arterial system.

> **Clinical Pearl**
>
> *When evaluating a patient with a history of CAVSD repair, the age at surgical repair and the presence and severity of residual lesions – most commonly LAVV regurgitation – can help in assessing the patient's risk of PH.*

How common is the combination of Down syndrome and a cardiac lesion including a L-to-R shunt?

Nearly 25% of children with Down syndrome also have an atrioventricular septal defect (AVSD), and of the population of children diagnosed with AVSDs approximately half also have Down syndrome. Therefore, when one of these diagnoses is observed, it is common or even likely for the other to be present as well.

What is the impact of this combination on the pulmonary vasculature?

Because Down syndrome and L-to-R shunts act through different mechanisms to produce PH, their effects on the pulmonary vasculature are synergistic. The risk of developing PH is therefore higher than if only one of these conditions were present alone and should raise a red flag when observed together.

In the child with repaired CHD and pulmonary hypertension, what are the determinants of anesthetic risk?

Risk assessment focuses on the following patient- and procedure-specific concerns:

- Patient age
- Severity of pulmonary hypertension
- Residual cardiac lesions of hemodynamic significance
- Presence of other significant comorbidities
- Procedural risk for hypotension or hypovolemia

The severity of PH can be described by the relationship or ratio between pulmonary and systemic arterial pressures. Anesthetic risk increases as pulmonary pressures exceed half-systemic and is highest in those with systemic or suprasystemic pulmonary pressures. The presence of right ventricular (RV) dysfunction in the setting of PH is also indicative of disease severity and reflects increased risk. Due to ventricular interdependence, RV dysfunction can also cause left ventricular (LV) dysfunction in an otherwise normal LV.

Disease severity and risk can also be inferred from the patient's functional status and the number of therapies being used to treat PH. For example, a patient who becomes dyspneic with minimal exertion or who has had syncopal episodes has more advanced PH than one who has minimal limitations in activity. Likewise, a patient on multidrug therapy would generally have more severe PH than one who is on monotherapy.

Younger age is associated with an increased risk of anesthetic complications, and patients with PH who are <2 years of age may be at increased risk compared to those older than 2.

Where should information regarding disease severity and residual cardiac defects be sought?

Common sources of information include:

- Clinic notes from the patient's cardiologist and pulmonologist
- Echocardiography and cardiac catheterization results
- Laboratory values: brain natriuretic peptide (BNP)

The patient's cardiologist and pulmonologist should be intimately involved in preoperative assessment and optimization. For those who have residual defects, the question of whether they should be addressed prior to proceeding with elective surgery should be discussed. Marked elevations in BNP suggest ventricular dysfunction and heart failure and are concerning for severe PH.

Based on the echocardiography report, does this child have PH?

While the echocardiographic findings presented are reassuring for preserved RV function, they do not comment on the presence or severity of PH. The body of the echocardiography report may be examined for additional data. Four observations are of particular importance:

1. ***Tricuspid regurgitation (TR) peak velocity***: If the patient has TR, its velocity can be used to calculate RV systolic pressure (which should equal PA systolic pressure in the absence of pulmonary stenosis). This value can then be compared to systemic blood pressure, which should be documented on the echo report. A TR velocity greater than 2.8 m/second is highly suggestive of PH. Using the modified Bernoulli equation:

   PA systolic pressure = 4(TR peak velocity)^2 + RA pressure,

   where PA = pulmonary artery; TR = tricuspid regurgitation; RA = right atrial.

2. ***Appearance of the interventricular septum during systole*** (a qualitative assessment of RV systolic pressure): The normal contour of the interventricular septum during systole is concave. That is, the septum extends slightly into the RV because LV systolic pressure normally exceeds RV systolic pressure. If RV pressure is elevated relative to LV pressure, however, the interventricular septum may be flattened, or in the case of suprasystemic RV pressures, it may bow *into* the LV during systole. LV filling may be compromised as a result.

3. ***Pulmonary regurgitation (PR) peak velocity***: This diastolic velocity can be used to calculate mean pulmonary artery pressure (mPAP):

   mPAP = 4(PR peak velocity)^2 + RA pressure,

where $mPAP$ = mean pulmonary artery pressure; PR = pulmonary regurgitation; RA = right atrial.

Mean PA pressures >25 mm Hg are concerning for PH.

4. **Size, thickness, and function of the RV**: RV dilation, hypertrophy, and/or depressed function are all suggestive of elevated PA pressure (assuming there is no pulmonary stenosis). Patients with depressed RV function and PH are at greater risk for periprocedural complications compared to those with preserved RV function.

Clinical Pearl

Echocardiographic findings consistent with PH can include:

- *Tricuspid regurgitant jet >2.8 m/second*
- *Interventricular septal flattening or bulging into the LV in systole*
- *Pulmonary regurgitant peak velocity > 2 m/second*
- *Right ventricular hypertrophy and/or dilation*
- *Diminished RV or LV function*

The patient's echocardiogram reveals the following information: TR peak velocity is 4.2 m/second and PR peak velocity is 1.99 m/second; the interventricular septum is flattened, there is mild RV dilation and hypertrophy with preserved RV function, and a systemic pressure measured during the study by noninvasive blood pressure cuff is 110/80 mm Hg. How can these findings be interpreted?

These findings are consistent with the known diagnosis of PH and can be used to risk stratify the patient.

- A TR peak velocity of 4.2 m/second would estimate a PA systolic pressure of 81 mm Hg assuming a CVP of 10.

PA systolic pressure = $4(4.2)^2 + 10 = 81$

- Given that the noninvasive systolic pressure was 110 mm Hg, this would suggest a PA (and RV) systolic pressure that is nearly 75% systemic. This would account for the interventricular septal flattening observed during systole and the presence of RV hypertrophy.
- The PR peak velocity of 2 m/second would estimate a mean PAP of 26 mm Hg assuming a CVP of 10.

mPAP = $4(2)^2 + 10 = 26$

Which data points are most relevant in evaluating catheterization data in a patient with pulmonary hypertension?

These variables (see Table 41.2) are first assessed at the patient's "baseline": most commonly at room air with normocapnia. Subsequently, these variables are repeated with exposure to 100% oxygen and 40 parts per million inhaled nitric oxide (iNO). These gases are both potent pulmonary vasodilators and should cause a decrease in PVR and mPAP. Such a response can help tailor therapy, and for the anesthesiologist, should underscore the need for iNO to be available when managing future anesthetics. Conversely, if the PVR does not change with these pulmonary vasodilators, then the patient has fixed pulmonary vascular disease. This occurs in the setting of long-standing PH and is often accompanied by significant RV hypertrophy and possibly dilation and decreased function. In these patients, oxygen and iNO provide no significant benefit, and anesthetic management focuses on maintaining cardiac output and avoiding further increases in PVR.

The patient's catheterization diagram and data are presented in Figures 41.1 and 41.2. What are the essential points?

Comparison of the pre- and post-iNO and hyperoxia cardiac catheterization data reveals that the child still has significant PH by mPAP and pulmonary vascular resistance indexed to body surface area (PVRI) criteria but is responsive to iNO and oxygen.

Clinical Pearl

Concerning findings on cardiac catheterization include

- *mPAP >25 mm Hg*
- *PVRI >3 Wood units/m²*
- *<20% decrease in mPAP following exposure to iNO and FiO₂ 1.0*

Table 41.2 Catheterization Parameters to Aid in Assessment of Pulmonary Hypertension

Variables	Abnormal Findings
mPAP	>25 mm Hg
PVR indexed to body surface area	>3 iWu
Pulmonary capillary wedge pressure (PCWP)	>18 mm Hg indicates left-heart disease as a contributor to PH while <15 mm Hg suggests a pre-capillary cause or pulmonary veno-occlusive disease
Response to increased FiO₂ and iNO: acute vasoreactivity testing	Lack of response pulmonary vasodilators defined as <20% decrease in mPAP

FiO₂, fraction of inspired oxygen; iNO, inhaled nitric oxide; iWU, indexed Wood units; mPAP, mean pulmonary artery pressure; PCWP, pulmonary capillary wedge pressure; PVR, pulmonary vascular resistance.

Given this functional information and the objective data from the echo and catheterization reports, how can the severity of this patient's PH be described?

See Table 41.3 for assessment of PH severity and anesthetic risk for this patient.

Using the framework noted previously and based on her moderate degree of PH, this patient is at increased risk for perioperative complications due to RV ischemia and/or PH crisis. While her functional status, surgical repair, and preserved biventricular function are all reassuring, they should not obscure this fact. The presence of moderate obstructive sleep apnea is also concerning for the potential for hypoventilation in the immediate postoperative period. Further assessment would be needed to ensure that the child's thyroid levels are normal and that the last episode of bronchitis was remote prior to proceeding. Of note, catheterization findings demonstrated that the patient still responds to iNO and oxygen, which should alert the

Table 41.3 Assessing Pulmonary Hypertension Severity and Anesthetic Risk for This Patient

Pulmonary hypertension severity	*Moderate:* PA pressures are 75% systemic in the setting of preserved right and left ventricular function; (+) response to vasoreactivity testing
Residual cardiac lesions of hemodynamic significance	No significant LAVV or RAVV regurgitation or stenosis, no LVOT obstruction
Presence of other significant comorbidities or end-organ dysfunction	OSA, GERD, hypothyroidism, and recurrent bronchitis
Procedural risk of hypotension or hypovolemia	Minimal expected hemodynamic fluctuations or fluid shifts for tympanoplasty
Age <2 years	No

GERD, gastroesophageal reflex disease; LAVV, left atrioventricular valve; LVOT, left ventricular outflow tract; OSA, obstructive sleep apnea; PA, pulmonary artery; RAVV, right atrioventricular valve.

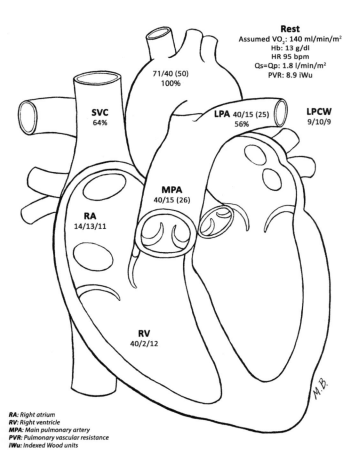

Figure 41.1 Baseline cardiac catheterization data pre-iNO and hyperoxia.

RA: *Right atrium*
RV: *Right ventricle*
MPA: *Main pulmonary artery*
PVR: *Pulmonary vascular resistance*
iWu: *Indexed Wood units*

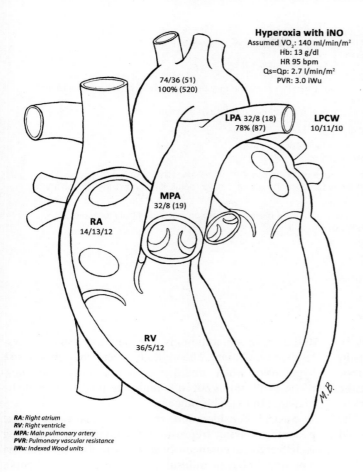

Hyperoxia with iNO
Assumed VO$_2$: 140 ml/min/m^2
Hb: 13 g/dl
HR 95 bpm
Qs=Qp: 2.7 l/min/m^2
PVR: 3.0 iWu

74/36 (51)
100% (520)

LPA 32/8 (18)
78% (87)

LPCW
10/11/10

MPA
32/8 (19)

RA
14/13/12

RV
36/5/12

Figure 41.2 Cardiac catheterization data post-iNO and oxygen.

RA: Right atrium
RV: Right ventricle
MPA: Main pulmonary artery
PVR: Pulmonary vascular resistance
iWu: Indexed Wood units

anesthesia team to have iNO readily available in the operating room when managing such a patient.

If the patient's most recent cardiology and pulmonary evaluations are a year old, would it be reasonable to proceed without updated information?

Contacting the patient's medical providers and discussing these issues is never wrong. While it is often assumed that the patient's medical team is aware of an upcoming procedure or anesthetic, that may not be the case. Factors that may suggest the need for an updated evaluation include the patient's risk (based on his or her history and the planned procedure) and any interval changes in clinical status that may have occurred since the last visit. For these patients, preoperative screening is critical not only for planning a safe intraoperative course but also an appropriate post-anesthetic disposition. At many institutions, surgeons refer

potential high-risk patients to a preoperative screening clinic so that these issues may be identified and the appropriate consultants can be notified in advance of the procedure.

What other comorbidities or perioperative issues may be present in children with Down syndrome?

See Table 41.4 for associated perioperative concerns in children with Down syndrome.

What additional information would be helpful prior to proceeding with surgery?

While the risk of bleeding with tympanoplasty is relatively low, clotting or coagulation defects could have a negative impact on surgical outcome given the confined space of the ear. As children with Down syndrome and PH may have abnormalities in platelet count or coagulation, a complete

319

Table 41.4 Perioperative Concerns in Children with Down Syndrome

Comorbidities or Perioperative Issues	Anesthetic Implications
Atlanto-axial instability	Cervical spine precautions or neurosurgical evaluation may be warranted in those who have clinical concerns for spinal compression Routine preoperative radiography is not recommended if asymptomatic
Difficult vascular access	Ultrasound may be helpful
Subglottic stenosis and/or small trachea	Smaller than expected endotracheal tube placement Potential for post-extubation stridor
Tendency toward profound bradycardia with inhalational induction	Close attention to heart rate and sevoflurane concentration during induction Rapid intravascular or intramuscular administration of anticholinergic if hemodynamically significant
Gastrointestinal anomalies Duodenal atresia Tracheoesophageal fistula Hirschsprung's disease Imperforate anus	Potential increased surgical time and risk of bleeding for subsequent abdominal procedures Potential risk of perianesthetic aspiration
Hematologic anomalies Increased risk of leukemia Thrombocytopenia	Potential increased risk of anemia and operative bleeding

blood count and coagulation panel would be reasonable to order. Specific to this patient who has had a CAVSD repair, an ECG would be helpful to identify any atrioventricular or intraventricular conduction delays that may influence the choice of anesthetic drugs used. First-degree atrioventricular block is particularly common in this subgroup. The patient's history of hypothyroidism also warrants thyroid function studies if not recently performed.

> **Clinical Pearl**
>
> *Children with Down syndrome and PH may have abnormalities in platelet count and coagulation. This may warrant laboratory evaluation prior to surgery. In children who have undergone CAVSD repair, some element of heart block may exist and can be identified with an ECG.*

Anesthetic Implications

How should the child's PH medications be managed perioperatively?

Though there are no pediatric studies to guide management, the tendency is to continue these medications perioperatively as their benefits exceed the risk. That is, they are not held preoperatively, and their scheduled administration is continued during surgery if an intravenous (IV) equivalent exists. A potential risk of pulmonary vasodilators such as the phosphodiesterase inhibitors (sildenafil or tadalafil) or the calcium channel blockers (nifedipine,

diltiazem, or amlodipine) is that they may also cause systemic vasodilation. Theoretically, then, they may cause hypotension when administered in proximity to an anesthetic. While this is not commonly observed, one should be prepared to treat this outcome.

Special consideration should be made for those patients receiving treprostinil (Remodulin®). This drug is delivered subcutaneously as a continuous infusion via a pump (similar to an insulin pump in diabetic patients). Depending on the procedure for which a patient is scheduled, conversion to IV treprostinil may be advisable to maintain a steady plasma concentration. At many institutions, the pulmonary service facilitates this transition preoperatively.

> **Clinical Pearl**
>
> *The benefits of perioperative continuation of PH medications likely exceeds the risks of the systemic vasodilation that they may cause.*

In addition to oxygen and iNO, what other rescue medications can be helpful to acutely reduce PVR intraoperatively?

For patients with severe PH or highly labile pulmonary pressures, the use of inhaled prostacyclin (Iloprost®) can be beneficial. It can be administered through an anesthesia circuit with the appropriate adapters and acts quickly due to its direct delivery to the pulmonary vasculature.

What vasoactive drugs should be immediately available?

Vasoactive drugs commonly used in the management of PH include epinephrine, norepinephrine, vasopressin, and phenylephrine. Epinephrine helps maintain or enhance RV function, while vasopressin and phenylephrine help maintain diastolic pressures to allow adequate RV perfusion.

> **Clinical Pearl**
>
> *When managing a child with PH available adjuncts should include:*
> - *Inhaled nitric oxide*
> - *Inhaled prostacyclin for patients with severe or labile PH*
> - *Vasoactive agents to increase systemic blood pressure*

Are there any anesthetic drugs that should be avoided in this patient?

The severity of the patient's disease should guide drug selection and dosing. Because **propofol** has the potential to cause myocardial depression as well as systemic vaso- and venodilation, hypotension can result with even small bolus doses in the high-risk patient. As such, it should be used with caution, if at all, in those with depressed RV function and/or moderate to severe PH. **Ketamine**'s effects on PVR and PAP have been the subject of controversy, but the drug is well tolerated assuming hypercapnea is avoided and the patient is exposed to pulmonary vasodilators such as oxygen or sevoflurane. Hemodynamically, ketamine is ideal in that it maintains blood pressure and therefore coronary perfusion pressure while also providing analgesia and sedation. **Dexmedetomidine** is thought to have a minimal impact on PVR. Caveats with this drug include its potential to decrease cardiac output by slowing the heart rate significantly or worsening the degree of heart block in a patient with existing conduction delays. Further, in patients with Down syndrome who are already prone to bradycardia, dexmedetomidine may cause hemodynamically significant decreases in heart rate.

Is invasive monitoring excessive for this procedure?

In this child with moderate PH, it would be reasonable to place an arterial line in order to monitor blood pressures more closely and draw blood gases to assess the adequacy of ventilation and oxygenation. A central line should not be needed for this procedure but could be considered if the hemodynamics were concerning following induction. If use of a vasoactive infusion appears likely, it is prudent to obtain central venous access.

How does a PH crisis present?

One of the common intraoperative triggers for a PH crisis is a painful stimulus, most commonly due to intubation or surgical incision. As a result, lung compliance may acutely worsen and blood pressure may fall in the absence of an atrial or ventricular level defect. If an atrial or ventricular level defect is present and provides a "pop-off" (the ability to shunt R-to-L when a PH crisis occurs), hemoglobin–oxygen desaturation could occur with resultant cyanosis but cardiac output would be maintained. If the PH crisis is sustained, ECG changes consistent with RV and LV ischemia often develop, leading to further hypotension and ultimately cardiac arrest.

Equally concerning in a PH crisis is the development of hypotension due to any combination of decreased SVR and/or hypovolemia. Hypotension results in a lower coronary perfusion pressure, and for a patient who already has an elevated right ventricular end diastolic pressure (RVEDP), this lessened gradient can result in RV ischemia.

RV myocardial perfusion = Aortic diastolic pressure – RVEDP

> **Clinical Pearl**
>
> *Factors that can acutely increase PVR and precipitate a PH crisis include*
> - *Painful stimuli (intubation or surgical incision)*
> - *Hypoxia*
> - *Hypercapnea*
> - *Acidosis*

What drugs are most helpful if such an event were to occur?

The main goals in this setting are dual and intertwined: decrease PVR and support RV perfusion. Depending on the etiology, the following drugs/maneuvers should be considered in rapid succession.

Treatment of a PH Crisis

- Phenylephrine to increase systemic pressure and decrease RV ischemia
- Administration of 100% oxygen and initiation of iNO
- Consider inhaled prostacyclin if available
- Analgesia and/or increased anesthetic depth
- Initiation of inotropic and pressor support

- Boluses of code dose epinephrine if no improvement with the above
- Rapid call for extracorporeal life support if these measures fail to resuscitate the patient

What issues specific to tympanoplasty are relevant in this patient?

The increased incidence of postoperative nausea and vomiting (PONV) associated with tympanoplasty may adversely affect respiratory dynamics as well as volume status. If PONV becomes severe, it may also affect the ability to continue oral PH medications in the post-operative period. Common antiemetics such as dexamethasone and ondansetron can be used to the decrease this risk. A low-dose continuous infusion of propofol may also be considered for PONV prophylaxis assuming the patient's blood pressure is being closely monitored.

Utilization of a pain control strategy that is not overly reliant on opioids can also aid in mitigating the risk of PONV. A multimodal plan including acetaminophen, ketorolac (in the setting of a normal platelet count and surgeon agreement), and ketamine can be useful.

What factors should be considered when determining postoperative disposition?

Perhaps the most important consideration is the patient's preoperative risk based on the aforementioned factors. If the patient is considered moderate- to high- risk, postoperative admission and monitoring in an intensive care setting may be warranted regardless of the stability of the intraoperative course. Discharge to the floor or home can be considered on postoperative day 1 if the patient is progressing as expected. For those who are lower risk, the decision point between floor admission versus discharge home after a period of observation in the recovery room may be considered. Any concerns regarding PONV, pain management, intraoperative hemodynamic instability, or the ability to resume medications should tilt the scales toward admission.

Suggested Reading

Adachi I., Uemura H., McCarthy K. P., et al. Surgical anatomy of atrioventricular septal defect. *Asian Cardiovasc Thorac Ann* 2008; **16**: 497–502.

Bush D., Galambos C., Ivy D. D., et al. Clinical characteristics and risk factors for developing pulmonary hypertension in children with Down syndrome. *J Pediatr* 2018; **202**: 212–19.

Hansmann G. and Apitz C. Treatment of children with pulmonary hypertension. Expert consensus statement on the diagnosis and treatment of pediatric pulmonary hypertension. The European Paediatric Pulmonary Vascular Disease Network, endorsed by ISHLT and DGPK. *Heart* 2016; **102**: ii67–ii85.

Shukla A. C. and Almodovar M. C. Anesthesia considerations for children with pulmonary hypertension. *Pediatr Crit Care Med* 2010; **11**: S7–73.

Twite M. D. and Friesen R. H. The anesthetic management of children with pulmonary hypertension in the cardiac catheterization laboratory. *Anesthesiol Clin* 2014; **23**: 157–73.

Pulmonary Hypertension and Prematurity

Sheila M. Rajashekara and Chandra Ramamoorthy

Case Scenario

A former 30-week preterm male, birth weight 1500 grams, presents at 40 weeks postconceptual age for a tracheostomy and laparoscopic Nissen fundoplication with gastrostomy tube placement. His history includes bronchopulmonary dysplasia, pulmonary hypertension, an unrepaired atrial septal defect, and failure to thrive. After delivery, he initially required continuous positive airway pressure and was ultimately intubated due to persistent oxygen desaturations below 85%.
A transthoracic echocardiogram revealed a small atrial septal defect, no ventricular septal defect, a dilated right ventricle, and normal biventricular function. Repeat echocardiogram at 7 days of life showed the development of interventricular septal flattening. Inhaled nitric oxide was initiated at 20 parts per million with an increase in SpO_2 to >92%.

Although now successfully weaned from nitric oxide and transitioned to sildenafil, he has failed multiple extubation attempts and is again experiencing frequent severe desaturation events. Current ventilator settings are peak inspiratory pressure 30 mm Hg, positive end-expiratory pressure 8 mm Hg, and FiO_2 0.4 to maintain acceptable tidal volumes and oxygen saturations. He has had poor weight gain with intolerance to increasing nasogastric feeds. His mother has also requested that he be circumcised.

Current vital signs are heart rate 164 beats/minute, respiratory rate 60 breaths/minute, noninvasive blood pressure 70/36 (mean 48), temperature 36.4°C, and SpO_2 93%.

Key Objectives

- Define pulmonary hypertension of prematurity and describe its pathophysiology.
- Describe the significance of the atrial septal defect in this patient.
- Discuss the combined effects of premature lung disease and pulmonary hypertension.
- Discuss anesthetic risk in this patient.
- Describe a perioperative plan including appropriate monitoring.
- Discuss management of a pulmonary hypertensive crisis.

Pathophysiology

How is pulmonary hypertension defined in preterm infants?

According to the 2018 Paediatric Task Force of the 6th World Symposium on Pulmonary Hypertension, pulmonary hypertension (PH) in preterm infants is defined by the same guidelines used for adults and children: mean pulmonary arterial pressure (mPAP) ≥20 mm Hg, pulmonary capillary wedge pressure (PCWP) <15 mm Hg, and pulmonary vascular resistance indexed to body surface area >3 Wood units/m^2 (iWu). Normal mPAP is 15 mm Hg.

What is bronchopulmonary dysplasia?

Bronchopulmonary dysplasia (BPD), the major cause of chronic lung disease in preterm infants, is defined as an ongoing supplemental oxygen requirement at 36 weeks postconceptual age in infants born at or prior to 32 weeks' gestation. It is most common in infants born prior to 28 weeks' gestation and <1000 grams at birth. Bronchopulmonary dysplasia results from a disruption of lung development at an early preterm age due to decreased surfactant supply and/or function, abnormal alveolar growth, and/or abnormal pulmonary vasculature. It is exacerbated by the need for mechanical respiratory support, supplemental oxygen administration, and fluid shifts. Although giving betamethasone to the mother can help reduce the incidence of acute respiratory issues, it has no effect on the development of BPD.

How is PH associated with BPD?

The disruption of growth and function of the pulmonary vasculature observed with BPD contributes to the failure of pulmonary artery pressures to decrease normally in the first few months of life. Abnormal pulmonary vasculature leads to a chronic elevation in mPAP and pulmonary vascular resistance (PVR) and over time the arteries become muscularized, hypertonic, and reactive. These alterations impede blood flow through the lungs and worsen hypoxemia, as fewer adequate blood vessels are available to participate in gas exchange. Additional mechanisms associated with persistent PH in the infant with BPD include oxygen toxicity, barotrauma, alveolar hypoxia, cardiac dysfunction, and pulmonary vein stenosis. As many as 20%–40% of patients with BPD have significant PH. The combination is accompanied by significant morbidity and mortality.

Clinical Pearl

The disruption of growth and function of the pulmonary vasculature observed with BPD contributes to the failure of pulmonary artery pressures to decrease normally in the first few months of life. As many as 20%–40% of patients with BPD will have PH. The combination is accompanied by significant morbidity and mortality.

What risk factors are associated with the presence of PH in an infant with BPD?

Risk factors associated with the presence of PH in an infant with BPD include extreme prematurity, birth weight <1500 grams, and respiratory factors including prolonged mechanical ventilation and prolonged oxygen therapy. Cardiovascular abnormalities, oligohydramnios, maternal preeclampsia, and intrauterine growth retardation are also risk factors, as are maternal infection and genetic abnormalities.

What screening is recommended in preterm infants with BPD and PH?

Early identification of PH in infants with BPD serves to improve patient management. Screening for PH with transthoracic echocardiography (TTE) is recommended in symptomatic patients or those with identified risk factors for PH. Patients with BPD can often show signs of PH on TTE as early as 7 days of life. If not previously performed, TTE is recommended at the time BPD is formally diagnosed. It is especially important to screen high-risk infants if they require general anesthesia, as PH is associated with an increased risk of adverse events under anesthesia.

Transthoracic echocardiography is recommended at least every 3 months for infants with BPD. However, if the infant maintains a persistent supplemental oxygen requirement or continues to display signs of respiratory distress such as increased work of breathing, more frequent examinations are indicated.

Laboratory values such as brain natriuretic peptide (BNP) or N-terminal pro-BNP (NT-proBNP) are not sufficient to formally diagnose or exclude PH; however, serial measurements may be used to observe trends which are helpful in assessing a patient's clinical status or response to treatment.

Clinical Pearl

Transthoracic echocardiography is recommended at least every 3 months for infants with BPD.

What information does TTE provide?

Transthoracic echocardiography has the advantage of being noninvasive and can evaluate alterations in the cardiac and pulmonary anatomy and pressures to diagnose or monitor PH. Depending on the quality of the TTE data, the following findings may be observed and monitored:

- Estimated right ventricular systolic pressure >40 mm Hg or mPAP >20 mm Hg
- Right ventricular: systemic systolic blood pressure ratio >0.5
- Intracardiac shunting with bidirectional or right-to-left flow
- Assessment of septal wall flattening

Assuming no RV outflow tract obstruction exists, the systolic PAP and right ventricular (RV) pressures can be estimated using tricuspid regurgitant jet velocity. If imaging results are nonconclusive, it can be difficult to determine if the etiology of persistent oxygen requirement is due to BPD, PH, or a combination of factors. If suspicion exists for undefined disease, providers may choose to utilize cardiac catheterization to assess hemodynamic values and the need for vasodilator therapy such as inhaled nitric oxide (iNO) or selective phosphodiesterase type 5 inhibitors such as sildenafil.

What cardiac catheterization findings signify the presence of PH?

Cardiac catheterization is the gold standard for diagnosis of PH but is less frequently performed in this patient population due to the patient's fragility and the need for general endotracheal anesthesia. For this reason, many providers choose to empirically treat preterm infants with iNO and/or oral vasodilators such as sildenafil and to assess treatments with serial TTE.

Cardiac catheterization findings indicating the presence of PH include

- PA systolic: systemic systolic blood pressure ratio ≥ 0.5
- PVR ≥ 3 iWu
- PVR: systemic vascular resistance (SVR) ratio ≥ 0.5
- Normal PCWP or normal LV end-diastolic pressure without significant evidence of pulmonary vein stenosis

Clinical Pearl

While cardiac catheterization procedures are the gold standard for diagnosis of PH, the majority of preterm infants are screened and diagnosed via noninvasive TTE. Clinical response to medical therapy is also monitored with serial TTE.

What are medical management goals in infants with BPD and PH?

The goals for management of PH in infants with BPD are focused on optimizing respiratory support to improve gas exchange, promoting blood flow to the pulmonary vasculature, minimizing further lung injury, and promoting growth of the lung parenchyma. This is accomplished with pulmonary vasodilators, supplemental oxygen, and conservative mechanical ventilation to avoid barotrauma.

Clinical Pearl

Medical management of PH in preterm infants utilizes pulmonary vasodilators such as iNO or sildenafil, supplemental oxygen, and optimizing respiratory support to avoid further lung injury and to promote gas exchange.

How does PH affect normal cardiac function? How do RV changes impact the LV?

Pulmonary hypertension causes increased RV afterload due to elevations in mPAP and PVR. Over time, increased afterload increases right ventricular end-diastolic volume (RVEDV) and right ventricular end-diastolic pressure (RVEDP) leading to RV hypertrophy. If untreated, RV dilation ensues. The morphologic RV changes secondary to increased RVEDV and RVEDP alter normal blood flow through the right coronary artery. In a normal heart the right coronary artery fills in systole and diastole; however, these pathologic changes impede flow, allowing filling only during diastole.

Elevated RV pressures can also displace the interventricular septum toward the LV, changing LV morphology.

This is often described on echocardiogram as "septal flattening" and results in impaired LV filling, decreased cardiac output and hypotension. These decreases in systemic pressures will further reduce coronary perfusion and risk complete cardiovascular collapse.

How does iNO affect the pulmonary vasculature?

Endogenous nitric oxide is produced by endothelial cells and released into the vascular system. Nitric oxide aids in the formation of cyclic guanosine monophosphate (cGMP), which allows smooth muscle relaxation in the pulmonary system. This relaxation allows PVR to decrease, potentially improving cardiac output and decreasing RV strain. Therefore, in patients with PH the addition of iNO may be therapeutic.

What is sildenafil and how does it help patients with PH? What side effects can occur with sildenafil?

Sildenafil is a selective cGMP phosphodiesterase inhibitor, thereby blocking the breakdown of cGMP. Cyclic guanosine monophosphate allows for the relaxation of smooth muscle, a primary component of the pulmonary vasculature. Relaxation of the pulmonary vasculature aids in reducing PH. Sildenafil should be continued without interruption throughout the perioperative period. Patients receiving sildenafil or iNO may develop hypotension from smooth muscle fiber relaxation, resulting in decreased brain, gastrointestinal, and renal perfusion.

What other medications are these patients frequently receiving?

Infants with BPD and/or PH also frequently suffer from gastroesophageal reflux and feeding intolerance. Increased airway reactivity may also result from gastroesophageal reflux and require medical treatment. Thus, medications such as ranitidine, omeprazole, furosemide, and albuterol are frequently administered as well.

How is the presence of a shunt significant in a patient with PH?

Intracardiac or systemic-to-pulmonary communications permitting left-to-right (L-to-R), right-to-left (R-to-L) or bidirectional intracardiac shunting are common in preterm infants and can include an atrial septal defect (ASD), patent foramen ovale, and/or persistent patent ductus arteriosus (PDA). A persistent L-to-R shunt leads to an increase in pulmonary blood flow (PBF), increasing the volume and pressure load to the vasculature. This results in increased shear stress, smooth muscle hypertrophy, and endothelial dysfunction which increase PVR and further worsen PH. As the RVEDP rises to equal RA pressures, the L-to-R shunt becomes bidirectional; it can eventually reverse to a R-to-L shunt through the ASD, increasing cyanosis. Most commonly the presence of a shunt means that with the abrupt rise of PVR blood can shunt bidirectionally, increasing cyanosis.

Clinical Pearl

The presence of a communication such as a patent foramen ovale, ASD, or PDA means that with an abrupt increase in PVR patients may shunt bidirectionally or R-to-L, maintaining cardiac output but increasing cyanosis.

Anesthetic Implications

What are the preanesthetic considerations for infants with BPD and PH?

The preoperative evaluation of infants with BPD and PH should include a thorough review of their current clinical status, including physical examination, medications, and clinical studies.

The gestational age at birth as well as the current post-gestational age are important factors for risk stratification. Preterm infants frequently experience multisystem organ disturbances beyond the cardiac and pulmonary systems. These include the inability to regulate body temperature, an immature central nervous system contributing to apneic spells, a predisposition to or a history of intraventricular hemorrhage (IVH), anemia, electrolyte imbalances, and retinopathy of prematurity. The preoperative examination should include ongoing measures to address these concerns in a systematic fashion.

Temperature: Heat is lost by radiation, conduction, convection, and evaporation. Patient temperature should be continually monitored and maintained above 36.5°C. Hypothermia can promote pulmonary vasoconstriction and worsen PH. Perioperative interventions can include the use of thin plastic wrap, utilizing a hat to reduce cranial heat loss, and forced air warming through warm air blankets and/or heat lamps.

Neurologic:

- *Central nervous system immaturity*: Predisposition to apneic spells can lead to bradycardia and desaturation

events requiring intervention. In patients not already dependent on mechanical ventilation this may indicate a need for postoperative mechanical ventilation.
- *Intraventricular hemorrhage*: Patients with various grades of IVH may have a seizure history requiring antiepileptics to be continued perioperatively. If anticoagulant medications are to be given during the procedure, a discussion about potential risks and benefits should occur with the medical teams and disclosed to the family.

Cardiac: Evaluation for the presence or absence of additional congenital heart disease should include an electrocardiogram and echocardiogram in addition to clinical examination. Coexisting congenital heart disease may worsen or even be the primary cause of PH in this patient.

Retinopathy of prematurity (ROP): A large percentage of preterm infants are at risk to develop ROP. While ROP is a concern in preterm infants, the risk: benefit ratio of supplemental oxygen administration must be considered and inspired oxygen concentration titrated to maintain adequate oxygen saturations.

Respiratory: The extent of respiratory support required (either via nasal cannula, continuous positive airway pressure, or endotracheal intubation) parallels disease severity. Oxygen flow and concentration, peak inspiratory pressure (PIP), inspiratory time, respiratory rate, tidal volume, and positive end-expiratory pressure (PEEP) should be evaluated to determine the optimal intraoperative ventilation management and respiratory support strategies. Intraoperative use of a neonatal intensive care unit (NICU) ventilator should be considered when an infant requires high levels of PEEP or maintains very low tidal volumes with increased PIP, and/or additional concerns exist about adequate ventilation. The goal is to maintain and optimize adequate ventilation and oxygenation. Insufficient ventilation leads to hypercarbia and will worsen PH. Respiratory therapies such as albuterol, sildenafil, and iNO should be continued perioperatively.

Hematologic: Neonates are frequently anemic due to decreased production of red blood cells and frequent blood draws. Determination of limits for allowable blood loss and appropriate transfusion thresholds allows optimization of oxygen delivery in patients with cardiorespiratory illnesses. Target hemoglobin levels may vary between patients with varied comorbidities but maintenance of hemoglobin levels above 9–10 g/dL is recommended.

Glucose: In preterm infants the liver is still developing; therefore, gluconeogenesis is not always sufficient. Thus, once fasting prior to surgery, infants should receive dextrose-containing maintenance fluids. Recent blood glucose levels and fluctuations in glucose levels should be accounted for and appropriately monitored. Hypoglycemia has significant neurologic affects that may adversely affect preterm infants. Alternatively, high serum glucose concentrations can lead to an osmotic diuresis and hypovolemia.

Vascular access: Vascular access should be adequate to appropriately manage PH and BPD perioperatively. The location and adequacy of peripheral intravenous (IV) access should be evaluated, along with the possible presence of a peripherally inserted central catheter (PICC). Patients with severe disease may benefit from central access in the event of cardiovascular compromise requiring intraoperative resuscitation.

Is anesthesia risk greater in patients with PH? What risks should be discussed with the family?

It is well documented that the presence of PH increases anesthetic risk and the risk of perioperative complications. The risk varies between patients and will correlate with individual disease severity. Patients with PH who are <2 years of age typically have the greatest anesthetic risk. Anesthetic risk increases as PA pressure becomes greater than half systemic pressure and is highest when PA pressure is suprasystemic. For patients with significant PH the potential role of extracorporeal membrane oxygenation (ECMO) rescue should be addressed in the preoperative assessment with the family and medical teams.

Clinical Pearl

Pulmonary hypertension is associated with an increased risk of adverse events under general anesthesia – especially for patients <2 years of age who have PA pressure greater than one-half systemic blood pressure.

Can all procedures be done safely at this time, and is there a suggested order?

The urgency and appropriate timing for each procedure should be considered for preterm infants, particularly in infants with PH. The patient's responsiveness to vasodilator therapies aids in presurgical planning, and continual reassessment of hemodynamic stability intraoperatively will help guide any necessary changes to the intraoperative plan. Clear communication between all surgical teams is essential to clarify parameters for successful completion of all procedures.

Laparoscopic Nissen procedures involve surgical conditions that may be disruptive to a fresh tracheostomy site. Therefore, if adequate ventilation can be maintained it may be best to proceed with the abdominal procedures prior to the tracheostomy. Alternately, significant issues with ventilation could increase the urgency of the tracheostomy and preclude performing the fundoplication during the same anesthetic.

Circumcision should be the last procedure performed providing the patient's cardiorespiratory status is stable. These expectations must be addressed with the parents and medical team in the preoperative period as ultimately patient safety should dictate the ability to proceed with all three procedures. The risk of increased anesthetic duration should be balanced against the risk of necessitating another general anesthetic in the future.

Are additional studies indicated prior to anesthetizing this patient?

As the last echocardiogram on this patient was performed at 1 week of age it is important to obtain an updated TTE to evaluate this infant's current cardiac status – specifically, the degree of PH and assessment of the therapeutic effect of the current medication regimen. If the patient's current cardiac condition has worsened, it would be reasonable to delay nonurgent procedures in order to optimize therapies for his PH. Additionally, other diagnostic or therapeutic interventions such as cardiac catheterization or PDA closure may be considered if PH has worsened in the interim.

What intraoperative monitoring and access should be considered?

Standard recommended American Society of Anesthesiologists monitoring should be utilized in addition to any additional monitoring indicated by the patient's cardiac disease and functional status. A 5-lead electrocardiogram is preferred to monitor for cardiac arrhythmias and ischemia, although in a small infant with multiple procedures leads will need to be carefully placed away from surgical areas. The need for additional vascular access and monitoring will depend on the size and scope of surgery, anticipated blood loss, fluid shifts, and degree of potential cardiac complications. Placement of an arterial line should be considered to allow for close monitoring of both hemodynamic and respiratory status if RV function is significantly compromised or risk of decompensation is anticipated.

The necessity of central access is dictated by the severity of PH and BPD. Often a PICC is present in this patient population. If present, a chest radiograph should be reviewed to evaluate location of the catheter tip as lines are not always centrally located. Even with a PICC line, a peripheral IV line should be placed if possible, particularly if the PICC line is a single lumen line. Although useful for administration of medications PICC lines are generally not as helpful should administration of blood or fluid boluses be necessary.

Is an uncuffed endotracheal tube acceptable? Should it be exchanged for a cuffed tube?

The presence of an uncuffed endotracheal (ETT) may contribute to difficulty ventilating during a laparoscopic procedure if a significant leak exists. This should be assessed prior to beginning the procedure. Previous documentation should be carefully reviewed for any issues with mask ventilation and recent ease of intubation, including the view on direct laryngoscopy. Options include exchanging the uncuffed ETT for a cuffed ETT or proceeding with the scheduled tracheostomy and rescheduling the laparoscopic Nissen fundoplication after appropriate recovery. Even if endotracheal intubation was previously easily accomplished, exchange of an ETT in a neonate with PH who requires significant ventilatory support carries significant risks even in experienced hands. Rapid desaturation and decruitment with loss of PEEP can at best require time to recover to baseline, and at worst can precipitate a PH crisis. Endotracheal tube position can also migrate as a result of insufflation. Through the insufflation process, frequent adjustments to inspired oxygen concentrations and minute ventilation may be required to prevent increases in end-tidal carbon dioxide ($ETCO_2$) levels or acidosis.

Clinical Pearl

Even if intubation was previously easily accomplished, exchange of an ETT in a neonate with PH who requires significant ventilatory support carries significant risks even in experienced hands. Rapid desaturation and decruitment with loss of PEEP can at best require time to recover to baseline, and at worst can precipitate a PH crisis.

What considerations exist for ventilation of this patient intraoperatively?

Depending on the capabilities of the anesthesia ventilator, consideration may be given to utilizing the NICU ventilator during surgery. This is particularly relevant in patients requiring a high level of ventilatory support when multiple procedures are being performed and the anticipated operating room time may be prolonged. Regardless of whether the anesthesia ventilator or the NICU ventilator is utilized iNO should be available for use if needed during the procedure.

How should anesthetic induction and maintenance be managed?

Performing a safe anesthetic induction in a patient with PH involves minimizing changes in SVR and PVR while ensuring adequate ventilation. Patients with PH are at risk for rapid hemodynamic decompensation on induction of anesthesia due to these effects. Slow titration of IV medications is preferred in preterm infants with PH with the addition of inhaled anesthetics as tolerated within desired hemodynamic parameters. Rescue medications (atropine, epinephrine, and phenylephrine) should be readily available prior to induction of anesthesia in the event of cardiovascular collapse.

Maintenance of general anesthesia can be continued with a balanced technique utilizing narcotics and inhaled anesthetics, with the goal of maintaining adequate analgesia and anesthesia to blunt the surgical stress response and avoid abrupt increases in PVR. As the patient will remain mechanically ventilated postoperatively opioids may form a significant part of the anesthetic plan to blunt stress responses. It is helpful to know the degree of exposure the patient has previously had to sedative and opioid regimens, as some neonates may require higher opioid dosing than expected to achieve the desired level of anesthesia due to prolonged preoperative exposure.

Factors that can negatively impact PVR such as hypoxia, hypercarbia, hypothermia, and acidosis should be avoided. Abrupt increases in PVR can reverse the shunt across the ASD, creating a R-to-L shunt and resulting in a drop in the systemic arterial oxygen saturation. Optimizing PVR via increased inspired oxygen concentration and initiation of iNO will facilitate L-to-R shunt flow and encourage PBF, enhancing cardiac output and coronary perfusion.

Clinical Pearl

It is helpful to know the degree of exposure the patient has previously had to sedative and opioid regimens as some neonates may require higher dosing ranges than expected to achieve the desired level of anesthesia.

What are the potential issues with a laparoscopic surgical approach?

Laparoscopic Nissen and gastrostomy tube (g-tube) procedures involve the imposition of surgical conditions that may not be well tolerated in small infants, particularly those with PH and BPD. Abdominal insufflation during laparoscopy and g-tube placement often significantly compromises ventilation.

This reduction in ventilation combined with insufflation of CO_2 leads to an increase in $ETCO_2$, thus necessitating a significant increase in ventilatory requirements. Prior to the start of surgery, laparoscopic surgical planning should be discussed. Utilization of the lowest acceptable intraabdominal insufflation pressure is recommended. A contingency plan should also be discussed should the patient fail to tolerate insufflation with consideration for expeditious conversion to an open surgical approach. (See Chapter 26 for discussion of laparoscopic surgery in an infant.)

Shortly after abdominal insufflation begins oxygen saturations drop to the mid-70s: what are the considerations?

Should gradual desaturation occur following insufflation, consideration should be given to manipulating ventilatory settings and decreasing insufflation pressures. With rapid desaturation the differential should also include secretions or a plug in the endotracheal tube, an endobronchial intubation, or the onset of a PH crisis. It is imperative to communicate openly with the surgical team for appropriate patient management and to stop surgical manipulation until the patient returns to his baseline oxygen saturations.

What is a pulmonary hypertensive crisis?

A pulmonary hypertensive crisis is an abrupt increase in PVR resulting in acute right heart failure and inadequate cardiac output.

A PH crisis is defined as two or more of the following changes in <10 minutes:

- Decrease in systolic blood pressure >20% from baseline
- Decrease in oxygen saturation to <90% in acyanotic patients and decline >10% in cyanotic patients in the absence of other causes
- Increase in central venous pressure >20% from baseline
- Change in baseline heart rate < or >20%

During a PH crisis hypotension develops due to impaired preload along with decreases in coronary blood flow and cardiac output. If the PH crisis is not treated expeditiously, bradycardia develops and can progress to cardiac arrest. Bradycardia can also be an ominous early sign accompanying or preceding oxygen desaturation. The goal of PH crisis management is to decrease PVR and increase SVR such that LV output and coronary perfusion are maintained.

Clinical Pearl

A pulmonary hypertensive crisis is an abrupt increase in PVR causing acute right heart failure and inadequate cardiac output; it may precipitate cardiovascular collapse.

How is a pulmonary hypertensive crisis treated?

Management of a PH crisis involves reducing RV afterload and increasing SVR expeditiously.

Although the following steps can be performed in the order listed, it is optimal to perform all actions in an expeditious fashion. (See also Chapter 40, Table 40.2.)

- **Respiratory interventions**
  - Increase FiO_2 to 100%
  - Increase minute ventilation
  - Avoid excessive PEEP, high inspiratory pressures and long inspiratory times
  - Initiation of iNO
- **Hemodynamic interventions**
  - Ensure adequate preload and inotropic support for LV
  - Maintenance of SVR to ensure coronary perfusion
  - Sedation or anesthetic strategies: consider neuromuscular blockade for intubated and mechanically ventilated patients
  - Correction of metabolic acidosis
- ***Early ECMO activation if the patient is a candidate***

Vasoactive drugs commonly used in the management of a PH crisis include epinephrine, vasopressin, and phenylephrine. Epinephrine helps maintain or enhance RV function, while vasopressin and phenylephrine help maintain diastolic pressures to allow adequate RV perfusion.

Clinical Pearl

Successful management of a PH crisis includes early recognition and treatment including oxygen, increased minute ventilation, iNO, and vasoactive medications (epinephrine, vasopressin, and phenylephrine), along with correction of any acidosis.

What are the postoperative considerations for this patient?

Anesthetic related risks for patients with PH continue postoperatively. It is imperative to maintain adequate pain control as well as appropriate ventilation and oxygenation to avoid acute elevations in mPAP and PVR following the procedure. Close monitoring is recommended so that adverse events may be averted, and in this case the patient would recover in the NICU.

Suggested Reading

Abman S. H., Hansmann G., Archer S. L., et al. Pediatric pulmonary hypertension: guidelines from the American Heart Association and American Thoracic Society. *Circulation* 2015; **132**: 2037–99.

Altit G., Dancea A., Renaud C., et al. Pathophysiology, screening and diagnosis of pulmonary hypertension in infants with bronchopulmonary dysplasia – a review of the literature. *Paediatr Respir Rev* 2017; **23**: 16–26.

Berkelhamer S. K., Mestan K. K., and Steinhorn R. An update on the diagnosis and management of bronchopulmonary dysplasia (BPD)-associated pulmonary hypertension. *Semin Perinatol* 2018; **42**: 432–43.

Bernier M. L., Jacob A. I., Collaco J. M., et al. Perioperative events in children with pulmonary hypertension undergoing non-cardiac procedures. *Pulm Circ* 2018; **8**: 2045893217738143. DOI: 10.1177/2045893217738143.

Hilgendorff A., Apitz C., Bonnet D., et al. Pulmonary hypertension associated with acute or chronic lung disease in the preterm and term neonate and infant. The European Paediatric Pulmonary Vascular Disease Network, endorsed by ISHLT and DGPK. *Heart* 2016; **102**: ii49–ii56.

Krishnan U., Feinstein J. A., Adatia I., et al. Evaluation and management of pulmonary hypertension in children with bronchopulmonary dysplasia. *J Pediatr* 2017; **188**: 24–34.e1.

Latham G. J. and Yung D. Current understanding and perioperative management of pediatric pulmonary hypertension. *Pediatr Anesth* 2019; **29**: 441–56. DOI: 10.1111/pan.13542.

O'Connor M. G., Cornfield D. N., and Austin E. D. Pulmonary hypertension in the premature infant: a challenging co-morbidity in a vulnerable population. *Curr Opin Pediatr* 2016; **28**: 324–30.

O'Connor M. G., Suther D., Vera K., et al. Pulmonary hypertension in the premature infant population: analysis of echocardiographic findings and biomarkers. *Pediatr Pulmonol* 2018; **53**: 302–309. DOI: 10.1002/ppul.23913.

Chapter 43

Pulmonary Hypertension and Moyamoya Disease

Timothy D. Switzer and Neil M. Goldenberg

Case Scenario

A 12-year-old boy with a history of moyamoya disease presents for surveillance brain magnetic resonance imaging. Transthoracic echocardiography at age 3 years revealed mild to moderate aortic coarctation for which he underwent balloon dilation with minimal improvement due to the stiffness of his aorta. At age 9 years he underwent cerebral revascularization surgery (temporal artery bypass) to address his moyamoya disease. Right and left heart catheterization at age 10 years demonstrated severe pulmonary hypertension with an initial pulmonary vascular resistance of 10.2 indexed Wood units; at that time, balloon dilation of his patent foramen ovale was performed. He is now taking tadalafil, ambrisentan, and treprostinil for his pulmonary hypertension. He also takes atenolol for systemic hypertension and uses nasal prong oxygen at 0.5–1 L/minute for hemoglobin–oxygen desaturations to the 80s noted during a 6-minute walk test.

Recent cardiac catheterization demonstrated the following:

- *Pulmonary vascular resistance of 6.1 indexed Wood units*
- *Right ventricular systolic pressure that is 60% systemic*

Key Objectives

- Describe the pathophysiology and treatment of moyamoya disease.
- Describe classification systems for pulmonary hypertension.
- Outline anesthetic management goals for patients with moyamoya disease.
- Describe medical therapy for pulmonary hypertension and potential anesthetic interactions.
- Outline anesthetic management options for patients with cerebrovascular disease and pulmonary hypertension.

Pathophysiology

What is moyamoya disease?

Moyamoya disease is a cerebrovasculopathy of unknown etiology characterized by chronic progressive stenosis of the arteries of the circle of Willis. An extensive collateralized circulation forms, giving rise to the smoky appearance seen on cerebral angiography (moyamoya is Japanese for "puff of smoke"). Primary clinical features of moyamoya disease, especially in children, are related to cerebral ischemia and include transient ischemic attacks and stroke. However, hemorrhagic strokes and seizures have also been described. Hyperventilation, crying, exercise, or fever can all trigger symptomatic ischemia in children.

> **Clinical Pearl**
>
> *Hyperventilation, crying, exercise, or fever can all trigger symptomatic ischemia in children with moyamoya disease.*

What other conditions are associated with moyamoya disease?

The characteristic angiographic appearance seen in moyamoya disease has also been described in other medical conditions, giving rise to the distinction between moyamoya disease and moyamoya syndrome, with the syndrome being associated with other medical conditions. These medical conditions may include chromosomal abnormalities (Down syndrome), neurocutaneous diseases (neurofibromatosis), connective tissue diseases (pseudoxanthoma elasticum), and extracranial vasculopathies.

How is moyamoya disease diagnosed?

Neuroradiology studies are the cornerstone of diagnosis for moyamoya disease. Commonly utilized imaging modalities include head computed tomography with angiography (CT, CTA), digital subtraction angiography, and magnetic resonance angiography (MRA). Although CT can show gross ischemic events, magnetic resonance imaging (MRI) is superior for the detection of smaller lesions. Noninvasive studies including magnetic resonance angiography and CTA can demonstrate the vascular abnormalities. Invasive cerebral angiography remains the gold standard in the diagnosis of the disease but is performed less frequently than either MRA or CTA.

The radiographic severity of moyamoya disease is graded on the Suzuki scale between 1 (least severe) and 6 (most severe), with grading based on the angiographic progression of the disease. Disease progression occurs in a proximal to distal manner with the internal carotid arteries affected first, leading to the eventual involvement of all cerebral arteries.

What is the effect of moyamoya disease on cerebral autoregulation?

The blood pressure limits of cerebral autoregulation in children are not known, but moyamoya has an impact on this autoregulation. A steal phenomenon may occur, leading to hypoperfusion of the areas most affected by moyamoya, as they are operating at full vasodilation and therefore dilation of other cerebral vessels will lead to decreased flow in these stenotic vessels.

What are the treatment options for moyamoya?

The goal of treatment is primarily to restore blood flow to the affected areas, either by direct or indirect bypass. There is no curative treatment for moyamoya disease. Direct bypass involves grafting of the superficial temporal artery to the middle cerebral or middle meningeal arteries (external carotid-to-internal carotid bypass). However, these procedures are technically difficult in children due to the small caliber of the vessels in this population. The indirect bypass method aims to promote the formation of a new vascular network over time by the placement of rich vascular tissue on the surface of the brain. Several procedures have been described, including encephaloduroarteriosynangiosis, encephalomyosynangiosis, and omental-cerebral transplantation. While outcomes are comparable with both direct and indirect revascularization techniques, it must be remembered that those who have had direct revascularization have an immediate postoperative improvement in cerebral blood flow (CBF), whereas those who have received indirect revascularization are dependent on angiogenesis and thus remain at risk for ischemia in the immediate postoperative period.

What is the underlying cardiac pathology in this patient?

The underlying cardiac pathology consists of a failed coarctation dilation with a residual aortic gradient. A patent foramen ovale (PFO) has also been ballooned and therefore in the setting of pulmonary hypertension (PH) the potential exists for bidirectional shunting across the PFO. Depending on the physiologic condition of the patient, flow across the PFO will be determined by the degree of PH, as the residual coarctation is a fixed afterload on the left ventricle (LV), unless acute LV failure occurs. The most recent investigations indicate that the right ventricular (RV) pressure is 60% that of the systemic arterial pressure. A right-to-left (R-to-L) shunt at the atrial level can result in a decrease in oxygen saturations, depending on the volume of blood being shunted. (See Figure 43.1.)

What are the implications of the failed coarctation repair in this patient?

The residual gradient after the unsuccessful balloon dilation of the aortic coarctation means that there is a hemodynamically significant persistence of fixed obstruction to flow in the

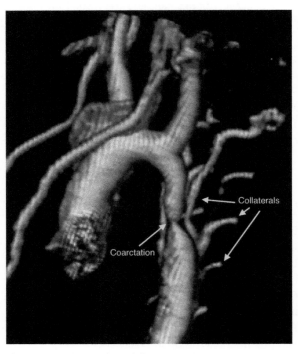

Figure 43.1 Coarctation of the aorta. 3D magnetic resonance imaging of juxtaductal coarctation of the aorta. There are multiple collaterals from the head and neck vessels that flow toward the descending aorta and effectively bypass the aortic narrowing. Courtesy of Michael Taylor, MD.

proximal descending aorta. There are several implications to this obstruction. The fixed increase in afterload may lead to LV hypertrophy and a subsequent increase in LV pressures, which will lead to increased myocardial workload, thus increasing myocardial oxygen demand. It will also lead to eventual diastolic dysfunction and altered lusitropy.

The rise in LV pressure will also be transmitted to the left atrium (LA), leading to two potential issues given the patient's intracardiac anatomy. First, an increase in LA pressure can act as an impediment to pulmonary blood flow, thus increasing the pulmonary arterial pressure. The second potential issue relates to the presence of the previously ballooned PFO. A rise in LA pressure may lead to an increased left-to-right (L-to-R) shunt across the PFO, which can contribute to RV volume overload and increased RV pressure. These factors increase myocardial workload and place the patient at risk for inadequate coronary perfusion.

The position of the residual aortic coarctation implies that the patient's cerebral vasculature has been exposed to relatively high perfusion pressures for a prolonged period of time. A blood pressure surge due to sympathetic activity, as might occur during laryngoscopy, has the potential to precipitate an intracerebral hemorrhage. It also means that the cerebral autoregulation limits for this child are likely to be higher than those for a similarly aged child without a coarctation, and therefore any decrease in blood pressure has the potential to compromise cerebral perfusion.

What are possible explanations for his intermittent desaturations?

Potential causes for this patient's desaturations during the 6-minute walk test include one or a combination of the following:

- Decreased diffusion capacity
- Ventilation-perfusion mismatch
- Decreased cardiac output (CO)
- The presence of intrapulmonary shunts

This patient has a known intracardiac shunt with the potential for R-to-L shunting.

How is pulmonary hypertension classified in children?

Pulmonary hypertension was first classified by the World Health Organization (WHO) in 1973 and this system has evolved over the years; it currently includes five groups. The aim of this classification system is to better understand the differing etiologies of each group and the natural history of the disease. However, it was recognized that the WHO classification system had some deficits when applied to the pediatric population given the significant developmental contribution to the disease. A consensus conference held in Panama in 2011 developed a new classification system for pediatric PH. (See Table 43.1.)

In this case the etiology of the PH is unclear but is most likely multifactorial.

Clinical Pearl

Understanding the etiology of PH is a critical step toward both risk stratification and appropriate acute and long-term management. Such understanding necessitates a multidisciplinary team, and investigations including imaging, invasive hemodynamic testing, and functional testing.

How is pulmonary hypertension graded?

There are several scales by which PH can be graded. The WHO uses a functional scale based on the level of physical activity that the patient can tolerate and is analogous to the New York Heart Association scale for heart failure. The consensus meeting in Panama also produced a functional classification of pediatric PH based on five different age groups: 0–0.5 years, 0.5–1 years, 1–2 years, 2–5 years, and 5–16 years. These provide child-specific measures of function such as play and school attendance. There is also a scale based on echocardiography and catheterization data that determines a patient's risk status depending on cardiac chamber size, ventricular function, measurement of pulmonary artery, and RA pressures and systemic venous saturations.

Table 43.1 Pulmonary Hypertension Classifications

WHO classification	Panama classification
1. Pulmonary arterial hypertension	1. Prenatal or developmental pulmonary hypertension
2. Pulmonary hypertension due to left heart disease	2. Perinatal vascular maladaptation (persistent pulmonary hypertension of the newborn)
3. Pulmonary hypertension due to lung disease	3. Pulmonary hypertension associated with congenital heart disease
4. Pulmonary hypertension due to thromboembolic disease	4. Bronchopulmonary dysplasia
5. Pulmonary hypertension associated with systemic disease/unclear etiology	5. Isolated pediatric pulmonary arterial hypertension
	6. Multifactorial in congenital malformation syndromes
	7. Pediatric lung disease
	8. Pediatric thromboembolic disease
	9. Hypobaric hypoxic exposure
	10. Pulmonary vascular disease associated with other disorders

What is the purpose of a right heart catheterization and what information should be sought?

The American Heart Association and American Thoracic Society have guidelines regarding the management of pediatric PH, including the performance and timing of cardiac catheterization. Right heart catheterization should include acute vasoreactivity testing (AVT), with a positive response defined as a 20% or greater decrease in pulmonary vascular resistance (PVR) without a decrease in CO. It is also recommended that patients undergo serial catheterizations to assess progress of the disease. After a change in therapy catheterization should occur within 3 to 12 months. Timing after this should be based on clinical judgment.

This patient's recent catheterization gives us the following important information:

- Pulmonary vascular resistance has decreased from 10.2 indexed Wood units (iWu) to 6.1 iWu, indicating significant responsiveness to the triple therapy of tadalafil, ambrisentan, and treprostinil that was initiated.
- The patient continues to have significant PH, as RV systolic pressure is 60% of systemic systolic pressure.
- The patient is not on a long-term calcium channel blocker, indicating that he most likely does not have AVT-positive PH.

A right heart catheterization also usually includes a pulmonary capillary wedge pressure (PCWP) measurement. This is helpful in determining whether there is increased LA pressure (PCWP >15 mm Hg), indicative of LV failure. This is important in the setting of an uncorrected coarctation of the aorta. Lastly, catheterization provides information regarding the size and morphology of the patient's pulmonary arteries and veins. If pulmonary artery or pulmonary vein stenosis is identified, he may be

a candidate for surgical correction of any hypoplastic or stenotic portions of these vessels.

What are mechanisms of action and potential side effects of pulmonary hypertension medications?

The mechanisms of action and potential side effects of pulmonary hypertension medications are given in Table 43.2.

Clinical Pearl

Intraoperative administration of PH medications requires planning regarding intravenous access, special delivery equipment, and interactions with anesthesia, particularly the risks of systemic hypotension and acute discontinuation syndromes.

Anesthetic Implications

What other investigations should be considered prior to proceeding?

Investigations can be broadly divided into imaging, blood/serum tests and functional tests. A review of previous cerebral MRI exams may provide information regarding the patient's cerebral reactivity, along with any evidence of ischemic or hemorrhagic lesions. An electrocardiogram (ECG) should be performed to ensure that no arrhythmias are present. In this patient, LV remodeling may have led to muscular hypertrophy and decreased cavity size. This, in turn, will reduce the passive filling of the ventricle during diastole, increasing dependence on the atrial kick. Pulmonary hypertension may have led to RA dilation, thus increasing the risk of

Table 43.2 Pulmonary Hypertension Medications

Medication	Mechanism	Side Effects
Conventional Oxygen Diuretics Anticoagulation	Prevent hypoxemia/hypoxic pulmonary vasoconstriction Optimize preload for right heart failure Prevent thrombosis in low flow states and hypercoagulable patients	Nasal prongs can dry out the nasal mucosa Intravascular depletion Bleeding potential
PDE$_5$ inhibitors Sildenafil, tadalafil	Reduce breakdown of cGMP to potentiate nitric oxide signaling, causing pulmonary vasodilation and decreasing vascular remodeling	Flushing, nausea, headaches Systemic hypotension in combination with other vasodilators
Endothelin receptor antagonists Bosentan, ambrisentan	Block actions of ET-1, a potent endogenous pulmonary vasoconstrictor	Hepatotoxicity, fluid retention
Prostacyclin analogues Iloprost (inhaled) Treprostinil (oral/inhaled)	Pulmonary and systemic vasodilators	Inhibit platelet aggregation, hypotension, flushing, rebound syndrome if discontinued

atrial fibrillation. Atrial fibrillation may make the patient unstable from a cardiovascular perspective, but this may only become evident when increased CO is required. Brain natriuretic peptide (BNP) or N-terminal proBNP can be useful serologic markers for tracking progressive heart failure, but it is necessary to have baseline values for the results to truly be meaningful.

If the patient has not been investigated for obstructive sleep apnea, it is advisable to do so, as this is a potentially reversible contributor to PH. Pulmonary function tests can also help to rule out a pulmonary disorder as a contributor to PH.

Functional tests include a 6-minute walk test, which was performed in this patient. Other examples include cardiopulmonary exercise testing, which has been correlated with PH prognosis in adults, and a dobutamine stress echo.

> **Clinical Pearl**
>
> *This child must be completely optimized from a cardiorespiratory standpoint before undergoing his surveillance MRI. Involvement of his entire care team in the timing of this procedure is critical.*

What unique issues does MRI present for the anesthesiologist?

Caring for patients undergoing MRI provides a number of challenges for the anesthesiologist. Many children find it a loud and claustrophobic environment, often resulting in movement during the procedure, interfering with image quality. The presence of the magnetic fields also disallows the use of any equipment that contains >2% ferromagnetic components. This impacts both anesthesia delivery systems and the monitoring used to ensure patient safety during the case. Anesthesia machines must be MRI safe, syringe pumps must be placed in a Faraday shield, and any emergencies require the prompt removal of the patient from the MRI scanning room given that the majority of resuscitation equipment is ferromagnetic. Monitoring can also prove challenging as the magnetic fields can induce artifacts on the ECG. There have also been reports of the pulse oximetry probe causing burns. Specialized pulse oximeters, blood pressure cuffs, and ECG electrodes must be used, and all suffer from artifacts during periods of scanning. High-fidelity monitoring of ST segments on ECG can be near impossible at times.

Magnetic resonance suites are often remote from operating room suites, limiting the availability of help should an emergency occur. This may also limit availability of certain pieces of equipment should a patient become unstable – in this case the availability of inhaled nitric oxide should the patient develop a pulmonary hypertensive crisis.

> **Clinical Pearl**
>
> *High-risk anesthesia in a remote location necessitates careful planning to ensure adequate support and equipment are available for crisis management.*

What anesthetic techniques may be utilized for MRI?

A range of possibilities exist for providing patient comfort and ensuring lack of movement to facilitate MRI. The first involves physical therapies such as parental presence and distraction devices such as audiovisual equipment. At the other end of the spectrum is a full general anesthetic. The advantages of a general anesthetic include complete immobility, guaranteeing image quality, but this approach suffers from the disadvantages of administering anesthetic agents, the majority of which have effects on systemic, pulmonary, and CBF. (See Table 43.3.) Between these two options is sedation, which allows delivery of lower doses of anesthetic agents, but also has a reported failure rate of up to 20%.

Ventilation during the procedure is also of critical importance. The presence of PH favors the patient spontaneously breathing, as this will decrease RV afterload. However, the administration of anesthetic agents may lead to hypoventilation in these circumstances, leading to potential hypoxemia and hypercapnia, which may in turn impact both pulmonary and CBF. It may be advisable to insert an airway, either a laryngeal mask airway (LMA) or an endotracheal tube (ETT), in order to ensure appropriate respiratory support.

What are the anesthetic management goals for patients with moyamoya disease?

The primary anesthetic management goal in patients with moyamoya disease is to match oxygen delivery with oxygen consumption. This involves maintaining the cerebral blood flow/cerebral metabolic rate (CBF/CMRO$_2$) relationship. A two-pronged approach can be taken toward this goal.

- *Minimize the cerebral oxygen requirement/CMRO$_2$.* This requires achieving an adequate depth of anesthesia for any procedure the patient is undergoing, avoiding hyperthermia, maintaining euglycemia and treating any seizures.

335

Table 43.3 Effects of Anesthetic Agents on Pulmonary Vascular Resistance and Cerebral Perfusion

Agent	Pulmonary Vascular Resistance	Cerebral Perfusion
Propofol	Decreased inotropy, no effect on pulmonary vascular tone	Decreases CBF due to decreased inotropy and vasodilation, decreased $CMRO_2$, preserves matching
Opiates	No direct effect on pulmonary vascular tone	No effect on CBF or $CMRO_2$
Volatile anesthetic agents	Inhibit HPV, decreasing V/Q matching	Increase CBF due to vasodilation, decrease $CMRO_2$
Dexmedetomidine	Mixed data regarding effect on PVR	Decreased HR but in low doses rarely clinically significant
Ketamine	Little change in PVR	Increases CBF and $CMRO_2$
Benzodiazepines	No change but potential for hypoventilation	No change CBF, decrease $CMRO_2$

CBF, cerebral blood flow; $CMRO_2$, cerebral metabolic rate of oxygen; HPV, hypoxic pulmonary vasoconstriction; HR, heart rate; PVR, pulmonary vascular resistance; V/Q, ventilation/perfusion.

- ***Optimize cerebral blood flow and oxygen delivery.*** This involves the avoidance of hypoxemia and maintenance of the patient's normal awake blood pressure while anesthetized. Maintenance of normocarbia is also vital. There are multiple case reports of pediatric patients with moyamoya who developed neurologic symptoms secondary to crying and subsequent hypocarbia, leading to cerebral vasoconstriction. Conversely, an increase in carbon dioxide (CO_2) may lead to a steal phenomenon with vasodilation of vessels in unaffected areas leading to ischemia in areas primarily affected by moyamoya, as these are operating at full vasodilation.

Patients who have undergone an indirect bypass procedure remain at risk for ischemia in the immediate postoperative period, as improved blood flow is dependent upon angiogenesis. This may take weeks to months to occur and these patients must be treated as high-risk during this time period. As this child has had a direct anastomosis involving the temporal artery, he should have had an immediate improvement in CBF postoperatively.

Clinical Pearl

The primary anesthetic management goal in patients with moyamoya disease is to match oxygen delivery with oxygen consumption. Blood pressure should be maintained at the patient's baseline awake level and normocarbia should be maintained.

What considerations exist in a patient with comorbid PH and moyamoya disease?

The dynamic phases of general anesthesia are the highest risk periods for patients with PH due to the sympathetic surge, which can precipitate a PH crisis, and they are also critical times for patients with moyamoya disease. If the child is upset and crying, this may lead to hypocapnia and subsequent hypoperfusion of the cerebral areas affected by the disease. While premedication may mitigate this risk, care must also be taken to avoid either hypoventilation or subsequent hypoxemia and hypercapnia, as these in turn may precipitate a PH crisis or neurologic deficits. Preoxygenation and the use of short-acting opiates prior to laryngoscopy can also aid in the prevention of sympathetic surge.

A balanced anesthetic will also aid in maintaining the PVR to systemic vascular resistance (PVR/SVR) ratio, along with the $CBF/CMRO_2$ relationship. This balanced anesthetic can involve the use of either a total intravenous anesthetic technique or the use of volatile anesthetic agents. However, if volatile anesthetic agents are used, the minimum alveolar concentration should be kept at ≤1% in order to maintain flow-metabolic coupling. This should be augmented with multimodal analgesia, the constituents of which should be determined by the nature of the procedure.

It may be necessary to control ventilation, necessitating the insertion of an LMA or ETT, should hypoventilation occur or seem likely, in order to maintain normoxemia and normocapnia. Blood pressure may also require augmentation via the use of vasopressors, positive inotropes, or both, in order to maintain preanesthetic induction levels. This is important to ensure maintenance of CBF, as cerebral autoregulation is impaired.

If general anesthesia is utilized for a procedure, consideration should be given to neuromonitoring, which could be used to guide positioning, as well as respiratory and hemodynamic management. Decisions surrounding neuromonitoring should involve (1) institutional availability and (2) the patient's baseline neurologic status, considering the possible presence of transient neurologic symptoms when awake. Should neuromonitoring be considered for this procedure, *MRI compatibility of all equipment must be assured.*

What monitoring is required to ensure safe anesthesia?

Standard recommended American Society of Anesthesiologists monitoring should be utilized, as for any procedure involving sedation or anesthesia. These include ECG monitoring for rate, rhythm, and signs of ischemia. This can be complicated by the effect of the MRI on the ECG waveforms. Hemoglobin–oxygen saturation monitoring is required to ensure that the patient does not become hypoxemic during the procedure. End-tidal CO_2 monitoring is also necessary to ensure that either hypoventilation or apneic episodes are not occurring, as the anesthesiologist is often remote from the patient. Blood pressure monitoring is also necessary given the cardiovascular effects of the sedative and/or anesthetic agents that are commonly employed. This generally takes the form of noninvasive blood pressure cuff measurements. While an arterial line may be employed if circumstances require it, standard arterial monitoring equipment must be modified to ensure that the transducer remains outside the magnetic field.

What is the optimal postprocedural disposition for this patient?

Decisions regarding postprocedural disposition of the patient are dependent upon the patient, the anesthetic technique used, and the center or location in which the procedure is being performed. From a patient perspective, the procedure itself is nonstimulating and there should be no postprocedural pain. The type of anesthetic technique utilized will inform postprocedural decision-making. Only patients who received no sedative or anesthetic drugs (physical therapies only) can be discharged immediately after the procedure, whereas patients who received sedation and general anesthesia may require a prolonged stay in the post-anesthetic care unit before eventual discharge to the ward or home. Once the patient has fully recovered from the anesthetic, they may be suitable for same-day discharge if the facility's protocols regarding same-day discharge support this course of action. There should be a mechanism by which patients with these comorbidities can be assessed and, if necessary, admitted should they become unstable in the postprocedural phase. The post-discharge destination of the patient is of importance also, as the patient should be within 1 to2 hours of the hospital should he/she require readmission.

Suggested Reading

Abman S. H., Hansmann G., Archer S. L., et al. Pediatric pulmonary hypertension. *Circulation* 2015; **132**: 2037–99.

Appireddy R., Ranjan M., Durafourt B. A., et al. Surgery for moyamoya disease in children. *J Child Neurol* 2019; 088307381984485.

Arlachov Y. and Ganatra R. H. Sedation/anaesthesia in paediatric radiology. *Br J Radiol* 2012; **85**: e1018–31.

Del Cerro M. J., Abman S., Diaz G., et al. A consensus approach to the classification of pediatric pulmonary hypertensive vascular disease: Report from the PVRI Pediatric Taskforce, Panama 2011. *Pulm Circ* 2011; **1**: 286–98.

Lammers A. E., Adatia I., Del Cerro M. J., et al. Functional classification of pulmonary hypertension in children: Report from the PVRI Pediatric Taskforce, Panama 2011. *Pulm Circ* 2011; **1**: 280–5.

Pritts C. D. and Pearl R. G. Anesthesia for patients with pulmonary hypertension. *Curr Opin Anaesthesiol* 2010; **23**: 411–16.

Chapter 44

Vascular Ring

Katherine L. Zaleski

Case Scenario

A 14-month-old boy weighing 8 kg with a history of frequent upper respiratory tract infections and gastroesophageal reflux presented to his pediatrician for a well-child visit. He has not been gaining weight and his reflux seems to be worsening, with frequent postprandial fussiness and increasingly frequent vomiting noted by his parents, especially with solid foods. Although he has always been a noisy breather, his parents have recently noticed increased wheezing with exertion. His pediatrician suspected a vascular ring and ordered a chest radiograph that demonstrated a right-sided aortic arch. The patient was referred to a pediatric cardiologist who is now requesting a computed tomography scan for anatomic delineation and potential surgical planning. Due to his respiratory symptoms, direct laryngoscopy and rigid bronchoscopy are also planned and will be performed in the operating room. These procedures have been scheduled as a single anesthetic, with a transthoracic echocardiogram to be performed in the post-anesthesia care unit while the patient is still sleepy.

Key Objectives

- Understand the anatomic implications of a vascular ring and the most common types.
- Describe anesthetic induction and management strategies for a patient with an unrepaired vascular ring for computed tomography scan and bronchoscopy.
- Understand the surgical approach for repair of vascular rings.

Pathophysiology

What is a vascular ring and what are the anatomic implications?

A vascular ring is a congenital malformation of the aorta and its branch vessels in which the esophagus and/or tracheobronchial tree are either completely (***complete***

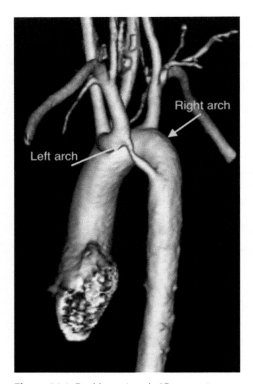

Figure 44.1 Double aortic arch. 3D magnetic resonance imaging of double aortic arch viewed from the left side. There is a dominant right arch and smaller left arch forming a vascular ring. The trachea and esophagus are contained within the ring. Courtesy of Michael Taylor, MD.

ring) or partially (***incomplete ring***) encircled by vascular structures and/or their atretic remnants, resulting in mechanical obstruction of these structures and resultant symptomatology. The term "vascular ring" was first used in 1945 when Robert E. Gross described the first successful surgical repair of a double aortic arch [1]. (See Figure 44.1.)

How commonly do vascular rings occur?

Vascular rings have a reported incidence of 1/1000 to 1/10,000 births, accounting for roughly 1%–3% of all congenital heart disease [2]. Because a large number of vascular rings are asymptomatic, it is likely that the actual prevalence is higher.

What are the most common types of vascular rings?

The most commonly diagnosed types of complete vascular rings are double aortic arch (DAA; 19%–60%) and right aortic arch (RAA) with aberrant left subclavian artery (LSCA)/ligamentum arteriosum (25%–79%), while the most commonly diagnosed types of partial vascular rings are left aortic arch (LAA) with aberrant right subclavian artery (RSCA) (16%–34%), pulmonary artery sling (2%–10%), and anomalous innominate artery (0.54%)[3–6]. The large variance in relative prevalence is reflective of the single-center nature of the published retrospective studies. To improve reporting, the Congenital Heart Surgery Nomenclature and Database Project has subclassified vascular rings as DAA, RAA/left ligamentum, pulmonary artery sling, and innominate compression since the overwhelming majority of vascular rings (>95%) are captured by this nomenclature system [7].

What is the underlying embryopathogenesis of a vascular ring?

The aorta begins to develop during the third week of gestation [7, 8] as blood passes from the endocardial tube through the aortic sac (distal truncus arteriosus) and into the paired dorsal aortae via a series of six paired aortic arches (pharyngeal arch arteries) that sequentially develop and regress in a cranial to caudal fashion [9]. As successive arches regress, portions of the first three are incorporated into the mature vascular structures of the head and neck (first – maxillary artery, second – stapedial and hyoid arteries, third – common and portion of internal carotid), while the fifth either regresses fully or doesn't form at all. The fourth and sixth arches contribute to the definitive aortic arch and the mediastinal segments of the pulmonary arteries as well as the ductus arteriosi, respectively [10]. Vascular rings result from abnormal segmental regression and/or persistence of portions of the embryonic aortic arch complex.

The normal morphology of the definitive aortic arch is left-sided, crossing the left mainstem bronchus at the level of the fifth thoracic vertebra and descending to the left of midline. In DAA, formation of two aortic arches (right and left) occurs due to the persistence of the distal right fourth arch. The rightward more cranially located arch is often dominant and the leftward arch is diminutive or atretic to a varying degree [4]. Each arch gives off their respective

common carotid and subclavian arteries. There is usually only one ductus arteriosus, generally located on the left side, and the descending aorta is most commonly located contralateral to the midline from the dominant arch. The right recurrent laryngeal nerve passes around the aorta rather than the RSCA [9].

> ### Clinical Pearl
>
> *Vascular rings result from abnormal segmental regression and/or persistence of portions of the embryonic aortic arch complex. In DAA, formation of two aortic arches (right and left) occurs due to the persistence of the distal right fourth arch.*

How and when do patients with a vascular ring typically present?

The timing and nature of patient presentation depends on the anatomy of the vascular ring and the degree of the resultant tracheobronchial and/or esophageal compression. Often symptoms are nonspecific, so a high index of suspicion for this diagnosis must be maintained. Most patients will present with respiratory symptoms (88%–95%) with or without esophageal symptoms; isolated digestive symptoms are relatively rare (11%)[11]. (See Figure 44.2.) Infants may present with recurrent upper respiratory infections (URIs) or pneumonia, wheezing, stridor, slow feeding, gastroesophageal reflux disease (GERD), vomiting, and/or failure to thrive. In children and older patients,

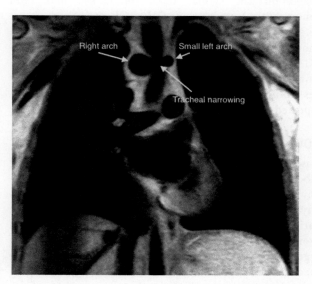

Figure 44.2 Double aortic arch. Coronal black blood magnetic resonance image showing left–right narrowing of the trachea by the double aortic arch. Courtesy of Michael Taylor, MD.

the symptoms are similar to those seen in infancy with the addition of dysphagia to solids (i.e., dysphagia lusoria secondary to the aberrant RSCA) and dyspnea on exertion.

Clinical Pearl

Tight rings with significant compression, as seen in DAA, may present early in the neonatal period with stridor, wheezing, respiratory distress, and apnea with feeds. Less restrictive rings may present later in life or may remain asymptomatic and be incidentally identified.

Are associated lesions and/or syndromes commonly seen?

While DAA and RAA with aberrant LSCA are isolated anomalies in the majority of cases, the reported incidence of concurrent cardiac lesions for all vascular rings is 12%–32% [3, 5]. The most common associated cardiac defect is tetralogy of Fallot; ventricular septal defect, atrial septal defect, aortic coarctation, transposition of the great arteries and complex single ventricle lesions have also been described [12]. In patients diagnosed with a pulmonary artery sling, coexisting complete tracheal rings can be present in as many as 65% of cases [13].

Aortic arch anomalies, including vascular ring, can be associated with a number of genetic syndromes, most notably 22q11.2 deletions (DiGeorge, CATCH-22, velocardiofacial syndrome, conotruncal anomaly face) and duplications [14]. Trisomy 21, VACTERL (vertebral defects, anal atresia, cardiac defects, tracheoesophageal fistula, renal anomalies, and limb abnormalities) association, CHARGE (coloboma, heart defects, atresia choanae growth retardation, genital abnormalities, and ear abnormalities) syndrome, and PHACE (posterior fossa brain malformations, hemangiomas of the face, arterial anomalies, cardiac anomalies, and eye abnormalities) syndrome have all been reported [14, 15].

How are vascular rings diagnosed?

Vascular rings can be diagnosed via numerous imaging modalities including chest radiography, echocardiography (including fetal), angiography, computed tomography (CT) scanning, magnetic resonance imaging (MRI), barium esophagography, and direct laryngoscopy and bronchoscopy [3, 11, 16]. The choice of imaging strategies is generally based on symptomatology, local expertise, the specialists involved, the availability of advanced imaging technology, and cost. There has been a trend away from barium esophagography and angiography toward CT and

MRI, with echocardiography and bronchoscopy also recommended for most patients [10, 11]. In patients diagnosed with a pulmonary artery sling, bronchoscopy should be performed to rule out the presence of complete tracheal rings. Although the optimal diagnostic imaging algorithm for vascular rings is unknown, the goal of imaging should be identification of the relevant vascular and airway anatomy causing the patient's symptoms to minimize unnecessary testing and allow for surgical planning.

How are vascular rings repaired?

Surgical division of a vascular ring is indicated when symptoms of airway and/or esophageal compression are present, and it is generally performed without delay once a diagnosis is made. The approach is dictated by the anatomy of the vascular ring and the presence of any intracardiac and/or tracheal anomalies requiring concurrent repair using cardiopulmonary bypass (CPB). Most commonly, repair is performed via a left posterolateral muscle-sparing thoracotomy (contralateral to the dominant arch) although a right-sided thoracotomy is necessary in the rare case of a left-dominant DAA or right-sided ductus arteriosus. Sternotomy and CPB are utilized for aortic uncrossing procedures for circumflex aorta, for cases when an intracardiac repair is also indicated, and for division/reimplantation of the left pulmonary artery with slide tracheoplasty in the case of complete tracheal rings with pulmonary artery sling. Thoracoscopic and robot-assisted approaches to vascular ring division have been described and are most appropriate in cases where the segment to be divided is not patent [17]. In all cases, the ligamentum arteriosum is divided.

- *Double aortic arch*: With DAA, the vascular ring is repaired by dividing the most diminutive (or atretic) portion of the nondominant arch. If there is not a clear target for division, it may be necessary for the surgeon to apply test clamps to the potential sites of division to assess for limb pressure gradients (there should be no pressure gradient with occlusion).
- *Right aortic arch with aberrant LSCA*: Classically, the surgery for RAA with aberrant LSCA is division of the ligamentum. In most patients with this anomaly, the LSCA arises from a remnant of the left fourth dorsal arch called the retroesophageal diverticulum of Kommerell. Increasingly, surgeons are resecting this at the time of vascular ring division and reimplanting the LSCA on the left carotid artery with the goal of preventing residual esophageal compression and the risk of late rupture [18].

Anesthetic Implications

What are the perioperative considerations for patients with unrepaired vascular rings undergoing diagnostic evaluation?

Patients with a suspected or known (but unrepaired) vascular ring that are undergoing diagnostic evaluation pose a challenge to the anesthesiologist. A detailed history and physical should be conducted with special attention paid to the cardiac, respiratory, and gastrointestinal systems. An overwhelming majority of patients with unrepaired vascular rings will present with some degree of obstructive airway symptoms. The type, severity, and time course of respiratory symptoms (including recurrent infections) should be established, as should the patient's current respiratory status and degree of optimization. Often, the anatomic nature and degree of the underlying airway obstruction are not known during the patient's initial workup. It should be appreciated that signs and symptoms from a concurrent cardiac abnormality may be masked by those of the patient's respiratory pathophysiology (tachypnea, intercostal retractions, nasal flaring, mild intermittent cyanosis), especially when chronic lung disease is present. Diagnostic procedures should be performed in a care setting that will allow for close postoperative monitoring and the ability to expeditiously escalate the level of care in the event that airway manipulation and/or residual anesthetic effects lead to an acute increase in airway obstruction during the postprocedural period.

Clinical Pearl

Patients with underlying genetic syndromes may have additional airway considerations such as subglottic stenosis or cleft lip/palate. Cardiac lesions should also be screened for given the significant incidence of intracardiac lesions in patients with genetic syndromes.

Should any other evaluation or optimization be considered prior to CT and bronchoscopy in this patient? Should echocardiography be performed first?

Even in the absence of concerning symptoms, it would not be unreasonable for a limited transthoracic echocardiogram to be performed without sedation given the relatively high incidence of concurrent congenital heart disease. The patient should also be optimized from a pulmonary standpoint and URIs or pneumonias aggressively treated. To

that end, a pulmonology consultation may be helpful. Because the signs and symptoms of 22q11.2 deletions can be subtle, laboratory screening for hypocalcemia and genetic testing should be strongly suggested in patients with vascular ring and conotruncal lesions.

Clinical Pearl

Symptoms of heart disease that cannot be explained by a respiratory etiology (e.g., murmur, pulmonary edema, hepatosplenomegaly, ascites, or four-extremity blood pressure differential) should prompt a preanesthesia echocardiogram and cardiology consult.

Should the case be delayed if the patient presents with a resolving respiratory infection?

The risks and benefits of proceeding with anesthesia in a patient with a vascular ring and a URI must be carefully weighed. Given the patient's respiratory symptomatology it would be best to allow recovery from an active URI prior to administration of an anesthetic if possible. Undue delays in surgery have the potential to hamper normal airway development and/or lead to progressive airway and lung injury [9].

Clinical Pearl

Although an attempt should be made to maximally optimize the patient's respiratory status ahead of a planned anesthetic, it must be appreciated that the definitive treatment strategy for recurrent infections in these patients is surgical repair of the vascular ring.

Should these procedures be bundled and performed at the same time?

The risk-benefit profile of performing multiple diagnostic procedures, potentially under the same anesthetic, should be approached in a patient-specific, team-based manner.

Important considerations include the following:

- Can adequate CT images be obtained without sedation or anesthesia, avoiding anesthesia in the out-of-operating room (OOR) setting and transport entirely?
- If the patient requires intubation, would it be safer to perform the bronchoscopy and intubation in the operating room (OR) prior to CT, allowing for careful endotracheal tube (ETT) placement proximal to the area of the obstruction, with return to the OR for extubation?

341

- If the CT protocol calls for a free-breathing patient, can the patient be safely induced in the OOR setting and then transferred sedated with an unsecured airway to the OR?
- If the patient is not intubated for the CT, can/should the bronchoscopy be delayed and instead performed intraoperatively during the vascular ring repair to avoid transport entirely?

Adequate airway support and vital signs monitoring during procedures in OOR settings and the transport to and from these locations is critical. According to the American Society of Anesthesiologists (ASA) Closed Claim Analysis Project, respiratory events (inadequate oxygenation and ventilation) are the most common type of adverse events in OOR locations and tend to be more severe in nature as compared to in-OR procedures [19]. A preponderance of respiratory events was also described by the Pediatric Sedation Research Consortium's multiple analyses of the adverse events encountered during sedation of pediatric patients in OOR settings [20, 21].

What are the major anesthetic considerations for this patient presenting for CT scan and bronchoscopy?

The overwhelming majority of patients with a vascular ring will present with some degree of respiratory symptoms and airway compromise due to an unknown combination of external obstruction, tracheobronchomalacia, and/or tracheal stenosis. Unfortunately, anesthetic goals for managing these various airway pathologies can be somewhat conflicting.

Specifics of the anesthetic plan will depend on

- The *degree of contribution of direct airway compression* and/or secondary airway disease (tracheobronchomalacia, interstitial lung disease) to the patient's symptoms
- The *imaging protocol* utilized (the need for breath-holding versus free-breathing during image acquisition)
- The *logistics of intubating the patient* in the OR versus an OOR setting

The choice of intravenous (IV) versus inhalation induction should be made after consideration of the severity of the patient's airway and/or gastrointestinal symptomatology; an inhalation induction is generally well tolerated. If the patient requires intubation for either respiratory or logistical reasons, the patient should be induced in a careful manner and the ability to ventilate with positive pressure ventilation should be confirmed prior to the administration of neuromuscular blockade. If necessary, intubation

and extubation should be performed in a controlled, familiar setting with adequate technical and material support including additional anesthesia personal, readily available airway equipment (e.g., smaller endotracheal tubes and appropriately sized suction catheters, bronchoscopy for endotracheal tube troubleshooting, noninvasive positive pressure ventilation devices), and rescue medications (e.g., dexamethasone, nebulized racemic epinephrine, albuterol, succinylcholine). If monitored anesthesia care is chosen, the provider should closely monitor oxygenation and ventilation and be prepared to rapidly treat episodes of desaturation, apnea, laryngospasm, and/or excessive airway or pooled oropharyngeal/esophageal secretions. Choices for titrated medications for monitored anesthesia care include midazolam, dexmedetomidine, and/or ketamine.

What anesthetic induction, monitoring, and airway management considerations exist for vascular ring repair?

The preoperative imaging and operative plan (sidedness, temporary or permanent vascular occlusion) should be carefully reviewed. A gentle mask induction with sevoflurane is generally well tolerated if gastrointestinal symptomatology does not preclude this and allows for the performance of bronchoscopy in a spontaneously breathing patient if further airway assessment is required. In addition to recommended standard ASA monitors, the placement of an arterial line is generally indicated, especially in cases when significant aortic manipulation is anticipated.

Clinical Pearl

The location of the noninvasive blood pressure cuff(s) and arterial line should be determined by the patient's anatomy and the type of repair to be undertaken:

- *DAA*: Bilateral upper extremity and unilateral lower extremity
- *RAA with aberrant LSCA*: Right radial arterial line if the LSCA is to be translocated or sacrificed
- *Vascular ring repair with concurrent anterior–posterior tracheopexy*: Upper and lower extremity arterial lines

At a minimum, there should be a way to reliably measure pressures in both an upper and lower extremity. The application of cerebral near-infrared spectroscopy monitors should be considered if vascular clamping is anticipated. A central venous line may be indicated for some cases to allow for the infusion of vasoactive medications and to provide additional access. Although blood loss is generally minimal, there is the potential for massive hemorrhage, so vascular access and blood product availability should be planned with this in mind. Transesophageal echocardiography is usually reserved for cases requiring CPB.

What is an appropriate emergence and extubation plan after vascular ring repair? What modalities can be considered for postoperative analgesia?

Most patients undergoing vascular ring division are candidates for early extubation in the absence of significant pulmonary disease, the performance of a complex intracardiac or tracheal repair, and/or significant residual lesions. Enhanced analgesia with neuraxial (thoracic epidural) or peripheral nerve blockade (paravertebral nerve block or erector spinae plane block +/– catheter placement) can aid in facilitating early extubation, as can the use of multimodal analgesia and intravenous acetaminophen.

What are potential immediate postoperative concerns?

Vascular ring division is associated with a very low perioperative mortality rate (0–5%) and a relatively low postoperative complication rate (2%–8%)[5, 6, 11]. Although repair results in the immediate relief of tracheal and esophageal compression in the overwhelming majority of patients, persistent tracheal obstruction due to residual lesions and/or tracheomalacia has been reported in >10% of patients [15]. Recurrent laryngeal nerve paresis/paralysis is seen in up to 8% in some series [11]. Other immediate postoperative concerns include bleeding, chylothorax, and pneumonia.

What is the expected long-term outcome for these patients?

Long-term mortality, freedom from reoperation, and complication rates are excellent with the majority of patients reporting either partial or complete relief of symptoms. In a certain percentage of patients, tracheomalacia does resolve at longer follow-up intervals [6]. Postoperative pulmonary function tests, however, have been shown to continue to demonstrate significant airway obstructive patterns even in asymptomatic patients. As the resection of retroesophageal diverticulum of Kommerell and aggressive surgical management of tracheomalacia become more commonplace at the time of vascular ring repair, the rates of residual and recurrent symptoms, long-term complications, and the need for reoperation may decrease further [22].

References

1. R. E. Gross. Surgical relief for tracheal obstruction from a vascular ring. *N Engl J Med* 1945; **233**: 586–90.

2. C. L. Backer and C. Mavroudis. Vascular rings and pulmonary artery sling. In Mavroudis C., Backer C. L. eds. *Pediatric Cardiac Surgery*, 4th ed. Oxford: Wiley-Blackwell, 2013; 234–55.

3. W. N. Evans, R. J. Acherman, M. L. Ciccolo, et al. Vascular ring diagnosis and management: notable trends over 25 years. *World J Pediatr Congenit Heart Surg* 2016; **7**: 717–20.

4. G. M. Lowe, J. S. Donaldson, and C. L. Backer. Vascular rings: 10-year review of imaging. *Radiographics* 1991; **11**: 637–46.

5. K. C. Kocis, F. M. Midgley, and R. N. Ruckman. Aortic arch complex anomalies: 20-year experience with symptoms, diagnosis, associated cardiac defects, and surgical repair. *Pediatr Cardiol* 1997; **18**: 127–32.

6. P. S. Naimo, T. A. Fricke, J. S. Donald, et al. Long-term outcomes of complete vascular ring division in children: a 36-year experience from a single institution. *Interact Cardiovasc Thorac Surg* 2017; **24**: 234–9.

7. C. L. Backer and C. Mavroudis. Congenital Heart Surgery Nomenclature and Database Project: patent ductus arteriosus, coarctation of the aorta, interrupted aortic arch. *Ann Thorac Surg* 2000; **69**: S298–307.

8. J. M. Schleich. Images in cardiology: development of the human heart – days 15–21. *Heart* 2002; **87**: 487.

9. B. D. Kussman, T. Geva, and F. X. McGowan. Cardiovascular causes of airway compression. *Paediatr Anaesth* 2004; **14**: 60–74.

10. K. Hanneman, B. Newman, and F. Chan. Congenital variants and anomalies of the aortic arch. *Radiographics* 2017; **37**: 32–51.

11. R. K. Shah, B. N. Mora, E. Bacha, et al. The presentation and management of vascular rings: an otolaryngology perspective. *Int J Pediatr Otorhinolaryngol* 2007; **71**: 57–62.

12. R. S. Loomba. Natural history of asymptomatic and unrepaired vascular rings: is watchful waiting a viable option? A new case and review of previously reported cases. *Children* 2016; **3**: 44.

13. W. E. Berdon, D. H. Baker, J. T. Wung, et al. Complete cartilage-ring tracheal stenosis associated with anomalous left pulmonary artery: the ring-sling complex. *Radiology* 1984; **152**: 57–64.

14. L. T. Nguyen, R. Fleishman, E. Flynn, et al. 22q11.2 microduplication syndrome with associated esophageal atresia/tracheo-esophageal fistula and vascular ring. *Clin Case Rep* 2017; **5**: 351–6.

15. A. Bonnard, F. Auber, L. Fourcade, et al. Vascular ring abnormalities: a retrospective study of 62 cases. *J Pediatr Surg* 2003; **38**: 539–43.

16. M. Etesami, R. Ashwath, J. Kanne, et al. Computed tomography in the evaluation of vascular rings and slings. *Insights Imaging* 2014; **5**: 507–21.

17. B. E. Kogon, J. M. Forbess, M. L. Wulkan, et al. Video-assisted thoracoscopic surgery: is it a superior technique for the division of vascular rings in children? *Congenit Heart Dis* 2007; **2**: 130–3.

18. D. Luciano, J. Mitchell, A. Fraisse, et al. Kommerell diverticulum should be removed in children with vascular ring and aberrant left subclavian artery. *Ann Thorac Surg* 2015; **100**: 2293–7.

19. R. Robbertze, K. L. Posner, and K. B. Domino. Closed claims review of anesthesia for procedures outside the operating room. *Curr Opin Anaesthesiol* 2006; **19**: 436–42.

20. J. P. Cravero, M. L. Beach, G. T. Blike, et al. The incidence and nature of adverse events during pediatric sedation/anesthesia with propofol for procedures outside the operating room: a report from the Pediatric Sedation Research Consortium. *Anesth Analg* 2009; **108**: 795–804.

21. J. R. Grunwell, C. Travers, C. E. McCracken, et al. Procedural sedation outside of the operating room using ketamine in 22,645 children: a report from the Pediatric Sedation Research Consortium. *Pediatr Crit Care Med* 2016; **17**: 1109–16.

22. C. Lawlor, C. J. Smithers, T. Hamilton, et al. Innovative management of severe tracheobronchomalacia using anterior and posterior tracheobronchopexy. *Laryngoscope* 2019; **130**: E65–74.

Suggested Reading

Backer C. L., Mavroudis C., Rigsby C. K., et al. Trends in vascular ring surgery. *J Thorac Cardiovasc Surg* 2005; **129**: 1339–47.

Backer C. L., Mongé M. C., Popescu A. R., et al. Vascular rings. *Semin Pediatr Surg* 2016; **25**: 165–75.

Hanneman K., Newman B., and Chan F. Congenital variants and anomalies of the aortic arch. *Radiographics* 2017; **37**: 32–51.

Herrin M. A., Zurakowski D., Fynn-Thompson F., et al. Outcomes following thoracotomy or thoracoscopic vascular ring division in children and young adults. *J Thorac Cardiovasc Surg* 2017; **154**: 607–15.

Kussman B. D., Geva T., and McGowan F. X. Cardiovascular causes of airway compression. *Paediatr Anaesth* 2004; **14**: 60–74.

Priya S., Thomas R., Nagpal P., et al. Congenital anomalies of the aortic arch. *Cardiovasc Diagn Ther* 2018; **8**: S26–44.

Chapter 45

Pericardial Effusion

Andrés Bacigalupo Landa, Matthew Careskey, and Lori A. Aronson

Case Scenario

A 3-year-old boy weighing 15 kg with acute lymphoblastic leukemia presents to the cardiac catheterization laboratory for drainage of a moderate to large pericardial effusion. He began induction chemotherapy with daunorubicin, vincristine, L-asparaginase, and prednisone 1 week earlier. He has a right tunneled subcutaneous internal jugular central line ("port-a-cath"). The medical response team was called to evaluate him this afternoon for down-trending blood pressure accompanied by worsening respiratory distress and admitted him to the pediatric intensive care unit for closer observation and evaluation. Recent vital signs are blood pressure 75/43 mm Hg, heart rate 144 beats/minute, respiratory rate 40 breaths/minute, SpO$_2$ 94% on room air, and temperature 36.8°C. On physical examination, the boy has mild suprasternal and intercostal retractions and is sitting upright. Lung fields are clear bilaterally, but heart sounds are muffled. Chest radiograph shows no pulmonary disease.

Bedside echocardiogram demonstrates the following:

- *Moderate–large circumferential pericardial effusion*
- *Right atrial collapse during early systole*
- *Right ventricular collapse during early diastole*
- *Inspiratory "bounce" of the interventricular septum toward the left ventricle*

Key Objectives

- Recognize the physiologic implications of symptomatic pericardial effusion.
- Describe the preoperative assessment for a patient with symptomatic pericardial effusion.
- Describe anesthetic management strategies for a patient with a pericardial effusion.
- Describe potential perioperative complications.

Pathophysiology

What is a pericardial effusion and what common causes exist in children?

A pericardial effusion (PCE) is an abnormal accumulation of fluid within the pericardial sac. The pericardial sac is the space contained between the visceral and parietal layers of the pericardium, and normally it can contain up to 50 mL of fluid, usually plasma ultrafiltrate. Any accumulation of fluid beyond this amount is considered a PCE. The hemodynamic consequences of this will depend on the pressure–volume relationship of the pericardial sac. Common causes of PCE in children include infection (mostly viral and gram-positive bacteria), neoplasm, inflammatory or immune-mediated response (including post-pericardiotomy syndrome, occurring in up to 15%–30% of open-heart cases and in <2% of closed procedures). Additional causes include hemopericardium (secondary to trauma, postoperative bleeding or iatrogenic), uremia, chronic renal failure, hyper- or hypothyroidism, and radiation therapy.

How is cardiac tamponade defined and what are the hemodynamic consequences?

A PCE is usually asymptomatic unless it causes cardiac tamponade. In tamponade, the external compression of the heart results in equalization of pressure in all cardiac chambers, causing reduced atrioventricular blood flow during diastole and biventricular stroke volume during systole. This, in turn, reduces cardiac output (CO) for both sides of the heart, causing signs and symptoms related to hypoperfusion. The patient may present with right-sided symptoms of hepatic congestion, peripheral edema, and jugular venous distension as well as left-sided symptoms of orthopnea, hypotension, sinus tachycardia, and cool extremities with prolonged capillary refill.

It is important to note that cardiac tamponade may also occur in cases of open pericardium. This usually happens in patients in whom the pericardium was used as an autologous patch during the surgical correction of their congenital heart disease, and so the pericardial sac was left "open." In these cases, the pericardial fluid will fill the mediastinum and again, once the extrinsic pressure compromises cardiac compliance, tamponade physiology will be seen.

In addition to PCE, cardiac tamponade physiology is also seen in other instances that are outside the scope of

345

this chapter, including pneumothorax, breath-stacking, mediastinal masses, pericarditis, and thoracoscopic insufflation.

How is cardiac tamponade diagnosed?

Cardiac tamponade is a clinical diagnosis that is supported by diagnostic studies. Classically, acute cardiac tamponade is defined by Beck's triad, which consists of the following:

- Jugular venous distension as a result of a noncompliant right ventricle (RV) with high filling pressures
- Muffled heart sounds secondary to the pericardial effusion or constriction
- Systemic hypotension due to diminished left ventricular filling

As all three findings occur simultaneously in only one-third of patients, the absence of any part of Beck's triad does not rule out tamponade. Other signs and symptoms may include right upper quadrant pain (due to hepatic congestion), orthopnea, dyspnea, tachypnea, and sinus tachycardia. Pulsus paradoxus, an abnormally large decrease in systolic blood pressure (>10 mm Hg) on inspiration, may also be present. It is important to note that patients may also have noncardiac symptoms related to the primary cause of the pericardial effusion.

> **Clinical Pearl**
>
> *Symptomatic pericardial effusion usually involves systemic hypotension, tachycardia, and high systemic venous pressures.*

What are the expected echocardiographic findings in a patient with cardiac tamponade?

Echocardiography is the gold standard for diagnosing PCE and detecting tamponade physiology, providing nearly 100% sensitivity. Furthermore, by allowing assessment of the site and characteristics of the effusion, it is a valuable tool to aid in determining and guiding the approach (percutaneous versus open) to drainage of the effusion.

In the case of PCE, echocardiographic images will show a hypoechoic fluid-filled pericardial sac. Effusions may be loculated or circumferential and are graded depending on the size of the hypoechoic space during diastole: small (<10 mm), moderate (10–20 mm), or severe (>20 mm).

In the case of cardiac tamponade, echocardiography will show collapse of cardiac chambers during various points in the cardiac cycle. Right atrial (RA) collapse

during systole is the earliest and most sensitive sign of cardiac tamponade physiology, with increased diagnostic accuracy when it persists for more than one-third of the cardiac cycle. Additionally, inspiratory "bounce" of the interventricular septum toward the left ventricle (LV) is commonly observed during diastole. Finally, inferior vena cava (IVC) dilation ("IVC plethora") and respiratory variation of the mitral, aortic, or tricuspid valve inflow peak velocity of >25% may also be seen.

What hemodynamic monitoring findings may be suggestive of symptomatic PCE?

In addition to systemic hypotension and sinus tachycardia, other findings can be suggestive of symptomatic PCE. Abnormal ECG findings, including electrical alternans and arrhythmias, are common. If an arterial catheter is in place, beat-to-beat pulse pressure variation and pulsus paradoxus may be observed. Respiratory variation of the pulse oximetry waveform may be present as well. With central venous pressure monitoring, a diminished *y descent* may also be seen secondary to elevated diastolic filling pressures. Symptomatic PCE is also reflected by elevated RA ("central venous") and left atrial pressures.

It is important to note that PCE can result in decreased coronary perfusion pressures due to the combination of systemic hypotension and elevated LV end-diastolic pressure. Consequently, ST segment changes (either depression or elevation, depending on the degree of myocardial compromise) may also be observed.

What is electrical alternans and what is its significance? What other electrocardiographic findings may exist?

Electrical alternans is the appearance of beat-to-beat amplitude changes of the QRS complex and axis observed in any or all leads on an electrocardiogram (ECG) with no additional conduction changes. The amplitude and axis changes are significant because they represent the position of the heart "shifting" within a full pericardial sac with each contraction.

Other possible ECG findings include sinus tachycardia, low-voltage QRS waveform, ST-T wave changes, and possibly atrial or ventricular ectopy or arrythmias.

> **Clinical Pearl**
>
> *Electrical alternans (amplitude changes of the QRS complex and axis) on ECG is suggestive of pericardial effusion.*

What are the cardiopulmonary interactions in symptomatic PCE?

Since the restrictive nature of PCE decreases diastolic filling and, in turn, stroke volume, CO becomes heart rate dependent.

$$CO = SV \times HR$$
$$SV = EDV - ESV$$

where CO = cardiac output; SV = stroke volume; HR = heart rate; EDV = end-diastolic volume; and ESV = end-systolic volume.

However, from these two equations, it may be inferred that another strategy to increase CO involves increasing EDV by increasing venous return and preload. This is important when considering the cardiopulmonary interactions with positive pressure ventilation (PPV), as PPV results in decreased venous return to the right heart and hence reduces CO. The change in intrathoracic pressure (from negative during spontaneous ventilation to positive during mechanical ventilation) decreases preload to a preload-dependent heart with restrictive physiology. For this reason, maintaining spontaneous (negative pressure) ventilation in this situation is of prime importance, particularly in a patient with a hemodynamically significant PCE.

Anesthetic Implications

What past medical history should be sought prior to induction of anesthesia?

The patient's comorbidities should be reviewed, particularly those that could be a contributing factor to formation of the PCE. Any history of recent bacterial or viral respiratory infections, presence of a mediastinal mass, or history of recent cardiac or thoracic surgery are important and help tailor the anesthetic plan accordingly.

Special concerns exist for oncologic patients. Prior exposure to cardiotoxic chemotherapeutic agents (i.e., doxorubicin, daunorubicin, or fluorouracil) is concerning for ensuing cardiomyopathy or QTc prolongation. Additionally, a recent complete blood count with platelets, a coagulation panel to assess hematopoietic effects of chemotherapy, and an electrolyte panel are indicated. If high dose or chronic steroids are part of the oncologic regimen, then stress dose steroids may be warranted as part of the anesthetic plan.

What physical examination findings correlate with symptomatic PCE?

Physical examination findings in symptomatic PCE are reflective of right and/or left-sided cardiac congestion.

A complete physical examination is required to determine the degree of cardiac involvement. As previously stated, right upper quadrant pain, abdominal distension, hepatomegaly, peripheral edema, and jugular venous distension are all signs of right-sided failure. Additionally, crackles, diminished breath sounds, intercostal muscle retractions with tachypnea and/or orthopnea, diminished peripheral pulses, and prolonged capillary refill all represent left heart compromise. All of these findings, associated with muffled heart sounds, hypotension, and sinus tachycardia, are supportive of cardiac tamponade.

What other information should be sought on physical examination?

Apart from the aforementioned findings, all indicative of symptomatic PCE, it is important for the anesthesia provider to evaluate any other systems affected by the patient's underlying condition. Additionally, a detailed assessment of the current vascular access lines (size, location, medications being delivered through them, and reliability), current invasive monitoring (presence of arterial and/or central venous catheters) and airway adjuncts or need for supplemental oxygen should be performed prior to going into the operating room or cardiac catheterization laboratory.

What are the fasting considerations for this case?

Fasting status is an important determinant in formulating the anesthetic plan to minimize the risk of pulmonary aspiration. If the patient is hemodynamically stable or the PCE is slowly progressing, the American Society of Anesthesiologists (ASA) preoperative fasting guidelines of 8 hours for a heavy meal, 6 hours for formula or a light meal, 4 hours for breast milk, and 2 hours for clear liquids may be followed. However, if the patient does not meet the preoperative fasting guidelines but is experiencing acute hemodynamic decompensation, one must weigh the risks of proceeding with the case assuming a risk for pulmonary aspiration against delaying the case with the risk of further circulatory collapse. Consideration should be given to performing the case with minimal sedation if possible, as performance of a rapid-sequence induction with initiation of PPV can be potentially life threatening.

What nonpharmacologic strategies are available to deal with separation anxiety?

A patient's developmental maturity and mental status are important factors when formulating a plan for child–parent separation. Most developmentally normal toddlers and small children experience extreme stress and fear near the time of separation. To the extent possible, nonpharmacologic interventions should be utilized first: age-appropriate videos or games on smart-devices, toys, and, if available, a child-life specialist or other staff member who can be solely dedicated to the patient's psychological needs.

What pharmacologic options for parental separation could be considered?

If pharmacologic anxiolysis is necessary, it is paramount to have ECG, blood pressure and oxygen saturation monitoring in place. Agents that avoid cardiac depressant effects and have minimal or no sympatholytic effects should be titrated in low doses. Intravenous (IV) midazolam is a reasonable choice and can be titrated in small aliquots (0.05 mg/kg or 0.5 mg boluses) to reach a desirable effect. Dexmedetomidine should be avoided as it predictably causes bradycardia, which can contribute to hemodynamic collapse as CO is primarily dependent on a fast heart rate. If a sedative/anxiolytic is given, exhibit patience while slowly titrating to clinical effect as CO is impaired.

Is it safe to use an existing in situ central venous catheter?

One potential complication of central venous cannulation is intrapericardial placement or migration, which can itself result in PCE. This uncommon yet dangerous complication should be ruled out prior to using an in situ central venous catheter, as further volume administration into the pericardial space will further worsen the clinical scenario. For this reason, it is advisable to carefully review the chart for evidence of difficulty with central venous line placement, as well as any recent chest imaging studies showing the catheter trajectory and tip position.

Is an invasive arterial blood pressure monitor indicated?

The need for invasive blood pressure monitoring depends on the degree of the patient's hemodynamic compromise, as well as on the type of procedure that will be performed. In the case of a symptomatic though hemodynamically stable patient in which a percutaneous ultrasound-guided drainage will be performed with sedation, analgesia, and local anesthesia, an arterial catheter is probably not necessary.

However, in a patient with an acute effusion and significant hemodynamic compromise, or recurrent pericardial effusions in which a pericardial window is planned, an arterial catheter would be useful as it would allow beat-to-beat blood pressure monitoring and rapid recognition of

hemodynamic changes both during induction of anesthesia and during the procedure itself. In this instance, multiple providers can be useful to help prepare the patient and expedite the procedure without delaying therapy. If there is no arterial line present, and the patient is in extremis, then it would not be advisable to delay definitive life-saving intervention for the placement of this monitor.

Additionally, placement of an arterial line in a young child without sedation or prior to induction of anesthesia is challenging and delays definitive treatment. In this scenario, other measures of perfusion (distal pulses, peripheral perfusion, capnography, and pulse oximetry waveform) can be closely monitored and treated to avoid delaying drainage of the PCE. Ultimately, the decision to place an arterial line is dependent on the entirety of the clinical scenario and should be made on a case-by-case basis.

What is the preferred anesthetic plan?

The ideal anesthetic plan depends on the patient's current status, as well as the type of drainage planned. When a percutaneous ultrasound-guided drainage will be performed, moderate sedation, analgesia, and local anesthesia should be sufficient and have minimal hemodynamic effects.

With either an acute severe effusion, or a recurrent pericardial effusion in which a pericardial window is planned, it may be beneficial to resuscitate the patient with IV fluids and start vasoconstrictor and inotropic agents prior to beginning the procedure. On the other hand, if the patient is unstable due to significant tamponade physiology and there is no time for preoperative optimization, a "staged" anesthetic and surgical plan can be proposed. While keeping the patient spontaneously breathing, moderate sedation, analgesia, and local anesthesia can be initially administered, allowing percutaneous drainage of the effusion and improving cardiac reserve before proceeding to induction of general anesthesia.

What precautions should be taken prior to initiation of sedation or general anesthesia?

Once in the procedure suite the patient is generally positioned with the head of the bed elevated at 30–45 degrees to alleviate orthopnea. With ECG, blood pressure, and oxygenation monitors in place, and after applying supplementary oxygen, the chest should be prepped and draped, and the procedural/surgical team should be scrubbed and ready to proceed before sedation or anesthesia is induced. Adequate communication and coordination between the various teams is of utmost importance. If sedation is planned, soft hand restraints should be applied to keep the patient from reflexively reaching during the intervention.

The induction of general anesthesia can precipitate circulatory collapse. For this reason, if general anesthesia is chosen, all ASA monitors should be applied, and emergency medications and airway resuscitation equipment should be ready prior to administration of any anesthetic medications. All team members should be available, including the sonographer and a cardiologist capable of quickly decompressing the PCE. It may be beneficial to increase preload with IV fluids and/or to initiate vasoconstrictor and inotropic agents prior to inducing anesthesia in order to ameliorate hemodynamic effects which can include loss of vascular tone and decreased preload. Additionally, it may be advisable to have packed red blood cells, a surgical team and in some cases availability of extracorporeal membrane oxygenation backup prior to starting the procedure.

What are the preferred sedative agents?

The ideal sedative/anesthetic agent is one that does not cause cardiac depression or decrease sympathetic outflow, while allowing the patient to remain spontaneously breathing. If sedation is the plan of choice, IV midazolam should be titrated (0.05 mg/kg boluses or 0.5 mg boluses), and after injection of local anesthetic, low-dose fentanyl may be given if needed (0.5 mcg/kg, slowly titrated as it may cause bradycardia).

It is crucial to keep in mind that given the low cardiac output state of the patient, the onset of action of the medications administered will be delayed. For this reason, the agents should be slowly titrated in order to avoid oversedation, drastic hemodynamic changes, and the potential need for PPV.

What if sedation is unsuccessful?

In cases in which additional deep sedation/anesthesia is required prior to drainage of the effusion, if sedatives and analgesics have already been administered, IV ketamine (0.2–1 mg/kg, in divided doses) may be cautiously titrated. Caution is indicated as ketamine has direct myocardial depressant properties which may be profound in patients who are catecholamine depleted or at maximal sympathetic drive. In most patients, ketamine will preserve sympathetic tone and spontaneous ventilation. Neuromuscular blockade should be avoided as the patient should be kept spontaneously breathing. If airway obstruction is an issue, placement of a laryngeal mask airway to maintain spontaneous ventilation may be an option.

If it is necessary to progress to a general endotracheal anesthetic, etomidate may be utilized for induction and low-dose sevoflurane may be used for maintenance. At this point, hypotension may be treated with volume expansion or medications as indicated. If necessary, the use of epinephrine, which has both α- and β-receptor effects, is preferred over phenylephrine, which has purely α-receptor effects. To help minimize the effects of PPV, increasing the expiratory time and utilizing minimal or no positive end-expiratory pressure should be considered to maximize venous return.

> **Clinical Pearl**
>
> *Positive pressure ventilation will reduce preload and hence CO. Maintenance of spontaneous ventilation is preferred until the PCE has been drained.*

What is the primary hemodynamic goal during induction of anesthesia?

The hemodynamic goal during induction of anesthesia is to maintain CO via the following:

- Avoid cardiac depression.
- Maintain sympathetic outflow: preserve vascular tone and an elevated heart rate.
- Avoid decreased preload either due to vasodilation and/or PPV.

Caution is advisable with cardiac depressant medications. Although ketamine preserves sympathetic tone, heart rate, and spontaneous ventilation, it also has direct cardiac depressant properties and can precipitate hemodynamic collapse. Similarly, although opioids have minimal cardio-depressant effects, they can decrease central sympathetic outflow and result in bradycardia. Maintaining normovolemia and spontaneous ventilation can help minimize hemodynamic changes.

> **Clinical Pearl**
>
> *The primary hemodynamic goal is to preserve CO by maintaining an elevated heart rate, high preload, and spontaneous ventilation.*

How is pericardiocentesis generally performed?

Percutaneous catheter drainage, or pericardiocentesis, is the most common method currently used for drainage of pericardial effusions. This is usually done under echocardiographic or fluoroscopic guidance in the cardiac catheterization laboratory. Echocardiographic imaging prior to starting the drainage allows the proceduralist to approximate the amount of fluid needing to be drained, as well as determining the most accurate location for the puncture site.

349

Common access points are apical (needle directed parallel to the LV long axis toward the aortic valve), parasternal (needle inserted 1 cm lateral to the left sternal border; >1 cm lateral will risk injuring the internal thoracic/mammary vessels), or subxiphoid (needle inserted 1 cm inferior to the left xiphoid-costal angle, aiming toward the left mid-clavicle).

Once the pericardial sac is accessed and fluid obtained, the Seldinger technique is utilized to insert a catheter connected to a three-way stopcock; this will be used for drainage, intrapericardial pressure monitoring and reinfusion if indicated. According to the 2015 European Society of Cardiology guidelines, fluid should be drained in small sequential aliquots to prevent acute RV dilation. If the aspirate is nonclotting blood, it can be reinfused directly to the patient to aid with resuscitation (peripheral or central access line connected to pericardial catheter via the three-way stopcock). The procedure is usually continued until the intrapericardial pressure is <5 mm Hg during inspiration. Figure 45.1 shows echocardiographic images of a pericardial effusion pre- and post-pericardiocentesis.

What acute complications can occur during pericardiocentesis?

Pericardiocentesis is considered a safe and effective procedure, with an incidence of major complications of 1.2%–1.6% in experienced hands. However, it is still important to be aware of the possible complications given the high morbidity and mortality associated with them.

During needle insertion, myocardial and coronary artery laceration may cause acute myocardial ischemia, generating ECG ST-segment changes, echocardiographic regional wall motion abnormalities, or a delayed presentation as persistent hemopericardium despite needle/catheter aspiration. Other vascular injuries to the intercostal or internal thoracic/mammary arteries may have a similar delayed presentation. Adequate and prompt communication with the procedural team is paramount as escalation to surgical intervention may be necessary.

Additionally, needle insertion can cause cardiac arrhythmias (supraventricular or ventricular) which usually resolve with retraction or redirection of the needle/catheter. Other potential complications include air embolism, pneumothorax (evidenced by worsening dyspnea), and intraabdominal organ injury, most commonly to the liver, by transperitoneal needle insertion.

The amount of pericardial fluid drained and the rate at which it is removed is also important. As referenced earlier, the 2015 European Society of Cardiology guidelines recommend that fluid should be drained in small sequential aliquots, as up to 25% of patients may have a vasovagal response secondary to pericardial decompression. This is evidenced by a sudden decrease in blood pressure and heart rate associated with a "fainting" sensation referred to by the patient (if conscious). Additionally, rapid pericardial decompression may cause acute left or right ventricular dilation and subsequent dysfunction, referred to as "pericardial decompression syndrome" (PDS). This has been reported in up to 5% of patients, and results in worsening hemodynamic instability, as well as pulmonary edema, following drainage. The best way to avoid PDS is to limit total initial drainage to <500 mL, continuing to drain the remaining fluid during the next

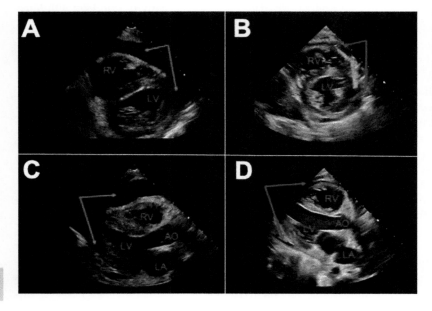

Figure 45.1 Echocardiographic images before and after pericardiocentesis. (A) Parasternal short axis view with large pericardial effusion (red arrows). (B) Parasternal short axis view post-pericardiocentesis showing resolution of pericardial effusion (blue arrows). (C) Parasternal long axis view with large pericardial effusion (red arrows). (D) Parasternal long axis view post-pericardiocentesis showing resolution of pericardial effusion (blue arrows). AO, aorta; LA, left atrium; LV, left ventricle; RV, right ventricle.

24–48 hours by leaving the catheter in place. The treatment for PDS is mainly supportive.

What additional perioperative complications need to be considered?

Other complications that may present in the postoperative period include the following:

- Cardiopulmonary edema secondary to aggressive fluid resuscitation, potentially worsened by the potential occurrence of PDS
- Pericardial decompression syndrome may manifest hours after the procedure
- Pneumopericardium secondary to a pleuro-pericardial fistula, causing tamponade physiology without pericardial effusion
- Persistent PCE, due to loculated effusions which may have been only partially drained
- Hemopericardium secondary to an initially "silent" vessel or myocardial injury
- Pericardial drain occlusion
- Infection

With this in mind, the postoperative disposition of these patients should be to a critical care unit.

Suggested Reading

Adler Y., Charron P., Imazio M., et al. ESC Guidelines for the diagnosis and management of pericardial diseases: the Task Force for the diagnosis and management of pericardial diseases of the European Society of Cardiology (ESC) endorsed by the European Association for Cardio-thoracic Surgery (EACTS). *Eur Heart J* 2015; **36**: 2921–64.

Azarbal A. and LeWinter M. M. Pericardial effusion. *Cardiol Clin* 2017; **35**: 515–24.

Ceriani E. and Cogliati C. Update on bedside ultrasound diagnosis of pericardial effusion. *Intern Emerg Med* 2016; **11**: 477–80.

Lee C. and Mason L. J. Pediatric cardiac emergencies. *Anesthesiol Clin North Am* 2001; **19**: 287–308.

Ozturk E., Tanidir I. C., Saygi M., et al. Evaluation of non-surgical causes of cardiac tamponade in children at a cardiac surgery center. *Pediatr Int* 2014; **56**: 13–18.

Prez-Casares A., Cesar S., Brunet-Garcia L., et al. Echocardiographic evaluation of pericardial effusion and cardiac tamponade. *Front Pediatr* 2017; **5**: 79.

Rawlinson E. and Bagshaw O. Anesthesia for children with pericardial effusion: a case series. *Paediatr Anaesth* 2012; **22**: 1124–31.

Vakamudi S., Ho N., and Cremer P. C. Pericardial effusions: causes, diagnosis and management. *Prog Cardiovasc Dis* 2017; **59**: 380–88.

Chapter 46

Kawasaki Disease

Wanda C. Miller-Hance

Key Objectives

- Define Kawasaki disease.
- Understand the clinical findings associated with Kawasaki disease.
- Describe the cardiac manifestations of this condition.
- Understand basic aspects of treatment in Kawasaki disease.
- Discuss the role of cardiac imaging modalities in Kawasaki disease.
- Describe the preanesthetic assessment of children affected with Kawasaki disease.
- Describe periprocedural and perioperative management considerations.

Pathophysiology

What is Kawasaki disease?

Kawasaki disease (KD), originally referred to as mucocutaneous lymph node syndrome, is an acute febrile illness affecting mostly infants and children, and, in particular, those under the age of 5 years. The condition, characterized by a systemic vasculitis, affects multiple organs and tissues.

What is the epidemiology of KD?

Kawasaki disease has been reported in children of all ethnic origins worldwide. In North America, the condition is estimated to affect nearly 25 out of 100,000 children under 5 years of age per year. In Asian countries, particularly Japan, the disease is substantially more prevalent, with an annual incidence approximately 10 times that of North America. There is a seasonal variation in the incidence of KD, with known peaks during the winter months and early spring.

What causes KD?

The etiology and pathogenesis of KD remain poorly understood despite its initial description many decades ago, an extensive clinical experience, and many years of research. Although no single infectious agent has been identified, an infectious cause has been strongly implicated. The current notion is that of a complex etiology likely influenced by an autoimmune process as well as genetic susceptibility.

What are the diagnostic features of KD?

The diagnosis of KD is established based on a constellation of clinical findings. The ***classic or complete form*** of KD is characterized by the presence of fever of five or more days in duration and at least four of the following five principal features as listed in Table 46.1.

The diagnosis of ***incomplete or atypical KD*** is considered in the presence of prolonged unexplained fever, fewer than four of the main clinical features, and compatible laboratory or echocardiographic findings.

Table 46.1 Diagnostic Clinical Features in Classic Kawasaki Disease

- Polymorphous generalized rash
- Cervical lymphadenopathy (at least 1.5 cm in diameter)
- Bilateral conjunctivitis without exudate
- Oral mucosal changes (erythematous mouth and pharynx, strawberry tongue, and red, cracked lips)
- Peripheral extremity changes (erythema of the palms and soles and firm induration of the hands and feet, often with subsequent periungal desquamation in the subacute phase)

What laboratory values are consistent with KD?

Laboratory tests in KD are nonspecific but may support the diagnosis. Most studies reflect systemic inflammation, particularly during the acute phase of the disease. Common findings include leukocytosis, anemia for age, thrombocytosis, and elevation of acute-phase reactants (erythrocyte sedimentation rate and C-reactive protein). Elevated D-dimer levels can reflect endothelial damage and fibrinolysis. Reported laboratory abnormalities also include hyponatremia, hypoalbuminemia, elevated transaminases, and sterile pyuria. Certain laboratory values can serve to monitor the effectiveness of therapy during early stages of the illness.

What are the known phases of the disease?

The clinical course in KD has been divided into three phases, reflecting the variable clinical features of the illness over time. The *acute* phase begins with fever and usually lasts approximately 7–14 days; the *subacute* phase begins from the end of fever until symptoms and signs resolve, usually until weeks 4–6. The *convalescent* phase is characterized by complete resolution of clinical signs, typically within 3 months of initial presentation. A fourth *chronic* phase has been described to focus on the cardiac complications of the disease.

What sequelae are associated with KD?

In most cases, KD is a self-limited condition, with signs and symptoms that resolve after the acute illness, even without treatment. However, serious cardiovascular manifestations and sequelae can develop, representing major contributors to morbidity and mortality in affected patients. The most common and threatening complication during the acute phase of the disease is the development of coronary artery abnormalities. This occurs in up to 25% of untreated children and a small proportion (3%–5%) of those who receive what is considered appropriate acute therapy. The proximal left anterior descending and right coronary arteries are the vessels most frequently involved, followed by the left main and left circumflex coronary arteries. Involvement of the coronary arteries can lead to myocardial ischemia, infarction, and sudden death.

Clinical Pearl

Coronary artery abnormalities occur in up to 25% of untreated children and a small proportion (3%–5%) of those who receive what is considered appropriate acute therapy. Kawasaki disease can lead to coronary artery ectasia and the formation of coronary aneurysms. The coronary pathology can result in myocardial ischemia or infarction, and in some cases, even death.

What is the pathophysiology of KD?

The vasculitis that characterizes KD affects mostly medium-sized muscular arteries, with a predilection for the coronary arteries. The pathology involving the coronary arteries ranges significantly in severity from minimal vessel dilation to the formation of giant aneurysms. The affected vessels may be at risk for thrombosis, calcification, progressive stenosis, occlusion, and rupture. Children with large or giant aneurysms, such as the toddler in this scenario, are at particularly high risk for coronary artery thrombosis.

What is the relevance of KD?

Kawasaki disease is the leading cause of acquired heart disease among children in the United States and other industrialized countries. In the developing world, rheumatic heart disease remains the main cause of cardiac-related morbidity and mortality.

Clinical Pearl

Kawasaki disease is the leading cause of acquired heart disease among children in the United States and other industrialized countries.

What are the recommendations for treatment in KD?

In a scientific statement published in 2017, the American Heart Association (AHA) provided detailed recommendations regarding diagnosis, management, and guidelines for treatment in KD. In the acute phase of the disease, the timely administration of intravenous (IV) immunoglobulin together with aspirin is the mainstay of therapy to reduce inflammation and arterial damage to the coronary vasculature and prevent cardiac sequelae. Adjunctive or alternate therapies for primary treatment that may be considered depending on the particular clinical setting include corticosteroids (more likely to be used in Japan), antibody therapy against cytokines (e.g., tumor necrosis factor-α), calcineurin inhibitors (cyclosporine), interleukin-1β receptor antagonists, cytotoxic agents, and plasma exchange. For prevention and treatment of thrombosis in patients with coronary artery aneurysms, drug therapy may include antiplatelet agents and anticoagulants. In some cases, thrombolytic drugs have also been used. Other drugs that may be considered for long-term treatment include β-blockers and statins.

What determines the prognosis in KD?

The prognosis in KD is dependent solely on the severity of the coronary artery involvement. Most of the morbidity and mortality is seen in patients with giant aneurysms. However, even in those patients considered to be low-risk survivors of KD, vascular abnormalities and serum markers have been identified, suggesting a potential increased risk for cardiac morbidity, such as the accelerated development of atherosclerotic coronary heart disease.

What information does echocardiography provide in KD?

Transthoracic echocardiography is highly sensitive and specific for the diagnosis of coronary artery involvement in KD. The study is considered essential during the acute phase of the disease and is key during long-term follow-up. Echocardiography can evaluate the coronary arteries for abnormalities (dilation, presence of aneurysms, and thrombosis) and serves to monitor for other cardiovascular manifestations during the acute episode such as myocardial dysfunction, valvular abnormalities, or pericardial effusion.

What is the role of other cardiovascular imaging modalities in these patients?

The need for additional cardiac imaging in KD is highly dependent on the severity of the coronary artery involvement and the expert opinion of specialists that routinely care for these patients. Imaging modalities that may be considered include transesophageal echocardiography, cardiac catheterization and angiography, computed tomographic angiography, cardiac magnetic resonance imaging (CMRI), and myocardial perfusion imaging. The selection of imaging technique considers factors such as the necessary information to be obtained, invasive versus noninvasive nature of the examination, radiation exposure, and need for sedation or anesthesia.

What information does CMRI provide? What are some of the risks associated with newer applications of the technique?

Cardiac magnetic resonance imaging represents an important noninvasive diagnostic technique in children with heart disease as it overcomes many limitations of alternate imaging modalities. Specific to KD, CMRI provides anatomic evaluation of the coronary arteries (see Figure 46.1), enables the measurement of cardiac chamber dimensions, and allows for estimates of ventricular function. In addition, the ability to provide detailed myocardial characterization offers clinically relevant information regarding the presence of inflammation, ischemia, and fibrosis.

Stress perfusion CMRI imaging facilitates the detection of vulnerable myocardium and hemodynamic reserve. This technology is increasingly being applied in children with KD and coronary artery involvement for surveillance, risk stratification, and to aid in decisions regarding the need for coronary interventions. Stress imaging involves the administration of a pharmacologic agent that causes coronary hyperemia or vasodilation, exaggerating the differences between healthy and diseased or obstructed arteries, so that flow differences can be assessed. Although the selection of these agents considers their safety profile, their use can be associated with side effects such as flushing,

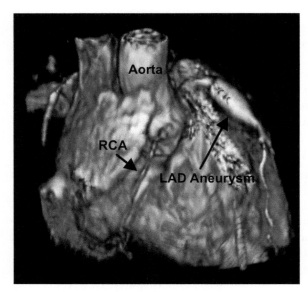

Figure 46.1 Left anterior descending coronary aneurysm in Kawasaki disease. Three-dimensional volume-rendered magnetic resonance image of the coronary arteries in a child with Kawasaki disease depicting a large fusiform aneurysm involving the left anterior descending (LAD) coronary artery. Note the normal appearing right coronary artery (RCA).

diaphoresis, nausea, and vomiting that may disrupt the study in a lightly sedated patient. Even more concerning is the fact that these drugs can trigger rhythm disturbances, alter hemodynamics (increase heart rate and lower systemic arterial blood pressure), and cause bronchospasm. Adequate preparation and a high level of vigilance are of utmost importance during these examinations.

> **Clinical Pearl**
>
> *Stress imaging involves the administration of a pharmacologic agent that causes coronary hyperemia or vasodilation, exaggerating the differences between healthy and diseased/obstructed arteries, so that flow differences can be assessed. These drugs can trigger rhythm disturbances, alter hemodynamics, and cause bronchospasm.*

Anesthetic Implications

What basic principles guide anesthetic care of children with KD?

In children with KD undergoing diagnostic testing or noncardiac procedures that require sedation or anesthesia, management plans should be formulated based on the following basic principles:

- Principles guiding sedation/anesthetic care in this age group in general
- Principles unique to the planned procedure
- Principles specifically related to the pathophysiology of the disease

The first set of principles should be familiar to most that provide sedation and/or anesthesia for infants and children on a regular basis. The second set, although well known to those acquainted with CMRI in children with heart disease, may present a challenge to those less accustomed to these types of studies, thus the need for communication and discussion with the radiologist, cardiologist, and/or technologist involved. The third set of principles requires individual assessment of the child, in particular a detailed appraisal of suspected or confirmed KD-associated cardiac manifestations and the extent of disease in order to identify patients with potential vulnerability for an acute coronary syndrome or cardiac decompensation.

What are key elements in the preprocedural assessment of patients with KD?

A detailed preprocedural/preoperative evaluation is critical for identifying and anticipating factors that may place a child with KD at potential increased risk during anesthesia care. The history and physical examination are essential components of this evaluation. During preanesthetic assessment specific information should be obtained regarding the clinical course of the illness and the nature and severity of cardiac disease, and most specifically, any involvement of the coronary arteries. Cardiac manifestations during the acute phase of the disease, such as myocardial dysfunction due to inflammation (i.e., myocardial edema, myocarditis, or heart failure), valvular regurgitation, or the presence of a pericardial effusion, can significantly impact the anesthetic plan, thus the relevance of ascertaining the phase of disease. In older children, exploration of signs and symptoms suggestive of myocardial ischemia is appropriate, but these are more difficult to investigate in young children. The preanesthetic evaluation should include a review of recent relevant studies such as a 12-lead electrocardiogram (ECG), echocardiogram, and any other relevant study. Recent cardiology evaluations should also be reviewed.

One of the initial steps in the preoperative assessment of this child, as with any patient with serious heart disease, is a consideration of the study indications and an appraisal of the risk-to-benefit ratio. In some cases, there may be a need for a multidisciplinary discussion in advance with appraisal of such factors as suitable study/procedural venue and appropriate area for patient recovery. The immediate preanesthetic evaluation will occasionally establish the need to delay or defer a diagnostic test, intervention, or elective noncardiac surgery in these children.

What issues exist regarding perioperative medication management in these patients?

It is well established that a number of regularly taken drugs can have perioperative effects or interact with anesthetic agents. This is relevant to patients with KD who may be receiving such medications on a daily basis. In most cases, there is no need to discontinue long-term medications prior to scheduled noninvasive cardiac imaging. There are, however, several unique issues in patients with KD to be considered. One is the fact that children may be taking medications that are unfamiliar to the anesthesia provider, and, in many cases, different than those regularly administered to children with other types of heart disease. A detailed review of all medications is suggested to assess for potential drug interactions. Even more important is the fact that some of these patients may be taking antiplatelet and anticoagulation agents routinely. Thus, the potential need exists for these drugs to be adjusted perioperatively. The patient may require preadmission to make changes in anticoagulation strategy, and preparation to manage potential bleeding complications may be necessary depending on the planned intervention or surgical procedure.

Would premedication be appropriate for this patient?

Premedication facilitates parental separation in children. Practical options include either oral or intranasal administration of these agents. Drugs most likely to be considered include midazolam, ketamine, and dexmedetomidine. In this toddler with KD and known coronary artery involvement, the use of premedication, in addition to allowing for smooth parental separation and anxiolysis, can also facilitate advanced placement of an IV catheter, enhancing the overall safety of anesthetic induction. The potential disadvantage of premedication in this setting is related to residual drug effects that could possibly result in delayed hospital discharge, if discharge is planned immediately after the procedure. Judicious dosing of premedication can circumvent some of these challenges and satisfy most needs.

Which procedural considerations influence anesthetic technique in this child?

Most infants and young children require sedation or general anesthesia for CMRI. A number of procedural factors can be taken into consideration when selecting the most appropriate anesthetic technique for these children as listed in Table 46.2.

Which anesthetic techniques are appropriate for children with KD undergoing CMRI?

Several different anesthetic agents and techniques have been safely utilized in children with heart disease undergoing CMRI, including children in high-risk groups. Selection should be guided by the patient pathophysiology and procedural requirements as mentioned. The patient's age and the length of the planned procedure are important factors to consider as well. In the specific case of this toddler undergoing CMRI with plans for inducible myocardial ischemia testing, potential advantages of general anesthesia with tracheal intubation, muscle paralysis, and controlled ventilation over deep sedation include the following:

1. Airway protection provided by endotracheal intubation, in contrast to potential airway obstruction and respiratory depression that may result from deep sedation in a setting of limited patient access
2. Reduced anesthetic depth requirements when neuromuscular blockade is part of a balanced technique, avoiding undesirable hemodynamic effects from higher doses of drugs needed for deep sedation
3. Ability to facilitate image acquisition through breath-holds when general anesthesia is used, reducing overall scanning time and increasing study efficiency

What monitors would be appropriate in this toddler?

As in all patients undergoing an anesthetic, oxygenation, ventilation, circulation, and temperature should be continually evaluated. In the care of this child, standard monitoring as recommended by the American Society of Anesthesiologists would be most appropriate and invasive monitors are likely not warranted. Reliable monitoring is essential, particularly in this toddler, in view of the cardiac disease implying potentially limited cardiovascular reserve. Given the MRI setting, suitable monitors should be utilized. There are several important considerations regarding CMRI and ECG monitoring worth highlighting.

Table 46.2 Procedural Considerations Influencing Selection of Anesthetic Technique for Cardiac Magnetic Resonance Imaging

• **Need for patient immobility**
Although stimulation related to this type of study is minimal, the goal of any anesthetic technique should be avoidance of patient movement in order to facilitate the acquisition of high-quality diagnostic images and to avoid image distortion.

• **Need for breath-holding sequences**
High spatial resolution coronary imaging may require respiratory pauses and periods of apnea to overcome artifacts related to respiratory motion. The combination of a respiratory navigator and availability of advanced software algorithms that integrate respiratory gating may circumvent the issue of lung excursion, allowing for free-breathing imaging techniques at some institutions.

• **Duration of the examination**
The extent of the information to be acquired in the study (anatomic, functional, ischemia assessment), directly influences the length of the examination. In some instances, concurrent imaging of extracardiac structures is planned, further lengthening the scan time.

• **Comfort level of the anesthesia provider**
Provider preferences are important in the selection of anesthetic technique given the particular type of study and unique issues associated with an MRI setting which can include a challenging environment, usually remote setting, limited access to the patient, and not uncommonly, monitoring and equipment issues.

• **Institutional preference**
The standard or usual approach of the facility regarding the conduct of the studies also impacts the anesthetic management plan.

- Sequence acquisition is synchronized to the cardiac cycle; therefore, reliable ECG monitoring that allows for gating is key.
- A number of obstacles within the magnetic environment prevent the acquisition of undistorted signals. Consequently, in most cases a special MRI-conditional ECG lead system is used with three or four electrodes placed at small distances from each other, with filters and settings adjustments primarily suitable for image acquisition synchronization but not for physiologic monitoring. This means that ECG-based ischemia detection, a highly desirable goal in this particular case, may not be feasible in most available CMRI systems.

What type of anesthetic induction and maintenance would be most suitable for this child?

The basic principles of anesthetic induction and maintenance for CMRI in this child do not differ significantly from those that guide care in infants and children with other types of severe heart disease. Minimizing acute changes in preload and afterload and preserving ventricular function are common themes. Maintaining a favorable myocardial supply to demand balance is an important goal in all patients, but particularly in those with a history of KD and coronary artery involvement due to their ischemic propensity. Similar management strategies to those that guide anesthetic care in adults with atherosclerotic coronary artery disease may be considered with the goal of preserving myocardial perfusion and ventricular function.

In general, the strategy for anesthesia induction (inhaled versus IV) in children with heart disease is primarily guided by their clinical status and the extent of cardiac reserve. In children with KD, the severity of cardiac involvement may be added to this appraisal. Inhalation induction with sevoflurane is usually favored in children considered to be at low risk. Conversely, an IV induction with carefully titrated drugs provides a larger margin of safety and is more appropriate in those with poor clinical status, significant cardiac manifestations or when there are concerns for hemodynamic instability during anesthetic induction. Given the presence of large coronary artery aneurysms in this child, options to be considered may include an IV induction with drugs such as etomidate, ketamine, or even carefully titrated very small doses of propofol (large doses are best avoided), or a combined inhaled/IV induction, with titrated doses of these agents. Both of these techniques assume the presence of IV access. Another less desirable option might be that of an inhalation induction, limiting the inspired concentration of the volatile agent, with early establishment of IV access.

This may avoid the stress associated with IV placement, particularly in the setting of difficult access. In most children anesthesia can be maintained with sevoflurane or isoflurane in a mixture of air and oxygen. Small doses of benzodiazepines, narcotics, or adjuvants such as dexmedetomidine may be administered. However, depending on the particular drug and dose, this may impact recovery times and discharge preparedness.

> ### Clinical Pearl
>
> *Maintaining an optimal myocardial supply to demand balance represents an important goal in the anesthetic management of the child with Kawasaki disease and coronary artery involvement due to their potential for myocardial ischemia.*

What special preparation, if any, is required for this type of case?

Given the cardiac disease in this child and potential risk, resuscitation drugs and equipment should be immediately and readily available. In the case of an acute event or emergency, the child should be immediately removed from the MRI scanning room for stabilization or resuscitation as indicated by the situation.

> ### Clinical Pearl
>
> *In children with a history of Kawasaki disease, advanced cardiovascular diagnostic imaging studies are usually performed for suspected or confirmed cardiac disease. In view of potential risks associated with anesthetic care, resuscitation drugs and equipment should be immediately available at all times.*

What data is available regarding risk in patients with KD?

The AHA Scientific Statement on KD proposed a risk stratification system for the development of long-term myocardial ischemia in affected patients based on the severity of past and current coronary involvement, in addition to other factors. As would be expected, the more severe the coronary pathology the higher the predicted risk, and consequently the greater the need for closer surveillance and more aggressive thromboprophylaxis and medical therapy. A similar risk estimation scheme can be applied to anesthesia care, implying a minimal risk level in the absence of coronary artery involvement or in the presence of only coronary artery dilation, and

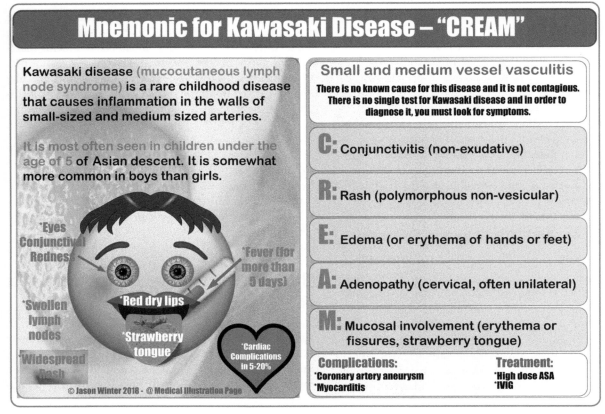

Figure 46.2 Mnemonic for Kawasaki disease: "CREAM." The graphic highlights the clinical features of Kawasaki disease and the diagnostic criteria utilized in an easy to remember mnemonic form. Illustration provided by Jason Winter and reproduced with permission.

greater risk for the development of myocardial ischemia if large or giant aneurysms are present or have persisted at the time that care is being provided.

Unlike the expanding literature addressing postoperative outcomes and risk assessment in the anesthetic care of patients with congenital heart disease undergoing noncardiac surgery, there is extremely limited data regarding anesthetic implications or outcomes in patients with KD. In fact, most of this literature is in the form of case reports. However, despite the small number of publications, the clinical experience to date has been favorable, indicating that despite potential risks, deep sedation or general anesthesia can be provided safely in most children with KD with a very low incidence of complications. An understanding of the disease process, as highlighted in Figure 46.2, and continued adherence to the basic principles discussed in this chapter will likely ensure the best possible outcomes in these children.

Suggested Reading

Daniels L. B., Gordon J. B., and Burns J. C. Kawasaki disease: late cardiovascular sequelae. *Curr Opin Cardiol* 2012; **27**: 572–7.

McCrindle B. W., Rowley A. H., Newburger J. W., et al. Diagnosis, treatment, and long-term management of Kawasaki disease: a scientific statement for health professionals from the American Heart Association. *Circulation* 2017; **135**: e927–99.

Odegard K. C., DiNardo J. A., Tsai-Goodman B., et al. Anaesthesia considerations for cardiac MRI in infants and small children. *Paediatr Anaesth* 2004; **14**: 471–6.

Son M. B. F. and Newburger J. W. Kawasaki disease. *Pediatr Rev* 2018; **39**: 78–90.

Sosa T., Brower L., and Divanovic A. Diagnosis and management of Kawasaki disease. *JAMA Pediatr* 2019; **173**: 278–9.

To L., Krazit S. T., and Kaye A. D. Perioperative considerations of Kawasaki disease. *Ochsner J* 2013; **13**: 208–13.

VACTERL Syndrome

Sana Ullah

Case Scenario

A 1-day-old neonate weighing 2.5 kg, born at 36 weeks estimated gestational age, is scheduled for esophageal atresia/tracheoesophageal fistula repair after initial feeding attempts led to choking, respiratory distress, and cyanosis. A Replogle tube could not be advanced and a chest radiograph showed the tube curled in the upper esophagus, with the presence of gas in the stomach.

An echocardiogram was obtained and showed the following:

- *Tetralogy of Fallot with severe infundibular stenosis*
- *Hypoplastic pulmonary arteries*
- *Right aortic arch*
- *Patent ductus arteriosus*

The pulse oximeter is consistently reading 85% with the patient breathing room air.

Key Objectives

- Describe the common anatomic forms of esophageal atresia/tracheoesophageal fistula.
- Understand the anesthetic implications of VACTERL association.
- Describe airway and ventilatory management strategies during surgical repair of a tracheoesophageal fistula.
- Understand the intraoperative management of ventilatory problems during tracheoesophageal fistula repair.
- Understand the perioperative management of patients with unrepaired tetralogy of Fallot undergoing noncardiac surgery.

Pathophysiology

What is the "VACTERL association"?

An "association" is a group of pathogenetically unrelated malformations occurring together more often than expected by chance without evidence of a single unifying cause. The original acronym Vertebral abnormalities, Anal atresia, Tracheoesophageal fistula with Esophageal atresia, Radial and Renal dysplasia was described in 1973 and later updated to VACTERL with the inclusion of Cardiac anomalies and Limb defects rather than radial anomalies. VACTERL association occurs in approximately 1 in 10,000 to 1 in 40,000 live births with the diagnosis confirmed by the presence of at least three of the aforementioned abnormalities [1]. Patients with VACTERL association frequently require surgery for anal atresia or repair of esophageal atresia/tracheoesophageal fistula (EA/TEF) in the first days of life.

While the cardiac anomalies most commonly associated with VACTERL association are ventricular septal defects (VSD) and tetralogy of Fallot (TOF), a variety of simple and complex cardiac defects are possible, and therefore multidisciplinary perioperative planning in conjunction with cardiac surgery and pediatric cardiology is necessary. Patients with a ductal-dependent cardiac lesion are the most critically ill. In this patient group severe obstruction to either systemic or pulmonary blood flow (PBF) exists, requiring maintenance of a patent ductus arteriosus (PDA) with prostaglandin E_1 (PGE$_1$) infusion and balancing of the pulmonary and systemic blood flows for survival.

> ### Clinical Pearl
>
> *Many of these neonates will require surgery in the first few days of life and will present significant anesthetic challenges, mostly due to cardiac anomalies, which occur in 40%–80% of patients with VACTERL syndrome.*

What is esophageal atresia and what is the most common subtype?

Esophageal atresia (EA) is a congenital malformation of esophageal continuity, associated in over 90% of cases with a fistulous communication of the esophagus with the

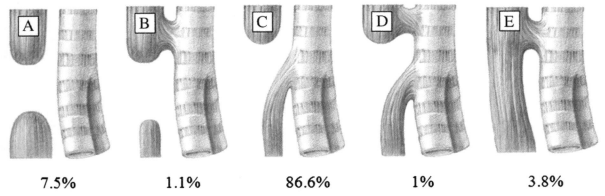

Figure 47.1 Gross classification and frequency of anomalies of the esophagus and trachea. (A) Isolated esophageal atresia without fistula. (B) Esophageal atresia with proximal tracheoesophageal fistula. (C) Esophageal atresia with distal tracheoesophageal fistula. (D) Esophageal atresia with proximal and distal tracheoesophageal fistula, "K-type." (E) Tracheoesophageal fistula without esophageal atresia, "H-type." From Parolini F., et al. *Esophageal atresia with proximal tracheoesophageal fistula: A missed diagnosis.* J Pediatr Surg 2013; **48**: E13–18. With permission.

trachea or a main bronchus. It occurs in approximately 1 in 2500 to 3500 livebirths [2]. Although two main classification systems (Gross and Voght) show the different subtypes, it is preferable to use descriptive language to avoid confusion. The most commonly occurring tracheoesophageal fistula (TEF) is Gross Type C (over 85%), consisting of a blind upper esophageal pouch and a distal tracheoesophageal fistula. (See Figure 47.1.) This results in pulmonary aspiration of upper pouch contents, with ventilation of the stomach via the fistula producing abdominal distension, increased ventilatory difficulty, and aspiration of gastric contents into the trachea via the fistula, producing aspiration pneumonitis. Embryologically, EA/TEF results from incomplete separation of the cranial part of the foregut into respiratory and esophageal parts during the fourth week of gestation. Most cases arise sporadically, but there is an association with certain major chromosomal abnormalities – specifically, trisomy 21, 18, and 13. Trisomy 18 has a very poor prognosis, and it may be necessary to rule out this chromosomal anomaly by urgent karyotyping before surgical planning. VACTERL association occurs in about 25% of EA/TEF infants.

> **Clinical Pearl**
>
> *Approximately 50% of patients with EA/TEF have additional congenital abnormalities. Congenital heart disease is common and can have a significant impact on survival.*

What is tetralogy of Fallot?

Tetralogy of Fallot (TOF) is the most common form of cyanotic congenital heart disease (CHD). The key morphologic abnormality producing the features of the tetrad is anterior and cephalad deviation and malalignment of the infundibular (or outflow) septum of the right ventricle (RV) resulting in the following:

- Right ventricular outflow tract (RVOT) obstruction
- Large, unrestrictive VSD
- Overriding of the aorta
- Right ventricular hypertrophy (RVH)

Right ventricular outflow tract obstruction may be subvalvular secondary to hypertrophied muscle bundles, valvular, or supravalvular due to variable degrees of hypoplasia of the pulmonary annulus and main/branch pulmonary arteries.

Echocardiography is the mainstay of diagnosis. The large VSD and the malaligned infundibular septum are easily demonstrated in the parasternal long axis view. The parasternal short axis and subcostal views are used to define the degree of RVOT obstruction. Additional findings may include an atrial septal defect (ASD), right aortic arch (RAA), left-sided superior vena cava (SVC), and coronary abnormalities. Cardiac catheterization is rarely required for diagnostic purposes and may be risky, as it may provoke a "tet spell" due to catheter manipulation in the RV. However, it is increasingly being used in selected patients for palliative procedures such as stenting of the PDA or the RVOT, as an alternative to surgical aortopulmonary shunt placement. (See Chapter 7 and Figure 7.1.)

What is an acceptable systemic saturation for a neonate with unrepaired TOF?

The systemic hemoglobin–oxygen saturation of a patient with unrepaired TOF can be quite variable, depending on the presence and size of the PDA and the degree of existing RVOT obstruction.

- *"Pink tets"* have normal systemic oxygen saturation due to their mild RVOT obstruction; they predominantly shunt from left-to-right (L-to-R) across the VSD, producing a picture similar to that of congestive heart failure.
- *If the PDA has closed,* systemic saturations will decrease as the RVOT obstruction worsens, and shunting across the VSD then becomes bidirectional. Systemic oxygen saturations in the mid- to high 80s are acceptable as long as they remain stable until the patient undergoes palliation or definitive repair. At the most severe end of the spectrum, shunting across the VSD is mostly right-to-left (R-to-L), producing severe cyanosis.
- *Patients with a PDA* should have adequate PBF and systemic oxygen saturations in the 90s even with RVOT obstruction, as the PDA also provides PBF.

Clinical Pearl

The systemic hemoglobin–oxygen saturation of a patient with unrepaired TOF can be quite variable, depending on the presence and size of the PDA and the degree of existing RVOT obstruction.

What is a "tet" spell? How should one be managed?

Infants can experience hypercyanotic episodes ("tet spells") resulting from infundibular spasm; these spells can occur even in "pink tets." These spells can be provoked by painful stimuli, feeding, or bowel movements, and unless treated promptly can lead to cardiovascular collapse due to severe hypoxemia and lack of PBF.

Treatment of a tet spell includes:

- *Airway*: Administration of 100% oxygen and tracheal intubation if necessary
- *Fluid*: Crystalloid or colloid boluses (15–20 mL/kg) to increase preload and promote antegrade PBF
- *Increase SVR (pharmacologic)*: Phenylephrine bolus(es) titrated to increase SVR and reduce R-to-L shunting across the VSD. Patients with severe RVOT obstruction and recurrent tet spells can require institution of a phenylephrine infusion.
- *Increase SVR (mechanical)*: Mechanical measures include bilateral femoral artery compression or placing the infant into a knee-to-chest position.
- *Sedation/anesthesia*: Intravenous (IV) sedation with morphine (0.05–0.1 mg/kg). If in the operating room,

or intubated, fentanyl (2–4 mcg/kg) can be used to reduce sympathetic overstimulation or increase anesthetic depth.

- *Reduce infundibular spasm*: Esmolol bolus(es) of 50–100 mcg/kg can be administered to reduce the heart rate and infundibular spasm via its negative inotropic effect. Infants who are prone to tet spells are frequently maintained on oral propranolol until surgical repair.

The frequent or continuing occurrence of tet spells resulting in severe hypoxemia and cardiovascular collapse is the main concern for unrepaired TOF patients. In this patient, if adequate PBF is maintained via a PDA maintained by PGE_1, then EA/TEF repair can be performed. After repair, PGE_1 can be stopped to assess whether PBF continues to be adequate without the PDA. If not, due to this patient's size and prematurity, he is most likely not currently a candidate for a complete TOF repair and therefore will require establishment of a stable source of PBF to allow time to grow and await complete TOF repair at 4–6 months of age. This initial palliative procedure can occur either in the cardiac catheterization laboratory in the form of a PDA or RVOT stent, or in the cardiac operating room via creation of a modified Blalock–Taussig shunt (mBT shunt). (See Figure 47.2.)

Clinical Pearl

The mainstays of treatment for a perioperative tet spell are phenylephrine and fluid boluses to increase PBF and reduce R-to-L shunting.

After EA/TEF repair, what is the impact of CHD on patient outcomes?

The two strongest predictors of morbidity and mortality in this patient population are low birth weight (<1500 grams) and the presence of major congenital anomalies. Spitz's prognostic classification from 1994 identified three groups: *Group 1* – birth weight >1500 grams and no major cardiac anomalies (98% survival); *Group 2* – birth weight <1500 grams OR major cardiac anomalies (59% survival); *Group 3* – weight <1500 grams AND major cardiac anomalies (22% survival). Although contemporary outcomes are improved, the overall trend is similar. Perioperatively, patients with CHD have significantly more complications, specifically, difficulties with ventilation and oxygenation, need for inotropic therapy, longer duration of mechanical ventilation, and longer intensive care unit (ICU) and hospital stay [3]. Patients with ductal-dependent cardiac lesions are an even higher risk group compared to non-ductal-dependent lesions [4].

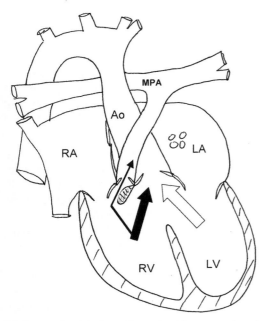

Figure 47.2 Tetralogy of Fallot. Malalignment of conal septum results in overriding aorta, subvalvular pulmonary stenosis, and VSD. With narrowing of RV outflow, desaturated blood flow will be divided (black arrows), a portion to the lungs and a portion across the VSD to the aorta, depending on the relative resistance of each pathway. Systemic saturation will be determined by the amount of desaturated blood mixing with fully saturated blood (white arrow). A right aortic arch is shown. Ao, aorta; LA, left atrium; LV, left ventricle; MPA, main pulmonary artery; RA, right atrium; RV, right ventricle. From Sommer R. J. et al. Pathophysiology of congenital heart disease in the adult. Part III: Complex congenital heart disease. *Circulation* 2008; **117**: 1340–50. With permission.

What is the significance of a RAA for surgical management in this patient?

The incidence of RAA is much higher in patients with CHD. It is commonly associated with TOF (approximately 25% of patients), vascular rings, prematurity, and lower birth weight. Because the RAA courses above the right mainstem bronchus, it can complicate surgical exposure of the TEF, making the repair more difficult. In these cases, the surgeon may prefer a left thoracotomy.

Anesthetic Implications

What are the most important aspects of preoperative workup in this patient?

- **Confirm the diagnosis of EA/TEF**: These patients are frequently premature and have low birth weights. The diagnosis may be suspected prenatally by the presence of polyhydramnios and a small or absent stomach

bubble, resulting from the inability of the fetus to swallow amniotic fluid, but this is not a specific finding. The first feed will result in choking, coughing and possibly cyanosis due to pulmonary aspiration. Attempts to pass a 10 Fr orogastric tube beyond about 10 cm will fail. A whole-body radiograph ("babygram") will reveal the tube curled up in the upper esophageal pouch, and the concomitant appearance of gas in the stomach will confirm the presence of a distal TEF. A "gasless" abdomen usually indicates EA without a fistula. The Replogle tube should be connected to low continuous suction, and the neonate kept nil per os after diagnosis.

- **Echocardiogram**: Every patient with VACTERL association or an EA/TEF needs an echocardiogram to rule out CHD and determine aortic arch sidedness, as both will influence intraoperative management. Repair of EA/TEF is usually done via a right thoracotomy, therefore the presence of a RAA significantly hinders surgical exposure, making the repair more complicated and riskier. In these cases, a left thoracotomy is usually preferred. A RAA, which passes over the right main bronchus, is present in approximately 4% of the normal population, but is much more common in patients with CHD. The presence of a ductal-dependent cardiac lesion (indicating severe systemic or pulmonary outflow obstruction) requires initiation of a PGE_1 infusion to maintain ductal patency until a more definitive cardiac palliation or repair is performed; this will significantly complicate intraoperative management and postoperative recovery for the patient.

Clinical Pearl

Every EA/TEF patient must have a preoperative echocardiogram both to determine aortic arch sidedness for the surgical approach and to define any existent CHD to aid in intraoperative management and prognosis.

What are the airway and ventilation management considerations in this patient?

Until the TEF is surgically controlled, management of intubation and ventilation present the biggest challenges for the anesthesiologist. *The main concerns are loss of tidal volume through the fistula leading to gastric distension and further difficulties in ventilation and oxygenation.* This is more likely to occur if the fistula is large and there is poor lung compliance due to preexisting lung disease secondary to prematurity or aspiration pneumonia. Massive gastric distension and rupture has been reported. Immediate needle decompression of the abdomen may be needed in this situation, followed by either immediate laparotomy and temporary ligation of the distal esophagus or rapid thoracotomy and ligation of the fistula.

What options exist for anesthetic induction in this patient? What intubation technique is preferable?

Awake intubation is traumatic and stressful to the neonate and does not provide optimal intubating conditions. In premature babies, it may also increase the risk of intraventricular hemorrhage due to the hypertensive surge associated with laryngoscopy. It is rarely practiced and cannot be routinely recommended.

Spontaneous ventilation, using a combination of sevoflurane and intravenous drugs (propofol, ketamine, or remifentanil infusion) is widely practiced and has many advantages. However, as propofol may reduce SVR and promote R-to-L shunting, it should either be avoided in this patient or utilized in reduced doses. Due to the negative intrathoracic pressure generated during spontaneous ventilation, inspired gas tends to favor the lungs rather than passing through the fistula into the stomach. As anesthesia is deepened gentle manual assistance with ventilation is usually needed, especially with low birth weight premature neonates. It is widely advocated to maintain spontaneous ventilation until the fistula is ligated, but in practice this is difficult to do with the chest open. Intravenous induction and the use of neuromuscular blockade allow rapid optimal intubating conditions even

though gentle positive pressure ventilation (PPV) is needed. It is the preferred technique in smaller, fragile infants with coexistent cardiac anomalies who may not tolerate deep inhalational anesthesia.

Is preoperative bronchoscopy necessary before surgery?

Routine pre-repair bronchoscopy is performed in only approximately 50%–60% of cases [5]. However, there are several strong arguments in favor of bronchoscopy [6, 7]. It can be done in less than 5 minutes, and in experienced hands, has minimal complications. It allows assessment of the position, size, and number of fistulas, which can be very helpful in correctly positioning the tracheal tube. Approximately 30% of TEFs are within 1 cm of the carina, so precise positioning of the tracheal tube is crucial. Intraoperative difficulties with ventilation or oxygenation can be managed more confidently if one knows the anatomy of the tracheobronchial tree. If the fistula is large or carinal (which can be diagnosed only with a bronchoscope), it can be helpful to occlude it with a Fogarty balloon catheter to improve intraoperative ventilation. A large fistula is also more likely to be inadvertently intubated during the procedure. This is especially important in premature babies with lung disease resulting in poor compliance that will preferentially result in inspired gas flowing into the fistula. Bronchoscopy can identify an upper pouch fistula and may indicate a long-segment atresia if the fistula is located higher in the trachea, which has potential surgical implications. (See Figure 47.3.)

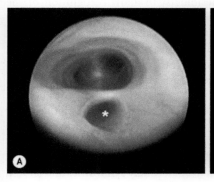
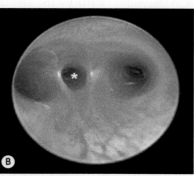

Figure 47.3 Bronchoscopic views showing distal TEF entering the trachea at different levels. (A) The fistula (asterisk) enters in the mid-trachea. (B) The fistula (asterisk) enters at the carina. These images emphasize the importance of preoperative bronchoscopy during airway management and repair. From Rothenberg S. Esophageal atresia and tracheoesophageal fistula malformations. In Holcomb G. W., Murphy J. P., and St. Peter S. D., eds. *Holcomb and Ashcraft's Pediatric Surgery*, 7th ed. Elsevier; 2020: 437–58. With permission.

How should the endotracheal tube be positioned?

The trachea should be intubated with a cuffed endotracheal tube (ETT) positioned below the fistula to seal the airway and minimize ventilation of the stomach. Presurgical bronchoscopy is extremely helpful in aiding accurate ETT placement and predicting ventilation difficulties during the procedure. Traditional teaching is to deliberately intubate the right main stem bronchus, and then, while auscultating over the left chest, slowly withdraw the tube until breath sounds are heard on the left side, indicating the tube position is just above the carina. Rotating the tube to place the bevel anteriorly may also help to occlude the fistula, which lies posteriorly. This will be satisfactory for most cases. However, in approximately 10% of patients, the fistula is located at the carina or the main stem bronchus. Positioning the tube just above the carina may cause gastric distension and ventilatory compromise. In these cases, deliberate endobronchial intubation may be needed to allow adequate ventilation. In cases with a large or a carinal fistula, a balloon catheter may also be employed via a rigid bronchoscope to occlude the fistula. This will improve ventilation and may prevent inadvertent intubation of the fistula during surgical manipulation.

After administration of muscle relaxant, the stomach is increasingly distended with mask ventilation, chest rise is diminished, and oxygen desaturation is occurring. What should be done next?

This scenario suggests loss of pulmonary ventilation through the fistula into the stomach and can rapidly lead to cardiorespiratory compromise. The trachea should be intubated immediately. If the abdomen becomes massively distended, there is a risk of gastric rupture and pneumoperitoneum. Needle decompression or opening the abdomen and placing a temporary ligature around the gastroesophageal junction may be required. If the clinical situation is stable, an immediate thoracotomy and ligation of the fistula may be required to stabilize the patient before proceeding with complete repair.

Is invasive monitoring necessary? What sites could be used for arterial and central access?

Umbilical arterial and venous access can be extremely useful but are not always possible. An arterial line should be placed in all cases, if possible, as there is significant lung retraction and manipulation of the great vessels. In patients with coexisting cardiac anomalies, it is essential for hemodynamic monitoring. The right arm should be avoided for IV and arterial access because it is positioned above the head and may be attached to a bar above the patient's head. Patients with VACTERL association can also have radial abnormalities which may preclude arterial line placement in the arms. In critically ill patients, or those with complex cardiac malformations, central venous access (internal jugular or femoral) is recommended in the event that administration of inotropes becomes necessary. Many neonates may have peripherally inserted central catheters placed prior to surgery.

Clinical Pearl

An arterial line should be placed in all cases, if possible, as there is significant lung retraction and manipulation of the great vessels. In patients with coexisting cardiac anomalies, it is essential for hemodynamic monitoring.

What are the pros and cons of thoracoscopic repair of TEF?

Thoracoscopic TEF repair requires significant technical skill and experience. Contraindications include prematurity, low birth weight, major cardiac defects, and significant abdominal distension. Advantages are avoidance of a thoracotomy with its associated risks of muscle and nerve damage to the chest wall, less pain, better visualization due to magnification, and less retraction on the lung and other mediastinal structures. Disadvantages are mostly due to carbon dioxide (CO_2) insufflation, which can result in significant acidosis that may not be tolerated in patients with delicately balanced pulmonary and systemic blood flows.

What are the key surgical steps in an open surgical repair of EA/TEF?

The patient is positioned for a right posterolateral thoracotomy in the fourth to fifth intercostal space with the right arm positioned above the head. A Replogle tube should be placed in the upper esophageal pouch and will be manipulated by the anesthesiologist to allow recognition of the upper pouch. Extrapleural dissection is carried out to the posterior mediastinum to reveal the azygous vein, which usually overlies the fistula. The azygous vein is usually (but not always) ligated and divided. A very important caveat to this is that the surgeon must be certain that there is no interrupted inferior vena cava (IVC) and azygous continuation that carries the venous drainage from the lower body to the SVC. In this situation, test clamping of the azygous will significantly and rapidly reduce cardiac output. An interrupted IVC with azygous continuation is a common finding in the heterotaxy syndromes and should be ruled out with preoperative echocardiography. The TEF is then identified, ligated, and divided. This usually improves ventilation significantly, and the subsequent surgery is then relatively uneventful. The two esophageal ends are then anastomosed to restore continuity over a feeding tube. Before chest closure, the chest cavity is irrigated with warm saline as positive pressure is applied to the tracheal tube to rule out an air leak.

During dissection, pulse oximetry rapidly decreases from 90% to 50%. What are the possible causes and management?

Problems with ventilation and oxygenation are common during TEF repair and require constant vigilance and close communication with the surgeon. It is important to emphasize that even with initially perfect ETT placement, patient positioning and surgical manipulation can frequently cause ventilatory difficulties. It is helpful to have a flexible fiber-optic bronchoscope immediately available in the operating room. Moderate hypoxemia (SpO$_2$ 80%–90%) usually results from lung retraction and may necessitate increasing inspired oxygen concentration and intermittent reexpansion of the lung to maintain oxygenation. Traction on the small pliant trachea can easily obstruct ventilation. Secretions, blood, or mucus can obstruct small tracheal tubes, and frequent suctioning may be necessary. A balloon catheter placed in the fistula may be displaced into the trachea and cause total obstruction of the airway. Deflation of the balloon and gentle withdrawal of the catheter may solve the problem. Sudden loss of the capnogram with severe desaturation may result from intubation of the fistula. If withdrawing the tube slightly does not restore oxygenation, the airway should be rapidly evaluated by passing the fiberscope through the ETT if time allows. Otherwise, the patient will need emergent reintubation.

In patients with ductal-dependent PBF undergoing a left thoracotomy due to a RAA, surgical retraction on the ductus or pulmonary arteries will cause hypoxemia due to diminished PBF. This may present as decreasing expired CO$_2$ on the capnogram. A tet spell is less likely to manifest in patients with a PDA, but acute infundibular spasm accompanied by hypotension and tachycardia may be enough to increase R-to-L shunting across the VSD causing profound desaturation. The surgeon should be asked to remove any retraction if possible. Manual ventilation should be used to reexpand the upper lung. If these measures do not restore appropriate oxygenation, phenylephrine and a fluid bolus should be administered to raise the SVR and reduce the shunting across the VSD. It is essential to check that the PGE$_1$ infusion has not been interrupted, as this may cause ductal closure.

Clinical Pearl

Mild intraoperative desaturation is common, but a complete loss of ventilation and oxygenation can be due to blockage of the ETT by blood or secretions, intubation of the fistula, or displacement of the Fogarty balloon into the trachea.

When should this patient be extubated?

Patients who undergo uncomplicated EA/TEF repairs can be extubated early, even in the operating room, to minimize trauma to the trachea from the ETT and suctioning. In unstable patients, and those with significant tension on the esophageal anastomosis, it may be beneficial to keep the patient intubated, sedated, and paralyzed for several days with the head in a slightly flexed position.

What modalities can be used for postoperative analgesia?

Opioids are the mainstay of analgesia. Caudal and thoracic epidural catheters can be placed if there are no vertebral or spinal cord anomalies. Intercostal nerve blocks and intrapleural catheters can also be used.

What are some common complications of EA/TEF repair?

Early complications include tracheomalacia, which may be severe enough to require reintubation or surgical aortopexy; anastomotic leaks, most of which can be managed conservatively; esophageal stricture requiring repeated dilations; and recurrence of the fistula. The major late complication is gastroesophageal reflux which may require surgical management if medical management fails.

Ten days later, the patient is extubated and progressing well. A trial of discontinuing PGE$_1$ resulted in severe hypoxemia. Based on size, the patient is not considered a candidate for complete TOF repair yet. What other management options exist?

Neonatal TOF repair, although feasible, is associated with higher morbidity and mortality [8]. In addition, several factors may mitigate against neonatal repair, including small patient size, gestational age, comorbidities, coronary anatomy, and inadequate branch pulmonary artery size and arborization. Repair is generally deferred until 3–6 months of age.

For ductal-dependent patients, there are several options. Recently, stenting the PDA or the RVOT in the cardiac catheterization laboratory has become a viable alternative with outcomes either equivalent or superior to surgical shunt placement. It is a less invasive procedure with shorter ICU and hospital length of stays. Surgical creation of a systemic-to-pulmonary shunt such as a mBTS can also be considered [9].

What anesthetic issues should be considered for ductal stent placement?

Although relatively simple in principle, this procedure requires significant experience and planning for a successful outcome [10]. The key points are outlined here.

Location: The procedure should be performed in a cardiac catheterization laboratory with general endotracheal anesthesia.

Pharmacologic: Inotropic infusions (dopamine or epinephrine, and phenylephrine) should be available. A heparin infusion will also be needed after stent placement to prevent in-stent thrombosis.

Monitoring: Invasive monitoring is usually not necessary.

Surgical team back-up including extracorporeal membrane oxygenation (ECMO) is essential in case of irreversible ductal spasm or ductal tearing.

Procedural considerations:

- Knowledge of ductal morphology is essential, including its origin (head and neck vessels, underside of aorta, descending aorta), length, and tortuosity.
- PGE_1 may be stopped several hours before the procedure to allow the PDA to shrink and allow a better assessment of the ductal size to choose the appropriately sized stent. It is important to leave the PGE_1 infusion in line so that it may be restarted immediately in case of ductal spasm during the procedure.
- Vascular access is chosen based on the site yielding the straightest route to the ductus. This may be the carotid or axillary artery.
- The most critical period occurs when the wire is being manipulated in the ductus, as this can cause sudden ductal spasm and rapid hemodynamic collapse, requiring rapid management with stent placement, resuscitation with inotropes and vasopressors, and reinstitution of PGE_1. ECMO rescue may be required if these measures fail.

Post-procedure: Heparin infusion and aspirin are usually started to prevent in-stent thrombosis and reduce thrombotic complication in the access vessel.

Complications: Vascular injury, stent thrombosis, and the need for reintervention for stent dilation or additional stent placement.

References

1. B. Solomon. VACTERL/VATER Association. *Orphanet J Rare Dis* 2011; **6**: 56.
2. L. Spitz. Esophageal atresia. *Orphanet J Rare Dis* 2007; **2**: 24.
3. L. K. Diaz, E. A. Akpek, R. Dinavahi, et al. Tracheoesophageal fistula and associated congenital heart disease: implications for anesthetic management and survival. *Paediatr Anaesth* 2005; **10**: 862–9.
4. K. Puri, S. A. Morris, C. M. Mery, et al. Characteristics and outcomes of children with ductal-dependent congenital heart disease and esophageal atresia/tracheoesophageal fistula: a multi-institutional analysis. *Surgery* 2018; **163**: 847–53.
5. D.R. Lal, S. K. Gadepalli, C. D. Downard, et al. Infants with esophageal atresia and right aortic arch: characteristics and outcomes from the Midwest Pediatric Surgery Consortium. *J Pediatr Surg* 2018; **54**: 688–92.
6. K. Taghavi and M D. Stringer. Preoperative laryngotracheobronchoscopy in infants with esophageal atresia: why is it not routine? *Pediatr Surg Int* 2018; **34**: 3–7.
7. P. Atzori, B. D. Iacobelli, S. Bottero, et al. Preoperative tracheobronchoscopy in newborns with esophageal atresia: does it matter? *J Pediatr Surg* 2006; **41**: 1054–7.
8. R. S. Loomba, M. W. Buelow, and R. K. Woods. Complete repair of tetralogy of Fallot in neonatal versus non-neonatal period: a meta-analysis. *Pediatr Cardiol* 2017; **38**: 893–901.
9. J. R. Bentham, N. K. Zava, W. J. Harrison, et al. Duct stenting versus modified Blalock–Taussig shunt in neonates with duct-dependent pulmonary blood flow: associations with clinical outcomes in a multicenter national study. *Circulation* 2018; **137**: 581–8.
10. V. Aggarwal, C. J. Petit, A. C. Glatz, et al. Stenting of the ductus arteriosus for ductal-dependent pulmonary blood flow: current techniques and procedural considerations. *Congenit Heart Dis* 2019; **14**: 110–15.

Suggested Reading

Knottenbelt G., Costi D., Stephens P., et al. An audit of anesthetic management and complications of tracheo-esophageal fistula and esophageal atresia repair. *Pediatr Anesth* 2011; **22**: 268–74.

Lal D. R., Gadepalli S. K., Downard C. D., et al. Perioperative management and outcomes of esophageal atresia and tracheoesophageal fistula. *J Pediatr Surg* 2017; **52**: 1245–51.

Puri K., Morris S. A., Mery C. M., et al. Characteristics and outcomes of children with ductal-dependent congenital heart disease and esophageal atresia/tracheoesophageal fistula: a multi-institutional analysis. *Surgery* 2018; **163**: 847–53.

Chapter 48

Hurler Syndrome

Kirk Lalwani and Erin Conner

Case Scenario

An 11-year-old girl with Hurler syndrome presents to the gastrointestinal suite for an aerodigestive evaluation including upper endoscopy and bronchoscopy. She has had two prior anesthetics. At the time of her first anesthetic for a Nissen fundoplication-gastrostomy tube placement at 3 years of age her airway was described as a Grade III view with a Wis-Hipple 1.5 blade utilizing direct laryngoscopy. She subsequently had another anesthetic at 8 years of age for open reduction of a supracondylar fracture, at which time a view was unobtainable on direct laryngoscopy with either a Miller 2 or Macintosh 2 blade. She required two-handed bag-mask ventilation; a laryngeal mask airway was ultimately placed, and the case proceeded without incident.

Echocardiography performed 6 months prior revealed the following:

- *Moderate-to-severe mitral regurgitation*
- *Dilated cardiomyopathy with mildly impaired ventricular function*

Key Objectives

- Discuss the pathogenesis of the mucopolysaccharidoses.
- Review the anesthetic considerations for patients with Hurler syndrome.
- Summarize hemodynamic goals for a patient with mitral regurgitation.
- Develop a plan to manage a known difficult airway in a patient with Hurler syndrome.
- Outline an anesthetic plan for aerodigestive evaluation.
- List potential airway management techniques.

Pathophysiology

What are the mucopolysaccharidoses?

The mucopolysaccharidoses (MPS) are a diverse group of lysosomal storage diseases caused by the genetic insufficiency of enzymes contributing to the degradation of glycosaminoglycans (GAGs). Glycosaminoglycans are then deposited in multiple organs of the body leading to widespread dysfunction, characteristic facies, and in some cases, early mortality. The constellation of signs and symptoms varies according to the specific enzyme deficiency.

These patients present multiple challenges to the anesthesiologist. Key features include difficult mask ventilation, difficult intubation, cardiac disease, coronary ischemia, obstructive sleep apnea (OSA), and skeletal abnormalities. Careful and thorough preoperative evaluation is crucial for safe management and anesthetic planning, and should be focused on airway management, as well as the cardiovascular, pulmonary, and neurologic systems. Cardiac valvulopathies and ventricular dysfunction are common and must be managed appropriately. Postoperatively, consideration should be given to caring for these patients in a high-acuity environment, depending on the type of surgery and severity of the disease.

What are GAGs?

Glycosaminoglycans are polysaccharides (dermatan, heparan, keratan, and chondroitin sulfates) that are degraded by lysosomal hydrolases. They have many functions in the body, including lubrication of joints, cell growth, regulation of proliferation, and adhesion to cell surfaces in molecules. When GAGs cannot be degraded, they accumulate and damage vital organs, bones, joints, and the central nervous system.

What is the classification system for MPS?

There are 7 types of MPS disorders (I, II, III, IV, VI, VII, and IX) and 11 subtypes. (See Table 48.1.)

What is the pathogenesis of Hurler syndrome, or MPS I?

Previously known as "gargoylism," MPS I is an autosomal recessive disorder caused by a deficiency of α-L-iduronidase, an enzyme required to break down dermatan sulfate and heparan sulfate, both of which accumulate

Table 48.1 Classification of Mucopolysaccharidoses

Type	Eponym	Defective Enzyme	Accumulated Product	Clinical Symptoms	Notes
IH IH/S IS	Hurler Hurler-Scheie Scheie	Alpha-L-iduronidase	Heparan sulfate, dermatan sulfate	Intellectual disability, micrognathia, coarse facial features, macroglossia, retinal degeneration, corneal clouding, cardiomyopathy, hepatosplenomegaly	The Hurlers form of type 1 is most severe, though all three may express these features
II	Hunter	Iduronate sulfatase	Heparan sulfate, dermatan sulfate	Intellectual disability, as well as the same symptoms as type I in more mild form	Only MPS that is X-linked recessive inheritance; all others are autosomal recessive
III A–D	Sanfilippo	A: Heparan sufamidase B: N-acetylglucosaminidase C: Heparan-α-glucosaminide, N-acetyltransferase D: N-acetylglucosamine 6-sulfatase	Heparan sulfate	Developmental delay, severe hyperactivity, spasticity, motor dysfunction	Most pronounced neurologic deficits of all MPS
IVA-B	Morquio	A: Galactose-6-sulfate sulfatase B: β-galactosidase	A: Keratan sulfate, chondroitin 6-sulfate B: Keratan sulfate	Severe skeletal dysplasia, short stature, motor dysfunction	
VI	Maroteaux-Lamy	N-acetylgalactosamine-4-sulfatase	Dermatan sulfate	Severe skeletal dysplasia, short stature, motor dysfunction, kyphosis, heart defects	
VII	Sly	β-glucuronidase	Heparan sulfate, dermatan sulfate, chondroitin 4,6-sulfate	Hepatomegaly, skeletal dysplasia, short stature, corneal clouding, developmental delay	
IX	Natowicz	Hyaluronidase	Hyaluronic acid	Nodular soft-tissue masses around joints with pain and swelling, short stature, normal intelligence	

in body tissues. Diagnosed at an average age of 9 months, MPS I is the most severe form of MPS. Without treatment, death occurs within the first decade of life. The manifestations grow progressively worse as the child gets older, and these patients have been described as some of the most challenging in all of pediatric anesthesia.

Clinical Pearl

Mucopolysaccharidosis I is the most severe form of MPS, with an average age at diagnosis of 9 months. Without treatment, death occurs within the first decade of life.

Are there any variants of MPS I?

Hurler–Scheie and Scheie syndromes are often referred to as the intermediate and mild forms of MPS I, respectively. Cognitive impairment is mild in Hurler–Scheie, but physical manifestations including growth retardation are severe.

Scheie syndrome patients have near-normal intelligence and close to normal life expectancy. Since physical manifestations are milder, these patients are often diagnosed later in life.

What are the characteristic features of Hurler Syndrome (MPS I)?

Patients with Hurler syndrome have characteristic coarse facies, macrocephaly, umbilical and inguinal hernias, angular thoracolumbar kyphosis (gibbus deformity), joint stiffness, progressive skeletal dysplasia (dysostosis multiplex), and growth retardation. They may also have ocular abnormalities, progressive neurologic disease, hydrocephalus, developmental delay, and hepatosplenomegaly. Cardiac and respiratory issues include macroglossia, airway compromise, obstructive sleep apnea (OSA), chronic and recurrent respiratory infections, restrictive lung disease, cardiac valvular disease, coronary artery disease (CAD), and cardiomyopathy.

What treatments are available for MPS?

Hematopoietic stem cell transplantation is effective at prolonging survival, preserving cognitive function, and reducing hepatosplenomegaly and sleep apnea. Weekly enzyme replacement infusion therapy with laronidase has also been effective at reducing liver volume, urinary GAG excretion, functional capacity, sleep apnea, joint flexion, visual acuity, and left ventricular (LV) hypertrophy. Enzyme replacement therapy allows minimal improvement in cognitive, skeletal, ocular, and heart valve function. However, most patients develop antibodies to laronidase that limit enzyme cell uptake.

What cardiac defects are commonly associated with MPS?

Cardiac defects are common in MPS, occurring in 60%–100% of patients. They are more common in syndromes where dermatan sulfate breakdown is affected (MPS I, II, and VI). Clinical signs and symptoms are uncommon despite the early development of cardiac lesions in severe forms of the disease, such as MPS I. Left-sided valvular lesions are more common as a result of thickened leaflets leading to regurgitation or stenosis. Progressive valvular disease ultimately leads to ventricular hypertrophy, overload, and dysfunction. Diffuse coronary artery narrowing or occlusion is most common in MPS I and II. Apical aneurysms have also been described along with diffuse narrowing of the great vessels, dilation of the aorta, and associated hypertension. Conduction defects are often seen in some types of MPS as well. Acute cardiomyopathy associated with endocardial fibroelastosis has been a presenting condition in some infants with MPS I at <1 year of age.

Clinical Pearl

Patients with MPS should have a full cardiovascular evaluation at time of diagnosis followed by regular monitoring (every 1–2 years for types I and VI and every 2–3 years for type II) as well as evaluation before any major surgical intervention. Full evaluation should include right arm and leg blood pressure measurements, careful auscultation, transthoracic echocardiogram, and 12-lead electrocardiogram.

Anesthetic Implications

What are the specific preoperative assessment concerns in a patient with MPS?

Cardiac: If the patient has MPS subtype I, II, or VI, a focused cardiovascular history and physical must be

performed. Many of these children will not overtly manifest significant cardiac clinical signs and symptoms (in part due to inactivity and communication difficulties), and therefore require additional evaluation by their cardiologist. A recent echocardiogram (within 6 months) should be considered a necessity. While not yet routine in MPS patients, a dobutamine-stress induced echocardiogram to assess LV function and areas of under-perfused myocardium should be considered. This may lead to evaluation for CAD, which can commonly exist in MPS patients. Unfortunately, MPS patients usually develop diffuse coronary disease, which is less easily detected but still carries significant risk.

Airway: Obstructive sleep apnea occurs in >80% of patients with MPS I and II. Details of polysomnography, previous airway surgeries or the use of continuous positive airway pressure (CPAP) should be investigated in detail. Severe OSA with chronic hypoxemia can also result in pulmonary hypertension; if suspected, pulmonary hypertension should also be assessed by echocardiography.

Pulmonary: While many MPS patients have restrictive lung disease and may have had pulmonary function testing done, these tests can be difficult to interpret given the lack of standardized data in patients who often have significantly shortened stature and skeletal abnormalities. Therefore, these results should be taken into consideration, but not solely relied on. Treatment for chronic infections, and optimization of any reactive airway disease or chronic bronchospasm should be noted. Consultation with a pulmonologist may be required.

Neurologic: A neurologic exam focusing on hyperreflexia or other signs of neurologic compromise from cervical spine stenosis should be done in patients with MPS type I, II, IV, and VI. Flexion/extension imaging studies may be indicated.

Which MPS variants are associated with a difficult airway? What features make their airway management difficult?

Most serious anesthetic complications in patients with MPS are airway related: these can include obstruction, difficulty with oxygenation and ventilation, and difficulties with advanced airway device placement. Airway-related difficulties can also lead to possible cardiopulmonary compromise, which is particularly concerning in patients who may also have cardiovascular involvement depending on their MPS subtype. Difficulty with airway obstruction and intubation are most pronounced in patients with MPS

I and II, though the overall difficult airway incidence for all subtypes of MPS is >75%.

- **Upper airway obstruction** may be obvious on induction, with sternal and intercostal retractions and a poor capnography trace. A precordial stethoscope is useful, simple, and easy to use for early detection of compromised breath sounds.
- **Bag-mask ventilation** may also be more difficult due to a flattened nasal bridge, midface hypoplasia, mandibular abnormalities, and/or a short, thick neck.
- **Tracheostomy** can be technically difficult due to a short, thick neck. In an emergency securing a surgical airway in these patients may take longer than anticipated, so if there is significant concern about the airway, having a surgeon and necessary surgical equipment available at induction may be prudent.
- **The internal upper airway** may be further obstructed due to narrowing caused by the accumulation of GAGs, resulting in macroglossia, adenotonsillar hypertrophy, and thickened pharyngeal tissues.
- **Laryngeal and tracheal** accumulations of GAGs may also occur, causing distortion of normal structures and making identification of the glottis difficult. Given their airway narrowing, these patients may not be able to accommodate the expected age-appropriate endotracheal tube (ETT) size. Multiple sizes should be available, and the first intubation attempt should be with a full size smaller cuffed ETT than the patient's age would predict.
- **Excessive and thick secretions** can affect visualization of the glottis, particularly with fiberoptic intubation. Treatment with an antisialagogue preoperatively is useful.
- **Cervical spine abnormalities** may be seen in patients with MPS type I, II, IV, and VI. Spinal canal narrowing can lead to spinal cord compression with even minor neck manipulation. Both MPS type IV and VI may have associated atlantoaxial instability due to odontoid hypoplasia. This must always be considered and included in the plan for airway management and positioning. Manual in-line stabilization during airway management should be planned for all MPS patients.

The degree of obstruction on induction and intubation portends difficulty with ventilation post-extubation and should alert the provider to consider having CPAP available postoperatively, or even electively keeping the patient intubated overnight or longer in the intensive care unit (ICU) depending on the difficulty of intubation, length of surgery, and the patient's respiratory reserve.

Clinical Pearl

All MPS patients should be considered a difficult airway until proven otherwise. Difficulty with airway obstruction and intubation are most pronounced in patients with MPS I and II. In an emergency securing a surgical airway in these patients may take longer than anticipated, so if there is significant concern about the airway, having a surgeon and necessary surgical equipment available at induction may be prudent.

What factors have been associated with pediatric airway complications?

In a prospective multicenter study from the Pediatric Difficult Intubation (PeDI) Registry, several factors were associated with any complication (severe or nonsevere):

- Multiple (>2) tracheal intubation attempts
- Weight <10 kg
- Short thyromental distance
- Abnormal airway physical examination
- Persistent direct laryngoscopy (DL) attempts, with an incremental increase in the occurrence of complications with each additional intubation attempt

The success rate of first intubation attempts was lowest for DL (3%), and similar for video laryngoscopy (55%) and fiberoptic bronchoscopy (54%). Early transition to a non-DL method (after the first or second DL attempt) was also associated with fewer complications than cases with late transition (>2 DL attempts). Hypoxemia was the most common nonsevere complication that occurred (9% of intubation attempts). Interestingly, only 10% of practitioners provided supplemental oxygen during intubation attempts, which could have contributed to interrupted attempts and additional attempts, thus increasing the incidence of complications. The incidence of cardiac arrest in children with difficult intubation in this study was 1:68, which is substantially higher than in the general pediatric population of 1–2 in 10,000, and hypoxemia was no doubt a contributory factor in most of these arrests.

In another PeDI Registry multicenter study investigators found that on the first intubation attempt fiberoptic intubation via a supraglottic airway was more successful than video laryngoscopy in children <1 year old. They also noted that the incidence of hypoxemia was lower when continuous ventilation through the supraglottic airway was used throughout the intubation attempt.

What strategies from the PeDI Registry can prove useful for optimizing airway management in MPS patients?

Three strategies can be utilized from these studies to improve the management of difficult intubation and reduce complications:

1. In a known difficult intubation, consider video laryngoscopy or fiberoptic bronchoscopy instead of DL on the first intubation attempt.
2. If DL is used initially, transition early (after two attempts) to an alternate method.
3. Insufflate oxygen continuously into the airway at a sufficient flow rate for passive oxygenation to occur during all intubation attempts to reduce hypoxemia and the number of interrupted intubation attempts.

Clinical Pearl

Use or transition early to methods other than DL for endotracheal intubation and insufflate oxygen continuously during intubation attempt(s).

What are the anesthetic considerations for patients with mitral regurgitation?

The regurgitant volume in mitral regurgitation (MR) depends on the size of the mitral valve orifice, the heart rate (HR) and the left ventricle–left atrial (LV–LA) pressure gradient. Major hemodynamic goals for anesthetic management of patients with MR include maintenance of relative tachycardia, reduced afterload, and avoidance of significant increases in preload. When HR is decreased the increased diastolic time allows the LV to overfill, further distending the valve annulus and worsening regurgitation. Caution must also be taken with volume administration, as excessive fluid administration can also worsen left ventricular dilation. Increased afterload increases the LV–LA pressure gradient, causing more regurgitant flow. (See Table 48.2.)

Clinical Pearl

Major hemodynamic goals for anesthetic management of patients with MR include maintenance of relative tachycardia, reduced afterload, and avoidance of significant increases in preload.

Table 48.2 Common Valvulopathies and Hemodynamic Goals

Lesion	Preload/Volume	Afterload/SVR	Heart Rate
Aortic stenosis	Increase	Increase	Decrease
Aortic regurgitation	Decrease	Decrease	Increase
Mitral stenosis	Increase	Maintain or Increase	Decrease
Mitral regurgitation	Maintain	Decrease	Increase

What other anesthetic concerns exist for patients with MPS?

Given the potential for difficult airway management in the setting of spinal pathology, it is worth considering whether a patient would benefit from spinal cord neuromonitoring with evoked potentials. While this would be expected in spinal surgery, it should also be considered in cases that require any significant head movement, or in particularly long cases requiring nonneutral head positions.

Patients with MPS often develop restrictive pulmonary disease secondary to thoracic cage abnormalities or compromised excursion of the diaphragm secondary to hepatosplenomegaly. Respiratory therapies to address possible elevations in inspiratory pressures and/or bronchospasm should be readily available.

Excessive secretions and gastroesophageal reflux disease (GERD) should be expected in all MPS patients. While a rapid sequence intubation would not be advisable for a patient with a difficult airway, these patients should be considered high-risk for aspiration and precautions to minimize this risk should be taken.

When is intraoperative neuromonitoring useful or required when caring for patients with MPS?

Mucopolysaccharidosis patients often suffer from angular thoracolumbar kyphosis/gibbus deformity, which may predispose their spinal cord to intraoperative injury. There are multiple case reports of MPS patients presenting with postsurgical neurologic deficits after nonspinal surgery, leading several institutions to employ somatosensory evoked potential and transcranial motor evoked potential monitoring intraoperatively for these patients. While there are no defined guidelines, expert opinion and available evidence suggest the use of intraoperative neuromonitoring (IONM) for MPS patients who meet the following criteria: significant kyphoscoliosis (>60 degrees), anticipated procedural duration >90 minutes, and/or expectation of extensive blood loss or hemodynamic fluctuations. In a recent report by Kandil et al. from Cincinnati Children's Hospital Medical Center, when these criteria were utilized to risk stratify patients, no new postoperative neurologic deficits were noted in patients who did not meet criteria for IONM, and when IONM was used for patients meeting criteria, 14% had significant changes detected with IONM which necessitated intervention.

Clinical Pearl

As the use of volatile anesthetic agents can significantly impact the reliability of IONM, total intravenous anesthesia (TIVA) with propofol and/or dexmedetomidine is the preferred anesthetic technique as these agents have the least effect on IONM signals.

What are the anesthetic considerations for these procedures?

Combined esophagogastroduodenoscopy (EGD) and bronchoscopy procedures are becoming more common as otolaryngology, gastroenterology, and pulmonology providers coordinate to simultaneously evaluate the anatomy of the upper airway, digestive, and respiratory systems in patients with complex issues during one anesthetic episode. Airway management may also require multidisciplinary coordination. However, if the patient is not having an airway evaluation and simply a combined bronchoscopy and EGD, these procedures could be performed with a natural airway, depending on the patient's anatomy and degree of airway obstruction. However, in a patient with likely obstructive airway disease and the potential for difficult intubation, this may not be an ideal way to ensure adequate ventilation.

Clinical Pearl

A preoperative discussion should be held with all proceduralists involved in a planned aerodigestive evaluation, focusing on the sequence of procedures, the airway management plan, and the management of potential complications.

Should this case be performed in a location that is remote from the general operating rooms?

Where an aerodigestive evaluation occurs is often dependent on the institution and the available resources. As patients with MPS are likely to have complex upper airway anatomy, OSA or other pathologies resulting in more challenging airway management and ventilation, deciding whether this case can safely be performed in a gastrointestinal suite depends on the proximity of the equipment needed for difficult airway management as well as the support personnel able to respond in case of difficult/impossible ventilation and/or intubation. The size and setup of the room in a possible emergent situation is also an important consideration.

How could induction and maintenance of anesthesia be managed in this patient?

Given the likelihood of difficult bag-mask ventilation and intubation, this patient should have an intravenous line (IV) placed preoperatively. Premedication such as oral midazolam can be given to facilitate IV placement, though caution should be taken with dosing to avoid significant respiratory depression and it may be advisable to reduce the premedication dose by 20%–30%. Cardiorespiratory monitoring should be established and maintained once medication has been administered. Induction agents should be chosen that meet the goals of maintaining both spontaneous ventilation and appropriate hemodynamics in a patient with MR and potentially reduced ventricular function. Ketamine will allow maintenance of spontaneous ventilation and hemodynamics, though an antisialagogue such as glycopyrrolate should be given to avoid increasing secretions. Dexmedetomidine may be considered but may induce excessive bradycardia; pretreatment with glycopyrrolate may assist in adequately maintaining HR. Dexmedetomidine may also prolong emergence in these patients. The use of a muscle relaxant in an unproven airway should be withheld if at all possible and is usually not necessary for a fiberoptic intubation or laryngeal mask airway (LMA) placement. The use of neuromuscular blocking agents is acceptable for MPS patients as indicated by their surgical procedure requirements once they are intubated.

Anesthesia may be maintained with inhalational agents but patients with moderate to severe MR may be very sensitive to volatile agents. A balanced technique allowing volatile agent to be used at a lower MAC is generally preferable. Continuous infusions such as remifentanil and/or ketamine and/or propofol can also be used to achieve anesthetic goals without hemodynamic compromise.

Can this case be performed without endotracheal intubation? Could these procedures be done with an LMA?

Both EGD and bronchoscopy can be performed with a natural airway and spontaneous ventilation. However, in an MPS patient, this decision should not be made lightly.

After induction, if the patient is able to maintain adequate ventilation and oxygenation while receiving TIVA with supplemental oxygen via nasal cannula, it may be safe to proceed with a natural airway. While the bronchoscopy portion of the procedure could be completed through the lumen of an LMA, the risk of LMA displacement with EGD exists. However, one could consider using an intubating LMA during bronchoscopy and placing an ETT for the endoscopy portion of the procedure if appropriate.

> **Clinical Pearl**
>
> *Consider early use of an LMA in MPS patients who do not require endotracheal intubation, or in MPS patients with difficult or failed intubation attempts.*

What are the considerations for extubation and postoperative management of these patients?

While early extubation is preferred to avoid significant airway swelling associated with ETT placement, this must be done cautiously. Patients should be fully awake, coughing vigorously, breathing adequately, and moving deliberately before they are extubated. All equipment should be available and ready for reintubation. Depending on the level of difficulty of initial intubation consideration can be given to leaving a tube exchanger in place. Transitioning the patient immediately post-extubation to CPAP is generally prudent. If extubation is delayed for any reason, the patient may benefit from a fiberoptic airway evaluation for swelling, debris, or bleeding prior to extubation. At the time of extubation the same precautions regarding available equipment and personnel should be followed even if the patient is no longer in the OR setting.

In some MPS patients with severe lung disease and/or challenging airway management it may be safer to keep the ETT in place and allow the effects of the anesthetic drugs and any iatrogenic airway edema to dissipate overnight in the ICU. This scenario is more likely with prolonged surgery and this decision should be made on a case-by-case basis.

If extubation occurs in the OR, the patient should be transitioned to CPAP immediately, and consideration should be made to continuing this in the ICU setting until the patient has fully emerged from anesthesia.

Should laryngospasm occur, how should it be managed?

The best cure for laryngospasm is prevention. Ensuring that the patient is wide awake (grimacing and making purposeful movements) and has a dry oropharynx (via suction and antisialagogue administration) makes laryngospasm less likely following extubation. The placement of an oral airway soon after extubation can also precipitate laryngospasm. Waking patients up following placement of an appropriately sized nasopharyngeal airway is extremely useful to avoid post-extubation obstruction and is far less likely to cause laryngospasm. Applying a jaw thrust in the "laryngospasm notch" may also be useful. If laryngospasm does occur, the use of CPAP and small doses of propofol may be sufficient to break the spasm without resultant apnea. If these measures are insufficient, administration of succinylcholine may be required, generally in a much smaller dose than needed for full paralysis.

If reintubation is required, serious consideration should be given to leaving the patient intubated overnight for the reasons mentioned earlier.

Suggested Reading

Braunlin E. A., Harmatz P. R., Scarpa M., et al. Cardiac disease in patients with mucopolysaccharidosis: presentation, diagnosis and management. *J Inherit Metab Dis* 2011; **34**: 1183–97.

Burjek N. E., Nishisaki A., Fiadjoe J. E., et al. Videolaryngoscopy versus fiber-optic intubation through a supraglottic airway in children with a difficult airway: an analysis from the multicenter Pediatric Difficult Intubation Registry. *Anesthesiology* 2017; **127**: 432–40.

Donaldson M. D. C., Pennock C. A., Berry P. J., et al. Hurler syndrome with cardiomyopathy in infancy. *J Pediatr* 1989; **114**: 430–2.

Fiadjoe J. E., Nishisaki A., Jagannathan N., et al. Airway management complications in children with difficult tracheal intubation from the Pediatric Difficult Intubation (PeDI) registry: a prospective cohort analysis. *Lancet Respir Med* 2016; **4**: 37–48.

Kandil A. I., Petit C. S., Berry L. N., et al. Tertiary pediatric academic institution's experience with intraoperative neuromonitoring for nonspinal surgery in children with mucopolysaccharidosis, based on a novel evidence-based care algorithm. *Anesth Analg* 2019: DOI: 10.1213/ANE.000000000004215, PMID: 31082970.

Osthaus W. A., Harendza T., Witt L. H., et al. Paediatric airway management in mucopolysaccharidosis 1: a retrospective case review. *Eur J Anaesthesiol* 2012; **29**: 204–7.

Sawamoto K., Stapleton M., Almeciga-Diaz C. J., et al. Therapeutic options for mucopolysaccharidoses: current and emerging treatments. *Drugs* 2019; **79**: 1103–34.

Stapleton M., Arunkumar N., Kubaski F., et al. Clinical presentation and diagnosis of mucopolysaccharidoses. *Mol Genet Metab* 2018; **125**: 4–17.

Walker R., Belani K. G., Braunlin E. A., et al. Anesthesia and airway management in mucopolysaccharidosis. *J Inherit Metab Dis* 2013; **36**: 211–19.

Chapter 49

Long QT Syndrome

Kelly L. Grogan and Susan C. Nicolson

Case Scenario

A 16-year-old female with congenital long QT syndrome presents for endoscopic nasal surgery due to multiple sinus infections requiring antibiotics and steroids. She was diagnosed with long QT syndrome at age 13 years after having a syncopal episode while running track. An electrocardiogram showed a heart-rate corrected QT interval of >500 ms while transthoracic echocardiography revealed a structurally normal heart with normal function. Genetic testing confirmed the diagnosis of long QT2. She was started on β-blockade and despite compliance experienced additional syncopal episodes. She underwent implantable cardioverter–defibrillator placement 18 months ago and had significant postoperative nausea and vomiting after that procedure. Since then, she has had no further syncopal episodes and continues on nadolol as her only medication. Her implantable cardioverter–defibrillator was last interrogated 6 months prior and was functioning normally at that time.

Key Objectives

- Understand the major subtypes of congenital long QT syndrome.
- Discuss the anesthetic implications of long QT syndrome.
- Describe the preoperative evaluation and perioperative management of a patient with a cardiovascular implantable electronic device.
- Describe the surgical implications for a patient with a cardiovascular implantable electronic device.

Pathophysiology

What is long QT syndrome?

Congenital long QT syndrome (LQTS), with an estimated prevalence of 1 in 2,000 to 2,500, is a group of genetically transmitted disorders characterized by abnormal cardiac repolarization resulting in QT interval prolongation that predisposes patients to the acute onset of ventricular arrhythmias, most notably torsades de pointes (TdP), which may cause syncope or sudden cardiac death (SCD) [1, 2]. The ion channel dysfunction that prolongs cellular repolarization is most often caused by decreased outward potassium current I_{Ks} (LQT1, LQT5) or I_{Kr} (LQT2, LQT6), or by enhanced activity of mutant inward sodium current (LQT3). Long QT syndrome is usually transmitted in an autosomal dominant pattern. Patients who carry two abnormal LQTS genes usually demonstrate a more severe clinical phenotype, characterized by longer QT interval prolongation and a higher risk of syncope and SCD.

How is a prolonged QT interval defined?

A corrected QT interval may be determined using Bazett's formula (QT interval divided by the square root of the R–R interval). The normal range of heart-rate-corrected QT intervals (QTc) varies by age and gender. Prolonged QTc is defined as >450 ms in males and >460 ms in females. With increasingly longer QTc values, the pretest probability of a patient having an LQTS-causing mutation also increases. Genetic testing for LQTS is a Class I indication for asymptomatic, postpubertal individuals if an otherwise idiopathic QTc ≥500 ms (≥480 ms prepuberty) is detected and persists on serial ECGs [3]. Increasingly prolonged QTc values portend a higher risk of potentially lethal arrhythmic events [4].

What are the presenting signs of LQTS?

Diagnosis remains challenging as roughly 40% of patients with genotype-positive LQTS do not demonstrate QT prolongation on resting ECG [5]. Clinical manifestations are heterogenous and include presyncope, syncope, aborted cardiac arrest, cardiac arrest, and SCD. Many patients are completely asymptomatic. The first clinical manifestation of LQTS is SCD in 10%–12% of patients. Left untreated, the prognosis is poor with a 21% mortality rate within 1 year of the first syncopal episode [1, 6]. Treatment dramatically reduces the risk of cardiac events and SCD.

What are the common types of LQTS and their clinical manifestations?

The first genes implicated in congenital LQTS were discovered in the mid-1990s and since that time more than 600 mutations in 14 susceptible genes have been identified. These mutations generally involve either *loss-of-function potassium channel* mutations or *gain-of-function sodium channel* mutations. With rare exception, LQTS is a pure "channelopathy" resulting from mutations in cardiac channel α- and β-subunits. Three genotypes, LQT1, LQT2, and LQT3, account for 75%–95% of cases of congenital LQTS [2, 7].

Long QT1 (LQT1) is associated with mutations in *KCNQ1*, the slowly activating component in the delayed rectifier potassium current channel (I_{Ks}). A properly functioning channel's current is induced by sympathetic activation and is essential for QT shortening with increases in heart rate (HR). Loss-of-function mutations in the *KCNQ1* gene create a substrate in which the defective channel is unable to adapt to β-adrenergic stimulation. Therefore, these patients classically have a broad-based T wave and are *most likely to suffer events triggered by stress, exercise, or sudden increases in sympathetic tone.* β-Blockade is very effective therapy for patients with LQT1 and can be instrumental in mitigating the risk of TdP in these patients. Compared to other genotypes, LQT1 is associated with a shorter, frequently normal QT interval; a lower cumulative cardiac event rate; and a lower incidence of cardiac arrest or SCD. With appropriate β-blockade, the cardiac event rate may be reduced to as low as 1.2%–2% annually [1, 2, 8].

Long QT2 (LQT2) is caused by a mutation in the *KCNH2* gene, which is responsible for the rapidly activating component of the delayed rectifier potassium current. These patients tend to have a notched or low-amplitude T wave and are *classically triggered by startle, fright, or emotion.* Sex hormones are also known to affect the risk of cardiac events in patients with LQT2, with females experiencing a significant increase in risk associated with puberty. β-Blockade is the first-line therapy in these patients but is not

as effective as in patients with LQT1. Long QT2 patients have a 6%–7% risk of cardiac arrest while on β-blocker therapy. These patients are also exquisitely sensitive to potassium levels, often requiring perioperative repletion, chronic potassium supplementation, or spironolactone therapy [1, 2].

Long QT3 (LQT3) differs from the previous two types in several ways. Although both LQT1 and LQT2 are associated with mutations in the same potassium channel, LQT3 is associated with mutations in *SCN5A,* a gene responsible for encoding an inward sodium current channel. Long QT3 is often associated with a gain-of-function mutation, whereas both LQT1 and LQT2 are associated with loss-of-function mutations. Patients with LQT3 have a long, flat ST segment, a tendency toward abnormal bradycardia, and are *most susceptible to cardiac events while sleeping or at rest,* as the QT interval prolongs excessively with slowing of the HR. Treatment in this subgroup can be very challenging, particularly in those who present at an early age [7]. β-Blockade remains a first-line therapy despite reduced efficacy and a 10%–15% rate of major cardiac events even with medical compliance. Sodium channel blockers, such as mexiletine and flecainide, have been shown to shorten the duration of QT interval in patients with LQT3; however, studies suggest that their clinical effectiveness may be mutation specific [2].

What are the genetics of LQTS and what is the role of genetic testing in LQTS?

Congenital LQTS is inherited in both an autosomal dominant and recessive pattern with variable penetrance. Whereas some gene carriers demonstrate QT prolongation, syncope, and even SCD, other gene carriers with the same mutation may show no prolongation and no symptoms. Therefore, while a family history of SCD may lead to a diagnosis of LQTS in a surviving family member, the survivor's individual risk is best predicted by his or her own history of symptoms and QT interval length [9].

Genetic testing should be performed if congenital LQTS is suspected after considering clinical features, family history, and ECG characteristics described earlier. Exercise or pharmacologic stress testing and Holter monitoring may increase the diagnostic yield in selective cases. Asymptomatic patients should be evaluated if they have an otherwise unexpected and persistently prolonged QT interval (QTc >480 ms for prepubertal patients and >500 ms for adults). In the presence of a clinical diagnosis of LQTS, the yield for genetic testing is about 75% [3].

Clinical Pearl

While a family history of SCD may lead to a diagnosis of LQTS in a surviving family member, the survivor's individual risk is best predicted by his or her own history of symptoms and QT interval length.

What is acquired LQTS?

Acquired QT prolongation is defined as QT prolongation and subsequent TdP caused by medications, electrolyte disturbances, or disease. Although most cases of acquired QT prolongation are not genetically based, the first manifestation of congenital LQTS may occur in the setting of acquired QT prolongation. Reversible causes of LQTS include medication, myocardial ischemia, hypothermia, and electrolyte abnormalities.

Are any clinical syndromes associated with congenital LQTS?

Timothy syndrome is a rare, often lethal form of LQTS. In addition to cardiac conduction abnormalities, including prolonged QT interval, atrioventricular block of varying degrees, and bradycardia, these patients may have syndactyly, facial dysmorphisms, and neurodevelopmental abnormalities such as autism. The most common cause of death is ventricular tachyarrhythmia at a mean age of 2.5 years. *Jervell and Lange–Nielson syndrome* is a rare, highly malignant autosomal recessive form of LQTS associated with bilateral sensorineural deafness [5]. *Anderson–Tawil syndrome* is a rare autosomal dominant disorder associated with periodic paralysis and developmental abnormalities including the face, skeleton, and limbs [10].

Clinical Pearl

Timothy syndrome is a rare, often lethal form of LQTS. Children with syndactyly should be evaluated for the presence of LQTS prior to anesthesia.

What is the overall mortality of LQTS? Are certain patient subsets at higher risk for SCD?

Annual mortality associated with LQTS is around 1% per year with highest risk subsets approximately 5%–8% per year.

Indicators of increased risk for SCD include:

- QTc >500 ms
- History of TdP-mediated syncope
- Specific genotypes
- Males and postpubertal females
- Cardiac events occurring during the first year of life

Sudden cardiac death risk in congenital LQTS patients varies by genotype: patients with LQT3 have the highest risk, followed by patients with LQT2 and finally LQT1. Patients with multiple mutations, including Jervell and Lange–Nielsen syndrome, have a particularly severe phenotype with markedly increased risk, even with treatment [11].

Patients who have their first event at <1 year of age belong to a particularly high-risk category, with a 2.3-fold increased risk of either aborted cardiac arrest (ACA) or SCD during the next 10 years compared with patients without events at less than 1 year of age [12]. Medication is less effective in this high-risk group, contributing to a poor prognosis. Alternative therapeutic interventions such as ICDs are also limited and are rarely implanted due to high complication rates in the very young.

What medications are typically used to treat LQTS?

The mainstay of therapy for congenital LQTS is medical management with β-blockade and avoidance of known triggers.

- *Long QT1*: β-Blockade (nadolol or propranolol) is extremely effective at reducing syncope, ACA and SCD [5]. With compliance, the mortality rate may be as low as 0.5%, with a rate of ACA near 1%.
- *Long QT2*: The risk of syncope despite β-blocker therapy is 40%. Cardiac arrest risk remains high at 6%–10%; however, most of these patients are able to be resuscitated.
- *Long QT3*: Patients are most refractory to β-blockers with a 10%–15% rate of cardiac arrest. Cardiac events in LQT3 patients are also more likely to be fatal. Sodium channel blockers may be considered as stand-alone or concomitant therapy with propranolol, as they markedly shorten the QT interval in some patients, reducing the cardiac event rate [8].

Do additional nonpharmacologic therapeutic options exist?

Permanent pacemaker (PM) placement may be considered in LQT1 or LQT2 patients experiencing clinically significant bradycardia while on β-blocker therapy. In addition, PM placement may be indicated in patients with LQT3 to provide HR consistency, decrease repolarization heterogeneity, and reduce the incidence of bradycardia- and pause-dependent TdP, which predisposes patients to TdP.

Left cardiac sympathetic denervation (LCSD) is an increasingly utilized surgical option for patients who either demonstrate recalcitrant symptoms or are unable to tolerate first-line medical management. This approach involves removal of the first four thoracic ganglia and may be performed either thoracoscopically or via extrapleural approach. Left cardiac sympathetic denervation may be suggested for patients with ventricular fibrillation (VF)-terminating implantable cardioverter–defibrillator (ICD) shocks, patients with cardiac events despite medical therapy, patients unable to tolerate β-blockade, and high-risk patients too small for ICD implantation who are inadequately protected with medical therapy [13].

What is CIED therapy?

Cardiovascular implantable electronic device (CIED) technology includes conventional PMs as well as ICDs with pacing capabilities. Creation of perioperative care algorithms for patients with CIEDs is complicated and perioperative advisories have been developed by the American Society of Anesthesiologists (ASA) and the Heart Rhythm Society (HRS) [14, 15].

Who should have an ICD placed?

Implantable cardioverter–defibrillator therapy should be considered in:

- History of an ACA, regardless of genotype
- Documented TdP or syncope despite adequate β-blocker therapy
- Intolerance of primary pharmacotherapy
- Prior LQTS-triggered cardiac event with excessive QT prolongation (>550 ms)
- Women with LQT2 and QT >500 ms [16]

Long QT3 patients also may benefit from ICD therapy [17]. Other high-risk subgroups include Jervell and Lange–Nielsen syndrome and patients with compound mutations. While ICDs may be lifesaving in children, inappropriate shocks and lead failures are common in this population, perhaps related to continued growth and activity placing a strain on leads.

Anesthetic Implications

What are specific preoperative considerations in LQTS patients?

Clarifying the severity of a patient's clinical presentation is essential to better assess their perioperative risk.

- *Mutation type*: *LQT1 and 2* patients are frequently triggered by increased sympathetic stimulation and will benefit from adequate premedication and a calm induction. *LQT2* patients are susceptible to sudden loud noises and should be kept in a quiet room. *LQT3* patients experience events at rest or during sleep and should be monitored closely during premedication and recovery from anesthesia.
- *Medications*: Continuation of β-blocker therapy may be the most important strategy for mitigating the risk of perioperative TdP in patients with LQTS. It is important to determine what medications patients are taking and to continue these medications perioperatively.
- *Longer QTc intervals*: These predict a higher likelihood of cardiac events. Patients should have an ECG performed prior to their procedure.
- *Electrolytes*: Patients with LQTS are exquisitely sensitive to metabolic derangements; hypokalemia, hypomagnesemia, and hypocalcemia may predispose patients to the development of ventricular arrhythmias [18]. Patients with LQT2 are sensitive to changes in potassium and should be monitored closely for hypokalemia.
- *Cardiovascular implantable electronic device*: For patients who have required CIED technology, understanding and planning management of their CIED is an important part of their preoperative assessment and will be discussed in the text that follows.

While medication interactions are the biggest consideration in LQTS patients, what other considerations exist?

Many of the medications administered during an anesthetic affect the QT interval; a list of medications and their effect on the QT interval may be found at www.crediblemeds.org.

Electrolyte derangements are poorly tolerated and should be monitored, particularly in procedures with significant volume shifts. It is reasonable to consider treatment with magnesium (30 mg/kg) given the low toxicity risk and stabilizing effect on the myocardium. Temperature should be monitored and modulated to keep the patient normothermic, as hypothermia has also been shown to prolong the QT interval and conversely, fever >39°C has been shown to develop TdP. Finally, because these patients are often receiving β-blockers, they may tolerate hypovolemia and fluid shifts poorly.

> **Clinical Pearl**
>
> *A list of medications and their effect on the QT interval may be found at www.crediblemeds.org.*

Are there special monitoring considerations in a patient with LQTS?

Ideally patients with LQTS should be fully monitored before induction of anesthesia, including a multiple-lead ECG tracing. The level of monitoring should be based on the severity of the patient's clinical condition and the procedure to be performed, with a low threshold for invasive monitoring. Central access may be helpful in the event that rapid institution of transvenous pacing is needed; however, the decision to place a central venous catheter remains largely based on procedural indications.

Are certain premedication agents safer than others in patients with LQTS?

Midazolam has not been implicated in QT prolongation. Ketamine has not been shown to prolong the QT interval; however, it is a sympathomimetic and should be avoided if possible in these patients [19]. Dexmedetomidine is being used with increasing frequency both for premedication and for sedation in the pediatric population. The risk profile of dexmedetomidine for LQTS patients is clouded by conflicting studies. One study performed in children demonstrated a prolongation of the QT interval [20], while other studies have reported a reversal of acquired and iatrogenic prolonged QT in adults and a protective effect in laboratory animals. The QT interval prolonging effect appears to be related to bradycardia, a known side effect that may be mitigated with dose adjustment and slow titration. Dexmedetomidine is likely safe when used cautiously in patients with LQTS; however, particular attention must be shown to those with LQT3 who are predisposed to cardiac events while at rest or with a slower HR.

> **Clinical Pearl**
>
> *Dexmedetomidine is likely safe when used cautiously in patients with LQTS; however, particular attention must be shown to those with LQT3 who are predisposed to cardiac events while at rest or with a slower HR.*

Are intravenous induction and maintenance agents safer than volatile anesthetic agents?

For induction, one must balance the potential stress associated with the placement of an intravenous (IV) line in an awake child against the potential risk of QT prolongation with a volatile anesthetic agent. Laryngoscopy and intubation can provoke profound sympathetic stimulation and prolong the QT if not appropriately blunted by adequate anesthetic depth. Propofol does not prolong the QT interval, does not accentuate the transmural dispersion of repolarization, and has been shown to reverse sevoflurane induced QTc prolongation in healthy patients. Etomidate has little effect on the QT interval [21].

Nitrous oxide has been used safely in case reports; however, it does possess sympathomimetic properties and should be used cautiously. When compared with commonly used IV agents, volatile agents have demonstrated the ability to prolong the QT interval when studied in healthy children. Whether this prolongation is enough to trigger an episode of TdP in LQTS patients is unclear [17]. QTc changes produced by sevoflurane are concentration dependent and can occur at clinically relevant concentrations. It has been suggested that perioperative continuation of β-blocker therapy may be sufficiently protective against volatile anesthetic agent induced QT prolongation and the development of TdP. However, LQT2 patients may be more susceptible to volatile agent induced arrhythmias than other genotypes, and volatile agents either should be avoided or used with great caution in these patients [22].

> **Clinical Pearl**
>
> *Long QT2 patients may be more susceptible to volatile agent induced arrhythmias than other genotypes, and volatile agents either should be avoided or used with great caution in these patients.*

Are nondepolarizing muscle relaxants safer than succinylcholine?

Succinylcholine should be avoided because of known QT prolongation and its propensity to cause abrupt potassium shifts. Vecuronium and rocuronium have been shown to have little effect on serum histamine concentration and do not prolong the QTc, making them the most suitable agents [23]. Anticholinergics such as atropine and glycopyrrolate prolong the QT interval in healthy patients and have been implicated in the development of TdP in patients with LQTS [17]. Bradycardia associated with neostigmine also can lead to QT prolongation and should be used with caution. With the availability of sugammadex, which does not prolong the QT interval, rocuronium now has the added advantage of easy reversibility with the avoidance of traditional reversal agents [24].

What is the appropriate management of TdP?

While TdP is the most common arrhythmia requiring treatment, LQTS patients may present with either brady- or tachyarrhythmias. Although most episodes of TdP are self-limited, prolonged episodes may be associated with hemodynamic instability, VF, and cardiac arrest. Rapid and short-acting β-blockers should be readily available to prevent and treat tachycardia in patients with LQT1 and 2. Cardiac pacing capabilities should be available to treat bradycardia in LQT3 patients. Magnesium sulfate is the first-line treatment for TdP; a 30–50 mg/kg bolus may be repeated after 15 minutes as needed, followed by an infusion. If TdP persists, temporary pacing may be attempted to terminate the arrhythmia. Defibrillation and cardiopulmonary resuscitation should be carried out swiftly should the patient deteriorate to VF. Amiodarone should not be used for VF, as it can prolong the QT interval. Lidocaine may be effective for refractory ventricular arrhythmias. While patients with acquired QT prolongation and TdP may benefit from isoproterenol or dobutamine to prevent bradycardia, these medications may worsen QT prolongation and increase the risk of arrhythmias in patients with congenital LQTS.

What is the best approach to pain management in patients with LQTS?

Fentanyl, alfentanil, remifentanil, and morphine have been used safely in patients with LQTS; however, methadone and sufentanil prolong the QTc. Commonly used local anesthetics including bupivacaine, ropivacaine, and lidocaine do not significantly affect QT interval. Lidocaine actually may shorten repolarization time [21] and may prevent QTc prolongation during intubation if given at induction. Epinephrine should be avoided as an adjunct to local anesthetics because it has been shown to prolong the QT interval in patients with LQTS. Spinal, epidural, and caudal anesthesia has been used successfully in patients with LQTS. Spinal anesthesia is associated with QT prolongation in healthy patients; however, it may be advantageous because it reduces the stress response and provides dense analgesia. Epidural anesthesia may be preferred because the onset of the block is more gradual, and the risk of abrupt hypotension is lower.

What antiemetics are safe to use in patients with LQTS?

Stress associated with postoperative nausea and vomiting can be severe enough to trigger an arrhythmia in patients with LQTS, but unfortunately many commonly prescribed antiemetics have been linked to prolonged QT. A black box warning for droperidol was issued by the US Food and Drug Administration (FDA) in 2001 because of the potential for cardiac arrest precipitated by QT prolongation. The 5-hydroxytryptamine type 3-receptor antagonists (i.e., ondansetron) are highly effective antiemetics, but they have been shown to prolong the QT interval. The clinical significance of this QT prolongation is unclear. Data are lacking on the specific safety profile of ondansetron in LQTS; however, current recommendations include cautious administration at the lowest effective dose with continuous cardiac monitoring [17]. The latest US FDA recommendations state that the QT prolongation associated with ondansetron is dose dependent and that no single IV dose of ondansetron should exceed 16 mg. Metoclopramide and dexamethasone can be safely administered as part of an antiemetic regimen.

Are there specific postoperative considerations for the patient with LQTS?

Long QTS patients should have continued ECG monitoring postoperatively. Whether they are monitored in the post-anesthesia care unit or intensive care unit must be determined on an individual basis, taking into account the severity of the patient's disease, the complexity of the surgical procedure, and the patient's intraoperative ECG. While there are no specific guidelines, it is reasonable to propose that these patients be monitored for at least 24 hours postoperatively. Patients need to understand the importance of resuming their home regime of medications following discharge.

Management of Implanted Devices

What are the indications for PM placement and what are the common lead configurations?

In 2008, the American College of Cardiology, American Heart Association, and HRS updated guidelines for PM implantation, including recommendations for pediatrics and congenital heart disease (CHD) [25]. Permanent PMs can be attached to the endocardium via a transvenous approach or to the epicardium via a surgical approach. The decision for a surgical approach is dependent on several factors including size of the patient and the cardiac anatomy. Regardless of the system used, it is generally believed that the greatest risk factor for damage to implanted leads is age at time of implant and the presence of CHD [26].

Pacemakers are either single chamber, dual chamber, or trichamber (cardiac resynchronization PMs) depending on the patient's size and device indication. Leads are typically placed in the right atrium (RA) and/or right ventricle (RV). In resynchronization systems, leads are usually placed in both the right and left ventricle. For endocardial systems, the LV lead is usually placed within the coronary sinus, but atypical configurations have been described in patients with CHD. In patients with single ventricle physiology, a resynchronization system may signify two epicardial leads on a single ventricle.

- **Single chamber devices** will sense intrinsic electrical activity from the corresponding chamber within a preset time limit, either inhibiting or triggering pacing of that chamber depending on device programming
- **Dual chamber devices** can sense and pace both in the atrium and ventricle, maintaining AV synchrony in patients without intact AV node function

How are the location and function of PMs described?

An internationally recognized code developed by the North American Society of Pacing and Electrophysiology (NAPSE) and the British Pacing and Electrophysiology Group (BPEG) [27] is used to describe pacemakers and is known as the NASPE/BPEG Generic (NBG) Pacemaker Code. (See Table 49.1.) The five-position code shown in Table 49.1 is often shortened to the first three positions. The dual-chamber mode is the most sophisticated and commonly used mode.

What is rate modulation?

Rate modulation, or rate adaptation, denoted by "R" in the fourth position of the NBG code, describes a pacemaker's ability to automatically change the pacing rate in response to certain monitored parameters in patients with chronotropic incompetence. This function is commonly used in patients who do not have intact sinus node function, and it enables the PM to automatically increase the HR to meet metabolic demands. Most patients with a permanent PM are programmed to the DDDR mode [28].

What is multisite pacing?

The fifth position of the NBG code conveys information regarding the performance and location of multisite pacing: pacing both atria, pacing both ventricles, or multiple pacing sites in a single chamber [28]. Biventricular pacing is a technique of using simultaneous or near simultaneous pace activation of one or both ventricles to improve ventricular dysynchrony and cardiac function.

What are the indications for ICD placement?

The first implantable cardioverter–defibrillator was implanted in 1980. Current indications include:

- Hemodynamically significant ventricular tachycardia
- Ventricular fibrillation
- Conditions associated with SCD (e.g., long QT syndrome, Brugada syndrome, arrhythmogenic RV dysplasia, and infiltrative cardiomyopathies)

Implantable cardioverter–defibrillators are also useful for primary prevention of SCD in patients with hypertrophic cardiomyopathy, post–myocardial infarction with an ejection fraction (EF) of <30%, or cardiomyopathy with an EF of <35%.

Table 49.1 Generic Pacemaker Code

Position I	Position II	Position III	Position IV	Position V
Chamber(s) paced	Chamber(s) sensed	Response(s) to sensing	Programmability	Multisite pacing
O = None	O = None	O = None	O = None	O = None
A = Atrium	A = Atrium	T = Triggered	R = Rate modulation	A = Atrium
V = Ventricle	V = Ventricle	I = Inhibited		V = Ventricle
D = Dual (A + V)	D = Dual (A + V)	D = Dual (T + I)		D = Dual (A + V)

How are ICDs coded?

ICDs also have an international generic code. (See Table 49.2.) In addition to tachyarrhythmia therapies, including defibrillation of tachyarrhythmias and pace termination of tachyarrhythmias, all transvenous ICDs are equipped with pacing capabilities. For complete identification, position IV is expanded to include all five pieces of information conveyed by its full pacemaker NBG code. For example, most devices with a rate responsive PM and ICD will be identified as VVE-DDDR.

What is important to determine during the preoperative evaluation in a patient with a CIED?

Preoperative assessment should include:

- Type of device
- Indication for placement and other coexisting cardiovascular pathology
- Determination of "pacemaker dependence"
- Determination of device function

The device identification card for the patient will include the make, model, and serial number of the device. Important information can also be obtained by referring to consult notes from the cardiologist or PM clinic.

The only reliable method of assessing battery status, lead placement, current settings, adequacy of PM/ICD function, and magnet mode is direct interrogation with a programmer.

What if the manufacturer's card or clinic notes are not available?

If no other data are available, a chest radiograph can often be utilized to identify an x-ray code that can help identify the manufacturer of the device. The chest radiograph can also help in determining the type of device (ICD vs. PM) and whether it is single, dual, or biventricular. It can also be used to determine the number, position, and integrity of leads as well as any unusual configurations of lead/

generator placement and tunneling that may impact the surgical approach.

> **Clinical Pearl**
>
> *If no other data are available, a chest radiograph can often be utilized to identify an x-ray code that can help identify the manufacturer of the device.*

What is meant by the term "pacemaker-dependent"?

Pacemaker dependence can be determined by one or more of the following:

- A verbal history or medical record indication that the patient has experienced a bradyarrhythmia that resulted in syncope or other symptoms requiring CIED implantation
- A history of successful AV node ablation resulting in CIED placement
- No evidence of spontaneous ventricular activity when the pacemaker function of the CIED is programmed to VVI pacing mode at the lowest programmable rate

Who should make recommendations regarding the management of a CIED during a procedure?

Current CIED recommendations from the ASA and HRS focus on an individualized, multidisciplinary approach driven by the primary CIED management team. The best perioperative care of a patient with a CIED will result from the patient's own CIED team (or another CIED team) providing a specific prescription for CIED management to the procedural team.

How close to surgery should the CIED be interrogated?

Pacemakers should be interrogated at least every 12 months. If the PM involves CRT therapy, then interrogation should be every 3–6 months. Implantable cardioverter–defibrillators

Table 49.2 Generic Defibrillator Code

Position I	Position II	Position III	Position IV
Shock chamber(s)	Antitachycardia Pacing chamber(s)	Tachycardia detection	Antibradycardia pacing chamber(s)
O = None	O = None	E = Electrogram	O = None
A = Atrium	A = Atrium	R = Rate modulation	A = Atrium
V = Ventricle	V = Ventricle		V = Ventricle
D = Dual (A + V)	D = Dual (A + V)		D = Dual (A + V)

should be interrogated every 6 months. Children and infants have higher resting and peak heart rates than adults, which will increase battery utilization and significantly impact the longevity of pulse generators.

> **Clinical Pearl**
>
> *Pacemakers should be interrogated at least every 12 months. If the PM involves CRT therapy, then interrogation should be every 3–6 months. Implantable cardioverter-defibrillators should be interrogated every 6 months.*

Once the device has been interrogated, what additional preoperative information will assist in management of the patient?

Preparation for patient safety and proper maintenance of the device during a procedure includes answering the following questions:

1. Is electromagnetic interference (EMI) likely to occur during the procedure?
2. Is preoperative reprogramming to asynchronous mode or disabling special algorithms (including rate adaptive functions) needed?
3. Do antitachyarrhythmia functions need to be suspended?
4. Can use of a bipolar electrocautery system or ultrasonic scalpel be considered to minimize EMI effects?
5. Are temporary pacing and defibrillation equipment available?

What is electromagnetic interference?

Electromagnetic interference can result from any device that emits radiofrequency waves between 0 and 10^9 HZ. The perioperative period is particularly problematic as patients are exposed to a number of energy sources and machinery that may generate EMI including, but not limited to, electrocautery, external defibrillation, electroconvulsive therapy, transcutaneous electrical nerve stimulation, and radiofrequency waves used in ablation procedures.

What are the potential problems associated with EMI and CIEDs?

The most common source of EMI is electrosurgical energy. Electrical current can be delivered in bipolar or monopolar configurations, and with a variety of power waveforms to produce these tissue effects. For bipolar electrosurgery, there appears to be minimal chance for an adverse CIED interaction. For monopolar electrosurgery, electrical current is applied via a small active electrode to the operative site and then flows through the patient's body to a large surface area return electrode. Monopolar electrosurgery is the most common source of EMI and CIED interaction in the operating room. Possible interactions include pacing inhibition; triggering of unneeded tachyarrhythmia therapy; damage at the lead–myocardial tissue interface causing an increase in pacing threshold; pulse generator damage; and the induction of electrical reset mode.

The most frequent CIED interaction with EMI is oversensing, which results in inappropriate inhibition of pacing output. Oversensing by an ICD has the additional problem of false detection of the tachyarrhythmia, possibly leading to inappropriate CIED therapy. The significance of oversensing is determined by a number of patient- and device-related factors. For example, ICDs require a certain duration of continuous high-rate sensing to fulfill arrhythmia detection criteria. For a patient with a robust underlying rhythm, pacing inhibition may be inconsequential, while a PM-dependent patient may experience a hemodynamically unstable underlying rhythm with prolonged pacing inhibition.

How can EMI risks be decreased?

The anatomic site of electrosurgery application, the duration of electrosurgery application, and the position of the return electrode determine the risk of oversensing. Management of potential sources of EMI associated with electrocautery includes:

- Assuring positioning of the cautery and current return pad to avoid the current pathway passing through or near CIED pulse generator and leads
- Avoiding proximity of the cautery's electrical field to the pulse generator or leads
- Use of short, intermittent, and irregular cautery bursts at the lowest feasible energy levels (less than 4 seconds, separated by at least 2 seconds)
- Use of a bipolar electrocautery system or an ultrasonic scalpel if possible

The risk is greatest if the current path crosses the CIED and/or leads and decreases when the presumed current path is kept at least 6 inches away from the CIED.

Who should have their CIED reprogrammed prior to their procedure?

Perioperative management largely relies on determining the patient's CIED dependence and EMI potential. The ASA task force recommends reprogramming to an asynchronous paced mode in patients who are PM dependent when there is a significant risk of EMI. Reprogramming to an asynchronous mode at a rate higher than the patients' intrinsic rate will overcome potential oversensing, or undersensing, from EMI.

Clinical Pearl

The ASA task force recommends reprogramming to an asynchronous paced mode in patients who are PM dependent when there is a significant risk of EMI.

Should rate adaptive functions be disabled?

Special algorithms such as rate adaptive function should be disabled. Pacemaker rate–response algorithms may cause unwanted HR elevation during a procedure. These algorithms are specific to the particular CIED model and manufacturer. For example, transvenous PMs that correlate an increase in respiratory rate and tidal volume with exercise and a need for increased cardiac output pose a challenge for anesthesiologists. Because of the monitored parameter (i.e., respiratory rate and tidal volume via thoracic impedance) the paced rate in these devices may increase inappropriately in response to mechanical hyperventilation.

What monitors need to be in place for a patient with CIED?

Primary activities associated with intraoperative management of CIED include the following:

- Monitoring the operation of the device
- Preventing potential CIED dysfunction
- Performing emergency defibrillation, cardioversion, or heart rate support if necessary

It is essential that ECG monitoring of the patient include the ability to continuously detect PM activity. A perfused peripheral pulse should be monitored with a waveform display such as pulse oximetry or invasive pressure monitoring. Temporary pacing and defibrillation equipment should be immediately available before, during, and after the procedure. Patients with disabled ICDs should have transthoracic defibrillator pads in place.

Clinical Pearl

Temporary pacing and defibrillation equipment should be immediately available before, during, and after the procedure. Patients with disabled ICDs should have transthoracic defibrillator pads in place.

How should a CIED be managed postoperatively?

Any PM that was reprogrammed for a procedure should be interrogated and the CIED function should be restored. This should occur while the patient is still being monitored in the post-anesthesia care unit or in the intensive care unit. Most manufacturers also advise reinterrogation of all devices postoperatively, especially if monopolar diathermy, significant fluid or blood component administration, or external defibrillation have occurred.

Can a magnet be used instead of reprogramming the CIED?

The appropriate role of magnets in the perioperative period remains controversial. Advisories and expert opinion statements caution against routine magnet use as a substitute for appropriate preoperative consultation and preparation. In emergency situations, where time may preclude reprogramming by qualified personnel, a magnet may be placed over the device.

How does a magnet affect a PM? Does a magnet affect an ICD differently than a PM?

Only an interrogation with a programmer can reveal current magnet response settings. However, the expected response for most PMs is the initiation of asynchronous pacing at a fixed, preset "magnet rate," as well as a fixed AV delay, which varies by manufacturer.

Although most ICDs will suspend antitachycardia therapy when a magnet is placed over the device, magnet response varies according to the manufacture and device program. While the ICD function will be suspended, the device will not be forced to revert to an asynchronous pacing mode. Patients with these devices who are PM dependent need to have their device reprogrammed to an asynchronous mode preoperatively if there is significant risk of EMI.

What are the potential disadvantages of using a magnet?

It is important to appreciate that a preset magnet rate may not be sufficient to meet the patient's metabolic demands, particularly for a pediatric patient. Cardiac function in any patient may be compromised, as asynchronous pacing may result in loss of AV synchrony, loss of CRT, loss of capture, or competition between the PM and the patient's intrinsic rate. A patient with an ICD who is PM dependent will still be at risk of

383

profound bradycardia or asystole if pacing is inhibited by EMI. It may be difficult to maintain the magnet in a stable position over the pulse generator of the device, particularly if the patient is lateral or prone. Although some devices emit a diagnostic tone when a magnet is applied, whether any sound is emitted, and its meaning depend on the device manufacturer.

Are there special considerations for performing defibrillation or cardioversion in a patient with a CIED?

If a life-threatening arrhythmia occurs, follow Advanced Cardiac Life Support guidelines to provide rapid cardioversion or defibrillation. If possible, attempt to minimize the current flowing through the pulse generator and lead system by the following mechanisms:

- Position defibrillator or cardioversion pads/paddles as far as possible from the pulse generator.
- Position defibrillator or cardioversion pads/paddles perpendicular to the major access of the CIED pulse generator and leads by placing them in an anterior–posterior location.

References

1. P. J. Schwartz, L. Crotti, and R. Insolia. Long-QT syndrome: from genetics to management. *Circ Arrhythm Electrophysiol* 2012; **5**: 868–77.

2. A. Barsheshet, O. Dotshenko, and I. Goldenberg. Genotype-specific risk stratification and management of patients with long QT syndrome. *Ann Noninvasive Electrocardiol* 2013; **18**: 499–509.

3. M. J. Ackerman, S. G. Priori, S. Willems, et al. HRS/EHRA expert consensus statement on the state of genetic testing for the channelopathies and cardiomyopathies: this document was developed as a partnership between the Heart Rhythm Society (HRS) and the European Heart Rhythm Association (EHRA). *Heart Rhythm* 2011; **10**: e85–108.

4. S. G. Priori, A. A. Wilde, M. Horie, et al. HRS/EHRA/APHRS expert consensus statement on the diagnosis and management of patients with inherited primary arrhythmia syndromes: document endorsed by HRS, EHRA, and APHRS in May 2013 and by ACCF, AHA, Paces and AEPC in June 2013. *Heart Rhythm* 2013; **10**: 1932–63.

5. J. R. Giudicessi and M. J. Ackerman. Genotype- and phenotype-guided management of congenital long QT syndrome. *Curr Probl Cardiol* 2013; **38**: 417–55.

6. S. G. Priori, P. J. Schwartz, C. Napolitano, et al. Risk stratification in the long-QT syndrome. *N Engl J Med* 2003; **348**: 1866–74.

7. J-E Ban. Neonatal arrhythmias: diagnosis, treatment, and clinical outcome. *Korean J Pediatr* 2017; **60**: 344–52.

8. P. J. Schwartz and M. J. Ackerman. The long QT syndrome: a transatlantic clinical approach to diagnosis and therapy. *Eur Heart J* 2013; **34**: 3109–16.

9. E. S. Kaufman, S. McNitt, A. J. Moss, et al. Risk of death in the long QT syndrome when a sibling has died. *Heart Rhythm* 2008; **5**: 831–6.

10. H. L. Nguyen, G. H. Pieper, and R. Wilders. Andersen-Tawil syndrome: clinical and molecular aspects. *Int J Cardiol* 2013; **170**: 1–16.

11. P. J. Schwartz, C. Spazzolini, S. G. Priori, et al. Who are the long-QT syndrome patients who receive an implantable cardioverter-defibrillator and what happens to them? Data from the European Long-QT Syndrome Implantable Cardioverter-Defibrillator (LQTS ICD) Registry. *Circulation* 2010; **122**: 1272–82.

12. C. Spazzolini, J. Mullaly, A. J. Moss, et al. Clinical implications for patients with long QT syndrome who experience a cardiac event during infancy. *J Am Coll Cardiol* 2009; **54**: 832–7.

13. H. E. Schneider, M. Steinmetz, U. Krause, et al. Left cardiac sympathetic denervation for the management of life-threatening ventricular tachyarrhythmias in young patients with catecholaminergic polymorphic ventricular tachycardia and long QT syndrome. *Clin Res Cardiol* 2013; **102**: 33–42.

14. American Society of Anesthesiologists. Practice advisory for the perioperative management of patients with cardiac implantable electronic devices: pacemakers and implantable cardioverter-defibrillator: an updated report by the American Society of Anesthesiologists Task Force on Perioperative Management of Patients with Cardiac Implantable Electronic Devices. *Anesthesiology* 2011; **114**: 247–61.

15. G. H. Crossley, J. E. Poole, M. A. Rozner, et al. The Rhythm Society (HRS)/ American Society of Anesthesiologists (ASA) Expert Consensus Statement on the perioperative management of patients with implantable defibrillators, pacemakers and arrhythmia monitors: facilities and patient management: executive summary. *Heart Rhythm* 2011; **8**: 1114.

16. W. Zareba, A. J. Moss, J. P. Daubert, et al. Implantable cardioverter defibrillator in high-risk long QT syndrome patients. *J Cardiovasc Electrophysiol* 2003; **14**: 337–41.

17. S. J. Kies, C. M. Pabelick, H. A. Hurley, et al. Anesthesia for patients with congenital long QT syndrome. *Anesthesiology* 2005; **102**: 204–10.

18. S. G. Priori, C. Blomström-Lundqvist, A. Mazzanti, et al. Task Force for the Management of Patients with Ventricular Arrhythmias and the Prevention of Sudden Cardiac Death for the European Society of Cardiology. 2015 ESC Guidelines for the management of patients with ventricular arrhythmias and the prevention of sudden cardiac death. *Europace* 2015; **17**: 1601–87.

19. G. E. Staudt and S. C. Watkins. Anesthetic considerations for pediatric patients with congenital long QT syndrome. *J Cardiothorac Vasc Anesth* 2019; **33**: 2030–8.

20. G. B. Hammer, D. R. Drover, H. Cao, et al. The effects of dexmedetomidine on cardiac electrophysiology in children. *Anesth Analg* 2008; **106**: 79–83.

21. R. Owczuk, M. A. Wujtewicz, A. Zienciuk-Krajka, et al. The influence of anesthesia on cardiac repolarization. *Minerva Anesthesiol* 2012; **78**: 483–95.

22. M. Kumakura, K. Hara, and T. Sata. Sevoflurane-associated torsade de pointes in a patient with congenital long QT syndrome genotype 2. *J Clin Anesth* 2016; **33**: 81–5.

23. M. Naguib, A. H. Samarkandi, H. S. Bakhamees, et al. Histamine-release haemodynamic changes produced by rocuronium, vecuronium, mivacurium, atracurium and tubocurarine. *Br J Anaesth* 1995; **75**: 588–92.

24. P-J de Kam, P. Grobara, J. Dennie, et al. Effect of sugammadex on QT/QTc interval prolongation when combined with QTc-prolonging sevoflurane or propofol anaesthesia. *Clin Drug Invest* 2013; **33**: 545–51.

25. K. E. Odening, G. Koren, R. I. Hospital, et al. HHS public assess 2015; **11**: 2107–15.

26. M. J. Shah. Implantable cardioverter defibrillator-related complications in the pediatric population. *Pacing Clin Electophysiol* 2009; **32**: S71–4.

27. A. D. Bernstein, J-C Daubert, R. D. Fletcher, et al. NAPSE Position Statement. The revised NAPSE/BPEG generic code for antibradycardia, adaptive-rate, and multisite pacing. *Pacing Clin Electrophysiol* 2002; **25**: 260–4.

28. B. Cronin and M. K. Essandoh. Update on cardiovascular implantable electronic devices for anesthesiologists. *J Cardiothorac Vasc Anes* 2018; **32**: 1871–84.

Suggested Reading

American Society of Anesthesiologists Task Force on Perioperative Management of Patients with Cardiac Implantable Electronic Devices. Practice advisory for the perioperative management of patients with cardiac implantable electronic devices: pacemakers and implantable cardioverter-defibrillators. An updated report. *Anesthesiology* 2011; **114**: 247–61.

Cronin B. and Essandoh M. K. Update on cardiovascular implantable electronic devices for anesthesiologists. *J Cardiothorac Vasc Anes* 2018; **32**: 1871–84.

Crossley G. H., Poole J. E., Rozner M. A., et al. The Rhythm Society (HRS)/American Society of Anesthesiologists (ASA) Expert Consensus Statement on the Perioperative Management of Patients with Implantable Defibrillators, Pacemakers and Arrhythmia Monitors: Facilities and Patient Management: Executive Summary. *Heart Rhythm* 2011; **8**: 1114.

Fazio G., Vernuccio F., Grutta G., et al. Drugs to be avoided in patients with long QT syndrome: focus on the anaesthesiological management. *World J Cardiol* 2013; **26**: 87–93.

Navaratnam M. and Dubin A. Pediatric pacemakers and ICDs: how to optimize perioperative care. *Pediatr Anesth* 2011; **21**: 512–21.

O'Hare M., Maldonado Y., Muro J., et al. Perioperative management of patients with congenital or acquired disorder of the QT interval. *BJA* 2018; **120**: 629–44.

Staudt G. E. and Watkins S. C. Anesthetic considerations for pediatric patients with congenital long QT syndrome. *J Cardiothorac Vasc Anesth* 2019; **33**: 2030–8.

Chapter 50

Marfan Syndrome

Destiny F. Chau

Case Scenario

A 16-year-old male, weighing 52 kg and 182 cm tall, presents for repair of pectus excavatum via Nuss procedure. The pectus deformity is severe, with a Haller index of 4.7, causing cardiac displacement and compression of the right atrium and right ventricle. Symptoms include worsening shortness of breath and chest discomfort during exertion. His medical history is also significant for Marfan syndrome, stable mild thoracolumbar scoliosis with 20-degree Cobb angle, mild ectopia lentis, and attention-deficit/hyperactivity disorder. The patient had a spontaneous left pneumothorax 2 years earlier that resolved with conservative treatment. Current medications include atenolol 25 mg and losartan 25 mg taken by mouth twice daily, and guanfacine ER 4 mg given once daily. Recent preoperative diagnostic studies include chest magnetic resonance imaging, chest computed tomography, pulmonary function studies, electrocardiogram, and an echocardiogram. Pulmonary function tests show moderate restrictive and mild obstructive pulmonary function. One small apical bleb in the left lung is seen on magnetic resonance imaging. Current vital signs are heart rate 62 beats/minute, blood pressure 106/71, SpO_2 98% on room air, respiratory rate 16 breaths/minute, and temperature 36.5°C. The surgeon is expecting to place two Nuss bars for correction of the pectus deformity.

A recent transthoracic echocardiogram reveals the following:

- *Stable aortic root dilatation measuring 3.7 cm (Z-score 3.8)*
- *Mild-moderate aortic insufficiency*
- *Mitral valve prolapse with mild mitral regurgitation*
- *Right atrial and ventricular compression with normal biventricular function*

Key Objectives

- Identify characteristic findings of Marfan syndrome.
- Define significant aortic root dilatation and the significance of the "Z-score."
- Describe medications used for management of cardiovascular pathology.
- Formulate anesthetic plans along with postoperative pain management strategies.
- Discuss the unique challenges of cardiopulmonary resuscitation in a patient with a pectus bar.

Pathophysiology

What is Marfan syndrome?

Marfan syndrome (MFS) is an autosomal dominant connective tissue disorder caused by *FBN1* gene mutations on chromosome 15, resulting in defective fibrillin-1 matrix glycoproteins manifesting as tissue abnormalities. Fibrillin-1, besides forming important structural tissue components, also impacts regulation of transforming growth factor β (TGF-β) which results in increased proteolytic activity and extracellular matrix degeneration. The aberrant protein expressions increase and worsen with age and are most notoriously manifested in the musculoskeletal, cardiovascular, and ophthalmic systems. Cardinal clinical features include aortic root dilatation and ectopia lentis. Other clinical manifestations may include pectus excavatum or carinatum, scoliosis, dural ectasia, pulmonary involvement (emphysema, lung cysts, spontaneous pneumothorax), retrognathia, malar hypoplasia, and joint abnormalities.

What cardiovascular abnormalities are commonly associated with MFS?

The most concerning cardiovascular abnormality is aortic root dilatation with progression to dissection and rupture. Aortic root dilatation is seen in approximately 50% of young children with MFS, with the risk of aortic rupture increasing during the teenage years. Aortic root rupture accounts for 50% of deaths by age 40 years in untreated patients with MFS. Dilatation can also involve the thoracic and abdominal aortic segments, the main pulmonary artery, and the carotid arteries. Other described cardiac findings are aortic valve insufficiency, mitral valve prolapse (MVP) and mitral valve insufficiency, ventricular arrhythmias, and dilated cardiomyopathy.

> **Clinical Pearl**
>
> *Aortic root dilatation is seen in approximately 50% of young children with MFS, with the risk of aortic rupture increasing during the teenage years.*

When aortic root dilatation is considered significant and what is the *Z-score*?

Aortic root size and rate of dilatation should be serially monitored. Per the 2010 Revised Ghent criteria for MFS, aortic root dilatation is significant when the aortic diameter (at the sinus of Valsalva) Z-score is 2 or greater. The **Z-*score*** conveys the deviation of a measurement from the population mean specific for body size and other factors, thus becoming a valuable tool for serial monitoring of a patient's aortic root diameter over time. Imaging modalities used for aortic root diameter measurement and correlation include echocardiography, computed tomography (CT), and/or magnetic resonance imaging (MRI). Yearly monitoring is recommended for stable rates of progression and more frequently for concerning findings. Risk factors for aortic dissection in MFS include aortic diameter 5 cm or greater, rapid rate of aortic dilatation, aortic dilatation progressing past the sinus of Valsalva, and family history of aortic dissection. Medical therapy aims to slow down the rate of aortic dilatation and delay surgical intervention. Delaying surgery until an adult-sized graft and valve can be utilized is highly beneficial for the pediatric patient; it also potentially lessens total lifetime replacements. Surgical therapy aims to improve survival via elective aortic root replacement for patients at high risk of rupture.

> **Clinical Pearl**
>
> *The Z-score conveys the deviation of a measurement from the population mean specific for body size and other factors, thus becoming a valuable tool for serial monitoring of a patient's aortic root diameter over time.*

What are the recommended treatment modalities for MFS?

Early therapy with β-blockers is the currently recommended treatment for all patients with MFS if tolerated. Dosage is adjusted to maintain a submaximal exercise heart rate of 110 bpm or less in children and 100 bpm or less in adults. It is thought that β-blockers' antihypertensive effect, reduction of myocardial contractility, pulse pressure, and aortic wall tension may delay the progression of aortic root dilatation. Atenolol is usually the drug of choice due to its long half-life and relative cardioselectivity. In patients intolerant to β-blockade, second-line therapy with an angiotensin receptor blocker (ARB) such as losartan is recommended. Currently, ARBs are the subject of ongoing research due to their action on reducing TGF-β activity, which is also implicated in tissue degeneration in MFS. Aortic root surgery is reserved for those patients at high risk of dissection and rupture; common approaches include use of a composite valve-graft or valve sparing aortic root replacement. Improved aortic root monitoring and elective aortic root surgery have decreased the rate of sudden death from aortic dissection, yielding improved life expectancies for patients with MFS. Careful monitoring of the aorta distal to the repair should continue after aortic root surgery because dilatation of the distal aorta continues to occur. Concomitant repair of MVP or replacement of the mitral valve is performed for those with severe mitral regurgitation.

What are the indications and possible surgical approaches for surgical correction of pectus excavatum?

The **Haller index** is the intrathoracic transverse diameter divided by the smallest anteroposterior diameter in a chest CT axial slice. Intrathoracic structures are commonly affected by the mechanical compression of the pectus deformity, leading to reduced thoracic volume with restrictive/obstructive lung disease, cardiac impingement or displacement, potential conduction abnormalities, and valvular disease. With chronically reduced chest compliance, cardiopulmonary function and symptoms may worsen with age. Surgical correction for pectus excavatum is indicated in the presence of cardiopulmonary symptoms, severity of deformity (defined by Haller index of 3.2 or greater), rapid progression of the malformation, cardiopulmonary compression or displacement, restrictive or obstructive pattern in pulmonary function tests (PFTs), and psychological disorders related to the chest deformity.

The Nuss procedure, a minimally invasive approach involving the placement of a retrosternal bar to correct the depressed anterior chest wall, has become the technique of choice for correction of pectus excavatum deformity. Compared to the open approaches, which are modifications of the original Ravitch procedure involving cartilage or sternal resection, the Nuss procedure is associated with shorter intraoperative times, significantly less blood loss, *increased* postoperative pain levels, and improved cosmetic results.

Anesthetic Implications

What are the primary goals of the preanesthesia visit?

Since this operation is elective, goals of the preoperative evaluation include a complete systemic review including anesthesia history, coexisting diseases, pertinent diagnostic studies and laboratory values, physical examination, preparation and optimization for this surgery along with discussion of anesthetic plans with the patient and family. Special attention is placed on the organ systems impacted by MFS and pectus excavatum, with careful documentation of symptoms and physical examination findings pertaining to the cardiopulmonary and musculoskeletal systems. A thorough airway examination should be performed. If the ophthalmologic history shows concerning deterioration, a consult may be warranted to rule out retinal involvement. Review of pertinent recent diagnostic studies with special consideration to the cardiopulmonary system is crucial. Discussion of specific anesthetic risks including the risk of aortic rupture and death, invasive monitoring, and plans for postoperative pain management should ensue with the patient and family. Emphasis on continuation of current medications is important.

What diagnostic studies are indicated in preparation for this surgery?

Recent evaluations of aortic and cardiopulmonary status for manifestations of MFS and pectus excavatum are needed for planning this elective procedure and should include the following:

- *Transthoracic echocardiogram* for assessing aortic root dimensions, evaluating valvular function, diastolic filling, and cardiac compression
- *Electrocardiogram (ECG)* for detecting the presence of conduction abnormalities due to MFS or cardiac compression
- *Magnetic resonance and CT imaging* to demonstrate the effects of the pectus excavatum on the intrathoracic

structures (including delineation of aortic size, morphology, and presence of dissection), lung parenchymal integrity, and to calculate the Haller index
- *Pulmonary function studies* for evaluating the degree of preoperative pulmonary impairment resulting from MFS, pectus excavatum, and kyphoscoliosis

In patients with MFS, if aortic root surgery seems impending, a multidisciplinary discussion is needed to determine the optimal timing of pectus correction and cardiac surgery.

What medications should be continued on the day of surgery?

It is very important to continue β-blocker therapy on the day of surgery to lower aortic wall stress and the risk of dissection throughout the case. The ARB can be held due to reports of hypotension under general anesthesia. Guanfacine, a central alpha-2 agonist, can be continued for treatment of attention deficit/hyperactivity disorder (ADHD) and for its concurrent effect of maintaining blood pressure control.

Clinical Pearl

β-Blocker therapy should be continued throughout the perioperative period to minimize the risk of aortic root dissection.

What postoperative pain strategies should be discussed for this patient?

The Nuss procedure is associated with significant levels of postoperative pain, reported to be much greater than pain from the open Ravitch procedure. No pain management technique has been demonstrated to be superior but varied multimodal techniques have been described as effective for postoperative pain management. The elevation of the sternum, new geometric chest wall configuration, and sternal pressure of the bars generate high-intensity pain in the patient's chest and spine. Many patients with MFS require more than one bar for correction of the pectus deformity. Pain management should start in the preoperative period. Continuous thoracic epidurals or bilateral paravertebral catheter infusions have been successfully utilized, and decision making regarding the use of regional techniques is institution dependent. Other components of postoperative analgesia management include intercostal nerve blocks, narcotic patient-controlled analgesia, subcutaneous infusion catheters of local anesthetic, nonsteroidal antiinflammatory drugs, intravenously administered acetaminophen, benzodiazepines for muscle spasms and anxiety, other muscle relaxants such as methocarbamol, and agents for neuropathic pain such as gabapentin. Postoperatively, the patient is mobilized early with physical therapy and encouraged to ambulate, which may acutely increase pain levels but is beneficial for long-term pain resolution. Preoperative education of the family and patient regarding expected pain levels is critical to create reasonable expectations and diminish anxiety.

Are there special concerns regarding regional or epidural anesthesia in this patient?

Dural ectasia, usually asymptomatic, has been associated with MFS. It results from the dilatation of the dural sac owing to pressure from the cerebrospinal fluid (CSF). Dural ectasia is most prominent in the lumbosacral area where the CSF also exerts the highest pressure. In general, neuraxial techniques have been described as potentially more challenging and less reliable in patients with MFS. Epidural catheter placement over the areas of degenerated dural sac may be associated with increased risks for dural puncture. Additionally, the dilated dura sac may hold an increased volume of CSF that would make appropriate dosing of spinal anesthesia more challenging. The presence of scoliosis in the patient with MFS may further complicate epidural catheter placement. Bilateral paravertebral catheters have been successfully used in patients with MFS. Placement under ultrasound guidance allows visualization of the pleura and may improve successful catheter placement. In the event of epidural placement in the postoperative period, the lateral decubitus position is contraindicated after surgery for fear of dislodging the recently placed Nuss bar.

Should premedication be utilized in this patient?

The patient's history of ADHD as well as the goal of avoiding a sympathetic surge leading to hypertension would favor the administration of premedication for anxiety with minimal risk.

What associated characteristics of MFS can cause airway concerns?

Patients with MFS have associated characteristics such as high-arched palate, retrognathia, and ligamentous hyperlaxity that can lead to joint subluxation during intubation maneuvers. The anesthesiology team should be prepared for a potentially difficult intubation owing to those factors.

What are the perioperative hemodynamic goals?

Maintenance of hemodynamic control and avoidance of hypertension both deserve special attention in order to minimize the risk of developing aortic dissection. β-blocker therapy should be continued until the day of surgery. In addition to adequate baseline levels of anesthesia and analgesia, various techniques are employed to blunt the hemodynamic response ahead of highly stimulating events such as laryngoscopy, intubation, and surgical maneuvers such as sternum elevation. Pharmacologic agents used to attenuate the hypertensive responses include short-acting opioid infusions and vasoactive agents such esmolol and nicardipine. Maneuvers or drugs that may lead to tachycardia or hypertension should be avoided.

Clinical Pearl

Maintenance of hemodynamic control with avoidance of hypertension deserves special attention during the entire perioperative period to minimize the risk of developing aortic dissection. Maneuvers or drugs that may lead to tachycardia or hypertension should be avoided.

What monitoring is appropriate for this patient?

In addition to the standard American Society of Anesthesiologists recommended monitoring for general anesthesia using a 5-lead ECG, invasive arterial blood pressure monitoring can be utilized for close monitoring and blood pressure management. The Nuss procedure is generally associated with minimal blood loss unless cardiac laceration occurs, an extremely rare complication (0.1% or less) with modern surgical techniques including thoracoscopy and sternum elevation for dissection. Although the risk of aortic dissection and rupture is present in this patient with MFS, the exact risk is unknown but presumed to be low in the setting of appropriate hemodynamic control. Transesophageal echocardiography can provide additional monitoring as needed to visualize the aortic root and cardiac status if unexplained or sudden changes in hemodynamics occur.

Clinical Pearl

In addition to invasive arterial blood pressure monitoring, transesophageal echocardiography can provide additional monitoring as needed to visualize the aortic root and cardiac status during unexplained sudden changes in hemodynamics.

If this patient had a prior history of mitral valve repair, how might that affect the anesthetic plan?

Previous surgeries (or inflammatory processes) in the intrathoracic cavity place the patient at a higher risk for cardiovascular or lung injury. Adhesions can obscure visualization of important mediastinal structures and make surgical dissection challenging. The risks of cardiovascular injury and bleeding are also increased in this setting. Some centers make this factor a contraindication for the closed chest approach. If the surgeon determines that the minimally invasive approach is feasible after thoracoscopic exploration, adequate blood availability with the cardiac team on standby until safe passage of the bars occurs should be arranged. The anesthesia team must prepare for and be able to respond quickly to adequately resuscitate the patient should catastrophic bleeding occur.

What anesthetic induction methods are appropriate?

Placement of a preinduction peripheral intravenous line allows the administration of pharmacologic agents for titrated induction and rapid control of hemodynamics. There is no superior anesthetic induction agent or technique as long as hemodynamic control is maintained during the process of induction and intubation. Significant hypotension during induction has been reported for patients with cardiac compression. Hypertension and tachycardia can occur during laryngoscopy and intubation. Blunting of sympathetic stimulation (i.e., use of lidocaine and opioids) and dose titration of induction agents with administration of short-acting vasoactive agents as needed can prevent detrimental hemodynamic swings while the airway is secured. If airway management proves difficult, having a separate person designated to monitor and control hemodynamics while the primary anesthesiologist's attention is placed on securing the airway is recommended.

What positioning concerns exist for this patient?

Proper positioning and support must be ensured, considering the scoliosis and joint hyperlaxity of patients with MFS. The arms are normally positioned 90° to the side to allow surgical access to both sides of the chest. The arms should not be hyperextended at the level of the brachial plexus, and proper support should be available at the elbows and wrists. Patients with MFS may have asymptomatic protrusio acetabuli (migration of the femoral heads into the pelvic cavity); there are no existing specific recommendations for positioning apart from the usual proper support of the hips, knees, and heels.

Does this patient need subacute bacterial endocarditis prophylaxis?

Per the current 2007 American Heart Association recommendations, this patient does not meet the current criteria to require prophylaxis for bacterial endocarditis. Antimicrobial prophylaxis for surgical site infection should be given per institutional guidelines.

What additional concerns exist during anesthetic maintenance?

Airway pressures during positive pressure ventilation must be kept as low as possible to reduce the risk of pneumothorax, especially if this patient has sustained a previous spontaneous pneumothorax and is known to have a current apical bleb. Pneumothorax must be kept high in the differential diagnosis if increased airway pressures or hemodynamic deterioration is noted. Although they are not routinely placed for uneventful Nuss procedures, chest tube(s) are often left in place for patients with MFS at risk of postoperative pneumothorax. Regarding the maintenance of anesthesia, since there is no anesthetic technique that has proven to be superior, anesthetic maintenance techniques are left to the discretion of the anesthesiologist while continuing to meet the hemodynamic goals for this patient.

Clinical Pearl

Airway pressures during positive pressure ventilation should be kept as low as possible to reduce the risk of pneumothorax.

New onset ectopy is observed during passage of the surgical introducer tool: what are the likely etiologies?

If the patient is otherwise stable and the arrhythmia coincides with surgical maneuvering of a tool inside the chest cavity, this is potentially a sign of contact with the myocardium and irritation of the conduction system. The surgeon needs to stop the maneuver and reassess the working distance to the heart. If the arrhythmia does not resolve or there are signs of hemodynamic instability, a detrimental cardiovascular event is occurring, and it must be quickly assessed and managed.

Ventricular fibrillation occurs during the placement of the pectus bar: what should the surgeon be asked to do?

If ventricular fibrillation (VF) occurs during placement of the pectus bar, the surgeon should immediately pull the pectus bar out of the thorax under direct thoracoscopic visualization while confirming again the absence of obvious structural injury. Removing the pectus bar will allow for improved chest compression and defibrillation efforts.

Clinical Pearl

If ventricular fibrillation occurs during the placement of the pectus bar, the surgeon must remove the pectus bar to allow for improved chest compression and defibrillation efforts.

What changes in chest compression strategy during cardiopulmonary resuscitation are recommended for patients with uncorrected pectus excavatum?

When performing cardiopulmonary resuscitation (CPR), patients with uncorrected pectus excavatum might benefit from compression at the level of the lower half of the sternum, with less compression depth required than for subjects with normal thoracic architecture. Evidence exists that standard compression depths might increase the risk of myocardial injury or other intrathoracic organ damage in these patients. Arterial tracings and end-tidal carbon dioxide waveforms are helpful to guide the effectiveness of chest compressions.

Clinical Pearl

If CPR is needed for patients with uncorrected pectus excavatum, compression at the lower half of the sternum with less compression depth than normally expected may decrease the risk of cardiac injury. Use arterial blood pressure tracings and end-tidal carbon dioxide waveforms to guide the effectiveness of chest compressions.

Should VF occur postoperatively, what changes during performance of CPR and positioning of defibrillating pads are recommended for patients with a sternal Nuss bar in place?

Stronger than usual chest compressions are recommended to achieve effective results when the sternal bar is in place.

Front-to-back defibrillation pad placement is recommended so that the electric current will better reach the heart and not be dissipated via the Nuss bar. At the time of hospital discharge patients should be given a medical alert bracelet about the Nuss bar to alert emergency medical and other healthcare providers about the recommended adjustments for resuscitative efforts should they ever be necessary.

Clinical Pearl

If CPR is needed on a patient with a pectus bar in place, stronger than usual chest compressions are recommended to achieve effective results. Front-to-back defibrillation pad placement is preferred, so that the electric current will better reach the heart and not be dissipated via the Nuss bar.

What are the anesthetic considerations for emergence and extubation?

Avoidance of agitation and coughing is highly desirable to minimize the risks of displacement of newly placed bars, to avoid hypertension placing stress on the aortic root and to minimize the risk of spontaneous pneumothorax.

What postoperative concerns are present during the early recovery period?

Adequate pain control can remain challenging once the patient regains consciousness despite the use of preemptive and continuing multimodal pain management strategies. Emphasis on adequate monitoring for blood pressure and heart rate thresholds needs to be clearly communicated to the healthcare team. Recommendations exist to maintain a heart rate of 110 bpm or less and blood pressure within 20% above baseline to reduce the risk of aortic dissection. In addition to aggressive pain management, continuation of preoperative β-blockade and ARB therapy is also important for control of hypertension during the entire postoperative period. Resumption of guanfacine, a central alpha-2 agonist, may be helpful both for treatment of ADHD and for its effects on modulation of blood pressure. The patient may benefit from admission to the intensive care unit for close monitoring. Follow-up transthoracic echocardiography can be performed postoperatively to assess for improvement in cardiopulmonary compression and assessment of aortic root status.

1

Suggested Reading

Ammash N. M., Sundt T. M., and Connolly H. M. Marfan syndrome: diagnosis and management. *Curr Probl Cardiol* 2008; **33**: 7–39.

Castellano J. M., Silvay G., and Castillo J. G. Marfan syndrome: clinical, surgical, and anesthetic considerations. *Semin Cardiothorac Vasc Anesth* 2014; **18**: 260–71.

Fraser S., Child A., and Hunt I. Pectus updates and special considerations in Marfan syndrome. *Pediatr Rep* 2018; **9**: 7277.

Mavi J. and Moore D. L. Anesthesia and analgesia for pectus excavatum surgery. *Anesthesiol Clin* 2014; **32**: 175–84.

Nuss D., Obermeyer R. J., and Kelly R. E. Nuss bar procedure: past, present and future. *Ann Cardiothorac Surg* 2016; **5**: 422–33.

Russo V., Ranno M., and Nigro G. Cardiopulmonary resuscitation in pectus excavatum patients: is it time to say more? *Resuscitation* 2015; **88**: e5–e6.

Wilson W., Taubert K., Gewitz M., et al. Prevention of infective endocarditis: Guidelines from the American Heart Association, by the Committee on Rheumatic Fever, Endocarditis, and Kawasaki Disease. *Circulation* 2007; **116**: 1736–54.

Wright M. J. and Connolly H. M. Management of Marfan syndrome and related disorders. UptoDate. 2018. www.uptodate.com/contents/management-of-marfan-syndrome-and-related-disorders (accessed July 4, 2019).

Index

393